Intracranial Tumors

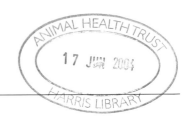

Intracranial Tumors
Diagnosis and Treatment

Lisa M DeAngelis MD
Chairman, Department of Neurology
Memorial Sloan-Kettering Cancer Center
New York, NY 10021
USA

Philip H Gutin MD
Chief, Neurosurgery Service
Department of Surgery
Memorial Sloan-Kettering Cancer Center
New York, NY 10021
USA

Steven A Leibel MD
Chairman, Department of Radiation Oncology
Memorial Sloan-Kettering Cancer Center
New York, NY 10021
USA

Jerome B Posner MD
Attending Neurologist, Department of Neurology
Memorial Sloan-Kettering Cancer Center
New York, NY 10021
USA

MARTIN DUNITZ

First published in the United Kingdom in 2002 by Martin Dunitz Ltd,
The Livery House, 7-9 Pratt Street, London NW1 0AE

Tel: +44 (0) 20 7482 2202
Fax: +44 (0) 20 7267 0159
E-mail: info@dunitz.co.uk
Webiste: http://www.dunitz.co.uk

A CIP record for this book is available from the British Library.

ISBN 1-90186-537-1

Although every effort has been made to ensure that all owners of copyright
material have been acknowledged in this publication, we would be glad to
acknowledge in subsequent reprints or editions any omissions brought to our
attention.

Distributed in the USA by
Fulfilment Center
Taylor & Francis
7625 Empire Drive
Florence, KY 41042, USA
Toll Free Tel: +1 800 634 7064
E-mail: cserve@routledge_ny.com

Distributed in Canada by
Taylor & Francis
74 Rolark Drive
Scarborough, Ontario M1R 4G2, Canada
Toll Free Tel: +1 877 226 2237
E-mail: tal_fran@istar.ca

Distributed in the rest of the world by
ITPS Limited
Cheriton House
North Way
Andover, Hampshire SP10 5BE, UK
Tel: +44 (0)1264 332424
E-mail: reception@itps.co.uk

Composition by Scribe Design, Gillingham, Kent, UK
Printed and bound in Spain by Grafos SA Arte sobre papel

Contents

Preface

This book is intended for clinicians who care for patients with tumors involving the brain. These tumors include meningiomas, pituitary, pineal and skull base tumors as well as tumors intrinsic to the brain – thus the title *Intracranial Tumors* rather than 'Brain Tumors'. The material in the book reflects our collective experience as: a radiation oncologist (Stephen Leibel), a neurosurgeon (Philip Gutin) and two neurologists (Lisa DeAngelis and Jerome Posner), working as a team in a cancer hospital. The book is divided into two sections. The first considers general principles of the biology, diagnosis and treatment of intracranial tumors whether 'benign' or 'malignant' and whether primary or metastatic. The second section deals with the biology, diagnosis and management applied to specific tumors.

Physicians from a wide variety of specialties (e.g. family practitioners, internists, neurologists, psychiatrists) are likely to be the first to encounter a patient with an intracranial tumor. Furthermore, neurosurgeons, oncologists, radiation oncologists or neurologists who do not specialize in intracranial tumors are those who treat most of these patients. This book was written primarily for these physicians and for aspiring neuro-oncologists. Accordingly, experienced neuro-oncologists may find sections of the book involving diagnosis and imaging overly simplistic, and medical or radiation oncologists may find the sections on radiation therapy and chemotherapy obvious. We

have reviewed the best current basic science and clinical evidence, compiled up-to-date references, and because the book expresses the opinions of a highly experienced team of neuro-oncologists working together in a cancer hospital, we hope that even seasoned neuro-oncologists will find the book useful in their own practice.

A word about the front cover. We chose this design to illustrate advances in the treatment of intracranial tumors. The figure on the left is from a chapter by Walter Dandy in Lewis (ed) *Practice of Surgery*, 1944. One is not surprised that in those days, before steroids and brain imaging, both morbidity and mortality were high. The figures on the right illustrate the use of frameless stereotaxy in the current surgical management of brain tumors, a technique that has substantially decreased both mortality and morbidity. Surgical and other treatments of intracranial tumors are discussed in Chapter 4.

The opinions expressed in this book are shared by many of our colleagues in neurology, radiation oncology and neurosurgery, but we bear the full responsibility for the statements and opinions in this monograph. Our approach to the patients, both diagnostically and therapeutically, has been a team approach, and the four of us generally agree on the opinions and approach expressed in this monograph. We take full responsibility for any omissions, errors or outrageous statements.

We had a lot of technical support in writing this monograph. Elenita Sambat and Judith Lampron typed the endless drafts, made more numerous by the availability of the computer. Carol D'Anella read the galleys and corrected the more egregious errors of syntax, grammar, and occasionally spelling that Spellcheck did not pick up. Amanda May and team at Martin Dunitz were extremely helpful in copyediting and putting the book together. They and Alan Burgess were very patient as we made last minute changes in both the text and the bibliography in an attempt to make the book as current as possible.

We would be happy to receive comments, corrections and opinions from any of the readers who may be so inclined. If this book has another edition we will certainly incorporate them. We hope all who read this book will enjoy it. If not, let us know.

Lisa DeAngelis
Philip Gutin
Stephen Leibel
Jerome Posner

I

General principles relevant to diagnosis and treatment

1

Classification, incidence and etiology of intracranial tumors

Introduction

Central nervous system (CNS) tumors are the most feared cancers. Although cancers not involving the CNS ('systemic' cancers, e.g. breast, lung, colon) can cause pain, substantial disability and even death, they attack the **body** whereas CNS tumors cause seizures, dementia, paralysis and aphasia, symptoms that attack the **self**. CNS tumors are also feared because many are intractable to therapies that are effective when applied to systemic tumors. There are several reasons why many CNS tumors resist treatment. For example, surgical techniques that allow complete removal of a breast or colon cancer along with a margin of surrounding normal tissue are not feasible in the brain. Radiation therapy that controls tumors elsewhere in the body often fails to do so in the CNS unless it destroys vital normal CNS tissue along with the tumor. Most CNS tumors are either intrinsically resistant to chemotherapeutic agents or develop resistance through genetic instability during treatment.

Adding to the public's concern is evidence that the incidence of several brain tumors is increasing. Brain tumors, long the second most common childhood cancer after the leukemias,[1] are now more common than acute lymphocytic leukemia and may soon surpass all leukemias as the most common childhood cancer.[2] Malignant brain tumors also appear to be increasing in adults, particularly in the elderly.[3]

Some of the apparent increase in CNS tumors may be due to better detection with powerful imaging techniques such as magnetic resonance imaging (MRI) or to the fact that most brain tumors occur in old age, a cohort whose numbers are increasing.[4] The proponderence of evidence indicates that most or all of the apparent increase in CNS tumor incidence in both adults and children is related to better diagnosis.[5] Primary CNS lymphoma is the exception (Chapter 11).

Despite the fear and pessimism about CNS tumors, progress in diagnosis (Chapter 3) and treatment (Chapter 4) is being made: better diagnostic techniques, such as MRI and stereotactic needle biopsy, have led to earlier diagnosis that in some instances improves therapy. New imaging techniques such as functional MRI[6] (fMRI) and intraoperative MRI[7] enable the surgeon to excise tumors more radically because brain structures vital for CNS function (e.g. motor, sensory, visual and language areas) can be accurately identified both prior to and during surgery, allowing more extensive and safer resection. These techniques are particularly important because, for most CNS tumors, **surgery** is the most effective treatment. New techniques of **radiation therapy** such as three-dimensional conformal radiotherapy, radiosurgery and fractionated stereotactic radiotherapy (FSRT) allow a more potent attack on tumors while sparing normal CNS tissue. New **chemotherapy** agents and novel

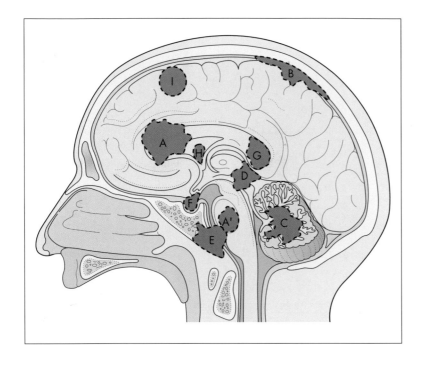

Figure 1.1
The general appearance and common location of several intracranial tumors, discussed in this book, are illustrated in this schematic: (A) A glioma of the anterior corpus callosum (Chapter 5). (A') A glioma of the brainstem (Chapter 5). (B) A meningioma compressing but not invading the brain (Chapter 6). (C) A medulloblastoma involving the vermis of the cerebellum (Chapter 7). (D) A pinealoma compressing the tectum of the brainstem (Chapter 8). (E) A chordoma of the clivus compressing the brainstem (Chapter 9). (F) A pituitary adenoma (Chapter 10). (G) A lymphoma involving the splenium of the corpus callosum (Chapter 11). (H) A colloid cyst of the Foramen of Monro. (I) A metastasis to the brain (Chapter 13).

combinations of established agents have demonstrated efficacy in certain brain tumors. Preliminary studies of gene therapy and anti-angiogenesis factors have generated much excitement, but still no cures. Thus, although CNS tumors remain largely intractable, survival has improved,[8–9] particularly in children[2] but also in adults.

This book is divided into two major sections. Part I (Chapters 1–4) discusses the general principles of diagnosis and treatment of CNS tumors. Part II (Chapters 5–13) discusses specific intracranial tumors. The reason for this division, despite the inevitable redundancy, is that many of the principles of diagnosis and treatment and many of the elements of fundamental biology of CNS tumors apply to all CNS tumors. Space considerations force us to concentrate only on major topics. Several much longer and, thus, more comprehensive books have been published recently.[10–14]

The term brain tumor, as most physicians use it, is a misnomer. Most of the time, when we use the term brain tumor we mean, instead, intracranial tumor (Fig. 1.1). Thus, meningiomas that compress but rarely invade the brain are considered to be brain tumors, as are tumors of the pituitary and pineal glands, which are not strictly part of the brain, but reside within the intracranial cavity. Furthermore, intracranial tumors can be classified into two major groups (Table 1.1): newly diagnosed tumors that arise de novo within the intracranial contents (**primary** CNS tumors) number about 30 000 in the United States each year; tumors that spread to the intracranial contents from a systemic cancer (**metastases**) number about 100 000 in the USA each year. In this book, the terms CNS and intracranial are used interchangeably; the much less common spinal tumors (also CNS) are not considered.

Table 1.1
Site of intracranial tumors.

Tumor type	Site	% of Primary brain tumors (approximate)[b]	Example(s)
I Primary intracranial tumors[a] (N = 30 000/year)			
Neuroepithelial tumors	Brain	36–45	Glioma, medulloblastoma, neurocytoma
Meningeal tumors	Dura	26–40	Meningioma
Pituitary tumors	Pituitary	6–10	Adenoma
Nerve sheath tumors	Cranial nerves	4–7	Acoustic neuroma
Pineal region tumors	Pineal, suprasellar cistern	0.3	Germinoma
Lymphocytic tumors	Brain	1–3[c]	Primary CNS lymphoma
Malformative tumors	Meninges	2	Dermoid, epidermoid
II Metastatic intracranial tumors[d] (N = 100 000/year)			
Cells from any organ	Brain, dura, meninges etc.		Breast, lung, melanoma

[a]After WHO Classification[15]
[b]Data from Radhakrishnan[16] and CBTRUS[17]
[c]See text
[d]From Posner[13] and Greenlee et al[18]

Primary intracranial tumors can arise from virtually any cell type (or its precursor)[17] found within the intracranial contents (Fig. 1.1); metastases can reach the intracranial contents from cancers of any organ or tissue. Although primary brain tumors are often classified as 'benign' or 'malignant', a classification by histologic grade (low-grade/high-grade) is preferable: Tumors that arise within the parenchyma of the brain are rarely truly benign, because surgery seldom cures and many that begin as low-grade tumors become more biologically aggressive over time. Most tumors arising outside the parenchyma of the brain, such as meningiomas and pituitary tumors, can be considered benign because they are often cured by surgery, although, at times, complete resection is not technically feasible, making the tumor less than 'benign'. Brain tumors are rarely truly malignant, in the sense of most systemic cancers, because they seldom metastasize to other organs. However, they can grow rapidly to destroy important surrounding normal tissues, extensively infiltrate the brain, and may seed virtually the entire neuraxis via cerebrospinal fluid (CSF) pathways. By contrast, metastases to the brain are truly malignant tumors (Chapter 13).

Classification

The World Health Organization (WHO) classifies CNS tumors by their patterns of differentiation and presumed cell of origin[15] (Table 1.2).

Table 1.2
Histological classification of tumors of the CNS.

Tumors of neuroepithelial tissue
    Astrocytic tumors
        Diffuse astrocytoma
        Anaplastic (malignant) astrocytoma
        Glioblastoma multiforme
        Pilocytic astrocytoma
        Pleomorphic xanthoastrocytoma
        Subependymal giant cell astrocytoma
    Oligodendroglial tumors
        Oligodendroglioma
        Anaplastic (malignant) oligodendroglioma
    Mixed gliomas
        Oligoastrocytoma
        Anaplastic oligoastrocytoma
    Ependymal tumors
        Ependymoma
        Anaplastic (malignant) ependymoma
        Myxopapillary ependymoma (spinal tumor)
        Subependymoma
    Choroid plexus
        Choroid plexus papilloma
        Choroid plexus carcinoma
    Neuronal and mixed neuronal-glial tumors
        Gangliocytoma
        Dysembryoplastic neuroepithelial tumor
        Ganglioglioma
        Anaplastic (malignant) ganglioglioma
        Central neurocytoma
    Pineal parenchymal tumors
        Pineocytoma
        Pineoblastoma
        Tumor of intermediate differentiation
    Embryonal tumors
        Medulloblastoma
        Primitive neuroectodermal tumor (PNET)

Tumors of cranial nerves
    Schwannoma
    Neurofibroma
Tumors of meninges
    Meningioma
    Hemangiopericytoma
    Melanocytic tumor
    Hemangioblastoma
Primary CNS lymphomas
Germ cell tumors
    Germinoma
    Embryonal carcinoma
    Yolk sac tumor (endodermal sinus tumor)
    Choriocarcinoma
    Teratoma
    Mixed germ cell tumors
Cysts and tumor-like lesions
    Rathke cleft cyst
    Epidermoid cyst
    Dermoid cyst
    Colloid cyst of the third ventricle
Tumors of the sellar region
    Pituitary adenoma
    Pituitary carcinoma
    Craniopharyngioma
    Granular cell tumor
Metastatic tumors
    From any primary source

*Abridged and modified from the WHO classification.[15]

For clinical purposes, it is often useful to classify a tumor by intracranial site, as in Fig. 1.1, as well as by cell of origin. Thus, in this book, tumors of the pineal region, whether neuroepithelial (e.g. pineocytoma) or germ cell in origin, are discussed together (Chapter 8), as are tumors of the pituitary and suprasellar regions (Chapter 10). Tumors considered by the WHO to be embryonal are discussed in Chapter 7, along with neuronal tumors, because the major embryonal tumor, the medulloblastoma, often expresses neuronal protein markers.

Approximately 70% of symptomatic primary CNS tumors arise within the parenchyma of the brain; although their exact lineage is unknown, they are believed to be of neuroepithelial origin, primarily from glial cells (usually astrocytes) or their precursors. The remainder arise from meninges, pituitary or other cell types (e.g. meningeal cells, pituicytes, lymphocytes, germ cells). That neuroepithelial tumors are among the most common brain tumors is not surprising because glia (from Greek for 'glue') constitute 90% of brain cells. Glia include astrocytes (from Greek for 'star' and 'cell'), oligodendrocytes (from Greek for 'few' and 'tree') and ependymal cells (from Greek for 'to place over' i.e. to line the ventricle). Neurons constitute less than 10% of brain cells; they number 100 billion and are mostly postmitotic in the adult CNS. They or their precursors are an uncommon source of CNS neoplasms.

Occasionally, CNS tumors arise from cells not normally found in the nervous system. These include germ cell tumors, histologically identical to those of the testis and ovary. Intracranial germ cell tumors grow in or around the pineal gland and the suprasellar area (Chapter 8). Primary lymphomas of the nervous system (Chapter 11) and metastases from systemic cancers (Chapter 13) can affect any part of the CNS. Tumors can also arise from faulty migration of embryonic tissues. These include craniopharyngioma (Chapter 10) and dermoid and epidermoid tumors (Chapter 12).

As Table 1.1 indicates, meningeal tumors and gliomas account for the majority of intracranial tumors. High-grade ('malignant') gliomas, such as glioblastoma multiforme and anaplastic astrocytoma, make up the majority of gliomas. Recent evidence suggests that oligodendrogliomas and their anaplastic counterparts may be more common than previously believed, an important observation because these tumors are chemosensitive and require different treatment (Chapter 5). Their increase in relative frequency among gliomas probably reflects changing pathologic criteria[19] rather than a true change in incidence. Primary CNS lymphomas are probably underestimated as a percentage of brain tumors because of their rapidly increasing incidence[20] (Chapter 11).

Incidence of intracranial tumors

The American Cancer Society (ACS) estimated the number of new 'brain and other nervous system' cancers (the term used by the ACS) in 2001 to be 17 200 (9800 males and 7400 females),[18] more than twice that of Hodgkin's disease and over half that of melanoma. These figures do not include metastases or 'benign' tumors. In 2001, primary CNS cancers killed approximately 13 100 persons. In women, the mortality caused by CNS cancers is about the same as that caused by uterine cancer. Brain tumors are the second leading cause of cancer deaths in children, the second leading cause of cancer deaths in men aged 20–39 and the fifth in women of that age.

Metastases to the CNS from a systemic (i.e. non-CNS) primary cancer are far more common than primary CNS tumors as a cause of disability and death. Exact data are not available, but one estimate suggests that over 100 000 individuals a year will die having suffered from **symptomatic** intracranial metastases.[13,21] CNS metastases usually appear late in the course of a patient's cancer, but in a significant number of patients CNS symptoms are the presenting complaint. Thus, the physician must always consider metastatic disease as a possible cause of neurologic symptoms and

Table 1.3
Primary brain tumors by histological type in Rochester, Minnesota, 1950 to 1989.

	Average age- and sex-adjusted incidence rate/100 000/year			
	All patients		Symptomatic patients	
Tumor type	% of total	Rate/100 000/year	% of total	Rate/100 000/year
All types	100	19.1	100	11.8
Malignant astrocytoma	18	3.6	26	3.3
Low-grade astrocytoma	7	1.3	8	0.9
Meningiomas	40	7.8	16	2.0

Modified from Radhakrishnan et al[16]

signs in any patient with cancer (Chapter 13), and include metastases in the differential diagnosis of intracranial mass lesions even in patients not known to have systemic cancer.

A major problem in epidemiologic studies of brain tumors is ascertainment. Incidence figures are affected by the quality of the clinical evaluation, record-keeping and autopsy rates. The most complete epidemiologic studies come from the Mayo Clinic[16] (Table 1.3). Table 1.3 includes only astrocytomas and meningiomas; other tumors including pituitary adenomas (Chapter 10) make up the remainder of the 100%.

This is because Olmstead County, Minnesota where the Mayo Clinic is based, is unique in that all medical records containing clinical and pathologic diagnosis and surgical procedures in the community, including those kept by private physicians, nursing homes, and chronic care facilities, are indexed through a centralized diagnostic registry. Thus, although the population of the county is small, the data are complete and include both clinical and autopsy data. Those data indicate that the age- and sex-adjusted incidence rate for primary intracranial tumors

was 19.1/100 000 persons/year for the period 1950–89. This includes incidences of 11.8 for symptomatic tumors and 7.3 for asymptomatic tumors. Gliomas (including oligodendrogliomas and ependymomas, not included in Table 1.3) represent 29% of all brain tumors but 42% of symptomatic tumors (malignant astrocytomas – 18% of all tumors but 26% of symptomatic tumors), meningiomas 40% and pituitary adenomas 10%. As indicated previously, primary CNS lymphomas, which are said to represent 1%, are probably underestimated with respect to current trends, as may be oligodendrogliomas. The age-specific incidence rates for malignant astrocytomas were highest in the 75–84-year age groups.

More recent but less complete data have been published from the Central Brain Tumor Registry of the United States (CBTRUS) that includes incidence data from 11 state cancer registries recording newly diagnosed cases of 'benign' and 'malignant' primary brain tumors.[17] The total number of patients in the registry is over 40 000 (Table 1.4). The overall incidence rate of 12.73 is similar to that of symptomatic patients from the Mayo Clinic

Table 1.4
Primary brain and CNS tumor incidence rates by major histology groupings and sex, CBTRUS 1992–97.

Histology	Male patients rate/10⁵/year	Female patients rate/10⁵/year	Total rate/10⁵/year (adjusted 2000)
Neuroepithelial tumors	7.50	5.20[a]	6.25
Cranial and spinal nerve tumors	0.90	0.87	0.89
Meningeal tumors	2.39	4.36[a]	3.45
Lymphomas and hematopoietic tumors	0.53	0.24[a]	0.38
Germ cell tumors and cysts	0.11	0.04[a]	0.07
Sellar region tumors	0.94	0.84	0.87
Skull base tumors	0.03	0.02[a]	0.03
Unclassified tumors	0.83	0.76	0.79
Total	13.23	12.33[a]	12.73

[a] $p < 0.05$ for difference between male and female patients.
Modified from CBTRUS[17]

study. This is expected, as state cancer registries are unlikely to include patients whose diagnosis was made at autopsy. The 14 state cancer registries represent a population of over 60 million people.

The National Cancer Data Base collects data from hospital tumor registries for both benign and malignant brain tumors. It now contains data from over 60 000 persons with primary brain tumors diagnosed between 1985–89 and 1990–92.[22] The data are similar to those of other databases.

A recent population-based study of all brain scans in two counties in England yielded a primary brain tumor incidence of 21.04/100 000 person years. About 1/5 of patients were not hospitalized. The incidence of neurepithelial tumors was 9.83 and of meningiomas 3.99. The sellar tumor incidence was also 3.99; the incidence of cranial nerve tumors was 2.38.[23] Because scans are more easily available in the USA, such a study here might find a higher incidence.

Factors affecting incidence of intracranial tumors

The incidence of intracranial tumors in general and of specific histologic types of intracranial tumors differs by racial and ethnic group, sex, age, geography and even social class.[24] Differences in brain tumor incidence by race and ethnic group include the findings that Jews now living in Israel who were born in Europe and America have a higher incidence of brain tumors than those now living in Israel who were born in Africa or Asia. The overall incidence of brain tumors (especially gliomas) is greater in whites than blacks. However, meningiomas are more frequent in blacks than in whites.[24] Pituitary adenomas are also more common in blacks than in whites.

Sex differences are striking. The male to female ratio is 1.7 for oligodendrogliomas, 1.6 for astrocytomas and 1.0 for malignant meningiomas. For benign meningiomas, the female to male ratio is 1.5 for intracranial meningiomas but 3.5 for spinal meningiomas. Nerve sheath tumors have an equal sex ratio. Lymphomas and germ cell tumors are more common in males. These data are from the National Cancers Institute's (NCI) SEER registry (Surveillance, Epidemiology, and End Results), which collects incidence and survival data on 'malignant' tumors from selected cancer registries across the USA (http://www-seer.ims.nci.nih.gov/Publications). The CBTRUS data[17] that include benign tumors, e.g.

meningiomas and pituitary adenomas, confirm the SEER findings.

CNS tumors can occur at any age. Both the overall incidence and the histologic type of intracranial tumors vary by age. Overall, there is a small peak before age 10 and a steady rise from 15 on. Some data indicate that intracranial tumor incidence flattens or even falls after age 75 (Fig. 1.2) but this finding may result from less vigorous evaluation of elderly

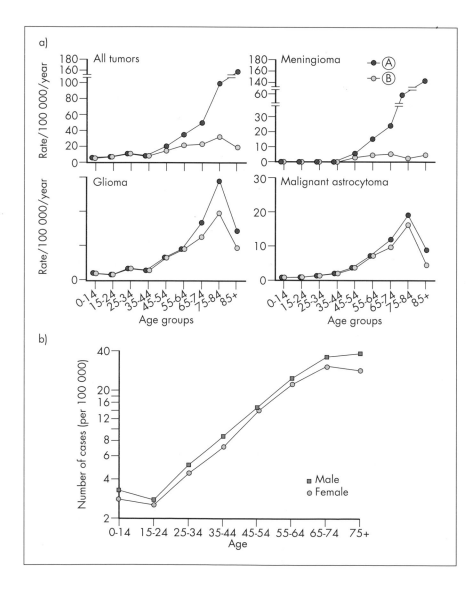

Figure 1.2
(a) Age-specific incidence rates of primary intracranial neoplasms in Rochester, Minnesota between 1950 and 1989. All primary intracranial tumors are indicated by the red circles. The green circles indicate those tumors that were identified in clinical evaluation of symptomatic patients. Note the fall-off in clinically diagnosed tumors at extreme old age. From Radhakrishnan et al[16] with permission. (b) Average annual age-specific incidence of intracranial tumors in white men and women in Los Angeles County from 1972 to 1993. Note in these 10 000 patients the leveling in incidence of tumors in old age. From Preston-Martin[25] with permission.

Table 1.5
CNS tumor incidence per 10^5 person-years by age at diagnosis.

Histology	Age at diagnosis (years)							
	0–19	20–34	35–44	45–54	55–64	65–74	75–84	85+
Total tumors	3.69	5.67	9.50	15.78	24.92	36.45	39.81	31.55
Glioblastoma	0.17	0.41	1.21	3.81	8.16	12.34	11.22	5.41
Meningioma	0.10	0.64	2.13	4.35	6.60	11.50	14.70	14.30
Lymphoma	0.01	0.26	0.47	0.41	0.65	1.09	1.22	0.47

Modified from CBTRUS[17]

patients with neurologic disability. Low-grade gliomas, such as astrocytomas, are more common in the young, and high-grade tumors, such as glioblastoma, are more common in the elderly. Medulloblastomas and germ cell tumors of the pineal region are tumors of childhood. SEER data from 1973–1991 report only 208 glioblastomas under age 20, compared to 3 479 over age 65. Conversely, pilocytic astrocytomas, a low-grade tumor (Chapter 5), was more common under age 20 ($n = 252$) than over age 65 ($n = 7$). There were 578 medulloblastomas under age 20 and only 3 over age 65. Pineal region tumors numbered 25 under age 20 and only 1 over age 65.[26] The lifetime risk of a CNS malignancy is 0.67% for men and 0.52% for women (SEER).

A recent population study from Japan[27] compared the incidence of intracranial tumors in those older and younger than age 70. Between 1989 and 1995, 1354 new primary intracranial tumors were diagnosed in Kumamoto, Japan. The overall age-adjusted incidence was $18.1/10^5$ for those older than 70 and $8.7/10^5$ for those younger. The CBTRUS data[17] show an increasing incidence in all intracranial tumors with age; the highest rate is in the 75–84-year-old age group.

Glioblastoma peaks between ages 65 and 74 and declines slightly after age 75. The meningioma rate also increases with age and does not decline after age 75 (Table 1.5).

Reported brain tumor incidence also varies by geography. The most developed countries report higher rates of primary brain tumors than less developed nations. The age adjusted incidence in Scandinavia is reported to be 31.4 per million, significantly higher than the US rates of 21.7 for blacks and 26.4 for whites. In the USA, Canada, western Europe and Australia, the rates are similar and greater than those of eastern Europe. The lowest incidences among developed countries are in Japan, India and Singapore.[24] Even though the overall incidence is low in Asia, specific tumors are more common. For example, germ cell tumors are much more common in Japanese boys than in any other group in the world (Chapter 8). Migrant populations usually have higher rates that are closer to those of natives of the adoptive country than those who remain in their country of origin, suggesting that environmental factors are important. How geographical differences are affected by diagnostic facilities and autopsy rates in individual countries is not known.

The reported incidence of intracranial tumors varies by social class (in some studies defined by occupation).[24] In several studies, the incidence of brain tumors increased with social class, this being more evident in men than in women. The differences between men and women would seem to rule out ascertainment as an explanation, as both sexes within each class should have equal access to medical care. The explanation of social class differences, if real, is not known.

Increasing incidence?

An important question is whether the incidence of brain tumors in general and certain specific tumors in particular is increasing. Some evidence suggests that the incidence is increasing, making most published data that consist of information from previous years unreliable with respect to the present situation.[23,28–30] For example, a study using data from the Florida Cancer Registry[29] comparing brain tumor incidence from 1981–84 with the incidence from 1986–89 indicates a consistently significant increase in all primary brain tumors in patients over age 65, with the largest increase in those over 85. An 'incidence density ratio' (IDR or risk ratio) was calculated by dividing age-adjusted incidence for the period 1986–89 by the corresponding age-adjusted incidence for 1981–84. When specific histologic types were examined, those patients aged 20–64 showed a statistically significant increase with an IDR greater than 3 for both anaplastic astrocytomas and primary CNS lymphomas. Those over 65 showed a statistically significant increase for anaplastic astrocytomas (IDR = 2.7), glioblastomas (IDR = 1.1) and lymphomas (IDR = 3.4) as well as total brain tumors.

Olney et al,[30] using the NCI SEER data compared year-by-year incidence of astrocytomas, anaplastic astrocytomas and glioblastomas from 1975–92. There was a decrease in astrocytomas but a sharp increase in both anaplastic astrocytomas and glioblastomas. Although it is possible that the decrease in astrocytomas and increase in anaplastic astrocytomas could be accounted for, in part, by differences in pathologic interpretation, it is unlikely that the same could be said for glioblastomas, where interpretation is fairly uniform among neuropathologists. A study using data from the French Cancer Registry from 1983 to 1989 indicates that malignant astrocytomas increased by 5% a year in individuals over age 65.[31]

A study of glial tumors identified in New York State between 1976 and 1995 revealed an increasing incidence of glioblastomas and anaplastic astrocytomas, especially in those over age 60. The reason for these statistically significant increases is not clear.[32]

Not all studies support an increasing incidence.[5,16] Furthermore incidence rates that were increasing seem to have stabilized.[33] Moreover, several problems complicate the epidemiologic data that appear to indicate that brain tumors are increasing in both adults[4] and children.[1] In adults, the major problem is ascertainment.[16] For example, studies of brain tumor incidence based on autopsy data differ substantially from those based on clinical evaluation. The differences occur in part because many brain tumors, particularly small meningiomas and pituitary tumors, are common but often asymptomatic and, thus, represent only incidental findings at autopsy. Furthermore, diagnosis even of clinically symptomatic patients, particularly those who are elderly, is often incomplete. Prior to the development of non-invasive brain imaging by computed tomography (CT) and MR scanning, many elderly patients with neurologic dysfunction were believed to have had strokes or dementing illnesses and were not further evaluated. We still encounter elderly patients who

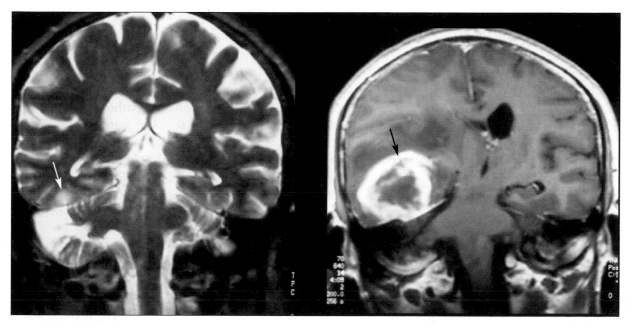

Figure 1.3
Failure to diagnose a brain tumor in an elderly woman. A 70-year-old woman presented with new-onset headache. A non-contrast MR T2 weighted (left image) scan revealed a right temporal lobe lesion (arrow) interpreted as representing ischemic vascular disease in this elderly patient. The headaches resolved, but when she developed personality change, confusion and weakness several months later, a contrast-enhanced MR scan (right image) clearly identified the previously small lesion as a now large glioblastoma (arrow).

suffer a sudden onset of neurologic symptoms and in whom a non-contrast CT scan or, more rarely, an unenhanced MRI is misinterpreted as cerebral infarction. Cerebrovascular disease is far more common than brain tumors (Fig. 1.3) and because a contrast study may have been omitted either to save costs or to save the patient 'side-effects', the true nature of the illness may not be discovered, and the patient's death attributed to a 'stroke'. If repeat imaging with contrast is never performed, the correct diagnosis is never established. This failure to identify tumors in the elderly has fostered the belief that the incidence of brain tumors peaks in late middle age and then declines in the elderly. As diagnostic techniques became less invasive, and therefore more widely used, and

as the general attitude toward the diagnosis and treatment of neurologic illness in those of advanced age has changed, accurate diagnosis has become more complete, making it clear that the incidence of primary brain tumors increases with advancing age. Whether the increase continues into very advanced age is not yet established.

Another consideration in evaluating the apparent increase in brain tumor incidence is a change in the age of the population.[4] As a population ages, its diseases change and the incidence of a particular disease in the population may rise. Genetic differences in elderly individuals who might in the past have died of premature cardiac or cerebrovascular disease, which are now treated effectively, may make them more susceptible later in life to brain tumors.[4] For example, one study found that individuals with a specific genetic variant of a hepatic metabolic gene were at increased risk for oligodendrogliomas.[34] If that same variant also conferred protection from heart disease and systemic cancers, enabling long-term survival, there would be more brain tumors in the elderly. Furthermore, when this factor is combined with the generally better health of the elderly population and more vigorous evaluation of neurologic complaints in these patients, the increase in brain tumors may not reflect an environmental factor. The advent of Medicare, giving many of the elderly better access to medical care, may also play a role.

Pediatric brain tumors also are reported to be increasing in incidence.[35] Data from SEER were analyzed for children 14 years of age or younger between 1974 and 1991. There was an average 2% increase in incidence per year for astroglial tumors. These increases were most apparent among children less than 3 years old.[36] A recent report from Ontario, Canada noted a 'small but significant trend toward increasing incidence' in persons under age 20.[35] Others interpret the data as showing a one time 'jump' in incidence, suggesting that the apparent increase represents either better detection methods, or more accurate reporting to tumor registries.[1,37]

Important for clinicians is a change in the relative frequency of specific tumors. For example, primary CNS lymphomas (lymphomas that arise in the nervous system and are not metastatic from systemic lymphoma) are increasing both in absolute incidence and in relative frequency when compared to other primary brain tumors (Chapter 11).[20] This increase is apparent in both the immunosuppressed (e.g. AIDS) and immunocompetent populations. The clinical result is that a tumor, once considered a curiosity and the subject of individual case reports, is now a clinical consideration in every patient who presents with a mass lesion in the brain. Furthermore, the relative increase of primary to metastatic brain lymphoma decreases the need, in appropriate clinical circumstances, for extensive, repeated searches for an extracranial primary lymphoma (Chapter 11). Because the diagnostic approach and treatment of primary CNS lymphomas differ from those of other brain tumors, the physician must consider lymphoma, even before the diagnosis has been established. Such patients should be evaluated for HIV infection or other immune-suppressing illnesses, and diagnosed by needle biopsy rather than craniotomy (Chapter 3).

A second clinical implication of the changing relative incidence of specific types of brain tumors relates to the apparent increase in the relative incidence of oligodendrogliomas (see Chapter 5). The apparent increase in incidence almost certainly represents a change in the criteria that neuropathologists use for diagnosis:[38] neuropathologic diagnosis is subjective and based on morphologic interpretation of the tumor tissue. A recently described transcription factor (OLIG2) may differentiate oligodendrogliomas from astrocytomas, the tumors most likely to be confused with each other.[39] However, because the treatment of oligodendrogliomas differs from the more common astrocytoma (Chapter 5), the clinician must work closely with the neuropathologist to determine the correct diagnosis, that will dictate therapy to some degree and predict prognosis. Luckily, genetic markers may soon solve the problem.[40]

Etiology

Many patients, when informed by their physician that they are suffering from a brain tumor, ask 'What caused it?' For the vast majority of patients, there is no adequate answer. In a small number of patients one can identify environmental factors that clearly cause or predispose toward the development of a brain tumor. In an even smaller number of patients, inherited genetic abnormalities are causal. For most patients, the physician cannot identify any factor that may have caused the tumor. Many patients, distressed over the diagnosis and our lack of knowledge concerning the cause, find this explanation unsatisfactory and search for potential causes. Some come up with what they believe to be satisfactory explanations: these include the use of cellular telephones, exposure to electromagnetic waves from power stations, head trauma, and various occupational or dietary exposures. Patients are often supported in their belief by anecdotal reports in the medical literature or by a single epidemiologic study.

Epidemiologic studies of risk factors for brain tumors are fraught with difficulty. Even when a large population is surveyed, the number of brain tumors is relatively small and statistically significant differences may not be reproducible. Furthermore, many studies consider 'brain tumors' as a group and do not stratify by histology. Stratification by histologic type is important because there are undoubtedly different risk factors for different tumor types, e.g. meningiomas compared to gliomas. Thus, two carefully done studies may yield conflicting results, one, for example, suggesting that exposure to high-tension wires increases the number of brain tumors, and another showing no such risk. Until more than one study clearly confirms the risk, the physician should withhold judgment. The paragraphs below consider the evidence for both environmental and familial risk factors.

Environmental risk factors

Although a large number of studies have examined the relationship between the environment and the occurrence of brain tumors

Table 1.6
Risk factors related to CNS tumors.[3]

Definitive
Ionizing radiation[41,42]
Immune suppression
HIV infection[43,44]
Iatrogenic (e.g. organ transplant)
Possible
Electromagnetic fields[45]
High tension wires[46]
Cellular telephones[47–49]
Diet[50]
N-nitroso compounds
Aspartame[30]
Occupation[51]
Petroleum industry
Agricultural pesticides[52]
Household chemicals
Hair dyes and sprays
Household pesticides[52,53]
Head injury[54,55]
Medications
Vitamins[56]
Infections
Cysticercosis[57]
Varicella-zoster[58]
SV40[59,60]

(Table 1.6), only two unequivocal risk factors have been identified.[24]

The first is ionizing radiation; the second is immune suppression. Low-dose irradiation to the scalp once given for the treatment of tinea capitus, a fungal infection of the scalp, has been shown to cause meningiomas,[42] many of which are anaplastic, and approximately a three-fold increase in the incidence of glial tumors. Nerve sheath tumors of the head and neck are increased an astounding 33-fold.[61]

Higher-dose irradiation for intracranial tumors, e.g. medulloblastoma or extracranial head cancers, including prophylactic irradiation for leukemia, increases the incidence of both gliomas and sarcomas seven-fold in those who survive more than 3 years. The cumulative relative risk of secondary brain tumors in patients treated with cranial irradiation for leukemia is 1.39 at 20 years; approximately two-thirds of the tumors are gliomas and one-third meningiomas.[62] High-grade gliomas have a shorter median latency (9.1 years) from the cranial radiotherapy than do meningiomas (19 years). The lower dose of prophylactic radiation now used for leukemia will probably decrease, but not eliminate, the incidence of secondary brain tumors. In one series, the use of antimetabolites during radiation therapy (RT) may have increased the number of brain tumors.[63] Prenatal radiographs may predispose to childhood brain tumors. Dental radiography[55] and cosmic rays do not appear to be risk factors, except for a possible increase in meningiomas in patients given the high-dose whole-mouth radiographs used decades ago.[64] Curiously, those dental X-rays appeared to protect against the later development of gliomas. That study also showed a similar unexplained decreased risk for glioma associated with exposure to amalgam fillings. Other studies have not found dental radiographs or amalgam to be either risk or protective factors.[65]

Acquired immune suppression, such as HIV infection[66] or the use of immunosuppressive agents after organ transplant, increases the incidence of primary lymphomas of the CNS; HIV infection may also increase the frequency of gliomas and intracranial leiomyosarcomas.[43] Congenital immune-suppressive illnesses such as the Wiskott–Aldrich syndrome are also associated with an increased incidence of cerebral lymphomas.

Primary CNS lymphomas in immunosuppressed patients are driven by pre-existing latent Epstein–Barr viral infection of B-lymphocytes. When a lymphoma occurs in an immunosuppressed patient, it is twice as likely to occur in the brain as elsewhere in the body. This is in contradistinction to the situation in the immunocompetent patient, where the brain is the primary site of lymphoma in only 1% of patients. The question of increased glial tumors in HIV-infected patients remains unsettled; reports suggested that immune suppression is a risk factor for glial tumors[44,67] but the incidence is not sufficiently high to classify glioma as an AIDS-defining illness.

Other studies of environmental risk factors are substantially less convincing than those of ionizing radiation and immunosuppression. Some investigators report that industrial exposure to polyvinyl chloride or dietary exposure to N-nitrosourea compounds could be risk factors[50] but others have failed to substantiate these findings. Some evidence suggests that consumption of cured meats, which contain N-nitroso compounds, may not only predispose to brain tumors in the consumer, but also in the children of mothers who consume the products during pregnancy.[68] Some evidence suggests that vitamins and other antioxidants[69] may protect against N-nitroso compounds. Prenatal or early childhood vitamin intake may protect children against brain tumors, but the data are equivocal.[56] Fruit and vegetable consumption may decrease risk. Other studies have tentatively identified high-protein diets and alcohol as risk factors, and a few studies have implicated parental exposure to these factors in causation of childhood brain tumors; the data are not compelling. Thus, the role, if any, of nutrition in either causing or protecting from brain tumors remains unknown. As a result, the physician is unable to give patients evidence-based advice.

Head trauma[55] has been reported as an environmental risk factor for the development of glial tumors and meningiomas but the evidence is unconvincing. One study relates acoustic trauma to the later development of acoustic neuromas (Chapter 9), but more studies are required to be certain.

There has been recent concern in the lay population that exposure to electromagnetic radiation, including high tension wires, computer terminals, and cellular telephones may cause brain tumors. Although cellular telephones cause headache,[70] and may cause death by increasing automobile accidents, evidence suggests that they do not cause brain tumors.[47,48] One doubts that we are going to see an epidemic of left temporal tumors whose incidence is related to telephone conversations.

Olney and colleagues[30] have proposed that the recent increase in malignant brain tumors may be due to ingestion of aspartame, a dipeptide sugar substitute consisting of phenylalanine and aspartic acid. Both of these amino acids are known to be active in the CNS but the evidence that they are a risk factor for brain tumors remains weak for at least three reasons: (1) brain tumors appear to be increasing predominantly in the elderly, the group least likely to use sugar substitutes; (2) these drugs have only been on the market for a few years and one would think that if they were a risk factor for brain tumors, it would take decades for this association to become apparent; and (3) women use aspartame-containing products more than men, but gliomas are more common in men. The first and second reasons apply to cellular telephones as well.

A few medical illnesses have been proposed as risk factors for brain tumors. Breast cancer may predispose to meningioma (Chapter 6). A past history of meningitis or epilepsy has also been reported to be associated with an increased incidence of brain tumor. Some studies have suggested that diabetes and allergic diseases protect against the development of gliomas. The cytochrome P-450 family of liver enzymes are required to metabolize drugs and other toxins. Many of the enzymes are polymorphic, with some forms metabolizing substances faster than others. There may be an increased risk of oligodendrogliomas in individuals who carry a poor metabolizer CYP2D6 variant allele (allele; from the Greek for reciprocally – the same gene location on paired chromosomes) and the GSTT1 null genotype.[34] The role, if any, of individual genetic differences in systemic enzymes in predisposing to brain tumors is not clear.

In other studies, hair dyes, pesticides, formaldehyde, and industrial or occupational substances have all been implicated as a cause of brain tumors, but in none has the hypothesis been confirmed. If any of these environmental factors are true risk factors, each can be responsible for only a small proportion of brain tumors, because only a small percentage of patients have been exposed to such substances.

Prior infection has also been reported to play a role in increasing or decreasing brain tumors. A recent report indicates that cysticercosis infection increases the incidence of gliomas.[57] Although the study was carefully done, the finding needs to be replicated. Cysticercosis is now so common in some parts of the USA that one would have expected to see almost an epidemic of gliomas if the infection were an important predisposing factor. Some reports[60] find SV40 large T-antigen sequences at high frequency in gliomas and medulloblastomas; others do not.[59] The role, if any, of that virus in the etiology of brain tumors is unclear. A recent study suggests that prior varicella-zoster infection, or absence of a serologic response to varicella-zoster with a history of prior infection, protects against glioma.[58] The mechanism is unclear and this study requires replication.

Genetic risk factors

Inherited genetic alterations are predisposing risk factors for brain tumors (Table 1.7). These genetic alterations are usually germline mutations that increase an individual's risk for a specific type or types of brain tumor and other malignancies. Because each mutation is found in every cell in the body, having been transmitted through parental DNA, the resultant brain tumor usually occurs as part of a syndrome that includes systemic cancers and

Table 1.7
Some hereditary syndromes associated with brain tumors.

Hereditary condition	Mode of Inheritance	Type of tumor(s)	Involved chromosomes	Gene	Reference
Li-Fraumeni	AD	Glioma Medulloblastoma	17p13	TP53	72
Tuberous sclerosis	AD	Subependymal giant cell astrocytoma, cortical tubers Glioma	9q34 16p13	TSC1 TSC2	73
Neurofibromatosis type 1 (von Recklinghausen's disease)	AD	Glioma (optic nerve) Astrocytoma, Glioblastoma	17q11	NF1	74, 75
Neurofibromatosis type 2	AD	Meningioma Schwannoma (bilateral acoustic neuroma) Ependymomas	22q12	NF2	76
Multiple endocrine neoplasia type 1	AD	Pituitary	11q13	Menin	77
Retinoblastoma	AD	Retinoblastoma	13q14	RB1	78
Basal cell nevus syndrome	AD	Medulloblastoma	9q22	PTCH	79
Turcot syndrome Hereditary nonpolyposis colorectal cancer syndrome (HNPCC)	AR or AD	Brain tumors of diverse histology, including glioblastoma and medulloblastoma	5q21 2p16 3p21 7p22	APC HMLH2 HMLH1 h85M2	80
von Hippel–Lindau disease	AD	Hemangioblastoma	3p25–20	VHL	81
Cowden's syndrome	AD	Dysplastic cerebellar gangliocytoma, meningioma, astrocytoma	10p23	PTEN (MMAC1)	82
Rhabdoid predisposition syndrome	AD	Choroid plexus carcinoma, medulloblastoma, primitive neuro-ectodermal tumors	22q11	hSNFS/INI1	83

AD, autosomal dominant; AR, autosomal recessive.

other malformations as well as CNS tumors (Chapter 12). Although these syndromes account for a small minority of brain tumors (about 5% of gliomas are familial and about 1% have a possible autosomal dominant inheritance),[71] the wide range of genetic abnormalities that can lead to CNS neoplasms suggests that there may be many genetic 'avenues' that can cause these tumors. Furthermore, the study of familial syndromes, where genetic abnormalities are more easily identified, may aid in finding similar defects in the more common sporadic brain tumors.

Interacting genetic and environmental factors

It is likely that for the vast majority of patients no single genetic or environmental factor is sufficient to explain the development of a brain tumor. Interactions among multiple factors may be necessary. For example, N-nitroso compounds clearly cause brain tumors in experimental animals. These compounds are found in the human diet in bacon, cured meats and other foods. Their role, if any, in the production of human brain tumors may be modified by the concomitant ingestion of vitamins and foods containing antioxidants that may decrease the carcinogenic properties of the N-nitroso compounds. In addition, genetic factors may play a role. For example, the genetically determined presence of the enzyme O^6-methylguanine-DNA methyltransferase (MGMT or AGT) is important in repairing DNA abnormalities caused by N-nitroso compounds.[84] A patient with a deficiency of this enzyme and poor intake of antioxidants may be more susceptible to N-nitroso compounds than another patient with a good intake of antioxidants and a relative excess of the enzyme. It will be very difficult for epidemiologists to dissect all of these multiple interacting factors, but such

investigations are necessary to clarify the etiology of brain tumors.

Biology of intracranial tumors

At their core, all tumors have a genetic origin.[85] In familial tumors, the defect is in the germ line; thus, the same genetic mutation is transmitted to all the somatic cells of the carrier's offspring. Acquired tumors begin when an environmental factor alters a gene, usually in a single somatic cell. However, a single genetic abnormality is insufficient to cause the altered cell to become a neoplasm. A series of genetic changes is required before the cell can exhibit unrestrained growth, outstrip the reproductive rate of its neighboring normal cells and develop into a tumor. The large number of genetic mutations in a cancer cell may result from an early mutation in a gene that is required for the maintenance of genetic stability.[86] However, genes need not be mutated to dysfunction. For example hypermethylation of a DNA promotor region can disrupt gene function.[87] Data from many cancers indicate that every tumor expresses a large number of genes not expressed in its counterpart normal tissue. Although the functions of most of these uniquely expressed genes are not known, most of their protein products appear to be involved either in regulating the cell cycle or regulating how the cell responds to environmental factors that promote differentiation, maturation and normal cell death, i.e. apoptosis. Apoptosis (from the Greek apo for 'off' plus ptosis for 'a falling') is a normal process of cell death. The process can occur as 'programmed cell death' that occurs in embryonic development or it can be induced by 'stress signals' arising within the cell or by signals elicited by binding of 'death ligands' to the cell. Apoptosis, as opposed to necrosis requires energy in order to synthesize proteins to initiate the process. Cells suffering damage to their DNA that cannot be repaired normally undergo apoptosis. Failure of the normal apoptotic process allows cells to accumulate further DNA abnormalities that can lead to the development of cancers. Several genes altered in cancer are involved either in initiating or inhibiting apoptosis. For example, as indicated below, the p53 tumor suppressor gene, and possibly the related genes p63 and p73,[88,89] have as one of their functions the initiation of apoptosis in a cell whose DNA damage is irreparable. Genetic abnormalities, such as mutation or deletion of p63 or related genes, prevent apoptosis and permit survival of damaged cells. Apoptosis is also necessary for radiation and chemotherapy to kill tumor cells.[90] Thus, failure of apoptosis protects the cancer cells from death by cancer therapies.

Two general kinds of genetic alteration usually cause CNS and other tumors. The first is a mutation that inappropriately activates a proto-oncogene. The second is a mutation that inactivates a tumor suppressor gene. Proto-oncogenes are normal cellular genes that regulate cell proliferation, differentiation and apoptosis. Proto-oncogenes can encode growth factors, e.g. basic fibroblastic growth factor (bFGF) or growth factor receptors, e.g. epidermal growth factor receptor (EGFR), or mediate

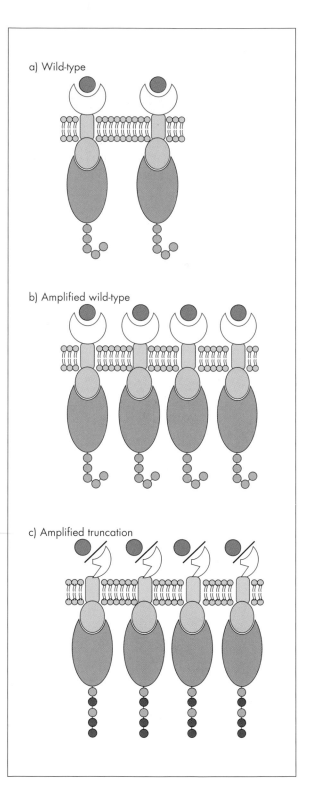

a) Wild-type

b) Amplified wild-type

c) Amplified truncation

Figure 1.4
An example of growth factor receptor abnormalities in a glioblastoma multiforme. (a) shows the wild-type epidermal growth factor receptor. The ligand (red circles) binds to the receptor, and forms a dimer, and signals to the cells to grow. In (b), when the normal receptor is amplified, excessive growth occurs. (c) shows a mutated receptor. The receptor no longer responds to circulating growth factors, but instead is constitutively active, signaling unrestrained growth downstream. Modified from Kleihues and Cavenee[15] with permission.

signaling pathways, e.g. protein kinase C (PKC), or regulate gene expression, e.g. c-myc. Proto-oncogenes become oncogenes by gene mutation, gene amplification, gene overexpression or chromosomal translocation. Mutations such as those that occur in the EGFR may lead to a receptor that is always turned on (constitutively active) and thus not subject to normal cellular control mechanisms (Fig. 1.4). Gene amplification refers to the expansion of the copy number of a gene within the genome. The process can occur through replication of genomic DNA or by homogenous staining regions or double minute chromatin bodies (pieces of extra chromosomal material) leading to increased expression of genes. Some brain tumors amplify EGFR; others amplify myc genes. Chromosomal translocations may activate proto-oncogenes. These abnormalities are often present in hematologic malignancies, including primary CNS lymphomas, and are found in some glioblastoma cell lines[91] but do not appear to play an important role in the development of brain tumors. Overexpression of proto-oncogenes without gene amplification plays an important role in many brain tumors. An example is platelet-derived growth factor (PDGF). Either the ligand, which is homologous to thymidine phosphorylase and thus stimulates DNA synthesis, or the receptor (PDGFR), or both, may be overexpressed.

Oncogenes

Oncogenes function in an autosomal dominant fashion, meaning that mutation of only one allele is necessary to transform the cell; oncogenes exert their malignant action through a gain of functional activity. One good example is the mutation of EGFR that occurs in 40% of glioblastomas. An in-frame deletion leads to a truncated protein that is constitutively active. The cells possessing this deletion are constantly

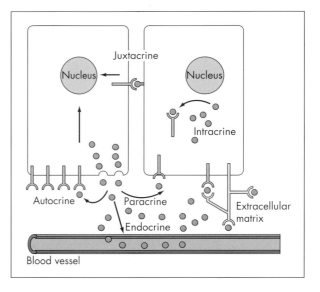

Figure 1.5
Examples of different modes of action of growth factors. Growth factors secreted by an individual tumor cell can stimulate the cell through either its surface receptor (autocrine – cell on left), or an internal receptor (intracrine – cell on right). The growth factor can stimulate neighboring cells by direct contact (juxtacrine), or by diffusing to nearby cells (paracrine), or the growth factor can be secreted into the systemic circulation to affect cells at a distance (endocrine).

stimulated to grow, even in the absence of the receptor ligands, transforming growth factor alpha (TGF-α) and/or epidermal growth factor (EGF) (Fig. 1.4).

Alterations of growth factors can lead to unrestrained growth not only of the cells possessing the alteration but of nearby cells and sometimes distant cells by autocrine, paracrine or endocrine stimulation (Fig. 1.5). One example of autocrine stimulation occurs when TGF-α stimulates EGFRs on the same cell from which the TGF-α is secreted. Sometimes the growth factor does not have to be secreted but can stimulate the receptor from within the cell, intracrine stimulation. One example of paracrine stimulation is when vascular endothelial growth factor (VEGF) secreted by some brain tumor cells stimulates receptors on nearby endothelial cells, causing the endothelial cells to form new blood vessels (angiogenesis; from Greek for 'vessel' and 'production') (Chapter 2). Endocrine stimulation does not appear to play an important role in many brain tumors. One possible example is TGF-β, which is secreted by glioblastoma cells into the bloodstream and may cause the immune suppression that accompanies many glioblastomas.

Many of the growth factors altered in brain tumors exert their function through reversible phosphorylation of tyrosine by tyrosine kinases.[92] Tyrosine kinases play a major role in both normal and neoplastic growth and cell cycle control as well as in differentiation. Growth factor receptors important in brain tumors that function as tyrosine kinases include the EGFR, VEGF, PDGFR and fibroblast growth factor receptor (FGFR).[93] For example, overexpression of the β-chain of PDGFR can cause brain tumors in mice[94] (Fig. 1.6).

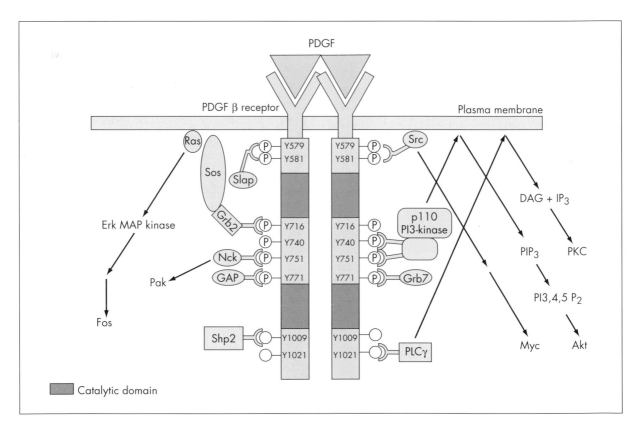

Figure 1.6
The PDGF receptor–tyrosine kinase signaling pathway. Both PDGF and its receptor are over-expressed in many brain tumors. Via autocrine or paracrine stimulation, the excessive activity of the PDGF-β receptor triggers a complicated pathway leading to transcription of genes that increase cellular proliferation. From Hunter[92] with permission.

Table 1.8
Some proto-oncogene abnormalities found in brain tumors.

Gene	Chromosomal location	Mechanism of activation
Oncogene EGFR	7p12	Amplification, rearrangement
PDGFR-A	5q31–q32	Rearrangement, amplification
bFGF	4q25	Overexpression
IGF-1/IGF-1R	12q23; 15q26.3	Overexpression
Ros-1	6q22	Overexpression
H-ras, N-ras	11p15; 1p13	Overexpression, point mutation
c-myc, N-myc	8q24; 2p23–p24	Amplification
gli	12q13–q14	Amplification
met	7q31	Overexpression
gsp	20q12–q13.2	Point mutation

Modified from Israel[95] with permission.

More than 100 different oncogenes have been discovered, most in experimental animal models of cancer. Some of these believed to be important in human brain tumors are detailed in Table 1.8.

Tumor suppressor genes

Tumor suppressor genes, the opposite of oncogenes, comprise the second common genetic alteration (Table 1.9). Normal tumor suppressor genes produce proteins that are involved in inhibiting cell growth or promoting cell differentiation. Unlike oncogenes, most tumor suppressor genes function in an autosomal recessive manner by a loss of function after both alleles are disabled. Many tumor suppressor genes have been identified. Tumor suppressor genes important in brain tumors include p53[96] (see below), PTEN/MMAC1[97] and CDKN2 A and B.[98]

Table 1.9
Tumor suppressor genes in brain tumors.

Gene or locus	Chromosomal location	Tumor type
P53	17p13.1	Astrocytoma
		Glioblastoma
PTEN/MMAC1	10q23	High-grade gliomas
NF1	17q11.2	Pilocytic astrocytoma
RB1	13q14	Glioblastoma
CDKN2 A and B	9p21	Glioblastoma
APC	5q21	? Medulloblastoma
Gorlin locus	9q31	Medulloblastoma
MEN1 locus	11q13	Pituitary adenoma
NF2	22q12	Meningioma

Modified from Israel[95] with permission.

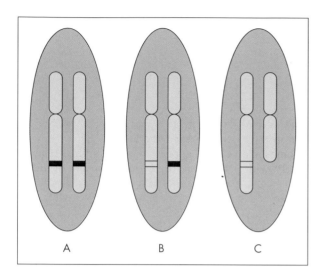

Figure 1.7
Knudson's two-hit therapy of oncogenesis due to loss of tumor suppressor gene function. (A) A normal somatic cell chromosome pair with two wild type alleles for a tumor suppressor gene. (B) Typical somatic cell chromosome pair in a patient with one wild type allele (black band) and one germ line mutant non-functioning allele (empty band). The cell has a normal phenotype. (C) Chromosome pair from a tumor cell arising in a patient with an inherited mutated non-functioning allele and a partial deletion of the chromosome on which the tumor suppressor gene is located. Neither allele of the tumor suppressor gene can function and a tumor develops.

Many of the abnormal or deleted genes in familial tumors are tumor suppressor genes.[99] The loss of a germline tumor suppressor gene on one chromosome may not cause a cancer. However, if through environmental factors a cell having only one normal allele undergoes a genetic mutation of the remaining allele, that cell escapes suppression of uncontrolled growth and grows as a tumor (Fig. 1.7). In individuals with a normal genetic complement, two 'hits', one on the tumor suppressor gene of each chromosome, are necessary before the cell can become transformed. This explains why hereditary retinoblastomas are usually bilateral: one allele is already absent in every cell because of the germline mutation and because single hits are relatively common, at least one cell in each eye is likely to suffer a mutation of the remaining allele. Non-familial retinoblastomas are usually unilateral because two hits in the same cell are rare.

Not all tumor suppressor genes require deletions of both alleles in order to cause tumors. Probably the most common tumor suppressor gene abnormality in cancer involves the p53 gene. This gene encodes a 53-kDa protein that modifies cellular function, including the cell cycle, DNA repair after radiation damage, genomic stability and induction of apoptosis. The protein product of the p53 gene prevents progression of the cell cycle beyond the G1/S checkpoint when damaged DNA is detected. If the DNA can be repaired, the cell cycle proceeds; if not, p53 directs the cell to die (apoptosis). If p53 does not function normally, cells with abnormal DNA can reproduce uncontrollably, causing a neoplasm. Some mutations of the p53 tumor suppressor gene on one allele can cause tumors through a so-called dominant negative mutation.[100] These p53 mutations lead to the synthesis of a defective p53 protein tetramer (the active form of the molecule) in which the mutated protein renders the entire complex inactive.

PTEN gene mutations are common in high-grade gliomas. The protein product of the gene, a protein tyrosine phosphatase, probably negatively regulates cell proliferation by inhibiting protein tyrosine kinase activity.[97]

Some genetic abnormalities are identified by examination of the chromosome on which the gene resides. Chromosomal abnormalities are abundant in CNS tumors. Comparative genomic hybridization (Fig. 1.8) is a technique to identify regions of chromosomal amplification and deletion by comparing normal DNA with tumor DNA. A profile is generated that

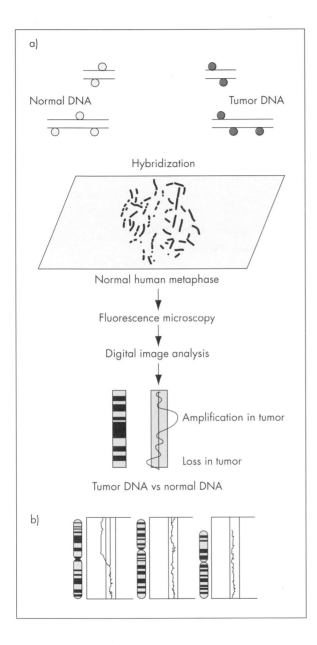

Figure 1.8
Comparative genomic hybridization. (a) Tumor DNA is labeled with a green flourescent dye and normal DNA with a red flourescent dye. Equal amounts are mixed with an excess of unlabeled DNA corresponding to highly repeated sequences and hybridized to a metaphase spread of chromosomes from normal human tissue. Areas of chromosome gain in the tumor appear red and areas of chromosome deletion appear green. (Modified from Israel[95] with permission. (b) A partial profile of an anaplastic astrocytoma showing loss of chromosomes 1p and 19q, gain of chromosome 1q and loss of chromosome 9p. (Modified from Bigner et al[101] with permission.)

9p. Many other chromosomal abnormalities are also found in anaplastic oligodendrogliomas[95,101] and other tumors. Furthermore, the genetic abnormalities may vary from area to area within a given tumor (heterogeneity).[102]

Chromosomal abnormalities found in brain tumors are usually characterized by a loss of all or a part of one arm of a chromosome containing a tumor suppressor gene. For example, loss of 22q deletes the tumor suppressor gene NF-2, leading to the development of neurofibromatosis type 2 (Chapter 12). Loss of chromosome 22 is also common in meningiomas and may also occur in anaplastic astrocytomas. What specific functional abnormality this deletion causes in these tumors is unclear.

Chromosomal deletions are not the only mechanism that can cause genetic dysfunction; a point mutation in a specific gene may lead to a similar change in the biology of the cell. For example, p53 abnormalities can occur either by deletions on the short arm of chromosome 17, or by point mutations at one or more of several sites in the gene, particularly at codon 273. Attempting to repair p53 abnormalities by inserting normal p53 into malignant cells is currently undergoing investigation as one form of gene therapy.

identifies all of the amplifications and deletions of chromosomes in a given tumor. The example of an anaplastic oligodendroglioma in Fig. 1.9 shows deletion of the short arm of chromosome 1 (1p), amplification of the long arm of chromosome 1 (1q), and deletion of 19q, and

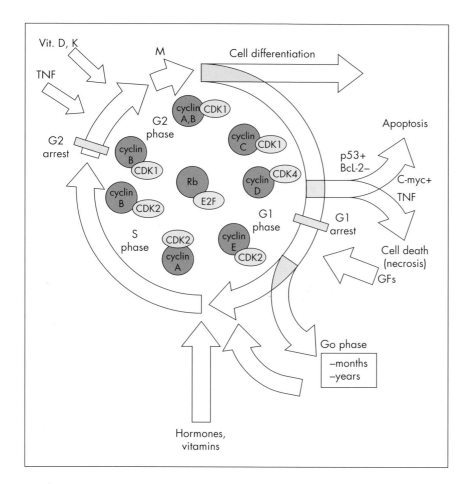

Figure 1.9
Cell cycle and its regulator factors. (Modified from Lupulescu[103] with permission.)

Gains in chromosomes may lead to amplification of oncogenes. For example, gene amplification can cause an increase in the EGFR. Overactivity of growth factor receptors transmits a signal to the cell which, over several steps, leads to excessive cellular reproduction. PKC, also involved in signal transduction, is expressed in many malignant gliomas. It is believed that high-dose tamoxifen, used to treat malignant gliomas, inhibits that enzyme.

As Fig. 1.9 illustrates, the cell cycle is complicated. Proteins called cyclins and cyclin-dependent kinases are essential at several steps in the cell cycle. Alterations in the genes coding for these proteins can cause either uncontrolled progression or inhibition of the cell cycle. For example, cyclin-dependent kinase 4 (CDK-4) phosphorylates RB protein, which, in turn, inhibits binding to transcription factors such as E2F, a factor that initiates cell cycle progression. Cyclin-dependent kinase p21 mediates p53 activity to induce cell cycle arrest; p16 also inhibits the cell cycle. Mutations in any of these proteins can lead to uninhibited progression of cellular reproduction. Abnormalities of cell cycle regulatory pathways are common in high-grade gliomas. Inactivation of CDKNA2A and B genes, inactivation of the RB gene and overexpression of CDK-4 dysregulate the normal cell cycle. While a variety of different and sometimes mutually exclusive genetic alterations have been documented in malignant gliomas, many lead to disruption of the same pathways that cause uncontrolled cell proliferation. For example, an inactivating mutation of p53 inhibits the cell's normal mechanisms of apoptosis in a manner identical to overexpression of MDM2.

The genetic alterations that play important roles in the pathogenesis of brain tumors, i.e. loss of tumor suppressor gene function, increases in growth factors, and mutation or amplification of growth factor receptors, represent not only a challenge but an opportunity. Each genetic alteration is a potential site for therapeutic intervention. For example, restoration of wild-type p53 may not only decrease growth of malignant cells, but might also cause those cells to undergo apoptosis. Inhibitors of a growth factor receptor may slow or even stop the growth of tumor cells. A particularly attractive site for therapeutic intervention is angiogenesis. Because newly formed tumor blood vessels are not neoplastic they are not genetically unstable as are tumor cells. Accordingly, unlike tumor cells, they lack the capacity to develop resistance to a therapeutic agent. Furthermore, recent experimental evidence suggests that tumor cells are not only incapable of developing resistance but, after time, they will fail to nourish a tumor even when the therapeutic agent is withdrawn.[104]

Because of their severe genetic instability, a major problem in the treatment of brain tumors, particularly gliomas, is their heterogeneity. The genetic changes shown in Tables 1.7 and 1.8 are not present in all brain tumors of a particular histologic type. For example, p53 mutations that are present in a majority of glioblastoma multiforme are not present in all glioblastomas, indicating that tumors that look identical under the microscope may have substantially different genetic origins. This implies that each individual tumor must be examined genetically before therapy directed at genetic alterations can be applied. To further compound the problem, even when a genetic change is identified in a tumor, not all tumor cells possess the same genetic change. EGFR overexpression is found in about 40% of all glioblastoma multiforme, but is not present in all of the tumor cells of the glioblastoma. The extreme heterogeneity of these tumors leads to different alterations in different portions of the tumor and in different cells in the same portion of the tumor. The result is that therapy applied to block growth of tumor cells might be effective in eradicating some tumor cells, but allows those that are not sensitive to the agent to continue to grow. It is likely that successful therapies applied to brain tumors will have to be multiagent rather than single agent and multimodality rather than single modality.

Other genetic alterations

One factor that perhaps plays a role in tumor heterogeneity is microsatellite instability. Microsatellites are simple, short, tandem repeats of di-, tri- or tetranucleotides occurring 5–30 times. Normally, the number of repeat units is highly conserved but when there are errors in DNA replication, the numbers may substantially increase or decrease. The term applied to this disorder is microsatellite instability or RER+ (replication error – positive) and it implies that the cell is genetically unstable, making it susceptible to more genetic changes that might eventually lead to cancer. The phenomenon was first observed in tumors associated with hereditary non-polyposis colorectal cancer (HNPCC), where mutations of DNA were due to dysfunction of mismatch repair genes.[105] These genes repair DNA altered by replication errors and environmental insults. Mutation of mismatch repair genes not only makes the cell genetically unstable, but also reduces the effects of certain chemotherapeutic agents. Methylating drugs such as streptozocin, temozolomide, cisplatin, 6-thioguanine, busulfan, etoposide and doxorubicin, all of which affect DNA at the O6 position of guanine, are substantially less effective against cells that have mutations of DNA mismatch repair genes. The resistance may be a result of failure of degradation of newly synthesized DNA opposite alkylation damage, or by an inability to detect the damage and cause apoptosis.[85,106] Microsatellite instability is more common in pediatric than adult CNS tumors.[107]

Other genetic alterations also affect cellular growth, proliferation and cellular immortality. For example, the enzyme telomerase maintains the size of the tandem hexamer repetitive sequences $(TTAGCG)_n$ at the ends of all chromosomes that are required for cell division. The number of repetitive sequences progressively decreases at approximately 50–100 base pairs per cell division as cells continue to divide. When the telomere (from the Greek telos = end, meros = part) becomes too short, the cell can no longer divide and becomes senescent; the cell may undergo apoptosis. Thus, telomere shortening functions as a mitotic clock, inexorably ticking to old age and death. Most normal cells, with the exception of germ cells, do not contain the enzyme telomerase and thus possess a 'built-in' senescence. Cancers, including many brain tumors contain telomerase, one mechanism that ensures cellular immortality. There is also a relationship between telomerase activity and histologic grade. Telomerase activity is not present in low-grade CNS tumors, but is present in more aggressive tumors and is an indicator of histologic progression from low to high grade.[108] Telomerase may also play a role in resistance of tumor cells to cytotoxic drugs; inhibition of telomerase activity can sensitize cells to cisplatin-induced apoptosis.[109]

Genetic abnormalities not only promote neoplastic growth and development, but may affect the sensitivity of tumor cells to therapy. Some normal genes and some genetic abnormalities may lead to the production of proteins that protect tumor cells against cytotoxic agents:

1. The enzyme MGMT repairs DNA damage caused by some chemotherapeutic agents, especially the nitrosoureas (e.g. 1,3-bischloro-(2-chloroethyl)-1-nitrosourea (BCNU)). Some tumors (about 75%) express increased amounts of MGMT, conferring resistance to nitrosoureas on the tumor cells.[110] The increased amount of MGMT does not appear to be related to proliferation per se, but does heighten the resistance of brain tumors to therapeutic alkylating agents. The presence of the enzyme in brain tumors appears to be associated with resistance to temozolomide as well as BCNU.[111]

2. P-glycoprotein is a membrane glycoprotein that is expressed in a number of brain tumors[112] and also at the luminal membrane of the brain capillary endothelial cell as a component of the normal blood–brain barrier (Chapter 2). The protein functions as a pump extruding a number of cytotoxic drugs from the cell, including vincristine and doxorubicin, one mechanism of resistance to chemotherapy. However, the agents that P-glycoprotein affects are not those usually active against brain tumors or even in brain tumor cell lines in tissue culture.

3. Metallothioneins (MT) are intracellular sulfur-containing proteins that have a high affinity for heavy metal ions such as zinc, cadmium, copper and mercury. Their normal function involves metabolism of trace metals and detoxification of toxic

metals. They also bind to cytotoxic agents containing a metal, e.g. cisplatin, and, when overexpressed, confer resistance to tumor cells that express these proteins.[113] The most likely mechanism of resistance to cisplatin is that the proteins enhance removal of platinum adducts from DNA, thus preventing damage by the cytotoxic agent. MTs are overexpressed in many brain tumors (66% of astrocytomas) and appear to be inversely related to survival of the patient.[113] The proteins are normally expressed at high levels during embryologic development and appear to have a role in cellular proliferation. MTs are normally active during the mitotic cell cycle and may serve as cellular proliferation markers.

4. Mutations in p53 also may confer drug resistance. One of the functions of normal p53 is to cause cell cycle arrest in the G1 phase when DNA is damaged. If the DNA cannot be repaired by the cell, p53 promotes cell death through apoptosis. Alterations in p53 function may allow cells with damaged DNA to continue to reproduce, thus conferring resistance to radiation therapy and cytotoxic agents including topoisomerase inhibitors, nitrosoureas and platinum compounds, all of which have DNA as their target. Tumor cell lines lacking the p53 protein are chemoresistant, particularly to paclitaxel and topotecan. When the wild-type p53 gene was introduced into these cells, the cells regained chemosensitivity.[114]

Prognosis

Several factors are important for predicting the prognosis of specific intracranial tumors (Table 1.10): histopathology, especially mitoses, vascular proliferation and necrosis, defines an aggressive tumor with a poor prognosis.

The location of the tumor determines symptoms, surgical resectability and, as a result of both, prognosis. For example, tumors of the non-dominant frontal lobe are often asymptomatic until they reach a large size, can often be completely resected, and have a better prognosis than tumors in highly symptomatic but surgically inaccessible regions such as the brainstem or basal ganglia. Tumors arising outside of the brain, such as meningiomas and pituitary tumors, even when histopathologically aggressive, generally have a better prognosis than tumors arising within the parenchyma of the brain. The age of the patient is an important prognostic factor. For certain tumors, such as high-grade gliomas,

Table 1.10
Some factors determining prognosis of CNS tumor.

Factor	Tumors in which the factor is particularly important
Histopathology	Astrocytoma, pineal tumors
Location	Meningioma
Age	Astrocytoma, lymphoma, glioblastoma
Extent of surgery	Glioblastoma
Performance status	Lymphoma, gliomas
Radiation and/or chemotherapeutic sensitivity	Oligodendroglioma

children fare better than adults and young adults fare better than older adults. In adults with high-grade gliomas, age is the single most important prognostic factor. On the contrary, adults with brainstem gliomas usually fare better than children. Race does not appear to influence survival.[115] Although controversial, most evidence suggests that the extent of surgery is an important prognostic factor.[116] In meningiomas, total surgical resection is curative. High-grade gliomas are never cured by surgery, but the less tumor that remains after resection, the better the prognosis. The patient's neurologic state before and after surgery (performance status) is also an important prognostic factor. Relatively asymptomatic patients have a better prognosis than those who are paralyzed or suffer other crippling

neurologic symptoms. The sensitivities of the tumor to radiation and chemotherapy are important prognostic factors.

Histopathologically malignant pineal region germinomas are cured by radiation, and an increasing number of CNS lymphomas appear to be cured by chemotherapy. It is poor sensitivity to radiation and chemotherapy that makes the high-grade glioma such an intractable tumor. The physician must consider all of these prognostic factors for each individual patient when prescribing treatment and discussing prognosis.

Data from CBTRUS tabulating 2- and 5-year survivals for specific intracranial tumors are tabulated in Table 1.11. Overall, the probability of a patient surviving a high-grade brain tumor is 36% at 2 years and 27% at 5 years. However,

Histology	% of Cases	% 5-year survival
Astrocytoma	18.7	30.3
Pilocytic astrocytoma	1.4	77.4
Anaplastic astrocytoma	5.2	21.9
Glioblastoma multiforme	29.6	2.4
Oligodendroglioma	2.4	59.6
Anaplastic oligodendroglioma	0.4	36.5
Ependymoma	1.7	68.1
Anaplastic ependymoma	0.2	54.3
Medulloblastoma	2.4	55.0
Germinoma	0.4	76.3
Pinealoma/pineocytoma	0.1	56.3
Pineoblastoma	0.2	35.6
Choroid plexus papilloma	0.1	70.8
Ganglioglioma	0.3	88.4
Meningioma	14.3	70.1
Malignant meningioma	1.2	54.6
Hemangioblastoma	0.5	83.6
Chordoma	0.2	62.0
Neurilemoma	2.5	84.9
Malignant neurilemoma	0.1	64.6
Lymphoma	4.3	12.9

Table modified from Surawicz et al[22] with permission.

Table 1.11
Prognosis of brain tumors from the National Cancer Data Base.

for those patients who survive 2 years, the likelihood of surviving 5 years is 76%.[117] Unfortunately, the quality of life for surviving patients, particularly children and the elderly is generally reduced from their premorbid state and not as good as that of most patients successfully treated for systemic cancer.[118]

References

1. Smith MA, Freidlin B, Ries LAG, Simon R. Trends in reported incidence of primary malignant brain tumors in children in the United States. J Natl Cancer Inst 1998; 90: 1269–77.
2. Bleyer WA. Epidemiologic impact of children with brain tumors. Child Nerv Syst 1999; 15: 758–63.
3. Davis FG, McCarthy BJ. Epidemiology of brain tumors. Curr Opin Neurol 2000; 13: 635–40.
4. Riggs JE. The biphasic pattern of age-specific malignant brain tumor mortality rates. Neurology 2000; 55: 750–3.
5. Gurney JG, Kadan-Lottick N. Brain and other central nervous system tumors: rates, trends, and epidemiology. Curr Opin Oncol 2001; 13: 160–6.
6. Schulder M, Maldjian JA, Liu WC et al. Functional image-guided surgery of intracranial tumors located in or near the sensorimotor cortex. J Neurosurg 1998; 89: 412–8.
7. Bohinski RJ, Kokkino AK, Warnick RE et al. Glioma resection in a shared-resource magnetic resonance operating room after optimal image-guided frameless stereotactic resection. Neurosurgery 2001; 48: 731–42.
8. Davis FG, Freels S, Grutsch J et al. Survival rates in patients with primary malignant brain tumors stratified by patient age and tumor histological type: an analysis based on surveillance, epidemiology, and end results (SEER) data, 1973–1991. J Neurosurg 1998; 88: 1–10.
9. Dickman PW, Hakulinen T et al. Survival of cancer patients in Finland 1955–1994. Acta Oncol 1999; 38: 1–103.
10. Levin VA. Cancer in the nervous system. 1st edn. New York: Churchill Livingstone, 1996: 1–474.
11. Black PM, Loeffler JS. Cancer of the nervous system. 1st edn. Cambridge, MA: Blackwell Scientific, 1997: 1–935.
12. Kaye AH, Laws ERJ. Brain tumors: an encyclopedic approach. 2nd edn. New York: Churchill Livingstone, 2001.
13. Posner JB. Neurologic complications of cancer. Philadelphia: F.A. Davis, 1995.
14. Vecht CJ. Neurooncology parts 1–3. New York: Elsevier, 1997.
15. Kleihues P, Cavenee WK. World Health Organization classification of tumours: tumours of the nervous system-pathology and genetics. Lyon: IRAC Press, 2000.
16. Radhakrishnan K, Mokri B, Parisi JE et al. The trends in incidence of primary brain tumors in the population of Rochester, Minnesota. Ann Neurol 1995; 37: 67–73.
17. CBTRUS (2000). Statistical report: primary brain tumors in the United States, 1992–1997. Central Brain Tumor Registry of the United States, 2000.
18. Greenlee RT, Hill-Harmon MB, Taylor M, Thum M. Cancer statistics, 2001. Ca Cancer J Clin 2001; 51: 15–36.
19. Coons SW, Johnson PC, Scheithauer BW, Yates AJ, Pearl DK. Improving diagnostic accuracy and interobserver concordance in the classification and grading of primary gliomas. Cancer 1997; 79: 1381–93.
20. O'Neil BP, Janney CA, Olson J et al. The continuing increase in primary central nervous system non-Hodgkin's lymphoma (PCNSL): a surveillance epidemiology, and end results (SEER) analysis. Proc Am Soc Clin Oncol 20, 53. 2001.
21. Cappuzzo F, Mazzoni F, Maestri A et al. Medical treatment of brain metastases from solid tumours. Forum (Genova) 2000; 10: 137–48.
22. Surawicz TS, Davis F, Freels S, Laws ER, Jr., Menck HR. Brain tumor survival: Results from the National Cancer Data Base. J Neuroncology 1998; 40: 151–60.
23. Pobereskin LH, Chadduck JB. Incidence of brain tumours in two English counties: a population based study. J Neurol Neurosurg Psychiatry 2000; 69: 464–71.

24. Preston-Martin S. Epidemiology of primary CNS neoplasms. Neurol Clin 1996; 14: 273–90.

25. Preston-Martin S. Descriptive epidemiology of primary tumors of the brain, cranial nerves and cranial meninges in Los Angeles County. Neuroepidemiology 1989; 8: 283–95.

26. Davis FG, Freels S, Grutsch J, Barlas S, Brem S. Survival rates in patients with primary malignant brain tumors stratified by patient age and tumor histological type: an analysis based on surveillance, epidemiology, and end results (SEER) data, 1974–1991. J Neurosurg 1998; 88: 1–10.

27. Kuratsu J, Ushio Y. Epidemiological study of primary intracranial tumours in elderly people. J Neurol Neurosurg Psychiatry 1997; 63: 116–8.

28. Ruiz-Tovar M, López-Abente G, Pollán M et al. Brain cancer incidence in the provinces of Zaragoza and Navarre (Spain): effect of age, period and birth cohort. J Neurol Sci 1999; 164: 93–9.

29. Werner MH, Phuphanich S, Lyman GH. The increasing incidence of malignant gliomas and primary central nervous system lymphoma in the elderly. Cancer 1995; 76: 1634–42.

30. Olney JW, Farber NB, Spitznagel E, Robins LN. Increasing brain tumor rates: Is there a link to aspartame? J Neuropathol Exp Neurol 1996; 55: 1115–23.

31. Fleury A, Menegoz F, Grosclaude P et al. Descriptive epidemiology of cerebral gliomas in France. Cancer 1997; 79: 1195–202.

32. McKinley BP, Michalek AM, Fenstermaker RA, Plunkett RJ. The impact of age and sex on the incidence of glial tumors in New York State from 1976 to 1995. J Neurosurg 2000; 93: 932–9.

33. Legler JM, Ries LA, Smith MA et al. Brain and other central nervous system cancers: recent trends in incidence and mortality. J Natl Cancer Inst 1999; 91: 1382–90.

34. Kelsey KT, Wrensch M, Zuo ZF, Miike R, Wiencke JK. A population-based case–control study of the CYP2D6 and GSTT1 polymorphisms and malignant brain tumors. Pharmacogenetics 1997; 7: 463–8.

35. Keene DL, Hsu E, Ventureyra E. Brain tumors in childhood and adolescence. Pediatr Neurol 1999; 20: 198–203.

36. Gurney JG, Davis S, Severson RK et al. Trends in cancer incidence among children in the US. Cancer 1996; 78: 532–41.

37. Linet MS, Ries LA, Smith MA, Tarone RE, Devesa SS. Cancer surveillance series: recent trends in childhood cancer incidence and mortality in the United States. J Natl Cancer Inst 1999; 91: 1051–8.

38. Giannini C, Scheithauer BW, Weaver AL et al. Oligodendrogliomas: Reproducibility and prognostic value of histologic diagnosis and grading. J Neuropathol Exp Neurol 2001; 60: 248–62.

39. Marie Y, Sanson M, Mokhtari K et al. OLIG2 as a specific marker of oligodentroglial tumour cells. Lancet 2001; 358: 298–300.

40. Ino Y, Betensky RA, Zlatescu MC et al. Molecular subtypes of anaplastic oligodendroglioma: implications for patient management at diagnosis. Clin Canc Res 2001; 7: 839–45.

41. Strojan P, Popovic M, Jereb B. Secondary intracranial meningiomas after high-dose cranial irradiation: Report of five cases and review of the literature. Int J Radiat Oncol Biol Phys 2000; 48: 65–73.

42. Sadetzki S, Modan B, Chetrit A, Freedman L. An iatrogenic epidemic of benign meningioma. Am J Epidemiol 2000; 151: 266–72.

43. Buttner A, Weis S. Non-lymphomatous brain tumors in HIV-1 infection: a review. J Neurooncol 1999; 41: 81–8.

44. Vannemreddy PSSV, Fowler M, Polin RS, Todd JR, Nanda A. Glioblastoma multiforme in a case of acquired immunodeficiency syndrome: investigating a possible oncogenic influence of human immunodeficiency virus on glial cells – Case report and review of the literature. J Neurosurg 2000; 92: 161–4.

45. Salvatore JR, Weitberg AB, Mehta S. Nonionizing electromagnetic fields and cancer: a review. Oncology 1996; 10: 563–74.

46. Wrensch M, Yost M, Miike R, Lee G, Touchstone J. Adult glioma in relation to residential power frequency electromagnetic field exposures in the San Francisco Bay area. Epidemiology 1999; 10: 523–7.

47. Muscat JE, Malkin MG, Thompson S et al. Handheld cellular telephone use and risk of brain cancer. JAMA 2000; 284: 3001–7.

48. Inskip PD, Tarone RE, Hatch EE et al. Cellular-telephone use and brain tumors. N Engl J Med 2001; 344: 79–86.

49. Zook BC, Simmens SJ. The effects of 860 MHz radiofrequency radiation on the induction or promotion of brain tumors and other neoplasms in rats. Radiat Res 2001; 155: 572–83.

50. Schwartzbaum JA, Fisher JL, Goodman J, Octaviano D, Cornwell DG. Hypotheses concerning roles of dietary energy, cured meat, and serum tocopherols in adult glioma development. Neuroepidemiology 1999; 18: 156–66.

51. Carozza SE, Wrensch M, Miike R et al. Occupation and adult gliomas. Am J Epidemiol 2000; 152: 838–46.

52. Bohnen NI, Kurland LT. Brain tumor and exposure to pesticides in humans: a review of the epidemiologic data. J Neurol Sci 1995; 132: 110–21.

53. Pogoda JM, Preston-Martin S. Household pesticides and risk of pediatric brain tumors. Environ Health Perspect 1997; 105: 1214–20.

54. Inskip PD, Mellemkjaer L, Gridley G, Olsen JH. Incidence of intracranial tumors following hospitalization for head injuries (Denmark). Cancer Causes Control 1998; 9: 109–16.

55. Wrensch M, Miike R, Lee M, Neuhaus J. Are prior head injuries or diagnostic X-rays associated with glioma in adults? The effects of control selection bias. Neuroepidemiology 2000; 19: 234–44.

56. Preston-Martin S, Pogoda JM, Mueller BA et al. Results from an international case-control study of childhood brain tumors: The role of prenatal vitamin supplementation. Environ Health Perspect 1998; 106: 887–92.

57. Del Brutto OH, Castillo PR, Mena IX, Freire AX. Neurocysticercosis among patients with cerebral gliomas. Arch Neurol 1997; 54: 1125–8.

58. Wrensch M, Weinberg A, Wiencke J et al. Does prior infection with varicella-zoster virus influence risk of adult glioma? Am J Epidemiol 1997; 145: 594–7.

59. Weggen S, Bayer TA, von Deimling A et al. Low frequency of SV40, JC and BK polyomavirus sequences in human medulloblastomas, meningiomas and ependymomas. Brain Pathol 2000; 10: 85–92.

60. Huang HT, Reis R, Yonekawa Y et al. Identification in human brain tumors of DNA sequences specific for SV40 large T antigen. Brain Pathol 1999; 9: 33–42.

61. Ron E, Modan B, Boice JD, Jr et al. Tumors of the brain and nervous system after radiotherapy in childhood. New Engl J Med 1988; 319: 1033–9.

62. Walter AW, Hancock ML, Pui CH et al. Secondary brain tumors in children treated for acute lymphoblastic leukemia at St Jude Children's Research Hospital. J Clin Oncol 1998; 16: 3761–7.

63. Relling MV, Rubnitz JE, Rivera GK et al. High incidence of secondary brain tumours after radiotherapy and antimetabolites. Lancet 1999; 354: 34–9.

64. Ryan P, Lee MW, North B, McMichael AJ. Amalgam fillings, diagnostic dental x-rays and tumours of the brain and meninges. Eur J Cancer B Oral Oncol 1992; 28B: 91–5.

65. Rodvall Y, Ahlbom A, Pershagen G, Nylander M, Spannare B. Dental radiography after age 25 years, amalgam fillings and tumours of the central nervous system. Oral Oncol 1998; 34: 265–9.

66. Camilleri-Broet S, Davi F, Feuillard J et al. AIDS-related primary brain lymphomas: histopathologic and immunohistochemical study of 51 cases. The French Study Group for HIV-Associated Tumors. Hum Pathol 1997; 28: 367–74.

67. Frisch M, Biggar RJ, Engels EA, Goedert JJ. Association of cancer with AIDS-related immunosuppression in adults. JAMA 2001; 285: 1736–45.

68. Bunin G. What causes childhood brain tumors? Limited knowledge, many clues. Pediatr Neurosurg 2000; 32: 321–6.

69. Schwartzbaum JA, Cornwell DG. Oxidant stress and glioblastoma multiforme risk: serum antioxidants, gamma-glutamyl transpeptidase, and ferritin. Nutr Cancer 2000; 38: 40–9.

70. Chia SE, Chia HP, Tan JS. Health hazards of mobile phones – Prevalence of headache is increased among users in Singapore. Br Med J 2000; 321: 1155–6.

71. Malmer B, Iselius L, Holmberg E et al. Genetic epidemiology of glioma. Br J Cancer 2001; 84: 429–34.

72. Tomlinson GE. Familial cancer syndromes and genetic counseling. Cancer Treat Res 1997; 92: 63–97.

73. Johnson MW, Emelin JK, Park SH, Vinters HV. Co-localization of TSC1 and TSG2 gene products in tubers of patients with tuberous sclerosis. Brain Pathol 1999; 9: 45–54.

74. Gutmann DH, Aylsworth A, Carey JC et al. The diagnostic evaluation and multidisciplinary management of neurofibromatosis 1 and neurofibromatosis 2. JAMA 1997; 278: 51–7.

75. Feldkamp MM, Gutmann DH, Guha A. Neurofibromatosis type 1: Piecing the puzzle together. Can J Neurol Sci 1998; 25: 181–91.

76. Pollack IF, Mulvihill JJ. Neurofibromatosis 1 and 2. Brain Pathol 1997; 7: 823–36.

77. Asa SL, Somers K, Ezzat S. The *MEN-1* gene is rarely down-regulated in pituitary adenomas. J Clin Endocrinol Metab 1998; 83: 3210–2.

78. Mulligan G, Jacks T. The retinoblastoma gene family: cousins with overlapping interests. Trends Genet 1998; 14: 223–9.

79. Wicking C, Bale AE. Molecular basis of the nevoid basal cell carcinoma syndrome. Curr Opin Pediatr 1997; 9: 630–5.

80. Foulkes WD. A tale of four syndromes: familial adenomatous polyposis, Gardner syndrome, attenuated APC and Turcot syndrome. Q J Med 1995; 88: 853–63.

81. Decker HJ, Weidt EJ, Brieger J. The von Hippel–Lindau tumor suppressor gene. A rare and intriguing disease opening new insight into basic mechanisms of carcinogenesis. Cancer Genet Cytogenet 1997; 93: 74–83.

82. Eng C. Genetics of Cowden syndrome: through the looking glass of oncology. Int J Oncol 1998; 12: 701–10.

83. Sévenet N, Sheridan E, Amram D et al. Constitutional mutations of the *hSNF5/INI1* gene predispose to a variety of cancers. Am J Hum Genet 1999; 65: 1342–8.

84. Spiro TP, Gerson SL, Liu L et al. O6-benzyl-guanine: a clinical trial establishing the biochemical modulatory dose in tumor tissue for alkyltransferase-directed DNA repair. Cancer Res 1999; 59: 2402–10.

85. Holland EC. Gliomagenesis: genetic alterations and mouse models. Nat Rev Genet 2001; 2: 120–9.

86. Loeb LA. A mutator phenotype in cancer. Cancer Res 2001; 61: 3230–9.

87. Esteller M, Corn PG, Baylin SB, Herman JG. A gene hypermethylation profile of human cancer. Cancer Res 2001; 61: 3225–9.

88. Simone NL, Bonner RF, Gillespie JW, Emmert-Buck MR, Liotta LA. Laser-capture microdissection: opening the microscopic frontier to molecular analysis. Trends Genet 1998; 14: 272–6.

89. Loiseau H, Arsaut J, Demotes-Mainard J. *p73* gene transcripts in human brain tumors: overexpression and altered splicing in ependymomas. Neurosci Lett 1999; 263: 173–6.

90. Villunger A, Strasser A. Does 'death receptor' signaling play a role in tumorigenesis and cancer therapy? Oncol Res 1998; 10: 541–50.

91. Chernova OB, Somerville RP, Cowell JK. A novel gene, LGI1, from 10q24 is rearranged and downregulated in malignant brain tumors. Oncogene 1998; 17: 2873–81.

92. Hunter T. The Croonian Lecture 1997. The phosphorylation of proteins on tyrosine: its role in cell growth and disease. Philos Trans R Soc Lond B Biol Sci 1998; 353: 583–605.

93. Yamada SM, Yamaguchi F, Brown R, Berger MS, Morrison RS. Suppression of glioblastoma cell growth following antisense oligonucleotide-mediated inhibition of fibroblast growth factor receptor expression. Glia 1999; 28: 66–76.

94. Uhrbom L, Hesselager G, Nister M, Westermark B. Induction of brain tumors in mice using a recombinant platelet-derived growth factor B-chain retrovirus. Cancer Res 1998; 58: 5275–9.

95. Israel MA. Molecular genetics of brain tumors. In: Martin JB, ed. Scientific American Molecular Neurology. New York: Scientific American, 1999: 95–114.

96. Maddalena AS, Hainfellner JA, Hegi ME, Glatzel M, Aguzzi A. No complementation between TP53 or RB-1 and v-*src* in astrocytomas of GFAP-v-*src* transgenic mice. Brain Pathol 1999; 9: 627–37.

97. Adachi J, Ohbayashi K, Suzuki T, Sasaki T. Cell cycle arrest and astrocytic differentiation resulting from *PTEN* expression in glioma cells. J Neurosurg 1999; 91: 822–30.

98. Simon M, Köster G, Menon AG, Schramm J. Functional evidence for a role of combined *CDKN2A* (p16–p14ARF)/*CDKN2B* (p15) gene inactivation in malignant gliomas. Acta Neuropathol (Berl) 1999; 98: 444–52.

99. Bodey B, Bodey B Jr, Siegel SE. Tumor suppressor genes in childhood malignancies: a review. Int J Pediatr Hematol Oncol 1999; 6: 47–64.

100. Chène P, Ory K, Rüedi D, Soussi T, Hegi ME. Functional analyses of a unique *p53* germline mutant (Y236Delta) associated with a familial brain tumor syndrome. Int J Cancer 1999; 82: 17–22.

101. Bigner SH, Rasheed K, Wiltshire RN, McLendon R. Morphologic and molecular genetic aspects of oligodendroglial neoplasms. Neuroncol 1999; 1: 52–60.

102. Jung V, Romeike BFM, Henn W et al. Evidence of focal genetic microheterogeneity in glioblastoma multiforme by area-specific CGH on microdissected tumor cells. J Neuropathol Exp Neurol 1999; 58: 993–9.

103. Lupulescu A. Cancer cell metabolism: its relevance to cancer treatment. Cancer Invest 1999; 17: 423–33.

104. Folkman J. Antiangiogenic gene therapy. Proc Natl Acad Sci USA 1998; 95: 9064–6.

105. Claij N, Te R. Microsatellite instability in human cancer: a prognostic marker for chemotherapy? Exp Cell Res 1999; 246: 1–10.

106. Fink D, Aebi S, Howell SB. The role of DNA mismatch repair in drug resistance. Clin Cancer Res 1998; 4: 1–6.

107. Alonso M, Hamelin R, Kim M et al. Microsatellite instability occurs in distinct subtypes of pediatric but not adult central nervous system tumors. Cancer Res 2001; 61: 2124–8.

108. Huang F, Kanno H, Yamamoto I, Lin Y, Kubota Y. Correlation of clinical features and telomerase activity in human gliomas. J Neurooncol 1999; 43: 137–42.

109. Kondo Y, Kondo S, Tanaka Y, Haqqi T, Barna BP, Cowell JK. Inhibition of telomerase increases the susceptibility of human malignant glioblastoma cells to cisplatin-induced apoptosis. Oncogene 1998; 16: 2243–8.

110. Esteller M, Garcia-Foncillas J, Andion E et al. Inactivation of the DNA-repair gene MGMT and the clinical response of gliomas to alkylating agents. N Engl J Med 2000; 343: 1350–4.

111. Friedman HS, McLendon RE, Kerby T et al. DNA mismatch repair and O6–alkylguanine-DNA alkyltransferase analysis and response to Temodal in newly diagnosed malignant glioma. J Clin Oncol 1998; 16: 3851–7.

112. Ashmore SM, Thomas DG, Darling JL. Does P-glycoprotein play a role in clinical resistance of malignant astrocytoma? Anticancer Drugs 1999; 10: 861–72.

113. Hiura T, Khalid H, Yamashita H et al. Immunohistochemical analysis of metallothionein in astrocytic tumors in relation to tumor grade, proliferative potential, and survival. Cancer 1998; 83: 2361–9.

114. Fueyo J, Gomez-Manzano C, Puduvalli VK et al. Adenovirus-mediated p16 transfer to glioma cells induces G1 arrest and protects from paclitaxel and topotecan: implications for therapy. Int J Oncol 1998; 12: 665–9.

115. Simpson JR, Scott CB, Rotman M et al. Race and prognosis of brain tumor patients entering multicenter clinical trials. A report from the Radiation Therapy Oncology Group. Am J Clin Oncol 1996; 19: 114–20.

116. Black P. Management of malignant glioma: role of surgery in relation to multimodality therapy. J Neurovirol 1998; 4: 227–36.

117. Davis FG, McCarthy BJ, Freels S, Kupelian V, Bondy ML. The conditional probability of survival of patients with primary malignant brain tumors – Surveillance, epidemiology, and end results (SEER) data. Cancer 1999; 85: 485–91.

118. Foreman NK, Faestel PM, Pearson J et al. Health status in 52 long-term survivors of pediatric brain tumors. J Neurooncol 1999; 41: 47–53.

2

Invasion, angiogenesis and the blood–brain barrier

Introduction

Once the genetic changes that lead to uncontrolled cellular reproduction have occurred, central nervous system (CNS) tumors must grow to a fairly large size (at least 1 cm) before causing neurologic symptoms. Most brain tumors grow both by increasing their core mass and by invading surrounding normal brain. In order to grow, a tumor requires nutrients that are supplied by the vasculature. After a tumor exceeds a few millimeters in size, it requires the production of new blood vessels (angiogenesis) to meet its metabolic demands. The newly formed blood vessels do not possess a normal blood–brain barrier and are thus a source of brain edema (see below), which contributes to the total tumor mass. The combined tumor mass and its edema not only cause neurologic dysfunction, but also raise interstitial fluid pressure, compromising blood flow and causing local hypoxia.[1,2] The combined size of a tumor and its edema necessary to cause symptoms depends, in part, on the location of the lesion (for example, a 1 cm lesion in the brainstem may be symptomatic, but a 5 cm lesion in the frontal lobe may be asymptomatic) and, in part, on the nature of the symptom(s) (e.g. small lesions may cause seizures but it requires a large lesion to alter cognition or personality).

Several mechanisms play a role in brain tumor growth and edema formation. These

Table 2.1
Sequential steps in growth of brain tumors.

1. Cellular gene mutation (multiple genes)
2. Uncontrolled cell division
3. Invasion into normal brain
4. Formation of a tumor blood supply, i.e. angiogenesis
5. Blood–brain barrier disruption
6. Edema

mechanisms (Table 2.1) include invasion of tumor cells into normal parenchyma (particularly true of glial tumors), angiogenesis (required for tumor growth beyond a few millimeters) and blood–brain barrier disruption leading to brain edema (a prominent feature of high-grade gliomas). This chapter describes some of these mechanisms and their clinical implications.

Invasion

Some CNS tumors are highly invasive (Fig. 2.1). Gliomas (Chapter 5) and primary CNS lymphomas (Chapter 11) are among the most invasive of cancers. During their migratory phase, brain tumor cells transiently exit from the cell cycle (see Fig. 1.9), making them relatively refractory to therapy because quiescent cells are less susceptible to radiation and

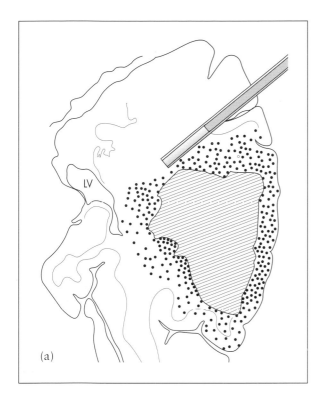

Figure 2.1
Invasion of brain by tumor. (a) A glioblastoma with a relatively sharp interface of the surrounding brain. A needle passing within millimeters of the neoplasm may obtain only normal tissue. However, there is infiltration of tumor beyond the enhancing edge. (b) and (c) – Greater and lesser degrees of differentiation that can be seen in the same glioma are illustrated in this untreated glioblastoma multiforme. The areas of low density marked by small closed and open triangles represent fibrillary and gemistocytic astrocytes respectively. The markedly cellular regions (small closed circles) represent small cell glioblastoma arising in the pre-existing better-differentiated tumor. A specimen obtained by needle biopsy from areas of lower density would indicate a well-differentiated astrocytoma (b), whereas a sample several millimeters more superiorly (c) would reveal the diagnostic features of a glioblastoma. (From Burger et al,[3] with permission.)

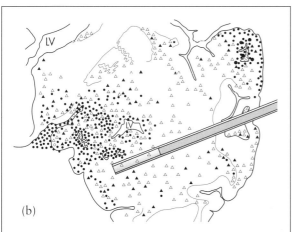

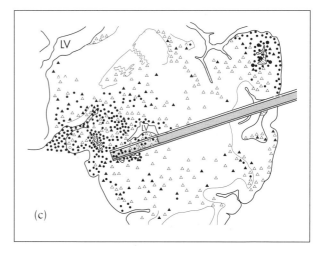

chemotherapy than are actively reproducing cells (Chapter 4). Invasive cells occur at the periphery of a tumor mass and can extend many centimeters away from the focal lesion identifiable on MRI.[4] Because individual cells migrate into normal brain, they derive their nourishment from normal cerebral blood vessels. Consequently, even when these cells may be intrinsically susceptible to chemical agents, they are sequestered behind a normal

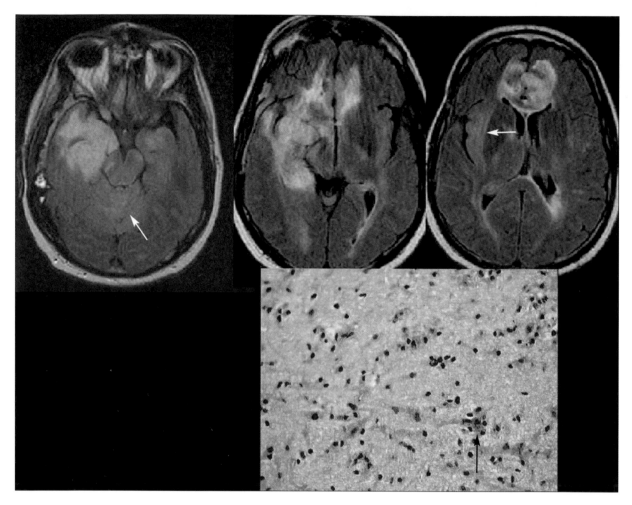

Figure 2.2
Diffuse tumor (gliomatosis cerebri). A 40-year-old man complained of dizziness and unsteadiness on his feet. Examination revealed nystagmus on left lateral gaze and a slightly ataxic gait. His mental state was normal. An MR scan (left panel) revealed increased signal in both medial temporal lobes, right greater than left, and cerebellum (arrow, left panel). Both frontal lobes and the right insula were also involved (arrow, right panel). A stereotactic needle biopsy of the right temporal lobe revealed increased cellularity and mildly atypical glioma cells infiltrating the parenchyma, some forming perineuronal satellitosis (arrow), consistent with a low-grade glioma. Whole-brain radiation therapy to 60 Gy partially relieved the symptoms. He was able to work effectively for 5 years, when he developed increasing ataxia and new cognitive changes. There was no significant change in the scan. Chemotherapy was begun.

blood–brain barrier (see below), making them inaccessible to most water-soluble chemotherapeutic agents. Sometimes a glioma may invade the entire neuraxis (gliomatosis cerebri), causing a diffuse increase in brain mass without evidence of a focal lesion (Fig. 2.2). Diffuse infiltration may be unaccompanied by any change in signal intensity on the

Table 2.2
Factors required for invasion.

- Tumor cell–cell interactions loosen
- Tumor cells bind to extracellular matrix
- Proteases degrade extracellular matrix
- Integrins promote cell motility
- Motility leads to invasion into normal brain
- Growth factors promote tumorigenesis

MRI. Other tumors such as meningiomas rarely invade normal brain but require angiogenesis in order to grow large enough to compress underlying brain and thus cause symptoms.

Several factors are required for tumor invasion of brain[5] (Table 2.2). These factors are not unique to brain tumors but are a general characteristic of most cancers. In the normal state, cells adhere to one another and to the underlying basement membrane using a diverse system of adhesion molecules and their receptors. These include: (1) cadherins,[6] (2) members of the immunoglobulin superfamily, including the neural cell adhesion molecule (N-CAM),[7] (3) integrins,[8] and (4) selectins.[9] Alterations in adhesion molecules play a dual role in tumor invasion. Downregulation of certain adhesion molecules loosens cell–cell interactions within the tumor.[10] Upregulation of adhesion molecules allows tumor cells to attach to the extracellular matrix (ECM), a requirement for cell migration.[11]

In most tissues, cadherins play a major role in cell–cell adhesion.[12] E-cadherin is expressed in endothelial cells and N-cadherin in neural cells. E-cadherin is downregulated in most carcinomas. Some data suggest that N-cadherin expression is decreased in high-grade neuroepithelial tumors and may correlate with tumor

invasion and dissemination of tumor into the CSF.[5] Another such molecule, possibly important in disaggregation of tumor cells, is N-CAM.

In order to migrate out from the core of the tumor, tumor cells must adhere to molecules of the extracellular matrix,[13] as well as break the adhesion between themselves. Brain extracellular matrix proteins differ from those of other tissues[4] and also differ from area to area in brain. Brain tumor cells in vitro adhere to several structures, including blood vessels, arachnoid, choroid plexus, ventricular ependyma and myelinated fiber tracts. The attachment of neuroepithelial tumor cells to blood vessels indicates that migration along blood vessels may be a guiding structure for dissemination of gliomas and perhaps lymphomas which grow around vessels. The major matrix proteins in small vessels, choroid plexus and ependyma are laminin, collagen type 4 and fibronectin. Arachnoid fibers contain various types of collagen, predominantly types 1 and 3. The only matrix protein in subependyma is fibronectin. The main ECM proteins of the brain paranchyma are hyaluronan, tenascin and brain enriched hyaluronan binding/brevican.[5] The last is upregulated in gliomas and its cleavage appears important for tumor invasion.[5]

Adhesion molecules, including integrins, are responsible for binding to extracellular matrix, whereas antibodies to adhesion molecules block binding. For example, antibodies to integrin block adhesion to arachnoid tissue, and anti-N-CAM antibodies inhibit attachment to cortex. Antibodies against CD44, adhesion molecules that permit binding to the brain's extracellular matrix, block intracerebral invasion in an experimental glioma model.[14] CD24, another adhesion molecule expressed on brain tumor cells, promotes invasion by glioma cells.[15]

The extracellular matrix not only serves as a site of attachment of cells but, when intact, may inhibit migration. Accordingly, tumor cells produce proteases that break down the extracellular matrix, allowing for invasion and migration.[16] Extracellular matrix proteins not only inhibit glioma cell proliferation, but also act as a chemoattractant for glioma cells in vitro. The inhibition of growth may be a requirement for cells to migrate. The situation along blood vessels appears somewhat different, because cells migrating along blood vessels appear to remain in the cell cycle and can proliferate, unlike invasive tumor cells elsewhere in the brain.

To break down the extracellular matrix, tumor cells secrete matrix metalloproteinases (MMPs), zinc-dependent endopeptidases that break down extracellular proteins.[17] Tumor cells not only secrete proteinases to break down the extracellular matrix, but also secrete proteinase inhibitors.[18] TIMP, a metalloproteinase inhibitor, has been detected in culture media from gliomas and meningiomas. The balance between the degrading proteinases and their inhibitors determines the extent of tumor growth and invasion. In addition, growth factors can play a role in extracellular matrix degradation. For example, some reports have suggested that transforming growth factor beta (TGF-β) can upregulate MMPs (MMP-2 and MMP-9) while downregulating TIMP-2. Some MMPs also participate in angiogenesis,[17] and perhaps in blood–brain barrier disruption, a phenomenon inhibited by dexamethasone.[19]

Many tumor cells are intrinsically mobile.[20] This should not be surprising for CNS cells because migration of neurons and glia is necessary for brain development and evidence suggests there is continued migration of non-neoplastic stem cells even into adulthood. Migratory routes along blood vessels, ependyma, and myelinated fiber tracts[21] may carry tumor cells long distances within the parenchyma of the brain. In addition, tumor cells may find their way into the ventricular fluid or the cortical subarachnoid space and disseminate along CSF pathways. Particular pathways that appear to be favored by invading brain tumor cells include growth across the corpus callosum and subependymal spread along the lateral ventricles (Fig. 2.3). Growth of a frontal lobe tumor across the anterior corpus callosum to the other frontal lobe (butterfly glioma) is a particularly common problem. Tumor growing across the splenium of the corpus callosum is somewhat less common but is encountered in both gliomas and lymphomas. Primary CNS lymphomas have a predilection for invading along blood vessels. This is particularly prominent at the microscopic level, where one may see cuffs of lymphoma cells surrounding blood vessels, with intervening parenchyma relatively spared. Inflammatory lymphocytes (T-cells) may also be present.[22]

The clinical implication of such widespread and extensive tumor invasion in the brain is that surgical cure is rarely possible. Past attempts at radical surgery to treat infiltrating tumors have failed. Even hemispherectomy, carried out to resect apparently localized tumor, usually results in recurrence of the tumor in the opposite hemisphere within a year. Although it is true that most gliomas that are treated locally[23] recur locally, this is probably due to the greater volume of disease immediately surrounding a large mass. Furthermore, a recent report indicates that radiation therapy, when sublethal, may actually promote invasion and migration of glioma cells.[24]

Frequently, lymphomas (Chapter 11) may be controlled by local treatment only to recur at some distance from the original tumor.[25] The implication is that tumor cells quiescent behind

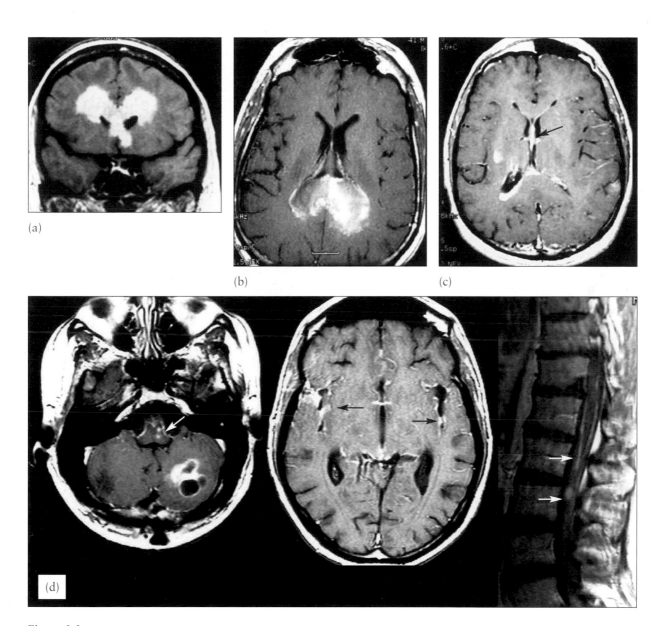

Figure 2.3

Pathways of tumor dissemination. (a) A patient with a butterfly glioma. The tumor presumably originated in one frontal lobe and grew across the corpus callosum to involve the other frontal lobe in the characteristic butterfly fashion. Tumors can cross the corpus callosum at any point but most commonly do so anteriorly. (b) Tumor spreading across the splenium of the corpus callosum. (c) Subependymal spread. A high-grade glioma is seen growing along the posterior horn of the lateral ventricle just below the ependyma as well as along the septum (arrow). (d) Distant metastases from a glioblastoma. The patient had a focal glioblastoma of the right cerebellum (left panel). The tumor infiltrated the leptomeninges of the cerebral hemisphere (middle panel, arrows) and diffusely infiltrated the lumbar subarachnoid space, forming small nodules as well (right panel, arrows). Two small metastatic lesions can be seen in the medulla as well as in the meninges surrounding the medulla (left panel, arrow).

the blood–brain barrier subsequently enter a growth phase and become detectable by imaging when angiogenesis leads to blood–brain barrier disruption (see below). A further clinical implication is that if cell invasion could be inhibited, local therapy might be more effective.

Angiogenesis

Brain tumors are among the most highly vascularized tumors. Glioblastomas, meningiomas, hemangioblastomas and primary CNS lymphomas demonstrate their impressive vascularity by the intense contrast enhancement seen on MR scans. Before the days when contrast-enhanced CT and MR scans were available, cerebral arteriography often revealed a blush of tumor vessels that identified the presence of neovascularity of the underlying brain tumor (Fig. 2.4).

Despite their vascularity, many areas of a tumor, especially high-grade tumors, are poorly perfused. Poor perfusion results in part from the tumor growing faster than new blood vessels can form, and in part from the fact that the newly formed capillaries are not normal brain blood vessels (see below) and have an increased intervascular distance. Furthermore, the tumor increases interstitial fluid pressure, which compresses the blood vessels within the tumor.[2] The result is that many tumors have areas that are ischemic, hypoxic and even necrotic. Even with a normal blood supply, tumor cells utilize anaerobic metabolism much more than normal brain, i.e. they use more glucose and less oxygen, and produce more lactate. These metabolic changes allow tumor cells to grow in a nutrient-deprived environment that also selects for tumor cells of a higher grade.[26] Furthermore, tumor hypoxia and hypoglycemia activate genes that lead to

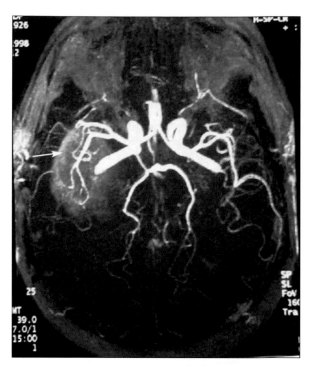

Figure 2.4
A tumor blush identified on magnetic resonance angiography. This elderly man presented with mental status changes. He was believed to have cerebral vascular disease and a magnetic resonance angiogram was performed which showed a blush representing the breakdown of the blood–brain barrier in a right temporal lobe tumor (arrow).

angiogenesis (see below) and also inhibit apoptosis, thus promoting tumor survival.[26]

Several angiogenic factors released by tumor cells react with receptors on normal endothelial cells to allow new vessel formation (Table 2.3). Perhaps the most important of these factors is vascular endothelial growth factor (VEGF),[27] which reacts with FLT-1 and FLK-1 receptors (Fig. 2.5).[28] The VEGF gene family has several members. Their relative roles are not fully established. VEGF not only promotes growth of new tumor, but also increases the permeability of normal capillaries and thus can

Table 2.3
Some factors implicated in angiogenesis and anti-angiogenesis

Promote angiogenesis	*Inhibit angiogenesis*
Vascular endothelial growth factors (VEGF-A-VEGF-D)	Thrombospondin
Placenta growth factor (PlGF)	Angiostatin
Fibroblast growth factors (aFGF, bFGF)	Endostatin
Angiopoietin-1	Angiopoietin-2
Transforming growth factors (TGF-α, TGF-β)	
Tumor necrosis factor (TNF-α)	
Hepatocyte growth factor/scatter factor	
Gelatinase-B	
Interleukin-8 (IL-8)	
Platelet endothelial growth factor-1 (CD31)	
Cyclooxygenase-2 (COX-2)	
Platelet derived growth factor (PDGF)	

lead to brain edema;[29] in fact, VEGF was first identified as vascular permeability factor (VPF). Hypoxia, which is often present in brain tumors, is an important stimulus to VEGF production.[30] The expression of TGF-β_1, bFGF, EGF, platelet derived growth factor (PDGF) and ganglioside in human gliomas can each stimulate VEGF, as can COX-2.[31]

A number of clinical trials are underway that are attempting to inhibit angiogenesis,[32] usually by blocking the endothelial cell VEGF receptor. These trials are predicated on the assumption that inhibition would have the effect of preventing tumor growth by depriving the tumor of adequate nutrition.[33] Furthermore, because endothelial cells are not neoplastic (a controversial point, because endothelial cells in

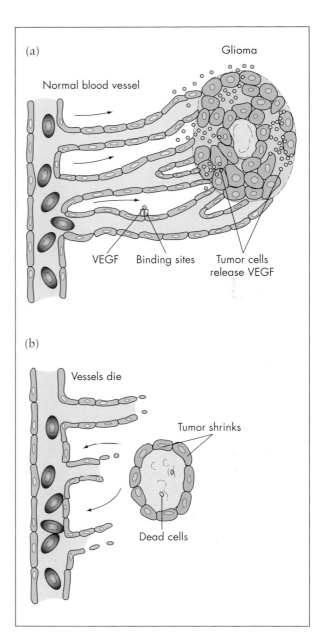

Figure 2.5
Angiogenesis in a malignant glioma. (a) Tumor cells produce a variety of angiogenic substances, including VEGF. VEGF binds to the receptors on endothelial cells of nearby blood vessels in a paracrine fashion and promotes the growth of new blood vessels into the tumor to nourish and sustain it. (b) Inhibition of VEGF causes the newly formed blood vessels to die. The tumor cells deprived of nutrients also shrink or die.

some glioblastomas show increased proliferative activity, suggesting they too may be neoplastic), and thus not genetically unstable, they should not develop resistance to agents that inhibit their development.[34]

Tumor cells secrete both angiogenesis and anti-angiogenesis factors.[35] Normal p53 protein promotes release of anti-angiogenesis factors. Mutated p53, a frequent abnormality in brain tumors, can confer an angiogenic gain of function. Such factors as angiostatin and endostatin, secreted by systemic tumors, have the effect of suppressing growth of tumor metastases. Clinically, one occasionally observes a marked increase in growth of metastases once the primary tumor is resected. One hypothesis is that the primary tumor secretes both angiogenesis and anti-angiogenesis factors. The angiogenesis factors promote growth in the primary tumor but are rapidly metabolized in the bloodstream, so they do not reach any metastasis which may not be synthesizing its own angiogenesis factor(s). The anti-angiogenesis factors are overwhelmed by the angiogenesis factors in the primary tumor, so that the primary tumor continues to invade and grow, but elsewhere in the body the circulating anti-angiogenesis factors dominate and suppress the growth of metastases. Larger primary tumors provide more inhibition of angiogenesis than the smaller metastases.[36] When the primary tumor is removed, growth of the metastases is no longer inhibited and the metastases become symptomatic. The converse has also been reported: rarely, surgical removal of the primary tumor leads to regression of metastases, presumably because growth or angiogenic factors secreted by the primary tumor were required to stimulate the metastases. This distant stimulation may explain the occasional finding of a large brain metastasis from a small, sometimes undetectable primary tumor (Chapter 13). A number of agents known to inhibit angiogenesis are undergoing early clinical trials. These include the drug thalidomide, a small molecule FLK-1 inhibitor, and an anti-VEGF antibody. Antisense VEGF has been reported to inhibit brain tumor growth in animal models.[37]

Factors other than VEGF are likely to play an important role in angiogenesis as well. A brain-specific angiogenesis inhibitor called BAI-1 is transcriptionally regulated by p53. This inhibitor is downregulated in brain tumors with p53 mutations. Its absence may play a role in brain tumor angiogenesis.[38] Fibroblast growth factor (FGF) binding protein mobilizes and activates locally stored FGFs and can serve as an angiogenic switch molecule. The gene is upregulated in a number of cancers.[39] Its role in brain tumor angiogenesis is unknown, but bFGF, as well as VEGF, is upregulated in many brain tumors. A recent study indicates that placenta growth factor (PlGF) mRNA is expressed in hypervascular but not hypovascular brain tumors; it is not expressed in metastatic tumors. VEGF and bFGF mRNA are also detected in hypervascular tumors. Making cells hypoxic increases PlGF levels, suggesting that it may play a role in angiogenesis in hypoxic brain tumors.[40] The extracellular matrix glycoprotein, tenascin-C, is enhanced in many brain tumors and correlates with angiogenesis. Expression of that protein may be associated with endothelial cell activation and play a role in angiogenesis.[41] Hepatocyte growth/scatter factor (SF), which is increased in high-grade gliomas, has been implicated both in motility of tumor cells, causing them to scatter in vitro, and motility of endothelial cells. SF also increases permeability of the blood–glioma barrier in some animal gliomas.[42] Thus, the protein may play a role both in tumor cell invasion[43] and in migration of endothelial cells necessary for angiogenesis;[44] it may also be responsible for the microglial infiltration found

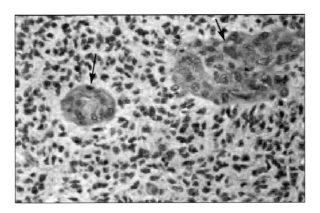

Figure 2.6
Endothelial proliferation in a high-grade brain tumor. Two foci of vascular endothelial hyperplasia (arrows) are surrounded by neoplastic glial cells.

Table 2.4
Steps in angiogenesis.

1. Endothelial cell (EC) and pericyte activation
2. Basal lamina degradation
3. Migration and proliferation of ECs and pericytes
4. Formation of new capillary lumen
5. Pericytes infiltrate new capillaries
6. New basal lamina forms
7. Capillary loops form
8. Involution and differentiation of new vessels
9. Capillary network formation
10. Formation of larger microvessels

in some high-grade gliomas.[45] Platelet endothelial growth factor is expressed in some anaplastic gliomas and favors angiogenesis.[46]

The overall result of angiogenesis is that the tumor develops a vasculature sufficient to sustain growth, even though areas of hypoxia in high-grade tumors are common. Microscopically, the tumors, particularly the high-grade ones, become hypervascular (Fig. 2.6). A study of vascularity in a number of brain tumors indicates a relationship between the microvessel density and the biology of the tumor. Meningiomas had a microvessel count (MVC; highest number of microvessels in three areas of highest vascular density at × 200 magnification) of 28, low-grade astrocytomas 14, anaplastic astrocytomas 42 and glioblastomas 50.[47] Furthermore, there are not only more blood vessels but they are different in anatomic structure. The capillaries induced by VEGF are fenestrated rather than non-fenestrated which contributes to permeability of the blood–brain barrier within the tumor.[48]

Angiogenesis makes a particularly appealing target for brain tumor therapy.[33,49] A major problem in the therapy of most brain tumors is tumor heterogeneity. Because tumor cells are genetically unstable, the tumor itself may consist of a large number of cells which differ from one another in their genetic expression. Therefore, some cells in the tumor are likely to be resistant to almost any agent or combination of agents used for treatment. Even if most tumor cells are sensitive, the resistant cells continue to reproduce and repopulate the tumor. Although endothelial cells in the tumor differ from those in normal brain, they are not, like tumor cells, genetically unstable. Accordingly, if one finds an agent to which endothelial cells are sensitive, they should remain sensitive and not develop genetic mutations[50] leading to resistance.

Table 2.4 summarizes the steps in angiogenesis.

Blood–CNS barriers

Under normal circumstances, the brain and the CSF do not permit the entry of most hydrophilic substances that circulate in the blood and easily enter other organs. Entry of hydrophilic substances such as peptides and proteins into brain is restricted by the blood–brain barrier, and entry into the CSF by the blood–CSF barrier. Glucose, some amino acids and some other vital compounds enter the brain or CSF by specific transport systems.[51] Water-soluble chemotherapeutic agents such as cytarabine and methotrexate enter the brain poorly,[52] although the physician can substantially increase the concentration of these substances in the brain by increasing the parenteral dose. Most lipid-soluble substances enter the brain rapidly. Some examples common in neuro-oncologic practice are phenytoin, methadone, and 1,3-bischloro-(2-chloroethyl)-1-nitrosourea (BCNU).

Blood–brain barrier

The blood–brain barrier resides in capillary endothelial cells.[53,54] Endothelial cells require the presence of astrocytes to maintain the blood–brain barrier,[55,56] and astrocytes are present in abundance in normal brain and even in most brain tumors. The characteristics of capillary endothelial cells that create the blood–brain barrier include (Fig. 2.7):

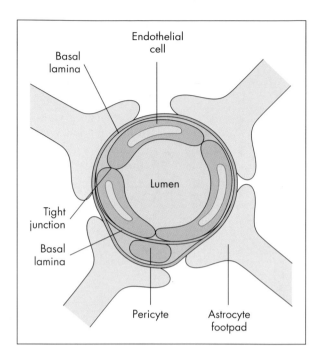

Figure 2.7
The blood–brain barrier is formed by capillary endothelium and supported by surrounding structures, including the basal lamina, astrocytes and pericytes. The pericyte process covers a substantial portion of the microvascular circumference including the endothelial tight junctions. (From Blabanov and Dore–Duffy[57] with permission.)

1. Capillary endothelial cells are connected by tight rather than gap junctions.[58] The aqueous channels through the tight junctions have diameters that are no larger than 0.6–0.8 nm, restricting free diffusion of most substances including water. Tumor capillaries of high-grade gliomas lack tight junctions; capillaries of low-grade infiltrating tumors may retain tight junctions.

2. Brain capillaries lack fenestrations within the endothelial cell, thus preventing the entry of large molecules, such as proteins, that find their way into the interstitial space of most organs. Brain tumor blood vessels are fenestrated.[48]

3. Pinocytotic vesicles transport plasma or interstitial fluid bidirectionally across the endothelium.[59] The density of pinocytotic vesicles in brain endothelium is about 5% of that in other organs, substantially limiting pinocytotic transport. Brain tumor and peritumoral capillaries are rich in pinocytotic vesicles.[60]

4. Mitochondria that supply the energy for active transport across the endothelium are 10-fold more abundant in brain endothelial cells than in the endothelium of other

organs. The increased mitochondria in the brain endothelium supply the energy for transport of water-soluble substances that cannot otherwise cross the blood–brain barrier and promote the expulsion of potentially toxic substances that accumulate as a result of brain activity (e.g. potassium, glutamate). Brain tumor vessels have a low density of mitochondria.[61]

5. P-glycoprotein, a unique membrane glycoprotein with a molecular mass of 170–180 kDa, is encoded by a multi-drug resistance gene (MDR).[62] P-glycoprotein is expressed either at the luminal membrane of cerebral endothelial cells or at astrocytic foot processes[62] and can be measured by PET scanning in rats.[63] Increased expression of P-glycoprotein has been associated with resistance of some systemic tumors to several chemotherapeutic agents. The protein 'pumps out' certain chemotherapeutic drugs, e.g. vincristine and doxorubicin. Unlike systemic tumors, brain tumor capillaries are characterized by the absence of P-glycoprotein, which contributes to the impaired blood–brain barrier seen in brain tumors.[64]

6. Capillary endothelial cells rest on a continuous basement membrane, which in turn is surrounded by astrocytic processes. At one time, this glial sheath was considered to be the site of the blood–brain barrier, but electronmicroscopy has demonstrated spaces of 200 angstroms between astrocytic processes, allowing for diffusion. Studies with horseradish peroxidase, a protein marker, have shown that the barrier resides at the tight junctions of endothelial cells. However, it is clear that normal astrocytes are essential for capillary endothelia to maintain an intact blood–brain barrier. Co-culture of non-brain endothelial cells with normal astrocytes or with glial cell line-derived neurotrophic factor[65] induces the endothelial cells to form a blood–tissue barrier. Abnormal glial cells, such as those lacking glial fibrillary acidic protein (GFAP), or neoplastic glial cells, are incapable of forming a normal barrier.

7. The extracellular matrix (ECM) also serves to support the blood–brain barrier. Disruption of ECM components may disrupt the blood–brain barrier.[66,67]

8. Peritumoral blood vessels also show morphologic changes that suggest to different investigators either increased permeability[68] or a role in edema resolution.[69]

9. Aquaporins, a family of water channels, regulate the brain's water content. They may play a role in formation of blood–CNS barriers and in development and restoration of brain edema.[70,71]

Blood–CSF barrier

The blood–CSF barrier differs from the blood–brain barrier in several respects.[72] It has a 5000-fold smaller surface area than that of the blood–brain barrier. The major sites of transport across the blood–CSF barrier are at the choroid plexus[73] (where a substantial portion of the spinal fluid is secreted and the composition of newly formed CSF is determined), and at the arachnoid villi (and, to a lesser extent, along nerve root sheaths), where spinal fluid is reabsorbed. Certain trace elements essential for brain nutrition, such as folic acid and vitamin B_{12}, that do not cross the blood–brain barrier may be transported into the nervous system via the choroid plexus and reach the brain by diffusion.[74,75] Certain acidic substances such as penicillin and methotrexate are transported out of the CSF to the blood by the choroid plexus, particularly in the fourth ventricle.

CSF is reabsorbed by bulk flow through the arachnoid villi and, especially when intracranial pressure is increased, through lymphatics that drain from the basal subarachnoid space into cervical lymph nodes.[76] The rate of CSF formation and absorption is about 0.35 ml/min. The CSF volume in the adult is approximately 150 ml, a volume achieved in children at about age 4 years. Therefore, the total CSF volume turns over approximately four times a day. A barrier does not exist between the CSF and the brain, because the ependyma lining the ventricles and the pia-arachnoid surrounding brain and spinal cord allow free diffusion of substances, including proteins such as albumin. However, the diffusion rate into and through brain parenchyma is considerably slower than that of bulk CSF flow. Furthermore, many substances are reabsorbed by the brain capillary bed into the systemic circulation once they have diffused a short distance into the parenchyma. Thus, most substances introduced into the CSF do not penetrate very far into the brain or spinal cord. The result is that drugs injected intrathecally, while exposing leptomeningeal tumor to high concentrations, usually fail to reach parenchymal lesions such as brain tumors in significant concentration. Consequently, administration of chemotherapeutic agents directly into CSF is unreliable for treating intraparenchymal lesions.[77] In experimental animals, an appreciable concentration of methotrexate has been shown to reach about 40% of the brain within an hour after intraventricular administration, but an adequate concentration cannot be achieved in the much larger human brain. In both experimental animals and humans, white matter adjacent to CSF contains the highest drug concentration, possibly explaining the tendency for drug-induced leukoencephalopathy to be periventricular.

The CSF also serves as the brain's lymphatic system although there are lymph channels around cranial nerves and perhaps around large arteries at the base of the brain as well. Substances that either cross the blood–brain barrier from the vasculature to enter brain interstitial space, or are secreted or excreted by neurons and glia, leave the nervous system by diffusing into the CSF and then being absorbed by bulk flow. In addition to diffusion, hydrostatic pressure may drive substances either toward or away from the CSF. A brain tumor and its surrounding plasma-derived edema cause increased tissue pressure; the pressure drives substances from the tumor through edematous brain and normal brain, and then to the subarachnoid space. Conversely, when subarachnoid pathways are blocked, pressure may drive substances from CSF into brain.

Disruption of blood–CNS barriers

Angiogenesis

Although angiogenesis leads to blood vessels that do not have a normal blood–CNS barrier, the degree of disruption in the barrier varies substantially from tumor to tumor, as well as within an individual tumor. Clinically, blood–brain barrier disruption is visualized by the passage of intravenously injected contrast material into the extracellular space of the tumor. In general, high-grade intrinsic tumors of the brain are associated with substantial disruption of the blood–brain barrier and lower-grade tumors with lesser or absent disruption (Fig. 2.8). There are, however, notable exceptions. Low-grade tumors, such as pilocytic astrocytomas, are often associated with significant blood–brain barrier breakdown and contrast enhancement. Meningiomas, benign tumors, characteristically intensely contrast enhance because their blood supply comes from the external carotid circulation, and they would not be expected to possess a

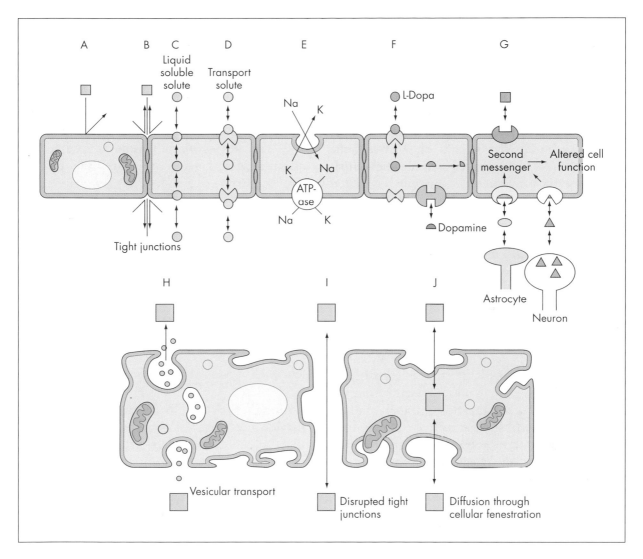

Figure 2.8

A schematic representation of the normal (top) and disrupted (bottom) blood–brain barrier. The endothelial cell lipid membrane (A) and tight junctions connecting endothelial cells (B) prevent the movement of polar molecules between the blood and the brain. Lipid-soluble molecules (C) and solutes for which the endothelial cell had transporters, such as glucose, some amino acids, and some micronutrients such as thiamine (D), cross from blood to brain by two-way transport systems. Other substances, such as potassium and sodium, are transported asymmetrically from either the blood to the brain or the brain to the blood (E). Some molecules that cross the luminal endothelial membrane, such as L-DOPA (F), are metabolized within the endothelial cell so that a metabolic product such as dopamine reaches the brain. Receptors on the endothelial surface, including selectrins and integrins, react with circulating messengers that affect the brain via a second messenger system (G). In patients with brain tumors or other lesions, the blood–brain barrier is disrupted. This occurs in part via increased vesicular transport (H), in part because the tight junctions are disrupted, allowing polar solutes to cross from the blood to the brain (I), and in part because fenestrations in the endothelial cell allow increased diffusion of polar solutes through the cell (J).

blood–brain barrier. Conversely, some high-grade tumors have little or no contrast enhancement, particularly early in the course of their development. Medulloblastomas, among the most high-grade of brain tumors, may sometimes be associated with minimal or absent contrast enhancement. Even when the tumor does contrast enhance, disruption of the barrier is rarely complete. Substantial variability is found in the degree of blood–brain barrier breakdown in primary brain tumors implanted into rats. Nitrosourea (ENU)-induced oligodendrogliomas have an almost normal blood–brain barrier, for instance, whereas avian sarcoma virus (ASV)-induced tumors are substantially leaky.[78] Although the clinician can use the degree of contrast enhancement as a clue to the histologic grade of the tumor, it is not sufficiently dependable to eliminate the need for biopsy to establish a definitive histology (Chapter 3).

Other sources of disruption

Tumor growth and its associated angiogenesis are not the only mechanisms that can disrupt the blood–brain barrier. An increase in hydrostatic pressure, such as that caused by severe arterial hypertension, can disrupt the barrier in tissue compressed by tumor.[79] Compression can also disrupt the barrier, interfering with venous drainage and increasing capillary hydrostatic pressure; this is possibly one mechanism of blood–brain barrier disruption caused by tumors such as meningiomas that compress the brain but do not directly invade it.

Peritumoral blood vessels

Vessels surrounding brain tumors may also show increased permeability. Peritumoral capillaries show an increase in endothelial surface-connected vesicles, a thicker basal lamina and

significantly reduced extension of pericytic and glial investments. The capillaries are rich in pinocytotic vesicles, which suggests increased capillary permeability although fenestrations and disruption of tight junctions have not been observed.[68] The increased permeability probably results from substances secreted by tumor cells that diffuse into surrounding brain; these substances can result from an inflammatory response to the tumor, or entry into the tumor via breakdown of the blood–brain barrier. VEGF is secreted by a variety of tumors and increases permeability of normal vessels.[37] Other substances, such as free radicals, bradykinins and arachidonic acid may be secreted by microglia or other cells in reaction to tumor formation. Vasoactive mediators such as glutamate, histamine and hormones may enter the tumor from the serum and diffuse into normal brain, increasing permeability of otherwise normal brain capillaries.

Brain edema

There is a close but incomplete correlation among the factors that cause angiogenesis and those that lead to disruption of the blood–brain barrier and production of brain edema.[80] The best example is the most important angiogenesis factor, VEGF. This factor was originally designated vascular permeability factor (VPF) because it increased the permeability of capillaries, both within the brain and elsewhere in the body. The increase in permeability may be mediated by nitric oxide.[81] In most circumstances, brain tumors that cause angiogenesis have a disrupted blood–brain barrier, producing contrast enhancement on MRI and substantial brain edema. However, the correlation among these three characteristics is not complete. For example, in some high-grade gliomas, angiogenesis, disruption of the blood–brain barrier

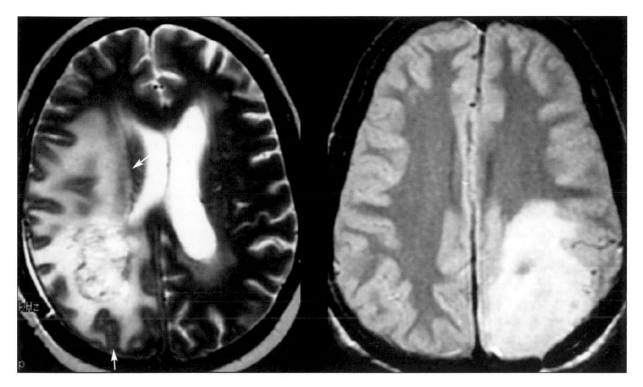

Figure 2.9
Edema versus infiltrating tumor. The panel on the left shows a tumor surrounded by edema, whereas the panel on the right shows a non-edematous low-grade tumor. The hyperintensity on the T2-weighted image seen on the left panel spares the cerebral cortex and the deep gray structures (arrows). The hyperintensity on the T2-weighted image on the right involves both the subarachnoid structures and the cerebral cortex.

and contrast enhancement may be present but edema may be minimal or absent (Fig. 2.9). Similarly, a meningioma, which also requires substantial angiogenesis, usually causes little or no edema of the underlying brain. When a meningioma does cause brain edema, it may result from secretion of VEGF by the tumor.[82]

When the blood–brain barrier is focally disrupted, water-soluble substances and large molecules such as proteins can enter the brain more easily. Because the brain has limited lymphatic drainage, these substances are not easily eliminated but are often driven into surrounding normal brain by increased hydrostatic pressure within the tumor. They may be eliminated by filtering through the white matter and then into the cerebral ventricles or subarachnoid space, to be reabsorbed by bulk flow of CSF.

The edema caused by brain tumors develops primarily in white matter rather than the more tightly packed gray matter with its interdigitating dendritic processes. The edema is extracellular, and follows low resistance white matter fiber tracts rather than diffusing in a spherical pattern.[83] Thus, a small occipital tumor may cause edema infiltrating along fiber tracts all the way to the tip of the temporal lobe. Edema fluid has more water and is less dense than normal brain, so it is relatively easy to image by MR or CT scans. Characteristically, edema fluid is hypodense on CT scan and T1 MRI and hyperintense on the T2-weighted MRI scan; typically, it extends like fingers into the white matter outlining the cerebral cortex (Chapter 3). Edema fluid does not contrast enhance, making it easy to differentiate from bulky tumor (Fig. 2.9); however, because some glial tumors are highly invasive, isolated tumor cells are often found in edematous brain areas, several centimeters from the main tumor mass. Edema has an elevated protein content, including albumin, and most studies suggest that vasogenic edema, no matter how produced, is similar in composition. However, one study of human tumors suggests that the mean serum protein content in tissues adjacent to tumor varies considerably, depending on the nature of the tumor; the serum protein content is high in peritumoral edema surrounding glioblastomas and low in edema surrounding a metastasis.[84]

The mechanism by which brain tumors cause vasogenic edema is complex and multifactorial. Increased vascular permeability to plasma constituents, including albumin, results in: (1) an increase in conductance of osmotically active solutes and a decrease in their reflection coefficients across the capillary wall; (2) an alteration of the normal concentration gradient of osmotically active solutes between plasma and brain extracellular fluid, by an increase in brain solutes, creating an imbalance between osmotic and hydrostatic pressures across brain and tumor capillaries, favoring fluid movement from blood to brain; (3) an increase in hydraulic conductivity across tumor vessels and through an expanded extracellular space between white matter fiber tracts, augmenting

the transcapillary movement of plasma-derived fluid from blood to tumor and from tumor into surrounding brain; and (4) hydrostatic pressure gradients within the extracellular tissue driving fluid movement from areas of blood–brain barrier breakdown into surrounding normal brain. The tissue hydrostatic pressure gradients and movement of edema fluid through the brain depend on arterial blood pressure and the hydraulic conductivity of the tissue itself (white matter to gray matter).

The formation within tumors of new vessels that do not have a blood–brain barrier is certainly important to the pathogenesis of brain edema, but new vessel formation (i.e. angiogenesis) may not be the only way that

Table 2.5
Some mediators of brain edema.

Mediator	Proposed mechanism
Oxygen-free radicals	Peroxidation of lipid membranes
	DNA strand breaks
	Depletion of cellular energy stores
	? Reaction with nitric oxide to form toxic peroxynitrite
Bradykinin	Dilation of cerebral vessels
Arachidonic acid	Dilation of cerebral vessels
	? Production of oxygen free radicals
Glutamate	Cellular energy depletion
	Dilation of cerebral vessels
Hormones	
Arginine vasopressin	Disruption of water and
Atrial natriuretic peptide	electrolyte homeostasis
Nitric oxide?	Vasodilatation
Histamine	

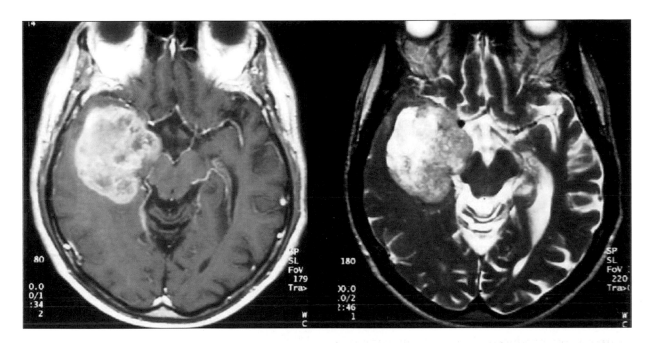

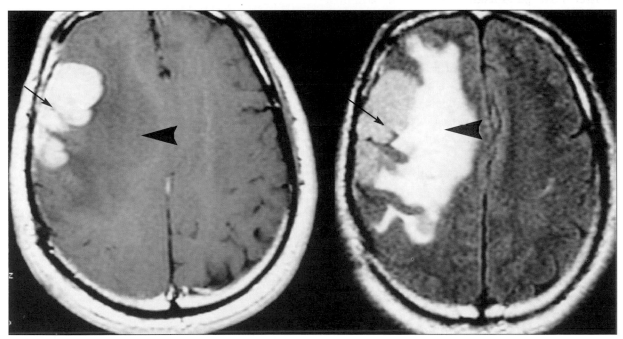

Figure 2.10

Not all intrinsic brain tumors cause significant edema nor are all tumors causing edema necessarily within the brain. The two panels on the top show the enhanced T1- and T2-weighted images of a patient with a large glioblastoma multiforme with no surrounding edema. Two panels (below) show the enhanced T1- and T2-weighted images of a patient with a meningioma (arrows) surrounded by substantial edema (arrow head) (Chapter 6).

edema is formed in brain tumors. Substantial evidence indicates that tumors secrete substances that not only promote angiogenesis of vessels lacking a blood–brain barrier, but also promote leakiness of normal brain capillaries in the brain immediately surrounding tumor (Table 2.5).[37,85,86]

The neurologic symptoms that result from brain edema are often more severe than those resulting from the tumor itself. However, not all intracranial tumors are accompanied by edema (Fig. 2.10); for example, most meningiomas (Chapter 6) do not cause edema. However, whether edema fluid in and of itself is toxic to the brain or whether all of its symptoms are a consequence of mass effect compressing and distorting normal tissue is not clear. No clinical or experimental evidence has defined whether or not symptoms are caused by the edema fluid itself. Edema differs from normal brain extracellular space because it contains substances normally excluded from the brain. For example, potassium, calcium and glutamate, all substances that affect neuronal function, are found at much lower concentrations in brain extracellular space and in CSF than in edema fluid. The normal CSF/plasma ratios are 0.62, 0.49 and 0.40, respectively. Disruption of the blood–brain barrier increases those ratios in the brain's extracellular space and could contribute to altered neural function. Positron emission tomography (PET) studies consistently show relative hypometabolism of edematous brain surrounding tumors that cannot be completely explained by a lesser cell density. The pragmatic issue is that there is no question that cerebral edema is instrumental in causing symptoms in patients with intracranial tumors; amelioration of the edema with steroids (see below) often substantially improves symptoms even before the tumor itself is treated.

Two additional aspects of the anatomy and physiology of the nervous system make it particularly vulnerable to the effects of tumors growing within the intracranial cavity:

1. The brain is enclosed in bone (the skull). As tumors grow, they distort and compress nearby normal brain and they raise tissue pressure both in the immediate area and at a distance (i.e. overall intracranial pressure), thus interfering with neural function remote from the tumor and sometimes giving rise to 'false localizing signs' (Chapter 3). Furthermore, tissue pressure is not equally distributed. Regional brain tissue pressure gradients develop, with the pressure highest near the lesion. These pressure gradients may further serve to shift tissue from its normal compartment.[87] Mechanical compression can initiate glial proliferation, possibly via a tyrosine kinase pathway. This may explain gliosis surrounding many brain tumors.[88] Increased tissue pressure in the tumor may retard entry of drugs into the tumor and may promote their diffusion away from the tumor.

2. The brain lacks lymphatics. Lymph channels positioned along cranial nerves, especially the olfactory nerve, and spinal roots may absorb some CSF, and macromolecules draining in this manner localize in cervical lymph nodes.[89] The amount, however, is not sufficient to prevent brain edema and the resultant increased intracranial pressure. The paucity of lymphatics may also play a role in preventing an immune response to some brain tumors. However, the lymphatic drainage into cervical lymph nodes appears sufficient in experimental animals to allow immune reactions. Because of the few lymphatics, most of the absorption of brain edema fluid can only occur by the long, tortuous route of convection or bulk flow through

the brain substance to the ventricular system or subarachnoid space, where it is eventually absorbed along with the CSF. Unfortunately, the tumor, with its increased intracranial pressure and elevated CSF proteins, often reduces the capacity of normal CSF absorptive pathways, thus compounding the problem of brain edema.

Consequences of barrier disruption and brain edema

Increased intracranial pressure, plateau waves and cerebral herniation

In those patients with mass lesions involving or compressing nervous system structures, the breakdown of blood–CNS barriers with the production of brain edema often leads to increased intracranial pressure. The pressure may be distributed evenly throughout the brain, such as when obstruction of the superior vena cava or sagittal sinus raises venous pressure and thus intracranial pressure uniformly, or pressure may be distributed unevenly, as exemplified in patients with focal mass lesions.[90] Evenly distributed increased intracranial pressure probably causes no symptoms until the intracranial pressure approaches the arterial blood pressure, resulting in cerebral ischemia. Focally increased tissue pressure causes herniation of portions of normal brain into areas of lower pressure. The most common sites of herniation, as illustrated in Fig. 3.2, include herniation of the medial frontal lobe under the falx cerebri, herniation of the medial temporal lobe through the tentorium cerebelli, and herniation of the cerebellar tonsils through the foramen magnum. The

clinical consequences of these herniations are described in Chapter 3. Focally increased tissue pressure can also cause symptoms by interfering with the local blood supply. Both mechanisms are probably responsible for many of the symptoms caused by brain tumors.

Some patients suffer intermittent episodes of neurologic dysfunction that result from sudden rises in intracranial pressure called plateau waves.[91–93] These episodes last 5–20 min and then cease. The waves, first described by Lundberg[92] in 1960 (Fig. 3.6), appear to result from an increase in cerebral blood volume due to a sudden decrease in cerebral vascular resistance;[94,95] blood flow may actually decrease as the blood volume rises. Patients with an intracranial mass and an elevated intracranial baseline pressure resulting in diminished CSF absorption are more likely to develop plateau waves than those with normal CSF absorption.[96]

Plateau waves can either occur spontaneously or be precipitated by certain activities. Common precipitating causes include tracheal suctioning, coughing or sneezing, and, particularly, rising from a lying or sitting position,[97] especially in the early morning after a night's sleep. Plateau waves are often asymptomatic even when they cause a dramatic increase in intracranial pressure. However, at times the symptoms can be dramatic and varied (Chapter 3). Plateau waves respond rapidly to relief of raised intracranial pressure either by steroids or other mechanisms.

Treatment of cerebral herniation

Immediate treatment of increased intracranial pressure is required to reverse or prevent cerebral herniation and to prevent death. The treatment of increased intracranial pressure and cerebral edema includes hyperventilation, hyperosmolar agents, and adrenocorticosteroids.

Hyperventilation

Hyperventilation is the most rapid technique for lowering intracranial pressure and reversing herniation, but its effect is short-lived. Hyperventilation lowers pCO_2, causing cerebral vasoconstriction and decreasing cerebral blood volume. If the patient is unconscious, an endotracheal tube should be inserted and the patient ventilated to a pCO_2 level between 25–30 mm Hg, which lowers intracranial pressure rapidly in most patients but only transiently, with a return to baseline blood volume in about an hour. Many patients with cerebral herniation spontaneously hyperventilate to these levels and require no additional respiratory intervention from the physician. However, intubation is advisable to protect the airway. Respiratory function must be monitored carefully, because brain herniation can cause respiratory failure. Mechanical ventilation can raise as well as lower intracranial pressure, and ventilated patients with brain lesions are at risk,[98] particularly when intrathoracic pressure is kept high, diminishing venous return. The increased intrathoracic pressure is transmitted to the superior vena cava and to intracranial vessels.

Osmolar therapy

Hyperosmolar agents decrease the water content of the brain by creating an osmolar gradient between the blood and that portion of the brain with an intact blood–brain barrier. The agent of choice is mannitol given intravenously over 10–20 min as a 20% solution at a dose of 0.5–2 g/kg.[99] This drug may also decrease CSF formation and volume.[100] In a few patients with severe and sustained increased intracranial pressure, pressure can be monitored and the dose tailored to maintain decreased pressure.[99] In patients with normal intracranial pressure, mannitol may actually increase the pressure briefly, probably due to a transient increase in cerebral blood flow and volume. This does not appear to occur in patients with increased intracranial pressure.[99,101] The mannitol effects are rapid and last several hours. Mannitol injections may be repeated in smaller doses if the patient first responds and subsequently relapses. Glycerol, urea and hypertonic saline[102,103] are less widely used. Repeated doses of mannitol can also cause a 'reverse' osmotic effect as the compound leaks into edematous brain. The addition of a diuretic (furosemide) enhances and prolongs the mannitol effect.[104]

Corticosteroids

Corticosteroids decrease the transfer across the disrupted blood–brain barrier of serum substances into brain. They lower intracranial pressure, diminish plateau waves and eventually decrease edema (see below). Dexamethasone (100 mg IV) is given immediately, followed by doses of 40–100 mg/24 h, depending on the patient's response to treatment. Some physicians add furosemide (40–120 mg IV) to the steroids and believe that the combination is better than steroids alone;[102] however, intravascular volume depletion must be closely watched. With such vigorous treatment, most patients who herniate from brain tumors can be stabilized, and many have complete amelioration of their symptoms within a few days.

Treatment of brain edema

Several drugs, including glutamate inhibitors, non-steroidal anti-inflammatory agents (e.g. indomethacin) and lazeroids (21-aminosteroids that have antioxidant but not glucocorticoid activity) have also been proposed for the treatment of brain and spinal cord edema,[105] but their clinical efficacy is unproved. Corticotropin-releasing factor (CRF) has proved effective in ameliorating tumor-induced brain edema in experimental animals; the mechanism of action is not known. The edema-ameliorating effects are not a result of CRF-induced cortisone release, because CRF is effective in adrenalectomized brain tumor-bearing animals.[106,107] An arginine vasopressin receptor antagonist may also prove useful.[86] However, at present, corticosteroids are the drug of first choice to treat tumor-induced brain edema.

Corticosteroids

The most widely used drugs in neuro-oncology are the synthetic glucocorticoids, commonly referred to simply as steroids.[108] They are the mainstay of treatment for nervous system edema and increased intracranial pressure. The optimum dose and best preparation of corticosteroids are not established.[109] The dosage probably should differ both with the nature of the problem and its severity.[110]

The steroid most widely used remains dexamethasone, largely because it was the drug whose usage was established by Galicich and French[111] to treat brain tumors. Dexamethasone may be preferred to other synthetic glucocorticoids for several theoretical reasons. First, it has no mineralocorticoid effect, and therefore is the least likely steroid to cause salt retention and systemic edema formation. Second, some investigators believe it is also less likely than other synthetic steroids to cause cognitive and behavioral dysfunction.[101]

Only a few experiments address a dose-response curve for CNS effects of corticosteroids. One such experiment in an animal model of spinal cord compression suggests that doses equivalent to 100 mg/24 h of dexamethasone may be superior to lesser doses both in decreasing edema and in ameliorating clinical symptomatology.[112] Because reports thus far give no indication that these higher doses given for a few days are deleterious, our practice is to use high doses in seriously symptomatic or deteriorating patients, tapering the dose after a few days to the lowest dose consistent with symptomatic control.[113]

Steroid treatment begins with the physician selecting a dose appropriate for the neurologic disorder and its severity (see below). Because of its long half-life, dexamethasone can be given twice daily, although most physicians give four divided doses. The drug is well absorbed from the gastrointestinal tract, but first-pass hepatic metabolism may decrease the effectiveness of an oral dose, especially in patients taking phenytoin. Because side-effects are numerous and often serious, patients should be maintained on the lowest dose of steroid that affords relief of symptoms. Thus, once symptomatic control is established and more definitive therapy (e.g. surgery, radiation, and chemotherapy) is underway, the steroid should be tapered to the lowest possible dose (see below).

Steroid taper

Because of the deleterious effects of corticosteroids (Chapter 4), patients should be treated with the smallest effective dose for the shortest time possible. Virtually all patients begun on corticosteroid therapy for brain tumors are treated subsequently with either radiation therapy (RT) or chemotherapy. Patients with brain tumors usually continue steroids during the course of RT, but the dose can be decreased after the first week and gradually tapered thereafter. Most patients can be off steroids by the completion of the RT, and the remainder should be weaned from the steroids entirely if possible. The steroid taper begins 3–4 days after surgery or during week 2 of RT and should be tapered gradually enough to prevent the development of steroid withdrawal symptoms, but rapidly enough so that the patient is not taking the drugs for an extended period. For patients receiving 16 mg dexamethasone, the drug should be tapered by 2–4 mg every fifth day. If at any time during the taper the patient develops symptoms of either brain tumor or steroid withdrawal, the drug is increased to the next higher dose for 4–8 days before tapering again. If, after the patient is withdrawn, brain tumor symptoms develop, it is probably wise to start the full regimen of 16 mg/24 h dexamethasone.

For patients who have been on steroids for many months, who fail the usual taper schedule, or who have large amounts of residual tumor, the drug is tapered more slowly (e.g. 1–2 mg/week) to the lowest dose tolerable. For patients taking large doses of steroids (e.g. 100 mg/24 h dexamethasone) who have stabilized and are receiving more definitive treatment, the dose can be halved every 4–5 days depending on the patient's clinical state. The dose should be raised again if the clinical condition deteriorates.

Weissman et al[114] propose a more rapid taper schedule, beginning at 16 mg/day (8 mg bid) for 4 days followed by 8 mg/24 h for 4 days and 4 mg/24 h until completion of RT. This procedure was well tolerated by their patients who had brain metastases.

Mechanisms of steroid action

The mechanisms by which steroids stabilize blood–brain, blood–spinal cord, and probably blood–CSF barriers are not entirely known, although several have been proposed. Glucocorticoids inhibit the production or release of a number of biochemical substances shown to increase vascular permeability and induce vasodilatation (an effect that, by increased hydrostatic pressure, also increases permeability). Glucocorticoids induce formation of lipocortins, which inhibit phosphorylase A_2, thus preventing the release of arachidonic acid.[115] Arachidonic acid and its metabolites increase vascular permeability; thus, the reduction of arachidonic acid by steroids might reduce brain edema. Nonetheless, other inhibitors of this pathway, such as indomethacin, do not stabilize the blood–brain barrier or ameliorate the symptoms of brain tumors as effectively as corticosteroids. Steroids inhibit the release of IL-1; whether the interleukins play a role in blood–brain barrier breakdown is not known. Steroids also appear to have a direct effect on endothelial cells, increasing resistance to transendothelial fluid flow and increasing the number of tight junctions.[116] In several organisms, steroids inhibit the increased permeability that results from endothelial cell interaction with a number of chemical agents.[117] Experimental evidence suggests that steroids can induce the synthesis of a protein that inhibits microvascular permeability, a direct action on the endothelial cell. It appears that the inhibitory protein is distinct from lipocortin and, thus, the effect is independent from the inhibition of phosphorylase A_2. Whatever their mechanisms, steroids appear to be unique in their ability to ameliorate clinical symptoms and stabilize the blood–brain barrier. Clinically, steroid-induced reconstitution of the blood–brain barrier can occasionally be visualized on neuroimaging.

Contrast enhancement can diminish in tumors after initiation of dexamethasone but before the start of definitive treatment. Sometimes, this is misinterpreted as a response to treatment if the steroid-induced diminution of enhancement is not appreciated or recognized.

In addition to restoring capillary impermeability,[118] dexamethasone also decreases cerebral blood flow and volume[119,120] and increases the fractional extraction of oxygen throughout the brain without affecting oxygen utilization. Reports suggest that the drug probably has a direct vasoconstrictive effect on cerebral blood vessels.[121] Dexamethasone treatment reduces or eliminates the filtration of plasma-derived fluid across tumor capillaries and the movement of albumin through the extracellular space by solvent drag. These effects may be mediated by reducing the size of the extracellular space or decreasing the pore size of tumor capillaries, which probably represents an important mechanism for corticosteroid control of peritumoral brain edema.[122] Although most studies have not demonstrated an effect of dexamethasone on the blood–brain barrier of normal brain, at least one study[123] suggests that dexamethasone may decrease the permeability to macromolecules of normal cerebral vasculature, possibly by interfering with vesicular transport.[123]

References

1. Milosevic MF, Fyles AW, Hill RP. The relationship between elevated interstitial fluid pressure and blood flow in tumors: a bioengineering analysis. Int J Radiat Oncol Biol Phys 1999; 43: 1111–23.

2. Boucher Y, Salehi H, Witwer B, Harsh GR, Jain RK. Interstitial fluid pressure in intracranial tumours in patients and in rodents. Br J Cancer 1997; 75: 829–36.

3. Burger PC, Scheithauer BW, Vogel FS. Surgical Pathology of the Nervous System and its Coverings, 3rd edn. Churchill Livingstone, New York, 1991.

4. Kelly PJ, Daumas-Duport C, Scheithauer BW. Stereotactic histologic correlations of computed tomography and magnetic resonance imaging-defined abnormalities in patients with glial neoplasms. Mayo Clin Proc 1987; 62: 450–59.

5. Gary SC, Hockfield S. BEHAB/brevican: an extracellular matrix component associated with invasive glioma. Clin Neurosurg 2000; 47: 72–82.

6. Asano K, Kubo O, Tajika Y, Takakura K, Suzuki S. Expression of cadherin and CSF dissemination in malignant astrocytic tumors. Neurosurg Rev 2000; 23: 39–44.

7. Tews DS. Adhesive and invasive features in gliomas. Pathol Res Pract 2000; 196: 701–11.

8. Tonn JC, Wunderlich S, Kerkau S, Klein CE, Roosen K. Invasive behaviour of human gliomas is mediated by interindividually different integrin patterns. Anticancer Res 1998; 18: 2599–605.

9. Hallahan DE, Staba-Hogan MJ, Virudachalam S, Kolchinsky A. X-ray-induced P-selectin localization to the lumen of tumor blood vessels. Cancer Res 1998; 58: 5216–20.

10. Sasaki H, Yoshida K, Ikeda E, et al. Expression of the neural cell adhesion molecule in astrocytic tumors – an inverse correlation with malignancy. Cancer 1998; 82: 1921–31.

11. Sehgal A, Boynton AL, Young RF et al. Cell adhesion molecule Nr-CAM is over-expressed in human brain tumors. Int J Cancer 1998; 76: 451–8.

12. Yap AS. The morphogenetic role of cadherin cell adhesion molecules in human cancer: a thematic review. Cancer Invest 1998; 16: 252–61.

13. Thorsen F, Tysnes BB. Brain tumor cell invasion, anatomical and biological considerations. Anticancer Res 1997; 17: 4121–6.

14. Gunia S, Hussein S, Radu DL et al. CD44s-targeted treatment with monoclonal antibody blocks intracerebral invasion and growth of 9L gliosarcoma. Clin Exp Metastasis 1999; 17: 221–30.

15. Senner V, Sturm A, Baur I et al. CD24 promotes invasion of glioma cells in vivo. J Neuropathol Exp Neurol 1999; 58: 795–802.

16. Nakada M, Kita D, Futami K et al. Roles of membrane type 1 matrix metalloproteinase and

tissue inhibitor of metalloproteinases 2 in invasion and dissemination of human malignant glioma. J Neurosurg 2001; 94: 464–73.

17. Forsyth PA, Wong H, Laing TD et al. Gelatinase-A (MMP-2), gelatinase-B (MMP-9) and membrane type matrix metalloproteinase-1 (MT1-MMP) are involved in different aspects of the pathophysiology of malignant gliomas. Br J Cancer 1999; 79: 1828–35.

18. Kachra Z, Beaulieu E, Delbecchi L et al. Expression of matrix metalloproteinases and their inhibitors in human brain tumors. Clin Exp Metastasis 1999; 17: 555–66.

19. Harkness KA, Adamson P, Sussman JD et al. Dexamethasone regulation of matrix metalloproteinase expression in CNS vascular endothelium. Brain 2000; 123: 698–709.

20. Fillmore HL, Shurm J, Furqueron P et al. An in vivo rat model for visualizing glioma tumor cell invasion using stable persistent expression of the green fluorescent protein. Cancer Lett 1999; 141: 9–19.

21. Bayer TA, Thier M, Roeb E et al. Migratory potential of transplantable neural tumor cell lines. Acta Neuropathol (Berl) 1999; 97: 607–12.

22. Molnar PP, O'Neil BP, Scheithauer BW, Groothuis DR. The blood–brain barrier in primary CNS lymphomas: ultrastructural evidence of endothelial cell death. Neurooncol 1999; 1: 89–100.

23. Hochberg FH, Pruitt A. Assumptions in the radiotherapy of glioblastoma. Neurology 1980; 30: 907–11.

24. Wild-Bode C, Weller M, Rimner A, Dichgans J, Wick W. Sublethal irradiation promotes migration and invasiveness of glioma cells: implications for radiotherapy of human glioblastoma. Cancer Res 2001; 61: 2744–50.

25. Loeffler JS, Alexander E, Hochberg FH et al. Clinical patterns of failure following stereotactic interstitial irradiation for malignant gliomas. Int J Radiat Oncol Biol Phys 1990; 19: 1455–62.

26. Dang CV, Semenza GL. Oncogenic alterations of metabolism. Trends Biochem Sci 1999; 24: 68–72.

27. Nishikawa R, Cheng SY, Nagashima R et al. Expression of vascular endothelial growth factor in human brain tumors. Acta Neuropathol (Berl) 1998; 96: 453–62.

28. Carroll RS, Zhang JP, Bello L et al. KDR activation in astrocytic neoplasms. Cancer 1999; 86: 1335–41.

29. Machein MR, Kullmer J, Fiebich BL et al. Vascular endothelial growth factor expression, vascular volume, and capillary permeability in human brain tumors. Neurosurgery 1999; 44: 732–40.

30. Zagzag D, Zhong H, Scalzitti JM et al. Expression of hypoxia-inducible factor 1α in brain tumors – association with angiogensis, invasion and progression. Cancer 2000; 88: 2606–18.

31. Joki T, Heese O, Nikas DC et al. Expression of cyclooxygenase 2 (COX-2) in human glioma and in vitro inhibition by a specific COX-2 inhibitor, NS-398. Cancer Res 19. 2000; 60: 4926–31.

32. Schirner M. Antiangiogenic chemotherapeutic agents. Cancer Metastasis Rev 2000; 19: 67–73.

33. Folkman J. Antiangiogenic gene therapy. Proc Natl Acad Sci USA 1998; 95: 9064–66.

34. Lund EL, Spang-Thomsen M, Skovgaard-Poulsen H, Kristjansen PE. Tumor angiogenesis – a new therapeutic target in gliomas. Acta Neurol Scand 1998; 97: 52–62.

35. Strik HM, Schluesener HJ, Seid K, Meyermann R, Deininger MH. Localization of endostatin in rat and human gliomas. Cancer 2001; 91: 1013–19.

36. Sckell A, Safabakhsh N, Dellian M, Jain RK. Primary tumor size-dependent inhibition of angiogenesis at a secondary site: an intravital microscopic study in mice. Cancer Res 1998; 58: 5866–9.

37. Oku T, Tjuvajev JG, Miyagawa T et al. Tumor growth modulation by sense and antisense vascular endothelial growth factor gene expression: effects on angiogenesis, vascular permeability, blood volume, blood flow, fluorodeoxyglucose uptake, and proliferation of human melanoma intracerebral xenografts. Cancer Res 1998; 58: 4185–92.

38. Shiratsuchi T, Nishimori H, Ichise H, Nakamura Y, Tokino T. Cloning and characterization of BAI2 and BAI3, novel genes homologous to brain-specific angiogenesis

inhibitor 1 (BAI1). Cytogenet Cell Genet 1997; 79: 103–8.

39. Czubayko F, Liaudet-Coopman ED, Aigner A et al. A secreted FGF-binding protein can serve as the angiogenic switch in human cancer. Nat Med 1997; 3: 1137–40.

40. Nomura M, Yamagishi S, Harada S et al. Placenta growth factor (PlGF) mRNA expression in brain tumors. J Neurooncol 1998; 40: 123–30.

41. Jallo GI, Friedlander DR, Kelly PJ et al. Tenascin-C expression in the cyst wall and fluid of human brain tumors correlates with angiogenesis. Neurosurgery 1997; 41: 1052–9.

42. Book AA, Ranganathan S, Abounader R, Rosen E, Laterra J. Scatter factor hepatocyte growth factor gene transfer increases rat blood–glioma barrier permeability. Brain Res 1999; 833: 173–80.

43. Welch WC, Kornblith PL, Michalopoulos GK et al. Hepatocyte growth factor (HGF) and receptor (c-met) in normal and malignant astrocytic cells. Anticancer Res 1999; 19: 1635–40.

44. Lamszus K, Schmidt NO, Jin L et al. Scatter factor promotes motility of human glioma and neuromicrovascular endothelial cells. Int J Cancer 1998; 75: 19–28.

45. Badie B, Schartner J, Klaver J, Vorpahl J. In vitro modulation of microglia motility by glioma cells is mediated by hepatocyte growth factor scatter factor. Neurosurgery 1999; 44: 1077–82.

46. Aroca F, Renaud W, Bartoli C, Bouvier-Labit C, Figarella-Branger D. Expression of PECAM-1/CD31 isoforms in human brain gliomas. J Neurooncol 1999; 43: 19–25.

47. Assimakopoulou M, Sotiropoulou-Bonikou G, Maraziotis T, Papadakis N, Varakis I. Microvessel density in brain tumors. Anticancer Res 1997; 17: 4747–53.

48. Roberts WG, Palade GE. Neovasculature induced by vascular endothelial growth factor is fenestrated. Cancer Res 1997; 57: 765–72.

49. Malonne H, Langer I, Kiss R, Atassi G. Mechanisms of tumor angiogenesis and therapeutic implications: angiogenesis inhibitors. Clin Exp Metastasis 1999; 17: 1–14.

50. Hanahan D. A flanking attack on cancer. Nat Med 1998; 4: 13–14.

51. Tamai I, Tsuji A. Transporter-mediated permeation of drugs across the blood–brain barrier. J Pharm Sci 2000; 89: 1371–88.

52. Habgood MD, Begley DJ, Abbott NJ. Determinants of passive drug entry into the central nervous system. Cell Mol Neurobiol 2000; 20: 231–53.

53. Drewes LR. What is the blood–brain barrier? A molecular perspective – Cerebral vascular biology. Adv Exp Med Biol 1999; 474: 111–22.

54. Li JY, Boado RJ, Pardridge WM. Blood–brain barrier genomics. J Cereb Blood Flow Metab 2001; 21: 61–8.

55. Schroeter ML, Mertsch K, Giese H et al. Astrocytes enhance radical defence in capillary endothelial cells constituting the blood–brain barrier. FEBS Lett 1999; 449: 241–4.

56. Kuchler-Bopp S, Delaunoy JP, Artault JC, Zaepfel M, Dietrich JB. Astrocytes induce several blood–brain barrier properties in non-neural endothelial cells. Neuroreport 1999; 10: 1347–53.

57. Balabanov R, Dore-Duffy P. Role of the CNS microvascular pericyte in the blood–brain barrier. J Neurosci Res 1998; 53: 637–44.

58. Kniesel U, Wolburg H. Tight junctions of the blood–brain barrier. Cell Mol Neurobiol 2000; 20: 57–76.

59. Stewart PA. Endothelial vesicles in the blood–brain barrier: are they related to permeability? Cell Mol Neurobiol 2000; 20: 149–63.

60. Vaz R, Borges N, Cruz C, Azevedo I. Cerebral edema associated with meningiomas: the role of peritumoral brain tissue. J Neurooncol 1998; 36: 285–91.

61. Coomber BL, Stewart PA, Hayakawa EM, Farrell CL, Del Maestro RF. A quantitative assessment of microvessel ultrastructure in C6 astrocytoma spheroids transplanted to brain and to muscle. J Neuropathol Exp Neurol 1988; 47: 29–40.

62. Golden PL, Pardridge WM. Brain microvascular P-glycoprotein and a revised model of multidrug resistance in brain. Cell Mol Neurobiol 2000; 20: 165–81.

63. Hendrikse NH, De Vries EGE, Eriks-Fluks L et al. A new in vivo method to study P-glyco-protein transport in tumors and the blood–brain barrier. Cancer Res 1999; 59: 2411–16.

64. Jolliet-Riant P, Tillement JP. Drug transfer across the blood–brain barrier and improvement of brain delivery. Fundam Clin Pharmacol 1999; 13: 16–26.

65. Igarashi Y, Utsumi H, Chiba H et al. Glial cell line-derived neurotrophic factor induces barrier function of endothelial cells forming the blood–brain barrier. Biochem Biophys Res Commun 1999; 261: 108–12.

66. Robert AM, Robert L. Extracellular matrix and blood–brain barrier function. Pathol Biol (Paris) 1998; 46: 535–42.

67. Yong VW, Krekoski CA, Forsyth PA, Bell R, Edwards DR. Matrix metalloproteinases and diseases of the CNS. Trends Neurosci 1998; 21: 75–80.

68. Vaz R, Borges N, Cruz C, Azevedo I. Cerebral edema associated with menin-giomas: the role of peritumoral brain tissue. J Neurooncol 1998; 36: 285–91.

69. Bertossi M, Virgintino D, Maiorano E, Occhiogrosso M, Roncali L. Ultrastructural and morphometric investigation of human brain capillaries in normal and peritumoral tissues. Ultrastruct Pathol 1997; 21: 41–9.

70. Venero JL, Vizuete ML, Machado A, Cano J. Aquaporins in the central nervous system. Prog Neurobiol 2001; 63: 321–36.

71. Nico B, Frigeri A, Nicchia GP et al. Role of aquaporin-4 water channel in the develop-ment and integrity of the blood–brain barrier. J Cell Sci 2001; 114: 1297–1307.

72. Saunders NR, Habgood MD, Dziegielewska KM. Barrier mechanisms in the brain, I. Adult brain. Clin Exp Pharmacol Physiol 1999; 26: 11–19.

73. Segal MB. The choroid plexuses and the barriers between the blood and the cerebrospinal fluid. Cell Mol Neurobiol 2000; 20: 183–96.

74. Ghersi-Egea JF, Strazielle N. Brain drug deliv-ery, drug metabolism, and multidrug resis-tance at the choroid plexus. Microsc Res Tech 2001; 52: 83–8.

75. Haselbach M, Wegener J, Decker S, Engelbertz C, Galla HJ. Porcine choroid plexus epithelial cells in culture: regulation of barrier properties and transport processes. Microsc Res Tech 2001; 52: 137–152.

76. Boulton M, Armstrong D, Flessner M, Hay J, Szalai JP, Johnston M. Raised intracranial pressure increases CSF drainage through arachnoid villi and extracranial lymphatics. Am J Physiol Regul Integr Comp Physiol 1998; 275: R889–R896.

77. Grossman SA, Reinhard CS, Loats HL. The intracerebral penetration of intraventricularly administered methotrexate: A quantitative autoradiographic study. J Neurooncol 1989; 7: 319–28.

78. Molnar P, Blasberg RG, Groothuis D, et al. Regional blood-to-tissue transport in avian sarcoma virus (ASV)-induced brain tumors. Neurology 1983; 33: 702–11.

79. Suzuki N, Sako K, Yonemasu Y. Effects of induced hypertension on blood flow and capillary permeability in rats with experi-mental brain tumors. J Neurooncol 1991; 10: 213–18.

80. Schilling L, Wahl M. Mediators of cerebral edema. Adv Exp Med Biol 1999; 474: 123–41.

81. Mayhan WG. VEGF increases permeability of the blood–brain barrier via a nitric oxide synthase/cGMP-dependent pathway. Am J Physiol Cell Physiol 1999; 276: C1148–53.

82. Goldman CK, Bharara S, Palmer CA et al. Brain edema in meningiomas is associated with increased vascular endothelial growth factor expression. Neurosurgery 1997; 40: 1269–77.

83. Geer CP, Grossman SA. Interstitial fluid flow along white matter tracts: A potentially important mechanism for the dissemination of primary brain tumors. J Neurooncol 1997; 32: 193–201.

84. Bodsch W, Rommel T, Ophoff BG, et al. Factors responsible for the retention of fluid in human tumor edema and the effect of dexamethasone. J Neurosurg 1987; 67: 250–7.

85. Strugar J, Rothbart D, Harrington W, Criscuolo GR. Vascular permeability factor in brain metastases: correlation with vasogenic brain edema and tumor angiogenesis. J Neurosurg 1994; 81: 560–6.

86. Bemana I, Nagao S. Treatment of brain edema with a nonpeptide arginine vasopressin V_1 receptor antagonist OPC-21268 in rats. Neurosurgery 1999; 44: 148–54.

87. Wolfla CE, Luerssen TG. Brain tissue pressure gradients are dependent upon a normal spinal subarachnoid space. Acta Neurochir Suppl (Wien) 1998; 71: 310–12.

88. Oishi Y, Uezono Y, Yanagihara N et al. Transmural compression-induced proliferation and DNA synthesis through activation of a tyrosine kinase pathway in rat astrocytoma RCR-1 cells. Brain Res 1998; 781: 159–66.

89. Weller RO, Engelhardt B, Phillips MJ. Lymphocyte targeting of the central nervous system: a review of afferent and efferent CNS-immune pathways. Brain Pathol 1996; 6: 275–88.

90. Weaver DD, Winn HR, Jane JA. Differential intracranial pressure in patients with unilateral mass lesions. J Neurosurg 1982; 56: 660–5.

91. Hayashi M, Handa Y, Kobayashi H, et al. Plateau-wave phenomenon (I). Correlation between the appearance of plateau waves and CSF circulation in patients with intracranial hypertension. Brain 1992; 114: 2681–91.

92. Lundberg N. Continuous recording and control of ventricular fluid pressure in neurosurgical practice. Acta Neurol Scand 1960; Supp 149: 1–193.

93. Rottenberg DA, Posner JB. Intracranial pressure control. In: Cottrell JE, Turndorf H. (eds) Anesthesia and Neurosurgery. C.V. Mosby Co., St. Louis, 1980.

94. Hayashi M, Kobayashi H, Handa Y, et al. Brain blood volume and blood flow in patients with plateau waves. J Neurosurg 1985; 63: 556–61.

95. Matsuda M, Yoneda S, Handa H, et al. Cerebral hemodynamic changes during plateau waves in brain-tumor patients. J Neurosurg 1979; 50: 483–8.

96. Hayashi M, Kobayashi H, Handa Y, et al. Plateau-wave phenomenon (II). Occurrence of brain herniation in patients with and without plateau waves. Brain 1991; 114: 2693–9.

97. Magnaes B. Body position and cerebrospinal fluid pressure. Part I: Clinical studies on the effect of rapid postural changes. J Neurosurg 1976; 44: 687–697.

98. Colice GL. How to ventilate patients when ICP elevation is a risk: Monitor pressure, consider hyperventilation therapy. J Crit Illness 1993; 8: 1003–20.

99. Ravussin P, Abou-Madi M, Archer D, et al. Changes in CSF pressure after mannitol in patients with and without elevated CSF pressure. J Neurosurg 1988; 69: 869–76.

100. Donato T, Shapria Y, Artru A, et al. Effect of mannitol on cerebrospinal fluid dynamics and brain tissue edema. Anesth Analg 1994; 78: 58–66.

101. Fishman RA. Cerebrospinal Fluid in Diseases of the Nervous System, 2nd Edn. W.B. Saunders Co., Philadelphia, 1992.

102. Rottenberg DA, Hurwitz BJ, Posner JB. The effect of oral glycerol on intraventricular pressure in man. Neurology 1977; 27: 600–8.

103. Qureshi AI, Suarez JI. Use of hypertonic saline solutions in treatment of cerebral edema and intracranial hypertension. Crit Care Med 2000; 28: 3301–13.

104. Pollay M, Fullenwider C, Roberts PA, et al. Effect of mannitol and furosemide on blood–brain osmotic gradient and intracranial pressure. J Neurosurg 1983; 59: 945–50.

105. Kondziolka D, Mori Y, Martinez AJ et al. Beneficial effects of the radioprotectant 21-aminosteroid U-74389G in a radiosurgery rat malignant glioma model. Int J Radiat Oncol Biol Phys 1999; 44: 179–84.

106. Tjuvajev J, Uehara H, Desai R et al. Corticotropin releasing factor as an alternative treatment of peritumoral brain edema. In Ito S (ed). Intracranial Pressure IX, Springer Verlag, Tokyo, 1994.

107. Villalona-Calero MA, Eckardt J, Burris H et al. A phase I trial of human corticotropin-releasing factor (hCRF) in patients with peritumoral brain edema. Ann Oncol 1998; 9: 71–7.

108. Weissman DE. Glucocorticoid treatment for brain metastases and epidural spinal cord compression: A review. J Clin Oncol 1988; 6: 543–51.

109. Oka K, Shimodaira H. Telepharmacodynamics to predict therapeutic effects of glucocorticoids. Letter to the Editor. Lancet 1991; 338: 385.

110. Renaudin J, Fewer D, Wilson CB, et al. Dose dependency of decadron in patients with

partially excised brain tumors. J Neurosurg 1973; 39: 302–5.

111. Galicich JH, French LA. Use of dexamethasone in the treatment of cerebral edema resulting from brain tumors and brain surgery. Am Practit-Dig Treat 1961; 12: 169–74.

112. Delattre J-Y, Arbit E, Thaler HT, Rosenblum MK, Posner JB. A dose-response study of dexamethasone in a model of spinal cord compression caused by epidural tumor. J Neurosurg 1989; 70: 920–5.

113. Lieberman A, LeBrun Y, Glass P, et al. Use of high-dose corticosteroids in patients with inoperable brain tumors. J Neurol Neurosurg Psychiatry 1977; 40: 678–82.

114. Weissman DE, Janjan NA, Erickson B, et al. Twice-daily tapering dexamethasone treatment during cranial radiation for newly diagnosed brain metastases. J Neurooncol 1991; 11: 235–9.

115. Chan PH, Fishman RA. The role of arachidonic acid in vasogenic brain edema. Fed Proc 1984; 43: 210–13.

116. Underwood JL, Murphy CG, Chen J et al. Glucocorticoids regulate transendothelial fluid flow resistance and formation of intercellular junctions. Am J Physiol Cell Physiol 1999; 277: C330–42.

117. Weissman DE, Stewart C. Experimental drug therapy of peritumoral brain edema. J Neurooncol 1988; 6: 339–42.

118. Williams TJ, Yarwood H. Effect of glucocorticosteroids on microvascular permeability. Am Rev Respir Dis 1990; 141: S39–S43.

119. Jarden JO, Dhawan V, Moeller JR, et al. The time course of steroid action on blood-to-brain and blood-to-tumor transport of 82Rb: a positron emission tomographic study. Ann Neurol 1989; 25: 239–45.

120. Tajima A, Yen M-H, Nakata H, et al. Effects of dexamethasone on blood flow and volume of perfused microvessels in traumatic brain edema. Adv Neurol 1990; 52: 343–50.

121. Leenders KL, Beaney RP, Brooks DJ, et al. Dexamethasone treatment of brain tumor patients: Effects on regional cerebral blood flow, blood volume and oxygen utilization. Neurology 1985; 35: 1610–16.

122. Nakagawa H, Groothuis DR, Owens ES, et al. Dexamethasone effects on [125I] albumin distribution in experimental RG-2 gliomas and adjacent brain. J Cereb Blood Flow Metab 1987; 7: 687–701.

123. Hedley-Whyte ET, Hsu DW. Effect of dexamethasone on blood–brain barrier in the normal mouse. Ann Neurol 1986; 19: 373–7.

3

Principles of diagnosis

Introduction

The diagnosis of central nervous system (CNS) tumors differs *quantitatively* but not *qualitatively* from the diagnosis of other neurologic diseases. The qualitative elements of history, general physical examination, neurologic examination and laboratory findings, especially imaging, are the same for all neurologic diseases. However, in most neurologic disorders, such as migraine, epilepsy and even, early in its course, multiple sclerosis, the history is by far the most important element, representing more than 80% of the information necessary for diagnosis. This is because most patients who present for neurologic evaluation have symptoms unaccompanied by neurologic signs or abnormal images. In patients with CNS tumors, the situation is different. This history is quantitatively far less important than the laboratory evaluation. Unless the patient presents with a focal seizure, symptoms may be vague and subtle and resemble those of many less serious neurologic syndromes. For example, one cannot easily distinguish, by history, the headache of brain tumor from that of migraine or tension-type headache (see below). Similarly, it is often hard to distinguish personality change associated with brain tumors from depression or other psychological disorders.

History

The duration of symptoms may be helpful in distinguishing brain tumors from other disorders and in distinguishing among histologic grades of brain tumors. Although seizures are sometimes present for many years before a brain tumor is identified[1] (this was much truer before current imaging techniques were available), a long duration of seizures usually indicates a diagnosis other than brain tumor. Neurologic symptoms other than seizures in patients with brain tumors usually evolve subacutely over weeks or months. A sudden onset of neurologic symptoms, followed by stability suggests cerebral infarction rather than brain tumor; a very slow onset over years suggests degenerative disease rather than brain tumor. More aggressive brain tumors, such as glioblastoma, metastases and primary CNS lymphoma, usually evolve rapidly over weeks, whereas lower-grade tumors, such as astrocytoma and oligodendroglioma, may evolve over months or a few years.

Neurologic examination

The general physical and neurologic examination is often not helpful, because many patients have no neurologic signs, and when signs are present they do not differ substantially from those of patients with cerebrovascular disease or other much more common neurologic disorders. Thus, unlike most neurologic disorders, the physician evaluating a patient with a possible intracranial tumor must depend on the laboratory, especially brain imaging.

Laboratory examination

By far the most important element in the evaluation of patients suspected of harboring an intracranial tumor is the magnetic resonance image (MRI). Often, MRI performed before and after the injection of contrast material (gadolinium) is the only laboratory test required prior to initiating therapy. At other times, more extensive evaluation is required, as indicated in the paragraphs below. With very few exceptions, a negative MRI in a patient suspected of harboring an intracranial mass lesion effectively excludes that diagnosis. This, of course, assumes that the scan is of high quality, that it has been read correctly and that it has been performed with injection of contrast. The clinician should review each MRI with the neuroradiologist, paying careful attention to the area, if any, of clinical interest suggested by the history or examination. Early in their course, tumors may be either missed or confused with ischemic changes, particularly in the elderly. We do not suggest that every patient with a headache receive an MRI[2] or that the history and physical findings not be meticulously reviewed before ordering an image, but we believe that, for most patients suspected of harboring an intracranial mass, MRI is the first and often the only step required for diagnosis.

This chapter considers symptoms, signs and laboratory tests necessary for the diagnosis of intracranial tumors. Specific laboratory tests necessary for the diagnosis of specific intracranial tumors are considered in the chapters on individual tumors.

Clinical findings

Introduction

Several factors determine the symptoms and signs in a patient with a CNS tumor (Table 3.1 and Fig. 3.1.)

Table 3.1
Factors determining symptoms and signs of CNS tumors.

- Location
  Supratentorial versus infratentorial
  Cortical versus subcortical
  Intraparenchymal versus extraparenchymal
  Eloquent versus non-eloquent
- Growth (histology)
  Rapid versus slow
  Infiltrative versus discrete
- Size
  Large versus small
- Secretions
  Angiogenic factors
  Pituitary hormones
  Immunosuppressive factors
  ?Melatonin
  Cytokines
  Neuropeptides

Figure 3.1
The impact of size, growth rate and location on clinical symptomatology. (a) The MR scan shows an enlarging right frontal tumor in 1995 (left) and 1999 (right) in a patient who had occasional focal seizures over 6 years characterized by sudden brief panic attacks. Despite the growth of the lesion, she has not had other neurologic symptoms and her clinical examination was normal. The diagnosis was oligodendroglioma. (b) The contrast-enhanced MRI of a 65-year-old man with progressive weakness of the left side over a 2-day period. A small enhancing tumor can be identified in the brainstem (arrow), probably a brainstem glioma. (c) The MRI of a 25-year-old woman with facial myokymia and slight facial weakness but no other neurologic symptomatology. A large mass infiltrated an enlarged pons, completely changing the signal in that structure without major neurologic symptoms. $\longrightarrow$

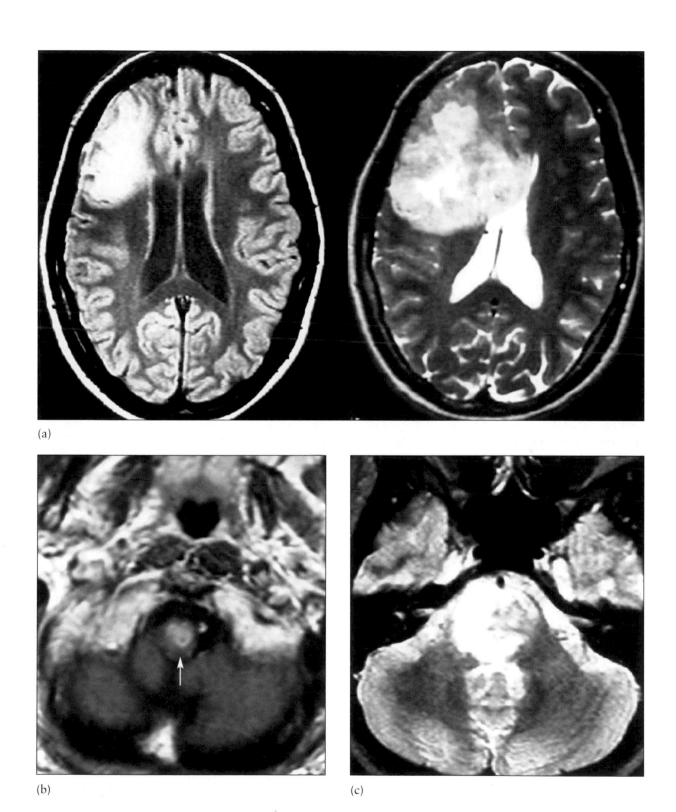

(a)

(b)

(c)

Location

A major factor determining symptomatology is brain location. Supratentorial tumors often present with seizures, whereas infratentorial tumors are more likely to cause headache and vomiting. Tumors involving the cortex (e.g. meningioma) are more likely to cause seizures as the only sign, whereas deep-lying tumors (e.g. lymphomas) are more likely to cause personality or cognitive changes. Tumors located in 'eloquent' areas (the term eloquent comes from the Latin for 'to speak' and is used by neurologists to indicate those vital cerebral structures necessary for language, e.g. Broca's and Wernicke's areas, or for movement or somatic sensory perception, e.g. sensorimotor cortex) usually present with either easily identifiable focal seizures or focal signs (e.g. speech arrest from frontal lobe tumors, hemiparesis from tumors involving the motor strip). Tumors in non-eloquent areas may present with what appear to be generalized seizures (actually seizures of focal origin in which the focal origin is unrecognized), or behavioral and cognitive changes. Tumors of the brainstem usually begin with cranial nerve palsies causing symptoms such as diplopia or facial weakness. Other posterior fossa or base of brain tumors often have headache as an early symptom, because they either involve pain-sensitive structures at the base of the brain, or cause early hydrocephalus (4th ventricular tumors). Infiltrating tumors are more likely to cause generalized symptoms of headache and personality change, whereas focal tumors are more likely to cause seizures, hemiparesis and other focal neurologic signs.

Growth rate

The growth rate of tumors also determines clinical findings. Slowly growing tumors (e.g. astrocytomas) usually present with seizures without other evidence of neurologic dysfunction, whereas rapidly growing tumors (e.g. glioblastomas) often present with focal neurologic signs, including paralysis and aphasia. Before modern imaging techniques, low-grade tumors often caused seizures for many years (20 years in one of our patients with an oligodendroglioma) before other symptoms developed.

Size

The size of the tumor also helps determine the neurologic symptoms. False localizing signs (see below) were first described in patients with meningiomas, where the large tumors in relatively silent areas caused major shifts of normal brain structures before the tumors were detected. Such false localizing signs are uncommon now, because other minor symptoms often lead to early neuroimaging and diagnosis.

Secretions

Intracranial tumors can cause symptoms not only by their size and location, but also by their secretions. Small tumors of the pituitary gland (Chapter 10) may secrete growth hormone and cause acromegaly associated with headache. Other tumors secrete prolactin, causing galactorrhea and amenorrhea in women or impotence in men. Adrenocorticotropic hormone (ACTH) secreting tumors cause Cushing's disease, also associated with behavioral change, usually depression. Larger tumors (macroadenomas) may cause pituitary failure with associated cognitive dysfunction. Pineal region tumors have been reported to interfere with normal melatonin secretion, leading to insomnia, sometimes with personality changes. Precocious puberty with behavioral changes may also complicate pineal region tumors (Chapter 8). Some tumors, e.g. high-grade gliomas and some meningiomas, secrete factors such as vascular endothelial growth factor (VEGF) and fibroblast growth factor (FGF) that cause angiogenesis and peritumoral edema (Chapter 2). The edema may cause more symptoms than the tumor itself. Some tumors secrete cytokines such as interleukins and tumor necrosis factor (TNF) and may alter brain neuropeptides,[3] which may affect cognitive function and behavior, e.g. anorexia.

Imaging

CT and MR imaging have substantially changed the symptoms at diagnosis of intracranial mass lesions. In the past, lesions often grew to considerable size and caused obvious signs and symptoms before the physician was willing to suggest such invasive and painful diagnostic tests as angiography or pneumoencephalography. Now patients present with more subtle symptoms that tax the clinical skills of the physician. The diagnosis of brain tumor is now often made long before intracranial pressure is substantially increased and sometimes made when the tumor is completely asymptomatic, the imaging having been procured for reasons unrelated to the tumor, such as minor head trauma or a syncopal attack. In one series of 1000 healthy, mostly young (average age 30), asymptomatic volunteers, 18% had some abnormal finding on MRI and 2 (0.2%) had a primary brain tumor.[4] The numbers would undoubtedly be greater if older volunteers were selected. Such 'unindicated' scans may reveal a tumor, leading to early diagnosis and treatment. However, all too often, they reveal a small meningioma that does not require treatment or show a structure misinterpreted as a tumor, e.g. a pineal cyst or enlarged Virchow–Robin space, leading to much patient anxiety.

Pathophysiology of symptoms and signs

CNS tumors cause neurologic symptoms by one or more of four mechanisms (Table 3.2, Fig. 3.2). These mechanisms include invasion, compression, CSF obstruction and herniation. Invasion and compression cause symptoms and signs suggestive of focal brain disease, i.e. signs referable to a particular region of the brain. CSF obstruction and herniation cause more generalized brain symptoms, such as diffuse headache and alterations of consciousness not ascribable to a specific brain area. When focal masses cause herniation, signs and symptoms may originate from portions of the brain distant from the tumor, so-called false localizing signs.

Invasion

The tumor invades and replaces or displaces normal brain. The underlying normal brain tissue may or may not be destroyed. Widespread brain invasion is particularly

Table 3.2
Pathophysiology of symptoms and signs of brain tumors.

Mechanism	Signs and symptoms	Example
Invasion	Focal	Hemiparesis, focal seizures
Compression	Focal	Hemiparesis
Cerebrospinal fluid obstruction	Generalized	Headache
Herniation	Generalized, false localizing	Confusion, stupor, abducens nerve paralysis

Figure 3.2
Pathophysiology of signs and symptoms in patients with brain tumors. This schematic coronal section of the brain enclosed in the skull illustrates the changes caused by a large brain tumor. The lesion itself (1) (green sphere) underlies the arm area of the motor strip and causes weakness of the contralateral arm. The edema (2) surrounding the mass involves most of the motor area and is likely to cause a contralateral hemiplegia. Because of the size of the brain tumor and the surrounding edema, the normal brain shifts, compressing itself and other normal brain areas. Herniation of the cingulate gyrus (3) under the falx cerebri compresses not only the contralateral frontal lobe but also the anterior cerebral arteries. Such herniation can cause bilateral frontal ischemia, with weak legs, urinary incontinence, and mental changes. The diencephalon (4) shifts toward the contralateral side, compressing itself, the third ventricle, and the opposite diencephalon. The resulting diencephalic dysfunction causes diminished consciousness. Herniation of the uncus and hippocampal gyrus (5) of the temporal lobe into the tentorial notch compresses the posterior cerebral artery, leading to infarction in the ipsilateral occipital lobe (Fig. 3.3). Uncal herniation also stretches the ipsilateral oculomotor nerve and compresses the brainstem and diencephalon, causing changes in the state of consciousness. Compression of the opposite cerebral peduncle (6) against the tentorium causes a hemiparesis that is ipsilateral to the side of the lesion (a false localizing sign). Downward displacement of the brainstem (7) alters consciousness and may cause

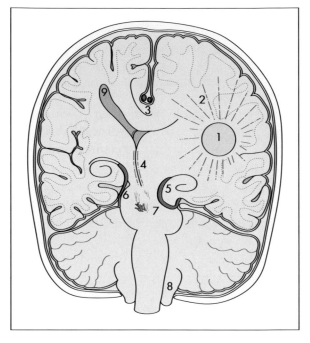

midbrain and pontine hemorrhages (Duret hemorrhages). Herniation of the cerebellar tonsils (8) through the foramen magnum compresses the lower brainstem and may cause respiratory arrest. Hydrocephalus (9) occurs in the contralateral lateral ventricle as a result of obstruction of the third ventricle and Sylvian aqueduct by compression. Any combination of the mechanisms illustrated in this figure may play a role in producing the symptoms caused by a brain tumor.

characteristic of infiltrating gliomas but sometimes occurs with meningiomas, pineal region tumors or metastases.

Compression

The tumor and surrounding edema compress normal tissue and its blood vessels, causing distortion and ischemia. Compression is a common mechanism in focal tumors such as meningiomas and metastases. Blood flow is reduced in peritumoral areas,[5] and capillaries may collapse, leading to brain ischemia.

Cerebrospinal fluid obstruction

The tumor obstructs cerebrospinal fluid (CSF) pathways, causing hydrocephalus. In some instances, the only symptoms of the tumor may be those of hydrocephalus. Examples include colloid cysts at the foramen of Monro, choroid plexus papillomas, intraventricular meningiomas, pineal region tumors, fourth ventricular ependymomas and occasionally intraspinal tumors.[6] In other instances, hydrocephalus may be a late complication of tumors that have caused preceding symptoms. These include large meningiomas at the base of the brain, intrinsic tumors of the hemisphere, such as glioblastomas and metastases, and brainstem gliomas.

Herniation

Large brain tumors with their peritumoral edema and sometimes hydrocephalus can herniate normal cerebral structures under the falx cerebri, through the tentorium cerebelli, or through the foramen magnum, often causing acute neurologic decompensation and at other times leading to false localizing signs (see below) (Fig. 3.3).

Symptoms and signs

As a result of these four mechanisms, neurologic symptoms and signs may be divided into one (or more) of three categories (Table 3.3). Patients may show: (1) generalized symptoms caused by raised intracranial pressure; (2) focal symptoms caused by invasion, ischemia and compression, or (3) false localizing symptoms caused by shifts of cerebral structures. Generalized or false localizing symptoms are particularly likely to be caused by slowly growing tumors that reach a large size in the relatively silent frontal lobe, whereas focal symptoms occur with even small tumors in more functionally important areas of the brain, such as the motor strip and brainstem.

Generalized symptoms and signs

Headache, the most common symptom of increased intracranial pressure, is the first symptom in about 30–40% of patients with a brain tumor.[7,8] Although headache may result from increased intracranial pressure, it occurs with almost equal frequency in patients without raised intracranial pressure. Conversely, many patients with elevated intracranial pressure, even to the point of

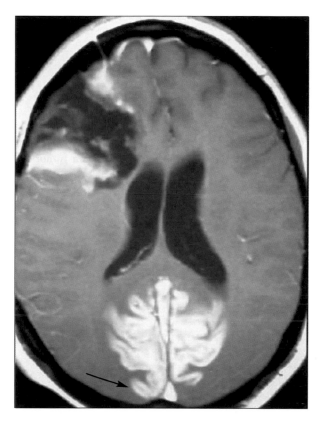

Figure 3.3
Cortical blindness caused by herniation. This 32-year-old woman was 9 months pregnant with a history of 6 weeks of progressive headache. An MR scan revealed a large right frontal tumor. She was admitted to the hospital for elective cesarean section and tumor removal. She became comatose shortly following admission, and an emergency cesarean section and craniotomy were performed. When she recovered from the surgery she was cortically blind. An MRI 2 weeks after the ictus revealed enhancing infarction in both occipital lobes (arrow) and the residual right frontal tumor. She eventually recovered macular vision, but peripheral fields remained abnormal and she had severe prosopagnosia.

developing papilledema, do not have headache. To cause headache, a tumor must stimulate pain-sensitive structures.[9] The brain itself is not pain sensitive. The dura over the cerebral convexity and the floor of the middle fossa are

Table 3.3
Some symptoms of signs of intracranial tumors.

Category	Symptoms	Signs
Generalized	Headache Vomiting Drowsiness Visual obscurations Personality change	Confusion Papilledema Apathy, abulia
Focal	Seizures Hemiparesis Paresthesias Cognitive changes Incoordination Diplopia Dysphagia	Postictal paralysis Focal weakness Sensory loss Aphasia, agnosia, ataxia Apraxia, ataxia Ocular muscle paralysis Aspiration
False localizing	Diplopia Tinnitus Visual loss	III, VI nerve paralysis Hearing loss Cortical blindness

also insensitive to pain, except immediately along or within a few millimeters of the meningeal arteries or dural sinuses. By contrast, the dura over the floor of the anterior fossa is sensitive over its entire surface. The superior surface of the tentorium, transverse and straight sinuses as well as the posterior portion of the superior and inferior sagittal sinuses are all pain sensitive, and like all of the supratentorial structures, are supplied by the first division of the trigeminal nerve, thus often referring the pain of a supratentorial brain tumor, no matter where above the tentorium it is located (e.g. occipital lobe), to the eye and frontal area of the head. Posterior fossa structures are supplied by lower cranial and upper cervical nerves, referring pain to the occipital area. The trigeminal nerve, in addition to being the sole source of supratentorial, dural and meningeal vessel sensory afferents, is also the source of sensory fibers to the vessels of the anterior circulation via the first or ophthalmic division of the trigeminal nerve. The common nerve supply to dura and vascular structures may explain the frequent similarity between brain tumor and migraine headaches.

Headache associated with brain tumor has several mechanisms: (1) traction on venous sinuses or their tributaries; (2) traction on meningeal arteries; (3) traction on large arteries at the base of the brain; (4) pressure on cranial and cervical pain-sensitive structures; (5) dilatation of intracranial arteries; and (6) inflammation of pain-sensitive structures. Interestingly, headache is more frequent in those patients with a prior history of non-tumoral headaches, suggesting an individual predilection for headache.

Most brain tumor headache is non-specific; however, a brain tumor should be suspected: (1) when mild to moderate headache is present on the patient's awakening from sleep but disappears within 1 h (severe headaches that awaken one from sleep are more probably due to non-tumoral causes); (2) when headaches begin in a middle-aged or older person who has not previously experienced them; (3) when the character or severity of headache in a chronic headache sufferer suddenly changes; (4) when a headache becomes progressively more severe over time (more often the result of brain edema rather than increasing tumor size[8]).

Localized headache is a reliable indicator of laterality but does not mark the precise location of the tumor. For example, a right frontal headache indicates that the tumor is on the right but does not indicate that the tumor is frontal; the tumor could be occipital or even cerebellar, the pain probably resulting from traction on the tentorium, the superior surface of which is supplied by the trigeminal nerve. Because intracranial tumors are progressive, headache is usually mild and intermittent at onset, and often relieved by over-the-counter analgesics. The headache becomes progressively more severe and more intractable as time passes. The headache can be either steady or throbbing, but is characteristically exacerbated by alterations of intracranial pressure, e.g. coughing, sneezing, bending, head-shaking or sexual activity. However, most cough or exertional headaches are not due to brain tumors.[10] Sudden short-lived episodic headaches may be associated with plateau waves in patients with raised intracranial pressure from a brain tumor (see below). As in patients with increased intracranial pressure from trauma, plateau waves are associated with acute vascular dilatation.

Because headache is such a common symptom and intracranial tumors are uncommon, even those headaches having the characteristics listed above are more likely to be caused by disorders other than brain tumors. Nevertheless, patients with these characteristics require careful evaluation. Most patients with headache due to brain tumors have other symptoms or neurologic signs suggesting brain tumor by the time they seek medical help.[11] Thus other symptoms, in particular, changes in memory, personality, behavior (see below) or language, should be carefully sought. A careful neurologic examination may reveal sensory or motor abnormalities unrecognized by the patient.

Vomiting with or without preceding nausea, particularly on awakening, and often described as 'explosive' or 'projectile', is a common symptom of brain tumor in children but is less common in adults. Vomiting with increased intracranial pressure is particularly frequent in children with medulloblastoma, ependymomas of the fourth ventricle and other posterior fossa tumors, probably because they directly compress the brainstem 'emetic center'. These tumors are common in children but rare in adults, explaining in part the high frequency of vomiting in children. However, that is not the entire explanation, because even with the same tumor, children are more likely to vomit than adults. Vomiting as an ictal event can occur in patients with tumors involving the insula (Latin for 'island'), an island of cortex deep within the Sylvian fissure.

Acute headache followed immediately by vomiting is characteristic of a brain tumor and indicates increased intracranial pressure; by contrast, a more prolonged headache followed several hours later by vomiting is characteristic of migraine. Vomiting in patients with brain tumors usually results from irritation of the vomiting center in the floor of the 4th ventricle. The emetic center can be activated either by increased intracranial pressure or by direct involvement by tumor. Accordingly, tumors of the posterior fossa and brainstem are most likely to cause vomiting, usually but not always preceded by headache. Vomiting in the absence of increased intracranial pressure has been reported in patients with brainstem tumors.[12]

Vertigo and dizziness. Vertigo occurs occasionally in patients with vestibular schwannomas (Chapter 9) because these tumors originate in the vestibular portion of the VIIIth cranial nerve. However, because the tumors grow so slowly, the vestibular system usually compensates, so that patients may have either no abnormal sensation or only a vague sensation of dizziness. Vertigo also accompanies tumors of the cerebellum and brainstem. In these cases, it is likely to be more severe and intractable. Many patients with brain tumors and increased intracranial pressure complain of a sensation of dizziness or light-headedness, possibly resulting from decreased blood flow to the brain causing mild brain hypoxia. The symptoms are non-specific. Patients who experience 'dizziness' may have a great deal of difficulty in precisely describing the sensation.

Papilledema occurs frequently in children and young adults but is less common in older patients and infants. (In older patients, brain atrophy gives a tumor more room to expand without raising intracranial pressure, and fibrosis of the optic nerve sheath may prevent pressure from being transmitted to the optic disk; in infants, the unfused skull bones can expand to accommodate the mass.) Papilledema itself is usually asymptomatic, often found by an ophthalmologist on a routine examination or when a patient complains of headache and consults an ophthalmologist for 'eye strain'. Papilledema always causes enlargement of the blind spot, because the optic disk produces the blind spot in the visual field, and when swollen the blind spot is enlarged; the patient is unaware of this change. In some patients, papilledema may cause constriction of the visual field or even loss of central vision. Many patients with pseudotumor cerebri (increased intracranial pressure without a tumor), but fewer patients with brain tumors (even with papilledema),

suffer significant visual abnormalities, including central scotomata.[13] More commonly in severe papilledema, there may be episodes of transient visual obscuration ranging from graying out of the visual field to complete blindness. These episodes are commonly associated with a plateau wave (see Chapter 2 and below). Visual obscurations associated with papilledema are not dangerous in themselves, as they do not presage a permanent visual abnormality.

Mental and cognitive abnormalities. Changes in mental and cognitive function are of two types. Specific cognitive abnormalities such as aphasia, alexia, agnosias and apraxias are a result of focal lesions in eloquent areas of brain. Less specific changes in behavior are often the presenting symptom of relatively large tumors in more silent areas of brain. These abnormalities vary from patient to patient, but often mislead the family and physician into believing the patient is suffering from a psychological rather than a neurologic disorder.

Non-specific mental changes begin with irritability and progress to apathy. Patients sleep longer at night, may fall asleep easily during the day, seem preoccupied when awake, and often fail to initiate activity, including conversation; however, if they are spoken to, they usually respond appropriately. In adults, psychiatric consultation for the treatment of what is thought to be depression is frequently obtained before a brain tumor is suspected. The astute psychiatrist will recognize the symptoms as being those of structural disease of the nervous system rather than depression. Although the patient usually first becomes irritable, in two of our patients with large, non-dominant frontal lobe tumors, the first alteration in behavior was a change from established irascibility to placidness. As their spouses put it, the patients suddenly 'became nice and easy to get along with'.

Episodic symptoms that include headache, visual loss, altered consciousness and sometimes transient weakness of the extremities are often precipitated by rising from a recumbent position, coughing, or sneezing. They are caused by plateau waves, abrupt increases in an already elevated intracranial pressure that last for 5–20 min (Table 3.4). Plateau waves are not seizures; they respond to

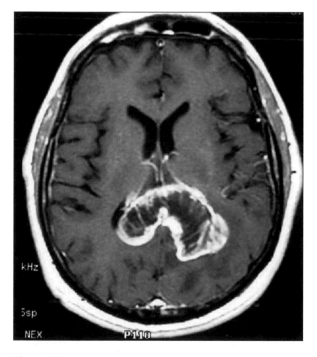

Figure 3.4
The MR of a patient with callosal amnesia. This man presented complaining of loss of recent memory. He had severe loss of recent memory but other cognitive functions were relatively intact and his segmental neurologic examination was entirely normal. The initial impression was that he was suffering from Alzheimer's disease, but an MR scan of the brain revealed a tumor that proved to be a glioblastoma.

Table 3.4
Paroxysmal symptoms from plateau waves in patients with intracranial space-occupying lesions.[14]

Impairment of consciousness
Trance-like state
Unreality/warmth
Confusion, disorientation
Restlessness, agitation
Disorganized motor activity
Sense of suffocation, air hunger
Cardiovascular/respiratory disturbances

Headache
Pain in the neck and shoulders
Nasal itch
Blurring of vision, amaurosis
Mydriasis, pupillary areflexia
Nystagmus
Oculomotor/abducens paresis
Conjugate deviation of the eyes
External ophthalmoplegia
Dysphagia, dysarthria
Nuchal rigidity
Retroflexion of the neck

Opisthotonus, trismus
Rigidity and tonic extension/flexion of the
    arms and legs
Bilateral extensor plantar responses
Sluggish/absent deep tendon reflexes

Generalized muscular weakness
Loss of muscle tone in the eyes
Facial twitching
Clonic movements of the arms and legs
Facial/limb paresthesias
Rise in temperature
Nausea, vomiting
Facial flushing
Pallor, cyanosis
Sweating
Shivering and 'goose flesh'
Thirst
Salivation
Yawning, hiccoughing
Urinary and fecal urgency/incontinence

Bold text indicates the more common symptoms

corticosteroids or a decrease in the intracranial pressure but do not respond to anticonvulsant therapy.

Focal symptoms and signs

Seizures are the most common focal sign of a brain tumor.[1] They affect at least 1/3 of brain tumor patients and are often the first and only symptom. They are more common in patients with low-grade gliomas than those with high-grade tumors.[15] Focal seizures are particularly common in patients who have tumors, such as meningiomas, that compress the cortex or arise in or near the motor strip or the temporal lobe. Focal seizures caused by frontal or temporal foci often cause episodic behavioral or emotional symptoms that are sometimes confused with panic attacks or psychological disorders. Episodic symptoms such as a hemiparesis or aphasia without clear seizure activity can last for hours to days, and then resolve. These episodes may respond to anticonvulsants. Generalized convulsions, without the patient experiencing an aura (Latin for 'breeze' – denoting the focal onset of a seizure as recognized by the patient), when caused by brain tumors, are not truly generalized at onset, but represent a focal seizure, arising from an asymptomatic focal discharge and then secondarily generalizing; the focal signature is not apparent either to the patient or an observer. Depending on the growth rate of the tumor, seizures may be present for months to years before other symptoms develop. Any patient with focal or generalized seizures that begin in adulthood should undergo diagnostic evaluation for a brain tumor (see below). However, only a minority of patients with adult-onset seizures have brain tumor as the cause. The figures vary from 2%–22% depending on the series.[16] The higher figures are probably the more accurate.

Other focal symptoms and signs of a brain tumor depend on the site of the lesion. These focal symptoms and signs are the same as those of CNS infection, stroke or other structural diseases of the brain. Table 3.5 lists some focal symptoms and signs of intracranial tumors in relation to their location.

Signs such as contralateral hemiparesis with basal ganglia or motor cortex tumors or ataxia and nystagmus with cerebellar tumors are obvious. A few other less obvious signs deserve comment. Tumors that arise posterior to the motor strip in the parietal and posterior temporal lobe may present with focal cognitive and behavioral changes that confuse both the patient and the physician. We have encountered several patients whose first symptom of a non-dominant parietal lobe lesion was dressing apraxia. The patients noticed that it took longer to get dressed because the visual–spatial relationship between the clothing and the patient's body seemed unclear. The family often noticed that the patient would wear clothes inside out or backwards.

A second perplexing problem is that of a visual field defect from an occipital tumor. The patient is usually unaware of the loss of peripheral vision but he or she suffers several minor car accidents, usually damaging the same side of the car in each accident. If the visual field defect is non-dominant, the patient may also complain of difficulty in reading, because as his eyes return to the beginning of the next line, he loses his place. With dominant visual field defects (right side), there is less difficulty in reading unless the lesion involves more anterior association areas, in which case the patient may develop alexia with or without agraphia.

Lesions of the posterior corpus callosum (splenium), probably due to invasion of hippocampal structures lying immediately below them, often present with memory loss[18] in the absence of other cognitive abnormalities.

Table 3.5
Focal symptoms and signs of intracranial tumors.

Frontal lobe
 Generalized seizures
 Focal motor seizures (contralateral)
 Expressive aphasia (dominant side)
 Behavioral changes
 Dementia
 Gait disorders, incontinence
 Hemiparesis

Basal ganglia
 Hemiparesis (contralateral)
 Movement disorders (rare)

Parietal lobe
 Receptive aphasia (dominant side)
 Spatial disorientation (non-dominant side)
 Cortical sensory dysfunction (contralateral)
 Agnosias

Occipital lobe
 Hemianopsia (contralateral)
 Visual disturbances (unformed)

Temporal lobe
 Complex partial (psychomotor) seizures
 Generalized seizures
 Behavioral changes
 Olfactory and complex seizures
 Visual auras
 Visual field defect

Corpus callosum
 Dementia (anterior)
 Behavioral changes
 Memory loss (posterior)
 Asymptomatic (mid)

Thalamus
 Sensory loss (contralateral)
 Behavioral changes (posterior)
 Language disorder (dominant side)

Midbrain/pineal
 Paresis of vertical eye movements
 Pupillary abnormalities
 Precocious puberty (boys)

Sella/optic nerve/pituitary
 Endocrinopathy
 Bitemporal hemianopia
 Monocular visual defects
 Ophthalmoplegia (cavernous sinus)

Pons/medulla
 Cranial nerve dysfunction
 Ataxia, nystagmus
 Weakness, sensory loss
 Spasticity

Cerebello-pontine angle
 Deafness (ipsilateral)
 Loss of facial sensation (ipsilateral)
 Facial weakness (ipsilateral)
 Ataxia

Cerebellum
 Ataxia (ipsilateral)
 Nystagmus

Modified from Vick.[17]

One of our patients with a lymphoma involving the posterior corpus callosum was unaware of the day, month, or year, but was able to determine the season by noting that he was wearing a summer-weight suit.

Truncal ataxia, sparing the limbs, is a common finding in lesions of the cerebellar vermis. Characteristically, the patient complains of ataxia and is found to be ataxic when walking, but point-to-point tests of both upper and lower extremities are performed well, sometimes leading the physician to believe that the ataxic gait is 'hysterical'. Hydrocephalus can cause gait abnormalities,

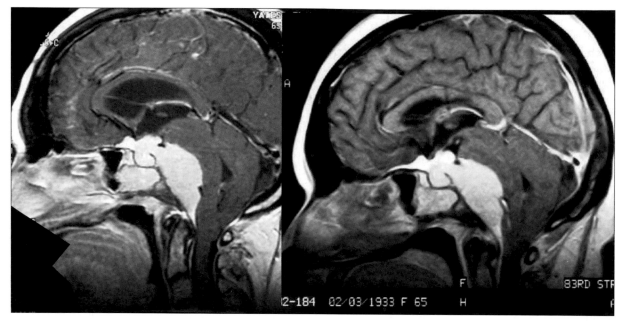

Figure 3.5
A patient with a large base of skull meningioma and secondary hydrocephalus. She presented with gait instability and ataxia, which were first believed to be secondary to compression of the brainstem by the tumor. However, despite the large tumor, the entire ventricular system was open, and communicating hydrocephalus (left) was evident. A ventriculoperitoneal shunt relieved her symptoms and the hydrocephalus (right). Note the decreased ventricular size after surgery. The tumor did not change in size.

so-called 'frontal ataxia', sometimes mistaken for cerebellar dysfunction (Fig. 3.5).[19]

As indicated above, prolonged episodic symptoms of a behavioral and cognitive nature may be the presenting complaint of a brain tumor. One of our patients suffering a dominant parietal lobe glioblastoma suddenly became unable to decide how to turn off the bath water that he had turned on a few minutes before. He then attempted to call his daughter, and although he remembered the phone number, could not dial it. There was no weakness, sensory loss, or other form of confusion. He eventually dialed the number. By the time he got to the emergency room, his neurologic examination was entirely normal.

On a few occasions, episodic transient global amnesia has been the presenting event of a brain tumor.[20] Most patients who have transient global amnesia caused by a brain tumor have some persistent abnormality of memory on careful neurologic evaluation.

False localizing symptoms and signs

False localizing symptoms and signs are caused by shifts of cerebral structures. Diplopia may result from displacement or compression of the abducens nerve at the base of the brain. Hemianopsia or even cortical blindness may be caused by tentorial herniation that compresses the posterior cerebral artery. A number of other cranial nerve palsies associated with shifts of brainstem structures may also occur. Table 3.6 lists some false localizing signs associated with brain tumors.

Most false localizing signs occur in patients with large, slowly growing brain tumors, e.g. meningiomas, but they have been reported in other situations as well. A few deserve comment.

Tinnitus, with or without hearing loss, is a common complaint in patients suffering increased intracranial pressure of any cause. At least one form of tinnitus appears to be due to turbulent flow through the transverse sinuses, which pass near the middle ear. The noise is heard as a 'venous hum'.[21] Increasing cerebral venous pressure, either by a Valsalva maneuver or by gently compressing the jugular vein in the neck, will often alter the tinnitus or make it disappear. In other patients, tumor compression of the acoustic nerve leads to hearing loss and more high-pitched tinnitus.

Diplopia. Increased intracranial pressure leads to compression of the abducens nerve, the cranial nerve that runs the longest intracranial course, causing horizontal diplopia on lateral gaze. The patient may complain only of diplopia when he looks into the distance and not notice it for near vision, when the abducens nerve is at rest. Abducens paralysis may be unilateral or bilateral. Less common, but more ominous, is involvement of the ipsilateral third nerve, compressed by the hippocampal gyrus as it herniates through the tentorium cerebelli (uncal herniation) (see Fig. 3.2). The first sign is ipsilateral pupillary dilatation followed by vertical and horizontal diplopia and sometimes ptosis. The patient may be fully conscious when the third nerve symptoms begin.

Ipsilateral hemiparesis. Unlike the contralateral hemiparesis that usually accompanies a supratentorial mass lesion, ipsilateral hemiparesis occurs when a supratentorial mass lesion

Table 3.6
Some false localizing signs associated with brain tumors.

Cranial nerves
    Anosmia
    Diplopia, ptosis, anisocoria
    Face pain, numbness, and weakness
    Tinnitus, hearing loss
 	
Parenchymal signs
    Ipsilateral hemiparesis
    Ipsilateral gaze palsy
    Visual field defect, cortical blindness
    Ataxia
 	
Other signs
    Nuchal rigidity

(usually extracranial, such as a meningioma) shifts the brainstem laterally, compressing the contralateral cerebral peduncle against the tentorium cerebelli (Kernohan's notch). The patient may have either ipsilateral hemiparesis only or bilateral hemiparesis.

Anosmia resulting from compression of the olfactory nerves by the overlying frontal lobe is a common false localizing sign, but is rarely noted by the patient or identified or tested for by the physician.

Cortical blindness and prosopagnosia. Cortical blindness (Fig. 3.3) results from compression of posterior cerebral arteries, a result of herniation of the bilateral hippocampus gyri through the tentorial notch. One of our patients with a large frontal oligodendroglioma herniated just prior to surgery and awoke cortically blind. Because the middle cerebral artery supplies macular vision, that vision returned, leaving her with a small area of central vision. Involvement of nearby association areas led to some memory loss and prosopagnosia (from Greek prosopon 'face' and gnosis 'recognition') so profound that she was unable to recognize her husband's face or her own face in the mirror. When looking into a mirror, she would protrude her tongue to be sure the image was hers.

Radicular pain can be a false localizing sign of increased intracranial pressure.[22]

Laboratory diagnosis

Imaging

All adults with new-onset seizures and all patients with papilledema or new focal motor or sensory signs require an MRI[23,24] with the injection of contrast material (gadolinium DPTA). Other presenting symptoms listed in Table 3.7 and discussed above should also prompt consideration of imaging. Once a tumor is identified, other imaging techniques, such as diffusion tensor MRI (to identify distortion of white matter near a tumor that appears normal on routine MRI[25,26]), positron emission tomography (PET) to measure glucose metabolism or amino acid uptake in the tumor, single photon emission computed tomography (SPECT),[24] magnetic resonance spectroscopy (MRS),[26,27] and functional MRI (fMRI),[24] may each prove useful in ascertaining histologic grade and in guiding surgical procedures.

MRI

MRI visualizes the entire intracranial contents clearly, unlike CT scans, where bone and teeth can obscure lesions, particularly in the posterior fossa and middle cranial fossa. A negative MRI almost always excludes a tumor as the cause of the patient's symptoms or signs. However, we had one patient who presented with confusion and whose MRI including a T2-weighted image was normal. As his symptoms progressed over the next month, a repeat MRI was obtained and a large enhancing glioblastoma was seen in the right temporal lobe.

MRI identifies tumors that CT misses, particularly in the posterior fossa, and distinguishes tumors from arteriovenous malformations. MRI often gives signal characteristics that suggest the histology (Table 3.7).[23] Except for biopsy (see below), other laboratory tests are usually unnecessary. MR scans can be performed relatively easily and repeatedly in most patients. Even in patients who are somewhat confused and therefore restless, 'fast' scans often suffice to give information that may not be easily detected on a CT scan. About 30% of patients are uncomfortable in the scanner because of claustrophobia. Most tolerate the procedure with encouragement from the technician or a companion sitting in the room with them. About 5–10% of patients require sedation. We use lorazepam 1–2 mg prior to the scan. Probably fewer than 1% of patients cannot tolerate the scan even with sedation. A cardiac pacemaker is an absolute contraindication, as are ferromagnetic foreign bodies (e.g. shrapnel) in the patient. For the claustrophobic patient who cannot tolerate a standard scan, imaging in an open scanner, although yielding an inferior scan, is preferable to CT.

Certain signal characteristics suggest a brain tumor (Table 3.7). The increased water content of brain tumors and their surrounding edema yield a hypointense (darker than normal brain) T1 image and a hyperintense (lighter than normal brain) T2 image. T1 and T2 refer to the proton relaxation time for the acquisition of MRI data. Disruption of the blood–brain barrier characteristically occurs in certain brain tumors (Chapter 2). A contrast agent (e.g. gadolinium) leaks across and enters the brain tumor's extracellular space, causing hyperintensity (enhancement) on T1 images.

Table 3.7
Imaging appearance of brain tumors.

	CT (MR)*		MR
	Non-Contrast (T1)	*Contrast (T1)*	*T2*
Malignant glioma	↓ Density	Irregular peripheral enhancement	↑
Low-grade astrocytoma	↓ Density	± enhances	↑
Oligodendroglioma	↓ to iso, ↑Ca²⁺ in 91% with blood	< 50% + enhances	↓↑ Heterogeneous if bleed
Lymphoma	↑ Density	Solid portion enhances	↑
Ganglioglioma	↓ Density, 33% Ca²⁺	50% enhances	↑
Ependymoma	↓ Density, Ca²⁺ > 50%	Irregular, enhances (often peripheral)	↑
PNET	Iso to ↑ density	Enhances	Mixed
Choroid plexus papilloma	Iso and Ca²⁺	+	Mixed
Choroid plexus carcinoma	Iso and Ca²⁺	+	Mixed
Germinoma	Iso to ↑	+	Iso to ↓
Embryonal carcinoma	Iso to ↑	+	↓
Teratoma	Mixed density	±	Mixed
Hemangioblastoma	↓	+	↑
Brainstem glioma	↓	±	↑
Cerebellar astrocytomas	↓	+ Largely cystic	↑
Meningioma	Iso to ↑	+	Iso to ↓
Schwannoma	↓ to iso	+	Iso to ↑
Metastases	↑ to ↓	+	Variable ↑ to ↓
CSF disseminated tumor	↓	+	Iso
Neurocytoma	Mixed cystic, Ca²⁺ 60%	+	Cystic inhomogeneous
Hemangiopericytoma	↑ or ↓	+	↑

*CT and T1-weighted MRI show similar changes
Modified from Zimmerman.[29]

Hemorrhages are best identified on gradient echo MRI.[30] They usually appear as hyperintense on non-contrast T1 images and hypointense on T2. However, these radiographic features vary depending on the age of the hemorrhage. Acute hemorrhage can be detected on MRI within 2 h.[31] In general, hemorrhage demonstrates low intensity to isointensity on T1 and low intensity on T2 during the first 3 days. The T1 image becomes hyperintense after about 3 days and may remain so for weeks to months. The T2 image becomes hyperintense, sometimes with a rim of low intensity after about a week and develops uniformly low intensity after months. Enhancement is absent acutely but the hemorrhage may develop a rim of enhancement after about a week. Earlier enhancement suggests hemorrhage into a pre-existing tumor.

Hemorrhage is hyperdense on CT scan. Calcifications are difficult to identify on MR, but are easily seen on CT scan as more dense than hemorrhage. On CT scan, calcification is a positive prognostic factor,[32] and enhancement a negative factor within each histologic grade of glioma.

Although both brain edema and the tumor appear hyperintense on T2, edema is usually more hyperintense (i.e. appears whiter). Sometimes, tumor and edema can be distinguished by the fact that edema spares the cortex, producing finger-like projections of T2 hyperintensity between normal-appearing cortical gyri. By contrast, infiltrating tumor involves the cortex, changing the cortical signal and often expanding gyri. Infiltrating tumor may have the appearance of a well-defined border on T2 MRI images, whereas edema typically has blurred and indistinct radiographic borders.

In low-grade gliomas, edema is often absent and there is usually no contrast enhancement. High-grade gliomas usually exhibit contrast enhancement on the T1-weighted image, showing an enhanced rim of irregular shape and thickness that surrounds a hypointense center; the T2 image shows only hyperintensity. Although the contrast enhancement does not encompass the entire infiltrating margin, it represents a clinically useful approximation of tumor volume. Fast fluid-attenuated inversion recovery (FLAIR) sequences provide prominent distinction between normal brain and brain tumor or edema and give high tumor-to-background contrast ratios;[33] however, tumor cannot be differentiated from edema on FLAIR images. Metastases have a regular and spherical rim because they grow by expansion and compression of adjacent brain tissue rather than by invasion and infiltration as gliomas do. Metastases are much more likely than gliomas to be multiple; 50% of patients with metastases

have multiple lesions, whereas only 5% of patients with gliomas have multifocal disease. Of patients with primary CNS lymphoma (PCNSL), 20–40% have multiple lesions that are located periventricularly, usually exhibit diffuse contrast enhancement, have poorly circumscribed margins compared with gliomas and metastases, and are usually surrounded by less edema than these other tumors. On T2, PCNSL has relatively low signal intensity compared with the high signal intensity of the surrounding edema. The MR scans of immunocompromised patients with PCNSL may not demonstrate enhancement or may show ring enhancement. Cortical and basal ganglia involvement is more common in these patients.

A separate technique, diffusion-weighted MR imaging, permits assessment of the mobility of water molecules, and may distinguish among: (1) ischemia; (2) cytotoxic edema within parts of the tumor; (3) radiation-induced gliosis; (4) vasogenic edema. However, the differences are relatively slight and have not been very clinically useful to date. Perfusion images measured during the first pass of contrast through the brain reflect blood volume and, thus, vascularity. The relative cerebral blood volume measured by the perfusion scan is a good indicator of tumor grade and correlates strongly with PET F[18]-deoxyglucose studies (see next section) of tumor grade.[34]

Serial MR scans can also be used to determine the effectiveness of treatment. The efficacy of treatment with radiation or chemotherapy is generally divided into four categories: a complete response (CR) indicates disappearance of the tumor; a partial response (PR) indicates a decrease in the size of the contrast-enhancing tumor to 50% or less of its former size; stable disease (SD) indicates no decrease, but also no increase, in the tumor size; and progressive disease (PD) indicates growth of the tumor. Some investigators include the term minor response (MR) to indicate tumor shrinkage by more than 25% but less than 50%. Although extremely useful in large series, these criteria are less useful in an individual patient. Because the patient's head is not fixed in the scanner, the orientation differs from one scan to the next, making exact measurements difficult. Furthermore, patients are often scanned on different machines using different computer settings and at different time intervals after contrast injection. Finally, unless quantitative measurements are made in all three dimensions and a volume calculated, differences of as much as 20% between scans may be missed. Even with quantitative measurements, 10% differences cannot be easily detected. The 50% difference required of a PR, however, is usually easily detectable.

Positron emission tomography (PET)

This procedure is performed by injecting substances such as glucose, an amino acid, or even a nucleotide labeled with a positron-emitting isotope (Fig. 3.6). These substances are taken up by cells and metabolized through normal biochemical pathways. Positron-emitting isotopes include O^{15}, C^{11}, N^{13}, and F^{18}. These isotopes have short half-lives of minutes to hours and disintegrate by emitting a positron, a positively charged electron, from the nucleus of the atom. The positron travels a very short distance before it encounters an electron. The two annihilate each other and convert a small amount of mass into a pair of photons that travel in opposite directions. The photons are recorded when they strike a crystal detection system (with a large circular array)

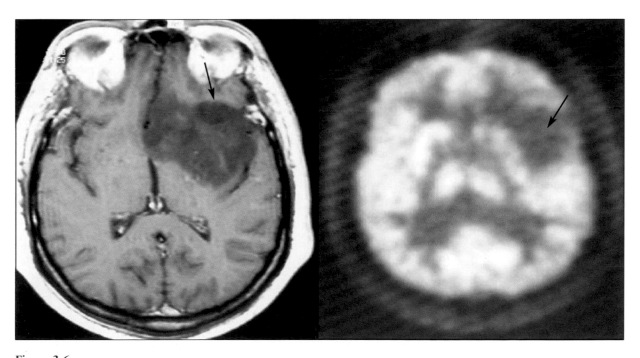

Figure 3.6
Comparison of MR and PET scan in a patient with a low-grade glioma. The MR scan (left) shows a lesion hypointense on the T1-weighted image (arrow). A coregistered PET scan reveals that the lesion is hypometabolic (arrow). A biopsy revealed a low-grade tumor.

and their location is identified by simultaneous detection electronics built into the tomograph. The number of reconstructed images reflects the emissions detected, which are proportional to the amount of isotope found in a particular volume of tumor or brain. If the arterial concentration of F18-deoxyglucose (FDG) radioactivity is measured to correct for isotope in the vascular compartment, the absolute metabolic rate of glucose utilization in specific brain tumor regions can be calculated. At present, FDG is the most common isotopically labeled compound used for evaluating brain tumors,[35] although C11-methionine can also be used, as can other amino acids.[36,37] The differential accumulation of a positron-emitting metabolite in normal brain compared with brain tumor tissue can provide information about the grade of the tumor.[38] For example, FDG imaging from glucose roughly defines the metabolic rate of the area being examined. Hypermetabolism (high FDG uptake) is common in high-grade tumors, and hypometabolism (low FDG uptake) is seen in low-grade tumors. Amino acid uptake is increased in high-grade tumors as well. The injection of nucleotides, such as iododeoxyuridine (IUDR), may help define DNA metabolism and thus the proportion of tumor cells progressing through the cell cycle.

PET scans are performed with FDG in some patients with putative low-grade diffuse astrocytomas prior to biopsy.[39] In a patient with a non-enhancing lesion who suffers only seizures controllable by anticonvulsants and has no other neurologic symptoms or signs, if the PET scan is hypometabolic (e.g. glucose metabolism less than normal white matter) we may elect to follow that patient clinically rather than biopsy or treat (Chapter 5). If an FDG PET scan that is generally hypometabolic shows an area of hypermetabolism, the neurosurgeon can direct the stereotactic needle biopsy to that area because treatment is determined by the highest grade in a heterogeneous tumor.

FDG PET scans are also useful, after radiation therapy, in helping to distinguish radiation necrosis from recurrent tumor. Both may appear similar on MRI, but radiation necrosis is usually hypometabolic and recurrent tumor is usually normometabolic or hypermetabolic. Unfortunately, this test is not completely reliable. Necrotic areas within recurrent tumor may result in a hypometabolic image and inflammation associated with radiation necrosis may result in a hypermetabolic image. Some reports suggest that FDG PET may predict the tumor response to irradiation or chemotherapy. Acute increases in glucose metabolism were associated with response to radiosurgery.[40]

Single photon emission spectroscopy (SPECT)

This procedure is less technically demanding, and is sometimes used to define blood flow and blood volume of tumors when compared with normal tissue. This method uses gamma cameras and computers. SPECT is widely available, whereas PET has limited availability. SPECT generally provides information similar to PET and has been called 'the poor man's PET scan'. The most commonly used agent is technetium-99m-labeled hexamethylpropyleneamine oxime (HMPAO), which is lipophilic and crosses the blood–brain barrier in proportion to blood flow. This agent identifies high-grade tumors by their increased blood volume due to extensive neovascularity. No increased uptake of technetium-99m-labeled-HMPAO is observed in low-grade, infiltrating tumors. One recent report,[41] using dual isotope SPECT with thallium-201 ion and technetium-99m-labeled HMPAO, accurately predicted histopathologic findings and survival after re-resection in patients treated with radiotherapy for glioblastoma. Thallium-201, a potassium analog, does not cross the intact blood–brain barrier but does cross an impaired blood–brain barrier, where it is taken up in proportion to the activity of the sodium–potassium ATP pump. Thus, necrotic tissue, which has a disrupted barrier, but does not take up much thallium, can be distinguished from viable contrast-enhancing tumor tissue. If the thallium uptake is more than 3½ times that of the scalp it suggests tumor recurrence, whereas if it is less than 2 times the scalp uptake, it represents necrosis. The technique has proved useful in differentiating radiation necrosis from recurrent tumor in patients who have been previously treated. It is also useful for following pediatric brain tumors after treatment.[42] Thallium can differentiate toxoplasmosis infection from tumor in patients with AIDS. Toxoplasmosis is largely necrotic and has a low thallium uptake, whereas tumor, usually a lymphoma or glioma, has a higher uptake. A recent report suggests that methyltyrosine SPECT is superior to glucose PET in grading tumor recurrence in patients treated for glioma[43,44] Technetium-99m-labeled sestamibi has been reported to detect recurrent tumor after radiation therapy.[45] Sestamibi imaging can also identify activity of the MDR gene and P-glycoprotein.[46]

Magnetic resonance spectroscopy (MRS)
This procedure is performed in a fashion similar to a standard MRI except that biochemical spectra from areas of interest are measured (Fig. 3.7). The major spectra assayed by proton MRS are N-acetyl aspartate (NAA), phosphocreatine, creatine, choline-containing compounds, myoinositol, several amino acids, including gamma-aminobutyric acid, lipids, lactate and glucose. NAA is a marker of neuronal and axonal density. Its presence is decreased with neuronal loss from tumor, ischemia, necrosis, infection and other processes that damage neurons. Creatine and phosphocreatine are markers of energy-depen-

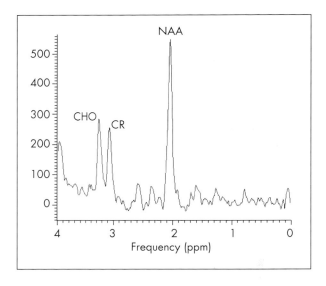

Figure 3.7
Magnetic resonance spectroscopy of normal brain. The choline (CHO) and creatine (CR) peaks are substantially the same size. The largest peak is made by N-acetyl aspartate (NAA), a component of normal neurons.

dent systems and choline marks cell membrane turnover. Choline levels are elevated with increased cell turnover. Lactate marks anaerobic metabolism and is never measurable in normal brain. Lipids may accumulate in areas of necrosis. The pattern of chemicals can help distinguish the grade of glioma, and sometimes the histologic type of glioma, and distinguish tumors from infections and demyelinating lesions.[47] However, these data are preliminary and the technique should still be considered experimental.

Current evidence suggests that NAA and gamma-aminobutyric acid are decreased in brain tumors, whereas choline is increased and lactate levels correlate with histologic grade (Fig. 3.8). Brain abscesses generally show absent creatine, choline and NAA with a large

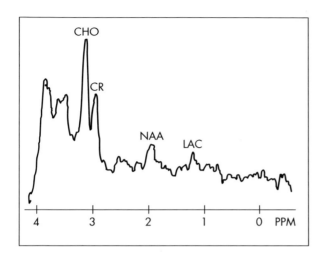

Figure 3.8
Magnetic resonance spectrogram of a high-grade glioma. Note that the choline peak (CHO) is higher than the creatinine peak (CR) and substantially higher than the N-acetyl aspartate (NAA) peak. NAA represents neurons and axons. The low peak indicates replacement of these structures by tumor. Lactate (LAC), not identifiable in normal brain, is also present, suggesting anaerobic metabolism.

lactate peak; amino acids are also elevated in an abscess. Demyelinating disorders are marked by normal or decreased NAA and increased choline. Meningiomas have no creatine and no NAA but show an increased choline and increased alanine peak.

Phosphorus MRS allows the measurement of varied phosphate-containing compounds, including phosphodiesters, phosphomono-esters, phosphocreatine, ATP, ADP and inorganic phosphate. Phosphorus MRS has been studied less, and its role in identifying brain tumors is uncertain. Preliminary evidence suggests that the phosphocreatine/inorganic phosphate ratio is reduced because the pH of brain tumors is alkaline, a counterintuitive observation.

Functional MRI (fMRI)

Areas of brain function can be identified. The fMRI technique takes advantage of the fact that when an area of the brain is activated, blood flow increases, and therefore proportionate oxygen extraction decreases in the activated region. The change in oxyhemoglobin to deoxyhemoglobin ratio results in an increased signal intensity on the MR scan.[48] This change can be imaged on a standard MRI without using contrast, although greater sensitivity is achieved by scanners with echoplanar capability. The technique is particularly useful for identifying language and motor areas. fMRI is clinically useful for presurgical planning, allowing the surgeon to maximally resect a tumor while avoiding areas that perform critical neurologic functions (Fig. 4.2).

Biopsy

Although MRI may suggest the histologic diagnosis (for example most low-grade tumors do not contrast enhance, whereas most high-grade tumors do), only biopsy is definitive.[49] An exception to this rule occurs in primary CNS lymphoma, in which lumbar puncture or, if the eyes are involved, vitrectomy, may yield malignant cells, obviating the necessity for brain biopsy (Chapter 11). In other tumors, lumbar puncture poses a risk of cerebral herniation and rarely contributes to diagnosis. Stereotactic (from the Greek word stereo for 'three dimensions' and the Latin term tactic for 'touch') needle biopsy is a technique used to obtain tissue in patients whose tumor location, extent or multiplicity precludes craniotomy and operative removal. The procedure can be done either under local or general anesthesia. The technique is usually performed by bolting a frame to the patient's head under local anesthesia and performing a CT or MR scan to localize the lesion. The frame defines the coordinates. Recently, frameless systems have become available which provide the same localizing information without requiring a frame to be secured to the skull. The needle is passed through a burr-hole to the appropriate spot and a core of tissue is removed. Several passes with the needle may be necessary to procure sufficient tissue to establish a diagnosis.[50] In experienced hands (both the surgeon and the neuropathologist), a diagnosis can be established in over 90% of patients (Fig. 3.9). Molecular genetic analysis can be performed on most samples,[51] although sampling error is a potential problem.

Stereotactic needle biopsy can cause problems. Although it is easily performed, the small sample retrieved may make it difficult for the neuropathologist to establish a diagnosis. Even when the pathologist can establish a diagnosis, he may not be able to accurately grade the tumor. The neurosurgeon performing a stereotactic needle biopsy should direct the needle to what appears to be the highest grade of the tumor. This can be established either by areas of contrast enhancement on the MR scan, or by areas of hypermetabolism on the PET scan.

Stereotactic needle biopsy can also cause two major complications. The first is bleeding. Although the overall rate of symptomatic bleeding in patients who undergo stereotactic needle biopsy is about 1%, the rate is substantially higher in patients with diffuse astrocytoma, particularly those with high-grade lesions. In one study, as many as 6% of patients with glioblastoma multiforme bled after stereotactic needle biopsy.[52] Complications are fewer in lower-grade tumors, but still greater than 1%. Asymptomatic small hemorrhages identified on post-biopsy scan may affect as many as 60% of patients.[53] In patients with AIDS, post-biopsy mortality (30 days) was 2.9% and morbidity was 8.4%.[54]

The second complication is that of neurologic worsening without bleeding. There is little in the literature on this complication, but we have found a significant number of patients (particularly those with widespread and diffuse tumors) whose neurologic condition worsens substantially after stereotactic needle biopsy in the absence of hemorrhage. Most recover over several days to a few weeks, but some do not. The neurologic worsening is of two types. One is an increase in focal signs (e.g. hemiparesis). The second is an alteration of mental status without focal signs. Some of our patients who demonstrate memory loss or personality change may, following a stereotactic needle biopsy, become and remain lethargic or confused without making a substantial recovery.

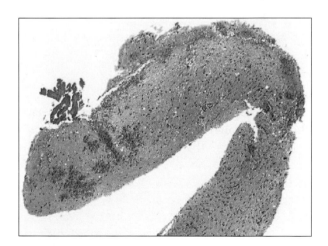

Figure 3.9
Stereotactic needle biopsy of a patient with a progressive hemiparesis. The tissue core obtained revealed increased cellularity with atypical cells, suggesting astrocytoma.

Differential diagnosis

Table 3.8 lists some lesions that must be considered in the differential diagnosis of intracranial lesions.

Three main non-neoplastic lesions should be considered in the differential diagnosis. The first is ischemic infarction. Older patients with intracranial tumors often present with transient symptoms presumably due to seizures. Unlike the short-lived focal seizures occurring with other epileptogenic lesions, these episodes may last many minutes to hours, are often associated with abnormalities of cognition and behavior, and typically cause 'negative' signs, e.g. hemiparesis, but not typical tonic–clonic seizure activity. Because of their length, they may be confused with transient ischemic attacks or even small resolving cerebral infarcts. A CT scan without contrast may show an area of hypodensity that is interpreted as cerebral infarction. However, CT hypodensity associated with intrinsic brain tumors is usually restricted to white matter and does not involve cortex. On the contrary, cerebral infarction is generally triangular-shaped with the base at the cortical surface. A contrast-enhanced MR scan often, but not always, establishes the diagnosis. Hyperintensity on a diffusion-weighted MRI is characteristic of acute ischemia, but we

Table 3.8
Differential diagnosis of brain tumors.[17]

- Hematoma
- Abscess[55]
- Granuloma
- Parasitic infections, e.g. Cysticercosis, histoplasmosis
- Vascular malformations
- Multiple sclerosis
- Cerebral infarcts

have often encountered a similar finding in brain tumors. Subacute infarcts that prominently enhance can also be difficult to differentiate from a tumor. Often, the clinical history, pattern of enhancement (i.e. ribbon-like following cortical gyri) and surrounding edema (little in subacute infarct, much in brain tumor) help clarify the diagnosis.

A second important distinction occurs in patients with large contrast-enhancing lesions caused by demyelinating disease that have the appearance of a high-grade diffuse astrocytoma. One distinction between demyelinating lesions and glioblastoma is that the contrast-enhancing ring is usually incomplete in demyelinating disease but complete in glioblastoma.[56] However, usually one cannot easily distinguish these lesions on MR scan, and biopsy may be necessary. It is the obligation of the neurologist and neurosurgeon to call to the attention of the neuropathologist the possibility of demyelinating disease, because the macrophages in a demyelinating lesion may be misinterpreted as tumor cells and patients subjected to major resection and radiation therapy. Radiation therapy appears to be particularly damaging in patients with demyelinating disease, and the distinction is therefore vital.[57]

Cerebral infection can mimic brain tumors. The diagnosis is often clinically obvious when the infection occurs in immune-suppressed patients or patients suffering from a severe systemic infection. Furthermore, certain MR characteristics (as indicated in a previous section) suggest infection rather than neoplasm, but often the diagnosis cannot be made clinically.[55] In those cases, biopsy either as part of resection of a single surgically accessible lesion, or by needle biopsy in patients who have inaccessible and multiple lesions, will establish the diagnosis. The clinician should indicate to the surgeon the possibility of an infection, so that appropriate cultures are performed on the surgical material.

Pathology

A correct pathologic diagnosis is essential to prescribe appropriate treatment and to predict prognosis. Examples abound. Meningiomas that can be completely resected need no further treatment; they do not metastasize. Hemangiopericytomas, once believed to be a variant of meningioma, have a much worse prognosis and often metastasize. Postoperative radiation therapy is required. Atypical or anaplastic meningiomas require focal radiation therapy even when 'completely' resected. Current evidence suggests that anaplastic astrocytomas are best treated with radiation therapy followed by chemotherapy, whereas anaplastic oligodendrogliomas are best treated by chemotherapy, perhaps even without radiation. The prognosis for intracranial germinomas and mature teratomas is excellent, whereas the prognosis for other intracranial germ cell tumors is poor.

Unfortunately, the histologic diagnosis of intracranial tumors is sometimes difficult for several reasons: (1) often the surgeon can supply only a very small biopsy sample because the location of the tumor prohibits a larger resection; (2) many intracranial tumors are quite heterogeneous with substantial variability in the histology of the tumor from area to area; (3) some relatively benign-behaving tumors can appear malignant under the microscope whereas some relatively clinically aggressive tumors can appear low-grade under the microscope. A few examples will suffice. A few mitotic figures in an otherwise benign meningioma do not alter the excellent clinical prognosis or the treatment. The relatively benign pleomorphic xanthoastrocytomas may contain a few mitoses, lymphocytic infiltration

and bizarre-appearing tumor cells often mistaken for glioblastoma multiforme.

The individual histologic characteristics of each tumor are discussed in the chapters on individual tumors in Part 2 of this book. A few general principles that apply to most intracranial tumors are listed here:

1. All tumor specimens should be reviewed by a neuropathologist. Neuropathology is as different from general pathology as neurology is from internal medicine, and expertise in the specialty is essential for making an appropriate diagnosis. That review should be completed before any postoperative treatment is undertaken.

2. The responsible physician should review the slides with the neuropathologist. Often, vital information, not available on the standard requisition form, is exchanged during a personal review of the slides with the neuropathologist. One example will suffice. One of our patients with a large contrast-enhancing mass that the neuropathologist was content to read as a glioblastoma had a history of a melanoma removed 2 years earlier. The patient was told that it was cured and did not report it to the surgeon. Only during the course of a postoperative physical examination, when a small scar was found on the patient's leg, was the history elicited. Once the neuropathologist was informed of this, he performed appropriate special stains to establish the diagnosis of a metastatic melanoma. It is often helpful to review the imaging studies with the neuropathologist, particularly when determining tumor grade or identifying rare variants of glial tumors (Chapter 5).

3. The surgeon should submit as large a sample as possible. This not only allows the neuropathologist sufficient material for making a diagnosis, but also allows an

estimate of the degree of heterogeneity. If the patient is not a candidate for resection, but only a stereotactic needle biopsy, the biopsy should include the area that appears most aggressive on preoperative imaging, such as any area of contrast enhancement on gadolinium MR scan or a region of hypermetabolism on FDG PET.

4. Utilize the most modern diagnostic techniques to identify the tumor. Several techniques beyond routine staining of pathologic specimens now aid in diagnosis. These include electron microscopy, immunohistochemical techniques and identification of genetic abnormalities. Molecular genetic analysis can be performed on needle biopsy specimens.[51] Electron microscopy of appropriately prepared tissue can distinguish central neurocytomas (neuronal tumors) with their synaptic vesicles from their almost identically appearing oligodendrogliomas, which lack synaptic vesicles. In similar fashion, microvilli and cilia identify an ependymoma that otherwise appears to be an astrocytoma. B-cell markers can distinguish primary CNS lymphoma from inflammatory diseases. Synaptophysin helps identify tumors of neuronal origin, and two recently described antibodies, anti-Hu[58] and Neu-N,[59] may prove to be even more effective in distinguishing neuronal and mixed glioneuronal tumors. Although there is no clear marker yet for identifying an oligodendroglioma, deletions of chromosomes 1p and 19q are common in oligodendrogliomas and not in astrocytomas.[60] Other genetic markers may prove to be equally valuable in the future.[61]

5. It is often wise to request a frozen section during the course of surgery. Immediate identification of histologic material can have several purposes. During the course of a stereotactic needle biopsy, a frozen section or a smear preparation can tell the surgeon that he has successfully biopsied a tumor, even if the exact nature of the tumor must await identification on permanent sections. During the course of open surgery, identification of the tumor may determine the course of surgery. For example, a lymphoma does not require extirpative surgery but is best treated by chemotherapy, whereas gliomas benefit from removal of as much tumor as is feasible. Often these two tumors are not distinguished preoperatively but only at the time of frozen section. The pathologist may also be able to tell on frozen section whether some tissue should be fixed for future electron microscopy to assist in definitive diagnosis. Finally, during the course of surgery the surgeon may want to sample the margins of his resection to determine whether tumor remains or he has reached normal white matter. Immediate histology can also be procured by smear or touch preparations.[62] In these preparations, cellular processes and nuclei are much better preserved than in frozen section although the tumor pattern is lost.[63]

6. CSF is sometimes useful to identify tumor cells, particularly if the leptomeninges have been seeded. In most instances, however, it is of no use in the evaluation of a brain tumor, and the risks of lumbar puncture far outweigh the benefits. In the case of suspected primary CNS lymphoma, however, examination of CSF can be fruitful in identifying lymphoma cells, obviating the necessity for brain biopsy. Immunohistochemistry for B-cells is particularly helpful, since most primary CNS lymphomas are B-cell lymphomas, whereas T-cells in the spinal fluid are generally associated with inflammatory states. It is

extremely rare for tumors arising outside of the substance of the brain, such as meningiomas, Schwannomas and neurofibromas, to exude cells into the CSF unless malignant variants of these tumors have seeded the leptomeninges.

7. Routine histology hematoxylin and eosin staining of formalin-fixed paraffin-embedded tissue still remains the most common histologic test for intracranial tumors. A variety of other stains are used for identification of particular abnormalities in individual tumors. Examples include reticulin stains, which are often positive in ganglioglioma, Masson's trichome stain to identify gliosarcoma, and a myelin stain to differentiate tumor from multiple sclerosis.

8. Immunohistochemistry tumors of glial origin are often positive for glial fibrillary acidic protein (GFAP). This stain is often positive in astrocytomas, particularly of higher grade, and in some oligodendrogliomas. Reactive astrocytosis also gives positive reactions. A recent report describes a specific marker for tumors of oligodendroglial origin.[64] Microglia are visualized by macrophage markers, such as CD68, which helps to distinguish demyelinating disorders from tumor. Antibodies against cytokeratins are helpful in distinguishing metastatic epithelial tumors from primary tumors. The HMB-45 stain identifies melanoma and differentiates it from primary gliomas. Immunohistochemistry can also help in grading tumors. Cell proliferation markers, such as Ki-67 (MIB-1), distinguish cells in all phases of the cell cycle save for G_o. The number of positive nuclei correlates well with the tumor grade and biological behavior in most studies.[65] Tumors with MIB indices over 5%, even with otherwise benign histology, should be viewed with suspicion by the clinician. Different isoforms of S100 protein are expressed in different tumors; recent reports indicate that modifications of S100 A3 protein expression distinguished pilocytic from diffuse astrocytoma.[65] The presence of p53 protein by immunohistochemical staining occurs in many astrocytomas, particularly of higher grade, but is rare in oligodendrogliomas.

Approach to the patient

Figures 3.10 and 3.11 describe the general approach to a patient who presents with seizures or other neurologic symptoms or signs. If after a history and physical examination the physician suspects a structural lesion, he should proceed to MR scanning both with and without contrast. If the scan suggests an intracranial tumor, further decisions will depend on whether the mass enhances or not. The algorithm does not apply to every patient with a brain tumor or every type of brain tumor, but describes a general approach which is most applicable to intrinsic intracranial tumors such as gliomas. Appropriate therapy depends on the clinical state of the patient and the type of tumor. The diagnosis and treatment of specific tumors are detailed in Chapters 5–13.

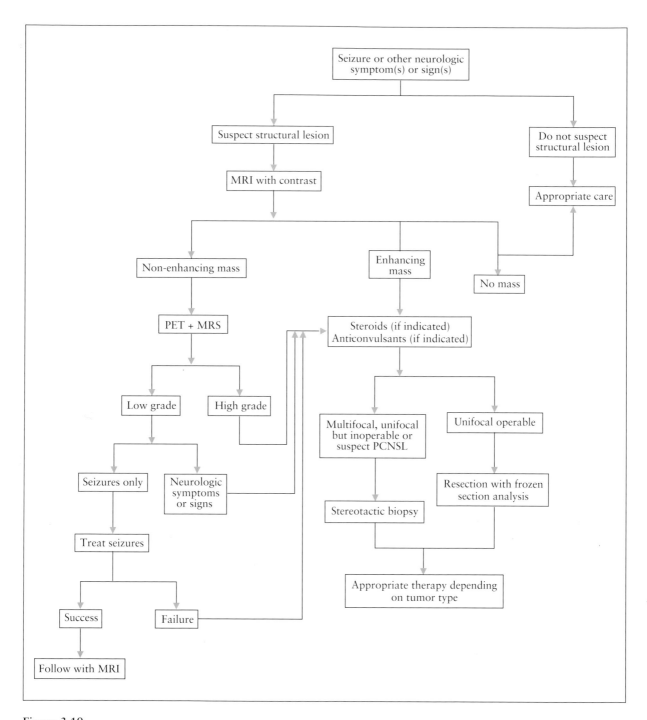

Figure 3.10
An algorithm describing the approach to a patient who presents with seizures or other neurologic symptoms or signs. The approach is a general one and does not apply to every patient or to every type of tumor. The indications for steroids and anticonvulsants are described in detail in Chapter 4.

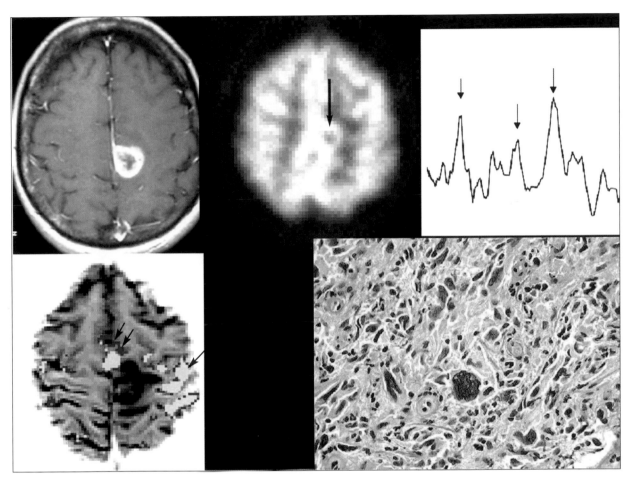

Figure 3.11
Evaluation of a patient with a suspected primary brain tumor. This 50-year-old woman presented with mild progressive weakness of the right leg. An MR scan (upper left panel) revealed a ring-enhancing mass in or near the motor strip. A PET scan (middle panel) revealed the ring enhancement to be hypermetabolic (arrow) and the center of the lesion to be iso- or hypometabolic, perhaps representing necrosis. An MRS (upper right panel) revealed a high choline peak (left arrow) with a smaller N-acetyl aspartate (NAA) peak (middle arrow). There was a high lipid peak (right arrow) compatible with necrosis. The patient was advised that the tumor was inoperable because of its proximity to the motor strip. However, functional MR (lower left) revealed that a posterior approach might successfully avoid both the laterally replaced sensorimotor areas (arrow) and the anteriorly placed supplementary motor area (double arrow). About 90% of the tumor was removed. The patient had a modest but transient increase in her weakness after the operation. The tumor proved to be a glioblastoma multiforme (lower right).

References

1. Liigant A, Haldre S, Oun A, Linnamägi Ü, Saar A, Asser T, Kaasik AE. Seizure disorders in patients with brain tumors. Eur Neurol 2001; 45: 46–51.

2. Frishberg BM. Neuroimaging in presumed primary headache disorders. Semin Neurol 1997; 17: 373–82.

3. Ilyin SE, Gayle D, González-Gómez I, Miele ME, Plata-Salamán CR. Brain tumor development in rats is associated with changes in central nervous system cytokine and neuropeptide systems. Brain Res Bull 1999; 48: 363–73.

4. Katzman GL, Dagher AP, Patronas NJ. Incidental findings on brain magnetic resonance imaging from 1000 asymptomatic volunteers. JAMA 1999; 282: 36–9.

5. Behrens PF, Ostertag CB, Warnke PC. Regional cerebral blood flow in peritumoral brain edema during dexamethasone treatment: a xenon-enhanced computed tomographic study. Neurosurgery 1998; 43: 235–40.

6. Kordas M, Czirjak S, Doczi T. The spinal tumour related hydrocephalus. Acta Neurochir (Wien) 1997; 139: 1049–54.

7. Forsyth PA, Posner JB. Headaches in patients with brain tumors: a study of 111 patients. Neurology 1993; 43, 1678–83.

8. Pfund Z, Szapary L, Jaszberenyi O, Nagy F, Czopf J. Headache in intracranial tumors. Cephalalgia 1999; 19: 787–90.

9. Fricke B, Andres KH, Von Düring M. Nerve fibers innervating the cranial and spinal meninges: morphology of nerve fiber terminals and their structural integration. Microsc Res Tech 2001; 53: 96–105.

10. Pascual J, Iglesias F, Oterino A, Vazquez-Barquero A, Berciano J. Cough, exertional, and sexual headaches: an analysis of 72 benign and symptomatic cases. Neurology 1996; 46: 1520–4.

11. Edmeads JG. Headache as a symptom of organic diseases. Curr Opin Neurol 1995; 8: 233–6.

12. Mann SD, Danesh BJ, Kamm MA. Intractable vomiting due to a brainstem lesion in the absence of neurological signs or raised intracranial pressure. Gut 1998; 42: 875–7.

13. Rowe FJ, Sarkies NJ. Assessment of visual function in idiopathic intracranial hypertension: a prospective study. Eye 1998; 12: 111–8.

14. Lundberg N. Continuous recording and control of ventricular fluid pressure in neurosurgical practice. Acta Neurol Scand 1960; 149: 1–193.

15. Lote K, Stenwig AE, Skullerud K, Hirschberg H. Prevalence and prognostic significance of epilepsy in patients with gliomas. Eur J Cancer 1998; 34: 98–102.

16. Holt-Seitz A, Wirrell EC, Sundaram MB. Seizures in the elderly: etiology and prognosis. Can J Neurol Sci 1999; 26: 110–4.

17. Vick N. Intracranial tumors. In: Bennett JC, Plum F, eds. Cecil textbook of medicine. Philadelphia: W.B. Saunders Co., 1996: 2125–30.

18. Rudge P, Warrington EK. Selective impairment of memory and visual perception in splenial tumours. Brain 1991; 114: 349–60.

19. Terry JB, Rosenberg RN. Frontal lobe ataxia. Surg Neurol 1995; 44: 583–8.

20. Shuping JR, Rollinson RD, Toole JF. Transient global amnesia. Ann Neurol 1980; 7: 281–5.

21. Meador KJ, Swift TR. Tinnitus from intracranial hypertension. Neurology 1984; 34: 1258–61.

22. Groves MD, McCutcheon IE, Ginsberg LE, Kyritsis AP. Radicular pain can be a symptom of elevated intracranial pressure. Neurology 1999; 52: 1093–5.

23. Gilman S. Imaging the brain. N Engl J Med 1998; 338: 889–96.

24. Hoffman JM. New advances in brain tumor imaging. Curr Opin Oncol 2001; 13: 148–53.

25. Wieshmann UC, Symms MR, Parker GJM et al. Diffusion tensor imaging demonstrates deviation of fibres in normal appearing white matter adjacent to a brain tumour. J Neurol Neurosurg Psychiatry 2000; 68: 501–3.

26. Pomper MG, Port JD. New techniques in MR imaging of brain tumors. Magn Reson Imaging Clin N Am 2000; 8: 691–713.

27. Lee PL, Gonzalez RG. Magnetic resonance spectroscopy of brain tumors. Curr Opin Oncol 2000; 12: 199–204.

28. Snyder H, Robinson K, Shah D, Brennan R, Handrigan M. Signs and symptoms of patients with brain tumors presenting to the emergency department. J Emerg Med 1993; 11: 253–8.

29. Zimmerman RA. Brain tumor imaging. In: Vecht C, ed. Neuro-oncology, Part 1. Amsterdam: Elsevier, 1997: 167–92.

30. Mitchell P, Wilkinson ID, Hoggard N et al. Detection of subarachnoid haemorrhage with magnetic resonance imaging. J Neurol Neurosurg Psychiatry 2001; 70: 205–11.

31. Linfante I, Llinas RH, Caplan LR, Warach S. MRI features of intracerebral hemorrhage within 2 hours from symptom onset. Stroke 1999; 30: 2263–7.

32. Lote K, Egeland T, Hager B, Skullerud K, Hirschberg H. Prognostic significance of CT contrast enhancement within histological subgroups of intracranial glioma. J Neurooncol 1998; 40: 161–70.

33. Essig M, Knopp MV, Schoenberg SO et al. Cerebral gliomas and metastases: assessment with contrast-enhanced fast fluid-attenuated inversion-recovery MR imaging. Radiology 1999; 210: 551–7.

34. Siegal T, Rubinstein R, Tzuk-Shina T, Gomori JM. Utility of relative cerebral blood volume mapping derived from perfusion magnetic resonance imaging in the routine follow up of brain tumors. J Neurosurg 1997; 86: 22–7.

35. Delbeke D. Oncological applications of FDG PET imaging: brain tumors, colorectal cancer lymphoma and melanoma. J Nucl Med 1999; 40: 591–603.

36. Shoup TM, Olson J, Hoffman JM et al. Synthesis and evaluation of [18F]1-amino-3-fluorocyclo-butane-1-carboxylic acid to image brain tumors. J Nucl Med 1999; 40: 331–8.

37. Inoue T, Shibasaki T, Oriuchi N et al. 18F α-methyl tyrosine PET studies in patients with brain tumors. J Nucl Med 1999; 40: 399–405.

38. Mineura K, Shioya H, Kowada M et al. Blood flow and metabolism of oligodendrogliomas: a positron emission tomography study with kinetic analysis of 18F-fluorodeoxyglucose. J Neurooncol 1999; 43: 49–57.

39. Sasaki M, Kuwabara Y, Yoshida T et al. A comparative study of thallium-201 SPET, carbon-11 methionine PET and fluorine-18 fluorodeoxyglucose PET for the differentiation of astrocytic tumours. Eur J Nucl Med 1998; 25: 1261–9.

40. Maruyama I, Sadato N, Waki A et al. Hyperacute changes in glucose metabolism of brain tumors after stereotactic radiosurgery: a PET study. J Nucl Med 1999; 40: 1085–90.

41. Schwartz RB, Holman BL, Polak JF et al. Dual-isotope single-photon emission computerized tomography scanning in patients with glio-blastoma multiforme: association with patient survival and histopathological characteristics of tumor after high-dose radiotherapy. J Neurosurg 1998; 89: 60–8.

42. Maria BL, Drane WE, Mastin ST, Jimenez LA. Comparative value of thallium and glucose SPECT imaging in childhood brain tumors. Pediatr Neurol 1998; 19: 351–7.

43. Bader JB, Samnick S, Moringlane JR et al. Evaluation of L-3-[123I]iodo-α-methyltyrosine SPET and [18F]fluorodeoxyglucose PET in the detection and grading of recurrences in patients pretreated for gliomas at follow-up: a comparative study with stereotactic biopsy. Eur J Nucl Med 1999; 26: 144–51.

44. Matheja P, Schober O. 123I-IMT SPET: introducing another research tool into clinical neurooncology? Eur J Nucl Med 2001; 28: 1–4.

45. Soler C, Beauchesne P, Maatougui K et al. Technetium-99m sestamibi brain single-photon emission tomography for detection of recurrent gliomas after radiation therapy. Eur J Nucl Med 1998; 25: 1649–57.

46. Hendrikse NH, Franssen EJ, van der Graaf WT, Vaalburg W, de Vries E.G. Visualization of multidrug resistance in vivo. Eur J Nucl Med 1999; 26: 283–93.

47. De Stefano N, Caramanos Z, Preul MC, Francis G, Antel JP, Arnold DL. In vivo differentiation of astrocytic brain tumors and isolated demyelinating lesions of the type seen in multiple sclerosis using 1H magnetic resonance spectroscopic imaging. Ann Neurol 1998; 44: 273–8.

48. Forster BB, MacKay AL, Whittall KP et al. Functional magnetic resonance imaging: the basics of blood-oxygen-level dependent (BOLD) imaging. Can Assoc Radiol J 1998; 49: 320–9.

49. Hall WA. The safety and efficacy of stereotactic biopsy for intracranial lesions. Cancer 1998; 82: 1749–55.

50. Soo TM, Bernstein M, Provias J, Tasker R, Lozano A, Guha A. Failed stereotactic biopsy in a series of 518 cases. Stereotact Funct Neurosurg 1995; 64: 183–96.

51. Müller MB, Schmidt MC, Schmidt O et al. Molecular genetic analysis as a tool for evaluating

stereotactic biopsies of glioma specimens. J Neuropathol Exp Neurol 1999; 58: 40–5.

52. Bernstein M, Parrent AG. Complications of CT-guided stereotactic biopsy of intra-axial brain lesions. J Neurosurg 1994; 81: 165–8.

53. Kulkarni AV, Guha A, Lozano A, Bernstein M. Incidence of silent hemorrhage and delayed deterioration after stereotactic brain biopsy. J Neurosurg 1998; 89: 31–5.

54. Skolasky RL, Dal Pan GJ, Olivi A, Lenz FA, Abrams RA, McArthur JC. HIV-associated primary CNS morbidity and utility of brain biopsy. J Neurol Sci 1999; 163: 32–8.

55. Klein CJ, DiNapoli RP, Temesgen Z, Meyer FB. Central nervous system histoplasmosis mimicking a brain tumor: difficulties in diagnosis and treatment. Mayo Clin Proc 1999; 74: 803–7.

56. Masdeu JC, Quinto C, Olivera C et al. Open-ring imaging sign – highly specific for atypical brain demyelination. Neurology 2000; 54: 1427–33.

57. Peterson K, Rosenblum MK, Powers JM et al. effect of brain irradiation on demyelinating lesions. Neurology 1993; 43: 2105–12.

58. Gultekin SH, Dalmau J, Graus Y, Posner JB, Rosenblum MK. Anti-Hu immunolabeling as an index of neuronal differentiation in human brain tumors-a study of 112 central neuroepithelial neoplasms. Am J Surg Pathol 1998; 22: 195–200.

59. Wolf HK, Buslei R, Schmidt-Kastner R et al. NeuN: a useful neuronal marker for diagnostic histopathology. J Histochem Cytochem 1996; 44: 1167–71.

60. Cairncross JG, Ueki K, Zlatescu MC et al. Specific genetic predictors of chemotherapeutic response and survival in patients with anaplastic oligodendrogliomas. J Natl Cancer Inst 1998; 90: 1473–9.

61. Firlik KS, Martinez AJ, Lunsford LD. Use of cytological preparations for the intraoperative diagnosis of stereotactically obtained brain biopsies: a 19-year experience and survey of neuropathologists. J Neurosurg 1999; 91: 454–8.

62. Slowinski J, Harabin-Slowinska M, Mrówka R. Smear technique in the intra-operative brain tumor diagnosis: its advantages and limitations. Neurol Res 1999; 21: 121–4.

63. Giannini C, Scheithauer BW, Burger PC et al. Cellular proliferation in pilocytic and diffuse astrocytomas. J Neuropathol Exp Neurol 1999; 58: 46–53.

64. Marie Y, Sanson M, Mokhtari K et al. OLIG2 as a specific marker of oligodendroglial tumour cells. Lancet 2001; 358: 298–300.

65. Camby I, Nagy N, Lopes MB et al. Supratentorial pilocytic astrocytomas, astrocytomas, anaplastic astrocytomas and glioblastomas are characterized by a differential expression of S100 proteins. Brain Pathol 1999; 9: 1–19.

4

Principles of therapy

Introduction

Intracranial tumor therapy can be directed at the tumor (definitive therapy) or at symptom control (supportive therapy) or, preferably, at both (Table 4.1). Definitive therapy includes the

Table 4.1
Therapy of intracranial tumors.

- Definitive therapy
  - Surgery
    Biopsy
    Resection
  - Radiation
    External beam
    Radiosurgery or stereotactic radiotherapy
    Heavy particles
    Brachytherapy
  - Chemotherapy
    Parenteral
    Local
  - Experimental modalities
    Angiogenesis inhibitors
    Growth factor inhibitors
    Differentiating agents
    Immunotherapy
    Gene therapy
    Antisense oligonucleotides
- Supportive therapy
    Anticonvulsants
    Corticosteroids
    Anti-thrombosis agents
    Psychotropic agents
    Physical therapy

three conventional therapeutic approaches – surgery, radiation and chemotherapy as well as several forms of experimental therapy. Supportive therapy encompasses management of tumor symptoms, e.g. seizures, and of complications of the tumor or its treatment, e.g. deep vein thrombosis, radiation necrosis. This chapter considers the principles of both definitive and supportive therapy. Therapy directed at individual tumors is considered in later chapters.

Principles of surgery

Introduction

Surgery is the most important single modality in the treatment of intracranial tumors.[1,2] Truly benign tumors, such as pituitary adenomas and meningiomas, are often cured by surgery. For those tumors that cannot be cured, almost all observers believe that surgery substantially enhances both the duration and quality of survival. The goals of surgery are several (Table 4.2).

The first goal of surgery is to establish a diagnosis, either by biopsy or more definitive tumor resection. Stereotactic needle biopsy is usually reserved for: (1) surgically inaccessible tumors such as those in the basal ganglia, corpus callosum or brainstem; (2) multifocal tumors; (3) diffuse gliomatosis (Chapter 5);

Table 4.2
Goals of surgery.

- Establish the diagnosis
- Cure the patient
- Decrease tumor burden
- Relieve symptoms
- Improve neurologic function
- Extend duration and quality of life

(4) putative primary CNS lymphomas, a tumor better treated by chemotherapy than surgery (Chapter 11). With these exceptions, surgery should remove as much tumor as feasible.

Stereotactic needle biopsy is performed under either CT or MR guidance.[3] Fiducials (Latin for 'trust', thus a fixed point of reference) or a frame is fixed to the head; a small incision is made in the scalp and a burr-hole drilled through the skull. A needle is inserted through the burr-hole, guided by the scan, into what appears to be the most 'malignant' area of the tumor, and a core taken for histologic evaluation. In some instances, several passes are made to ensure an adequate sample. Stereotactic needle biopsy and its complications are discussed in Chapter 3.

Needle biopsies have several limitations. The limited tissue sample procured often makes diagnosis difficult, especially when attempting to grade tumors such as gliomas. For example, samples taken from the tumor edge may suggest low-grade glioma or even gliosis, whereas deeper samples may demonstrate a higher-grade histology. Stereotactic needle biopsy is preferred for deep-seated lesions, such as those in the brainstem or basal ganglia, or those where direct inspection will not assist the surgeon. A biopsy performed under direct inspection allows the surgeon to procure a larger and thus more easily diagnosed specimen and to control bleeding.

A second aim of surgery is cure. Meticulous attempts to remove the entire tumor sometimes result in cure without additional therapy. When cure is not possible, the goal is to remove as much tumor as possible without compromising neurologic function. Removal of substantial amounts of even infiltrative tumors has several salutary effects:

1. It reduces the number of tumor cells that must subsequently be eliminated by radiation therapy and/or chemotherapy. RT and chemotherapy exert their effects by killing a percentage of tumor cells regardless of tumor volume (see below). Thus, these modalities are more likely to improve survival when a smaller rather than a larger number of cells remain after resection.
2. Reducing tumor size decreases areas of hypoxia, thus increasing radiation sensitivity.
3. Because small tumors often grow exponentially, but larger tumors grow more slowly, with many tumor cells in a quiescent phase, surgical cytoreduction puts more cells into the cell cycle, making them susceptible to RT and chemotherapy. Therefore, even with high-grade tumors such as glioblastoma, most evidence suggests a direct correlation between extent of surgery and improved duration and quality of survival.[4–6] Extent of surgery is now recognized by most observers to be an important prognostic factor.

Because virtually no tissue is removed by needle biopsy in patients with large tumors, postoperative brain swelling often worsens neurologic symptoms; however, a substantial resection of tumor provides space for any postoperative cerebral swelling to occur safely without causing clinical deterioration. Several studies indicate that patients undergoing gross total resection of intrinsic brain tumors have less postoperative morbidity and better neurologic function than do those undergoing only biopsy or subtotal resection.[7]

(a)

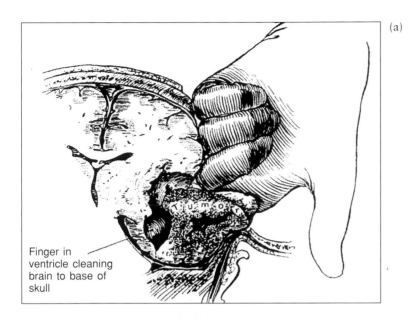

Finger in ventricle cleaning brain to base of skull

(b)

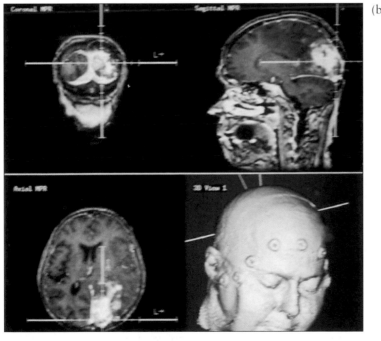

Figure 4.1
Old and new techniques for brain tumor surgery. (a) A figure redrawn from an illustration by neurosurgeon Walter Dandy, indicating the surgical approach used for brain tumors in the first half of last century. Corticosteroids were not available. The trauma of the finger removing the tumor engendered severe brain edema. Mortality and morbidity were high. (b) Illustration of modern computerized imaged-guided therapy. The 'viewing wand' is a fully computerized, frameless MR-guided system that directs the surgeon toward the target by continually providing the location of the operating site. A mechanical arm is freely mobile and is attached to a computer that contains the patient's preoperative image data.

Because of improved ability to identify functionally important areas of brain, e.g. by fMRI, the neurosurgeon is now able to remove more tumors safely than in the past, without compromising neurologic function.[8]

As Fig. 4.1 illustrates, the surgery of intracranial tumors has improved substantially because of technical improvements over the past several decades.[9] The result has been dramatic reduction in both mortality and morbidity resulting from neurosurgical procedures. In the days of the early neurosurgical giants, Dandy and Cushing, surgical mortalities of 25–30% were common, and many patients who were operated on for brain tumors suffered substantial neurologic disability after the procedure. Of course, because of limited diagnostic techniques, the tumors were usually larger than those operated on today. Improvements in diagnostic, neuroanesthetic and surgical techniques have lowered operative mortality in the best centers to 3% or less and postoperative neurologic worsening to less than 10% (see below).

Preoperative evaluation

As indicated in Chapter 3, an MRI is usually sufficient for the neurosurgeon to plan the procedure. The day prior to surgery, a contrast-enhanced MR scan is performed and fiducial markers placed upon the scalp to allow use of frameless stereotactic guidance apparatus during the procedure. In some instances, other imaging techniques give the surgeon additional information (Table 4.3).

A CT scan of a skull base tumor may help the neurosurgeon evaluate the anatomy of the

Table 4.3
Preoperative evaluation.

All patients	Some patients
Localizing MRI	CT scan
Discontinue aspirin	Functional MRI
Give anticonvulsants	Angiogram
Start steroids	PET
Evaluate general physical and neurologic condition	Tumor embolization

bone and determine if the bone is eroded or invaded by tumor. An **angiogram** may be required of some tumors both to evaluate the vascularity of the tumor and to identify normal arterial and venous structures that may help dictate the neurosurgeon's approach to the tumor. Sometimes MR angiography or MR venography will suffice to identify the anatomy, obviating the need for more invasive arteriography. For a few highly vascular tumors, including some meningiomas, hemangioblastomas and metastases, preoperative **embolization** may allow a better and safer resection.

If the tumor is in or close to a functionally important area, a **functional MRI** will reliably identify language, motor and sensory areas (Fig. 4.2) and allow the surgeon to plan his approach to avoid those regions.[10,11] Identification of language areas is particularly important when operating on dominant temporal lobe lesions, since they are quite variable.[12] Some surgeons prefer awake craniotomy to map language areas during surgery.[13] For patients undergoing needle biopsy, an FDG **PET scan** will identify any areas of hypermetabolism and perfusion MRI will identify areas of increased blood flow, both of which presumably represent the most rapidly growing tumor, allowing the neurosurgeon to target that area for biopsy.

The preoperative workup should also include, depending on the patient's age and general medical status, an evaluation of cardiac and pulmonary function. Aspirin or aspirin-containing compounds (there are about 400 of them) should be discontinued 7–10 days prior to surgery. Non-steroidal anti-inflammatory drugs (NSAIDs) also inhibit platelet function but do so reversibly and can be discontinued 48 h prior to surgery. Except in the case of primary central nervous system lymphomas (PCNSL), corticosteroids in a dose equivalent to 16 mg dexamethasone a day should be given

(a)

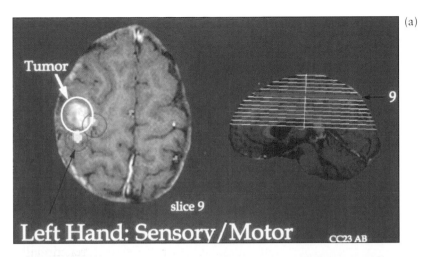

(b)

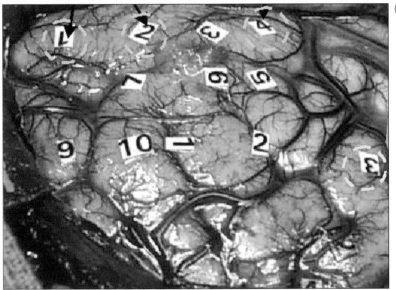

Figure 4.2
The usefulness of functional imaging in planning surgery. (a) This 16-year old girl had intractable seizures and a non-enhancing mass in the right posterior frontal lobe. Several neurosurgeons refused surgery because they believed that the tumor was too close to the sensorimotor strip. Functional MR scan revealed sensory and motor activity posteriorly and medially to the tumor. A gross total resection was carried out without postoperative weakness. The seizures ceased. (b) At the time of surgery, areas close to the sensorimotor strip are marked with numbered tags. Motor areas are identified by stimulation of the cortex and sensory areas by peripheral stimulation.

for at least 48 h prior to the operative procedure. Other medications, except aspirin, should be continued. Controversy exists concerning the use of prophylactic anticonvulsants in those patients who have not previously had a seizure. Two studies disagree. One shows protection during the first postoperative week;[14] the other does not.[15] We give glioma patients a loading dose of phenytoin (15 mg/kg) or fosphenytoin just prior to surgery. The anticonvulsants can be continued for 2 months, and then if the patient has not had prior seizures, tapered or discontinued (see below). For standard, clean neurosurgical procedures, we give a broad-spectrum antibiotic such as cefazolin 1 g every 8 h for three doses, the first just before the skin is incised. Anticoagulants are discussed on page 137.

Operative procedures

Specific operative procedures differ depending on the location and size of the tumor and the goal of the surgeon (e.g. biopsy, subtotal resection, total resection). These factors are considered in the chapters on individual tumors.

For all patients undergoing craniotomy, during induction of anesthesia an arterial catheter is placed in the radial artery for continuous monitoring of blood pressure. Some measure jugular bulb oxygen saturation to ensure adequate cerebral perfusion.[16] Pneumatic compression boots are placed on each calf. The patient is given 1–1.5 g/kg of a 20% solution of mannitol over 20–30 min. This hyperosmolar substance extracts water from normal, non-edematous brain. In some instances, a lumbar drain is placed to drain cerebrospinal fluid (CSF). Both mannitol and CSF drainage serve to slacken the brain for easier and safer retraction. If the patient is being operated on in the sitting position, a central venous line and a cortical Doppler are used to monitor for air emboli.

Once the patient is positioned and prepared, an incision is made in the scalp as defined by the location of the tumor on MR scan and dictated by frameless stereotactic localization. The stereotactic apparatus links the preoperative scan to landmarks on the surface of the head, providing continuous information on the relationship of the surgeon's instruments to the intracranial tumor. Both CT and MR stereotactic systems are accurate to within a few millimeters.[17] Unfortunately, as the surgery proceeds, shifts of intracranial structures decrease the reliability of the information that was based on the preoperative scan. Intraoperative MRI remedies this problem.[18] The incision should provide optimal exposure of the tumor but maintain an adequate blood supply to the scalp. The overlying skull is removed. If it is involved

Table 4.4
Operative tools.

- Frameless stereotaxy
- Ultrasound
- Microscope
- Cortical mapping
- Ultrasonic aspirator
- Laser
- Endoscope
- Intraoperative MRI

by tumor, it may have to be discarded and later replaced by an acrylic prosthesis.

Modern neurosurgical techniques include several tools that allow better access to and identification of a tumor once the skull has been opened (Table 4.4).

Frameless stereotaxy, ultrasound and microscope

Frameless stereotactic systems, based on preoperative imaging, allow precise placement of the bony opening, accurate planning of the trajectory to the tumor, and feedback about the extent of resection. Some surgeons prefer, instead or in addition to frameless stereotaxy, to localize and approach the tumor using intraoperative ultrasound applied directly to the cortical surface. This modality also provides 'real time' feedback about the presence of residual tumor and helps the surgeon to gain more complete resections. The operating microscope will sufficiently magnify to allow good visualization of blood vessels and other critical structures and, when combined with microdissection using micro-instruments, improves the safety of surgical resections.

Cortical mapping

If the tumor is in or near functionally important areas, such as language, primary motor or sensory cortex, cortical mapping may complement fMRI (Fig. 4.2).[19] Cortical mapping of language can be carried out only by direct cortical stimulation in an awake patient being operated on under local anesthesia.[20] Motor and sensory cortex can be mapped by cortical stimulation or by somatosensory evoked potentials in patients being operated on under general anesthesia.[19] Somatosensory evoked potentials or nerve stimulation are also very useful in assessing cranial nerve function during surgery on the skull base.

Ultrasonic aspirator, laser and neuroendoscope

An ultrasonic aspirator utilizes high-frequency vibrations to shatter tumor cells with sound waves before suctioning the debris away. The technique inflicts minimal damage on surrounding normal structures and blood vessels and is especially effective in firm tumors such as meningiomas and acoustic neuromas. Additional operative tools include an operating laser, sometimes useful in removing tumor in tight working places, and a neuroendoscope, a tool that can be used to explore the ventricular system, remove intraventricular masses, and even explore the posterior fossa to aid acoustic neuroma surgery.[21]

Intraoperative pathology

Intraoperative consultation with a skilled neuropathologist establishes the diagnosis in most instances.[22] Frozen sections help guarantee that appropriate tissue has been obtained for diagnosis. It may also help the surgeon decide whether to proceed with further tumor removal. For example, if a lymphoma is seen on a frozen section, there is no need for a gross total excision, which could lead to neurologic deficits.

After the tumor has been resected to the maximum extent possible and hemostasis has been secured (in some instances by raising the systolic blood pressure to 140 mm Hg to ensure there is no bleeding), the wound is closed and the patient monitored in a recovery room for several hours before being returned to the neurosurgical unit.

Postoperative care

At Memorial Sloan–Kettering, we return patients from the recovery room to a small, constant-observation unit, where they remain for 24–48 h (Table 4.5).

The monitoring includes careful neurologic evaluation with particular attention to state of consciousness, blood pressure via the arterial catheter until the morning postsurgery (i.e. 12–14 h), and careful measurement of urine output via Foley catheter placed at the time of surgery. Depending on the extent of surgery and degree of preoperative edema, corticosteroids in doses of 16–40 mg a day are prescribed for several days following the surgery and then tapered to the patient's tolerance. Pneumatic pressure boots are maintained until the patient is fully ambulatory. Most patients are able to eat and are mobilized the morning after surgery, first to a chair and then to ambulation.

Table 4.5
Postoperative care.

- State of consciousness
- Pupillary reactions
- Segmental neurologic exam
- Cerebral perfusion pressure = blood pressure–venous pressure
- Intravenous fluids
- Corticosteroids
- Anticonvulsants
- MRI

For most neurosurgical procedures, one can anticipate the patient's neurologic examination will be the same or improved over the preoperative examination in the immediate postoperative period. Because the brain swells 24–48 h after the surgical manipulation, some patients become drowsy or lethargic, or have worsening focal signs after having initially appeared wide awake, with improved neurologic function. In most instances, this disappears after 24–36 h and, if it does not, can usually be obviated by increasing the dose of corticosteroids. Rarely, the swelling can cause herniation and/or permanent neurologic disability.

A postoperative gadolinium-enhanced MR scan is performed 24–72 h after surgery to determine the extent of residual tumor, if any. The pre-contrast T1 image is compared with the post-contrast image (Fig. 4.3). Blood appears hyperintense on both (the reason blood appears hyperintense so early after the surgery is probably because the exposure of the tumor bed to room air, i.e. oxygen, has promoted the early development of paramagnetic methemoglobin), but contrast enhancement indicates residual tumor. After about 72 hours, normal brain structures surrounding the tumor bed begin to enhance and may remain enhanced for weeks to months following the surgery, thus precluding accurate identification of residual tumor.

For certain tumors, particularly those at the skull base or tumors operated on after radiation therapy or prolonged use of steroids, a CSF leak may develop in the postoperative period. Bedrest and placement of a lumbar drain to lower CSF pressure are usually effective treatments. Other complications that may occur include hyponatremia and postoperative seizures. Cerebral infarction may be caused either by arterial occlusion or spasm or by

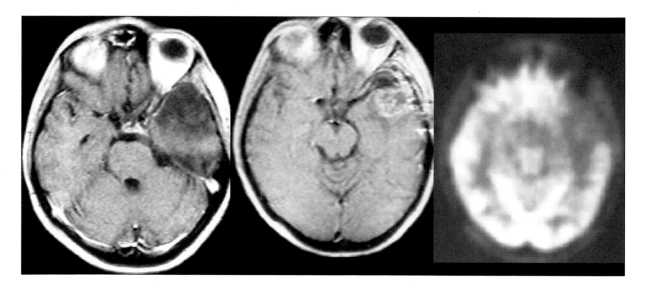

Figure 4.3
The value of immediate postoperative scans. This patient had a non-enhancing left temporal lobe tumor (left panel). His physicians did not order an immediate postoperative scan. When the scan was repeated some weeks later, the physicians became concerned that the enhancement represented a change in the biology of residual tumor (middle panel). However, a PET scan (right panel) shows that the area was hypo- not hypermetabolic, and after several months the enhancement disappeared. The tumor was a low-grade glioma.

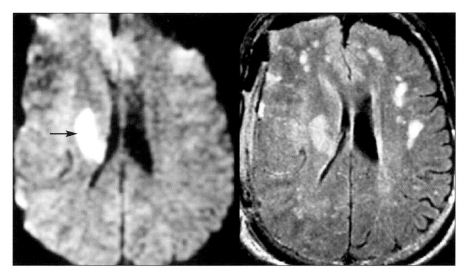

Figure 4.4
A postoperative infarct causing weakness of the left face and arm. This 62-year-old man with a long history of hypertension had a single generalized seizure. The MR scan (not shown) showed a tumor involving the right temporal lobe and the insula. Some of the tumor was in the sylvian fissure. His neurologic examination was normal. A partial resection was carried out, and in the postoperative period his face and arm were paralyzed, with the leg being relatively normal. The diffusion-weighted image (left) showed evidence of an acute infarct (arrow). The T2-weighted image (right) showed the recent infarct plus multiple hyperintensities in the white matter related to hypertensive small vessel disease.

venous occlusion. Arterial occlusion or spasm causes bland infarction (Fig. 4.4). Tumors involving the sylvian fissure, through which the middle cerebral artery passes, or meningiomas abutting veins that enter the sagittal sinus, are at particularly high risk for postoperative vascular complications.

Another cause of neurologic deterioration after surgery may be the development of a hematoma in the operative bed. In any patient whose neurologic condition worsens significantly in the postoperative period, an urgent unenhanced CT scan should be performed to look for a hematoma. Hematomas usually develop within the first 24 h postoperatively. Those of sufficient size to cause neurologic symptoms require evacuation.

Infection following clean craniotomy is rare, especially when prophylactic antibiotics are used. Infection is more likely after second surgery in a patient who has been treated with steroids and who has received RT, as both treatments interfere with wound healing. Interestingly, long-term remissions of high-grade tumor have been reported in several patients after intracranial infection,[23] perhaps a result of inhibition of angiogenesis.[24]

Future developments

As indicated above, surgical technology has improved dramatically. New techniques promise to improve the neurosurgical approach to tumors even more in succeeding years.

Intraoperative MRI, robotic equipment and endoscopic surgery

Intraoperative MRI[18] allows the surgeon to stand in an MR machine and, using ceramic rather than metal tools, to monitor the tumor in real time as it is resected.[25] This eliminates the errors that occur because of slight shifts of the brain as the procedure is being carried out that change the position of the tumor from the preoperative MR scan. This technique is already in place in some centers. Robotic equipment and virtual reality techniques may, in the future, replace the hands of the neurosurgeon. Endoscopic surgery has already proved useful in the treatment of vestibular schwannoma (Chapter 9)[26] and colloid cysts (Chapter 12)[27] for some neurosurgeons.

Principles of radiation therapy

Introduction

For most CNS tumors, RT is the second most important treatment modality. For some tumors, such as germinomas, RT is curative; for others it substantially prolongs survival or at least retards progression. Techniques of radiation have improved over the years, allowing higher doses to the tumor and sparing normal brain (Fig. 4.5). For example, in the original Brain Tumor Study Group prospective randomized trial of high-grade gliomas,[28] the median survival of patients treated by surgery alone was 14 weeks, whereas those receiving postoperative whole-brain RT of 50–60 Gy had a median survival of 36 weeks. A direct relationship between dose and survival was also demonstrated. Patients receiving 50 Gy had a median survival of 28 weeks, and those treated with 60 Gy had a median survival of 42 weeks.[29] RT is usually delivered after the histologic diagnosis has been established and in most cases after surgical debulking or gross total resection. The goal of the radiation oncologist is to deliver radiation in a precise fashion to the tumor, usually defined by the area of contrast enhancement on MR scan with a margin of 2–3 cm, sparing as much as possible the surrounding normal tissue.

Physics of radiation

X-rays and γ-rays represent two forms of electromagnetic radiation used conventionally in clinical practice to treat cancer.[30] X-rays are generated by an electrical device known as a linear accelerator, which accelerates electrons to high energies so that they emit X-rays when they encounter a metal target. γ-Rays, produced by cobalt-60 teletherapy units, arise through the decay of the radioactive isotope. Electromagnetic radiation can be considered either as a wave or a quantum of energy, called a photon. When X-rays of sufficient energy are absorbed in biological material, a photon may encounter an atom within a target molecule, leading to the release of an energetic electron from its orbit around the nucleus and a secondary energy-attenuated photon. The atom, having lost an electron, is now an ion. Hence, X-rays are also referred to as ionizing radiation. The ejected electrons and the secondary photons interact with other cellular molecules, leading to a chain of reactions which dissipates the original photon energy within the cell and produces a variety of short-lived, chemically unstable free-radical species. Other atomic particles used to deliver radiation therapy include electrons, produced by linear accelerators, and neutrons, protons, α-particles and heavy charged particles such as helium ions, which are generated by cyclotrons.

When radiation is absorbed, ionizing events are usually localized along tracks of individual charged particles with a pattern that is dependent

(a)

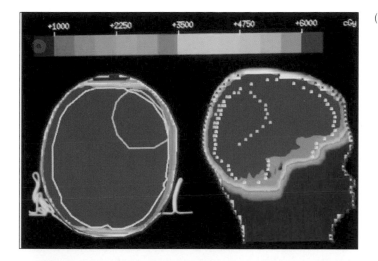

(b)

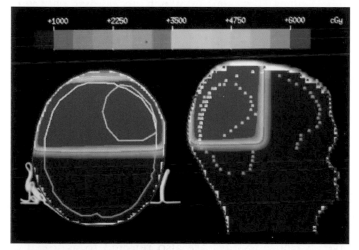

(c)

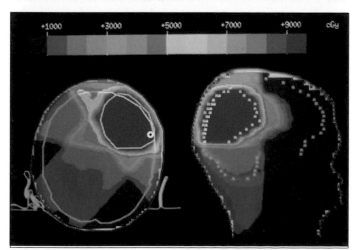

Figure 4.5
The evolution of radiation therapy for brain tumors. Up to early 1980, most patients with primary and metastatic tumors of the brain received whole-brain irradiation to lateral opposing ports (a). In the early 1980s, when it was discovered for most primary brain tumors that recurrences were local rather than elsewhere in the brain, the treatment was modified to give 40 Gy to the whole brain and an additional 20 Gy to the tumor (b). This was further modified to deliver only partial brain irradiation through bilaterally opposing ports. This treatment nevertheless irradiated a substantial portion of normal brain. The development of conformal field radiation (c) now allows one to treat the tumor and a surround that is probably infiltrated by microscopic disease, but spares most of the normal brain. The color bar indicates the dose that that area received.

on the type of radiation involved. The energy deposited per unit length of the track is referred to as the linear energy transfer (LET). Densely ionizing radiation with higher LET (e.g. neutron radiation) causes more biological damage than sparsely ionizing, low-LET radiation (e.g. X-rays).

Mechanisms of radiation damage

The predominant mechanism by which radiation kills mammalian cells is the reproductive (also known as clonogenic) pathway of cell death. The target is DNA, and double-strand breaks are regarded as the specific lesion that initiates the lethal response. Most radiation-induced DNA single-strand and some double-strand breaks, particularly if both strands are broken at the same site, are rapidly repaired by constitutively expressed repair mechanisms (known as sublethal damage repair). Residual unrepaired or misrepaired breaks result in genetic instability, increased frequency of mutations and chromosomal aberrations, and, thus, carcinogenesis. Lethal mutations or dysfunctional chromosomal aberrations eventually lead to cell death at the first or a subsequent attempt of the damaged cell to reproduce. When radiation is directed at the brain, cellular damage may become apparent only months or years later, because glial and Schwann cells reproduce slowly.

Because DNA uncoiled during the reproductive cycle is more susceptible to radiation damage than DNA coiled in the more quiescent phases of the cycle, cells are more radiosensitive at particular times in the cell cycle (Chapter 1). Cells are most sensitive in the mitotic (M) stage of the cell cycle and most resistant in the latter part of the S phase. G_1 and G_2 show intermediate sensitivity, although G_2 is more sensitive than G_1. If G_1 is long, the early phase is resistant and the latter phase

more sensitive. Cells in G_0 are resistant. Although these rules hold in general, there are a number of exceptions.

Ionizing radiation damages DNA either directly or indirectly. When a photon strikes the DNA itself, ionizing that molecule, the damage is direct. This type of interaction is relatively rare with X-rays, but it represents the dominant process of high-LET radiation such as neutrons. Alternatively, if the radiation interacts with other atoms or molecules within the cell, especially water, to produce highly reactive free radicals that secondarily damage the DNA, the action is indirect. Indirect action is the predominant mechanism in conventional external beam photon irradiation. The presence of molecular oxygen prolongs the life of the reactive species that attack DNA, making oxygenated cells more susceptible to radiation damage than hypoxic cells. On the other hand, sulfhydryl compounds neutralize and reduce the lifespan of free radicals, and analogs of these agents are being investigated as radioprotectors. Radiation also causes apoptosis, although significantly less frequently than clonogenic cell death. Ionizing radiation also attacks lipids, proteins and RNA, causing cellular damage and probably cell death.

Radiation dose and fractionation schedules

The unit of measurement that describes the amount of radiation energy absorbed per unit mass or the absorbed dose was previously called a rad (for radiation absorbed dose). A rad is equal to 100 ergs of energy absorbed per gram of tissue. The currently used unit of absorbed dose is the Gray (after Louis Gray, a British radiologist). One Gray is equal to 100 rad. The term centiGray (cGy) is frequently used to equate the dose with the rad. For example, 6000 cGy is equal to 6000 rad.

Radiotherapy is usually given in a series of equal-sized fractions, either daily or more than once a day for several weeks.[31] Each fraction kills a similar proportion of tumor cells, resulting in a logarithmic decline in the number of surviving cells as the number of fractions increases. Thus, smaller tumors are more susceptible than larger ones at any given dose.

The biological basis for fractionation is that dividing a dose into a number of fractions spares normal tissues, because sublethal damage of normal cells is repaired between dose fractions, whereas tumor cells are not repaired. Cellular division also allows repopulation of normal cells if the overall treatment time is sufficiently long. At the same time, dividing a dose into a number of fractions increases damage to the tumor by allowing time for cells that were quiescent and thus resistant to radiation to re-enter the cell cycle and become more sensitive. In addition, each fraction selectively kills cells in the more radiosensitive phases of the cell cycle. The remaining cells progress into the more radiosensitive phases of the cycle, where they can be killed by the next fraction (known as reassortment). Furthermore, tumors contain hypoxic cells. Oxygenated mammalian cells are 2.5–3 times more sensitive to radiation than hypoxic cells. Fractionation permits the shrinking tumor to reoxygenate, thus making the tumor cells in a previously hypoxic area more sensitive to radiotherapy. These phenomena also apply to normal cells, but they can repair themselves.

A course of external beam irradiation is described in terms of the total dose delivered, the amount of radiation given at each treatment session (known as fraction size), the frequency of dose fractions, and the overall time in days over which the course of radiation is given. For example, in the treatment of malignant gliomas, a typical treatment course is 59.4 Gy delivered in 33 daily fractions of 1.8 Gy each, five days per week, given over 45 days. Together, these factors constitute a fractionation schedule. The ability to cure a tumor without excessive complications depends on a complex interplay of these factors. Late complications of radiotherapy are influenced by the total dose, the size of the dose per fraction, and the time interval between fractions when they are closely spaced. Acute reactions are most affected by the fraction size and the overall time taken to deliver the treatment. In acute-reacting tissues such as skin, mucous membranes, bone marrow and, hopefully, tumor cells, injury occurs early but regeneration occurs quickly. In late-reacting tissue such as the CNS and probably many CNS tumors, injury may not occur for months or years, and recovery, if it occurs at all, occurs late. However, prolonging the overall treatment time excessively allows surviving tumor cells to divide more quickly, and some tumors may actually proliferate during the treatment.

Most brain tumors are treated with doses ranging from 45–60 Gy in daily fractions of 1.8–2.0 Gy. Higher doses per fraction have been associated with an increased incidence of late radiation injury to the CNS (see below). The dose used for each tumor type is discussed in the chapters reviewing the management of specific tumors.

Changing the conventional fractionation parameters of time and dose can lead to differential effects on the tumor and normal tissues. This has stimulated the design of altered fractionation schedules that deliver more than one dose fraction per day. These schemes seek to reduce the size of the dose per fraction or reduce the overall time of treatment.

Hyperfractionated irradiation differs from conventionally fractionated irradiation in that two or more treatments are given daily with fraction sizes that are smaller than the standard fractions of 1.8–2.0 Gy. The goal is to deliver a higher total dose (10–15%) in the same overall time as a conventional treatment schedule (6–6.5 weeks) without increasing toxicity, by exploiting differences in the capacities of normal and tumor tissues to repair radiation damage. The ability of normal neural tissues to repair sublethal radiation injury increases if the dose per fraction is small.[32] Hence, the risk of late complications can be reduced by using smaller individual fractions. Because rapidly proliferating tumor cells are less efficient at repairing damage from reduced dose fractions, and because tumor cell death is influenced more by total dose than by fraction size, there should be a therapeutic advantage to using a larger number of smaller fractions. It is necessary to administer more than one fraction per day to prevent tumor repopulation from negating the potential gain in tumor control.[33] The 6–8 h interval between doses allows sufficient time for normal tissues to repair sublethal radiation damage. However, the repair process may require more than 8 h in the CNS, making hyperfractionation less safe than some dosage formulas suggest. Proliferating tumor cells progress into more radiosensitive phases of the cell cycle during the interval between fractions, increasing the opportunity for tumor cell killing. Target cells for late sequelae proliferate slowly, so for these tissues little cell cycle reassortment or 'self-sensitization' occurs during irradiation. Studies using white matter changes on MR imaging as an endpoint demonstrate that morbidity is decreased in patients receiving doses in excess of 70 Gy with hyperfractionated schedules, compared to conventional fractionation regimens. However, studies of RT administered in multiple doses per fraction to treat brain tumors have failed to demonstrate superior efficacy over single daily dose RT.[34] In vitro studies indicate that hyperfractionation may prove useful for tumors expressing wild-type p53.[35]

Accelerated fractionation attempts to improve radiation-induced tumor cell killing in rapidly proliferating tumors by reducing the length of time needed to complete the treatment course.[33] Conventional dose fractions (1.6–2.0 Gy) are given two or three times daily. This treatment schedule may further improve the therapeutic ratio by overcoming the effects of accelerated tumor cell repopulation during treatment, thereby increasing the probability of tumor control for a given dose level.[31] However, trials using different accelerated fractionation regimens for brain tumors have not shown a survival benefit over conventional irradiation.[36,37]

Radiation therapy treatment planning and delivery approaches

Conventional treatment planning
Ionizing radiation can be delivered to a brain tumor in several ways (Table 4.6).

The most common technique, external beam radiotherapy, aims several radiation beams at the tumor to maximize the dose while minimizing the dose to normal tissue outside of the target. Recent advances in external beam radiation therapy techniques have

Table 4.6
Radiation therapy of brain tumors.

Conventional	Experimental
Conformal fields	
Intensity-modulated radiotherapy[38] (Fig 4.6)	Charged particles[39]
Radiosurgery	Boron neutron capture[40]
Stereotactic radiotherapy	Radioprotectors
Interstitial radiation[41]	
Radiosensitizers	

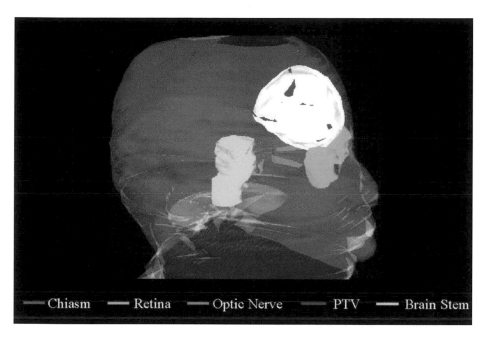

Chiasm — Retina — Optic Nerve — PTV — Brain Stem

Figure 4.6
Three-dimensional dose display for a four-field treatment plan designed using intensity modulation. The dose cloud, which represents the prescription isodose level, conforms closely to the shape of the planning target volume (PTV), while avoiding nearby optical structures, including the chiasm (orange), bilateral optic nerves (pink), retinas (green) and brainstem (blue).

improved the efficacy and lowered the toxicity associated with the treatment of brain tumors. To plan and carry out a course of radiation therapy, the radiation oncologist must determine the volume of the brain to treat based on neuroimaging studies, the operative findings and the patterns of tumor spread. The target volume is made up of three components: (1) the tumor visible on neuroimaging studies; (2) a margin of surrounding tissue considered to be at risk for microscopic tumor spread; and (3) an additional 0.5–1.0 cm margin to account for daily variations in positioning the patient on the treatment machine and patient motion. The radiation beam energy and field arrangements are selected after consideration of the location of the target volume within the brain and its geometry. Beam energies produced by linear accelerators range from 4 MV (million electron-volts) to 25 MV. The more energetic

the beam, the more energy it carries to greater depths within the brain. Beams with energies of up to 10 MV are typically used in the treatment of brain tumors. Cobalt-60 γ-rays, used less often to deliver brain irradiation, have an average energy of 1.25 MV. The total radiation dose to be administered and dose given at each daily treatment are based on the histology of the tumor.

In the past, especially for gliomas, radiation was directed to the entire brain (Fig. 4.5). This was in part because of the recognition that many brain tumors were diffusely infiltrative, but was mainly because imaging techniques which clearly defined the location of the tumor were not available. Whole-brain irradiation at doses that affect most brain tumors causes substantial toxicity. In addition, most primary brain tumors are unifocal at the time of initial diagnosis and they relapse at their original location after either whole-brain or limited-field irradiation. Accordingly, as imaging techniques improved, radiation was delivered only to the part of the brain encompassing the tumor and its surrounding microscopic extensions. An exception is the treatment of tumors such as medulloblastomas (Chapter 7), which often disseminate via CSF pathways. Such tumors are treated with a 'shrinking field' approach, in which the entire craniospinal axis is treated and a smaller field, encompassing the site of the primary tumor, receives a higher dose.

Treatment planning begins on a simulator. Simulators are X-ray machines designed to duplicate the geometry and configuration of a treatment machine, but they produce standard radiographs, rather than therapeutic X-rays. Specialized CT simulations are now available that permit three-dimensional reconstruction of tumors and normal tissues. During the simulation, patient positioning (supine or prone) is determined and an individualized custom-designed immobilization device is constructed. Such devices allow daily reproduction of patient position on the treatment couch and prevent patient movement during each radiotherapy session.

For conventional treatment planning, lateral or 90° orthogonal simulator radiographs are obtained. The target volume is reconstructed directly on the simulation film from the CT and/or MR images. For more complex field arrangements, an outline of the target volume is drawn on a contour of the head, taken through the central axis of the proposed treatment portals. The contour is digitally transferred to a treatment planning computer, radiation beams are defined, and radiation dose distributions (known as isodose distributions) are generated. The goal of treatment planning is to cover the target in its entirety while minimizing the dose to normal brain tissue, especially the retina, optic nerve, and optic chiasm.

Three-dimensional conformal radiation therapy. The development of modern three-dimensional conformal radiation therapy (3D-CRT) treatment planning techniques permits the design of treatment plans which match the high dose of radiation to the three-dimensional contour of the target volume while the dose to surrounding tissues is reduced to a minimum (Fig. 4.5). Conformal treatment planning not only decreases the risk of normal tissue injury, but also allows higher than traditional doses to be safely administered to selected patients with malignant gliomas[42] and other intracranial tumors.

Intensity-modulated radiation therapy (IMRT) recently has been introduced as an advanced form of 3D-CRT[43] (Fig. 4.6) to produce an additional refinement of dose configuration. Dose distributions generated in this fashion exquisitely conform to the shape of the target volume and sculpt around adjacent critical normal tissues. As with all focal RT techniques, great care and expertise are required to ensure accuracy of field alignment. Errors in treatment planning or delivery may reduce the efficacy or increase the toxicity to the normal brain.[44]

Stereotactic radiosurgery is a technique for delivering highly focal, external irradiation to a clearly defined small target[45] (Fig. 4.7). It requires the use of a stereotactic frame, identical to that used for neurosurgery, to precisely localize the tumor within the intracranial cavity. Image-guided robotic radiosurgery may eliminate the need for fixing the head in a stereotactic frame.[46] Multiple radiation beams intersect at one (or sometimes more) point(s), known as isocenters, within the skull after entering through numerous points or arcs distributed over the head. The technique delivers a high radiation dose to an intracranial target in a single session without delivering

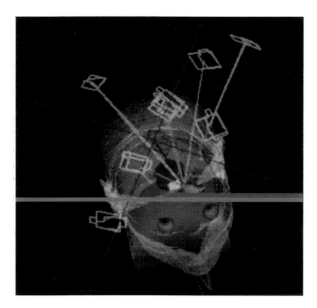

Figure 4.7
The concept of radiosurgery. Multiple beams are aimed at the tumor from several angles and the normal brain receives only a small amount of radiation. Maximal radiation can be delivered to the tumor.

significant radiation to adjacent normal tissues. To maintain a steep dose gradient at the edges of the field, the target volume must be small. Furthermore, because the volume is limited, the application of radiation in effective single doses is restricted to lesions 4 cm or less in diameter. Stereotactic radiosurgery originally found its greatest usefulness in treating small vascular malformations in the brain, but it is now being widely used to treat metastatic tumors, meningiomas, acoustic neuromas, pituitary adenomas and other relatively small tumors (see appropriate chapters).

Stereotactic radiosurgery by Gamma Knife[47] uses 201 cobalt-60 sources positioned such that the long axis of each source is oriented along the radius of a sphere and aimed precisely at the central point of the unit. Some sources may be selectively blocked to alter the shape of the dose distribution. Radiosurgery by linear accelerator[48]

(Fig. 4.7) requires rotation of the gantry, the couch, or both. In either approach, a single large radiation fraction is delivered to the pathologic tissue. For larger tumors, micro-Multileaf Collimators provide superior dose distributions for the linear accelerator compared to the Gamma Knife, eliminating the need for multiple overlapping isocenters, which leads to dose inhomogeneity and an increased risk of morbidity. The amount of radiation that most normal tissue receives is minimal, except to the area immediately surrounding the tumor. This is a particular problem when the tumor abuts the brainstem or optic nerve. Calculations of late effects on normal tissue relative to fraction size are available.[49]

Stereotactic radiotherapy. The terms 'stereotactic radiotherapy' and 'fractionated radiosurgery' refer to several fractions delivered stereotactically, allowing for a larger total dose to the pathologic tissue with minimal exposure to surrounding brain.[50] Stereotactic radiotherapy combines the focal advantages of radiosurgery with the radiobiological advantage of fractionation. Fractionation improves the therapeutic ratio, allowing larger tumors and those located within or near critical intracranial structures to be treated. Fractionated stereotactic radiotherapy is accomplished using head frames that can be relocalized daily in a non-invasive, reproducible fashion. This approach is being applied to the treatment of malignant gliomas, craniopharyngiomas, pituitary adenomas, and small tumors of the optic tracts, and as a boost for medulloblastomas.[51] Recent reports have suggested that fractionated radiosurgery is superior in some instances to single-dose radiosurgery.

Interstitial brachytherapy. The surgical implantation of radiation isotopes into a brain tumor is called brachytherapy (from Greek for 'short').[52] This conformal technique allows maximal radiation to the tumor, while surrounding tissues receive considerably lower doses. This approach has been applied to the treatment of newly diagnosed and recurrent malignant gliomas in the USA and has been used in Europe for low-grade gliomas arising in functionally critical areas of the brain.[52] Because of the requirement for high-activity sources for malignant brain tumors, stereotactic techniques have been devised to place afterloading catheters that are removed after the prescribed dose has been delivered. Controlled trials using high-activity iodine-125 sources plus external beam irradiation for high-grade gliomas have failed to show efficacy over external beam irradiation alone.[53] Other radioisotope sources such as iridium-192 have also been used but less frequently. In some instances, interstitial radiation has been coupled with hyperthermia for the treatment of gliomas.[54] Low-activity iodine-125 sources have been implanted directly into the tumor bed as an intraoperative boost in patients with meningiomas and gliomas and as retreatment for patients with previously resected skull base tumors.

Experimental approaches in radiation therapy

As with surgery, recent developments in radiation therapy have made that treatment modality both more effective for some tumors and less toxic to the brain (Table 4.6).

Heavy particle irradiation. Protons, neutrons and heavy charged particles have been used to treat CNS tumors.[55] For malignant gliomas, neutrons successfully eradicated tumor tissue, but caused diffuse white matter degeneration, probably because the relative biological effectiveness of neutrons was underestimated. No known dose of neutrons eradicates tumor without unacceptable injury to normal tissue.

Proton beams interact with the nuclei of atoms rather than their orbital electrons. Like conventional radiation, protons are sparsely ionizing as they enter tissue. However, they become more densely ionizing as they decelerate in tissue, whereupon the dose deposited reaches a sharp maximum, after which it falls to zero. The region of the sharp rise and fall in dose is called the Bragg peak, allowing large doses of radiation to be deposited in one area while dramatically sparing adjacent tissues. Because of this feature, protons and heavy charged particles such as helium ions, which behave in a similar fashion, have been used for radiosurgery as well as to deliver fractionated treatments. The depth of penetration can be controlled by varying beam energy or by placing brass or plastic absorbing material in the beam path. Charged particle beams can be made to stop in front of a critical structure, and in combination with other lateral or oblique beams, can be wrapped around a critical structure.[56] This form of radiation is ideally suited for the treatment of skull-base tumors such as meningiomas, chordomas and low-grade chondrosarcomas that are located adjacent to critical structures such as the optic nerves, chiasm, and brainstem. Pituitary adenomas and choroidal melanomas are also treated with this modality. Note that the biological properties of protons are similar to those of X-rays and that it is only the physical dose distribution that provides an advantage over conventional photon radiotherapy.

Boron neutron capture therapy (BNCT). This technique has been utilized off and on for over 50 years. It has gained renewed prominence, in part because it is theoretically so satisfying and in part because new techniques for delivery of boronated agents have been developed. The patient is injected with a boron-10-containing compound that, because of blood–brain barrier disruption, finds its way to the tumor but not to normal brain. The tumor is then irradiated with low-energy epithermal neutrons. The boronated compound captures the neutron, releasing an α-particle, which travels only a short distance, approximately the diameter of a cell. In theory, if the boron is within the cell, the α-particle should destroy no more than the cell itself. The procedure is being used to treat gliomas and other brain tumors but is still experimental.[57,58] This approach cannot reach microscopic disease that resides behind the blood–brain barrier. The problem of getting sufficient quantity of the boronated compound into the tumor[59] may be helped by the use of blood–brain barrier opening, but this will also expose normal brain.

Chemical modifiers of the radiation response
Radiosensitizers. Oxygen assists in the DNA damage induced by radiation. Hypoxia protects cells from the effects of low-LET radiation (X-rays). The radiation dose must be increased by a factor of three to obtain in hypoxic cells the same effect achieved in cells that are fully oxygenated. Even when only 2–3% of such resistant cells are present, a two-fold increment in radiation dose may be required to completely eradicate a tumor. The radioresistance of glioblastoma multiforme may, in part, be due to the presence of radiobiologically hypoxic but viable tumor cells within necrotic areas.

Nitroimidazoles are electron-affinic compounds that mimic oxygen in damaging DNA by free radicals. They are ineffective in the presence of oxygen. Unfortunately, no survival improvement was observed in malignant glioma patients receiving the most extensively tested compound, misonidazole, along with radiation in any of the dose-fractionation or drug schedules tested.

Halogenated pyrimidine analogs are radiosensitizers that become incorporated into the DNA of dividing cells because of their similarity to the DNA precursor, thymidine;[60] they enhance the number of DNA strand breaks by dissociating hydrogen atoms from adjacent deoxyribose moieties.

Radiosensitization appears to be directly related to an increased production of unrepaired double-strand breaks in drug-exposed cells. Sensitizer enhancement ratios of 1.5–3 have been observed, and the degree of enhancement is dependent on the percentage of thymidine replaced. Two analogs, bromodeoxyuridine (BrdU) and iododeoxyuridine (IdU), have been tested in patients with malignant gliomas and in brain metastases. These studies have not demonstrated an improvement in outcome.[37] Further, tumor biopsies obtained in some patients showed relatively low levels of drug incorporation.

Motexafin gadolinium may enhance radiation therapy of brain metastases.[61] Trials in primary brain tumors are underway.

The Herpes thymidine kinase gene and a dominant-negative epidermal growth factor receptor may also be radiosensitizers.[62,63]

Radioprotectors. Because the limiting factor in radiating brain tumors is toxicity to normal brain, a number of attempts have been made to find substances that protect normal brain against the effects of radiation but do not affect tumor tissue. Agents containing sulfhydryl groups will help return a free radical to its normal state. Omega fatty acids and bioflavonoids may be protective.[64] Some thiophosphate compounds such as amifostine (WR2721), when transformed by enzymes inside the living cell, do give some protection but have not yet been shown to be clinically effective. In cell culture experiments, neurons are protected against damaging effects of radiation by the additional presence of astrocytes as well as by free-radical scavengers.[65] However, clinical efficacy has not been demonstrated for any putative radioprotectors.[66]

Radiation toxicity

The goal of RT is to cause as much damage to the tumor with as little damage to the nervous system as possible (Fig. 4.8). Several isoeffect formulas exist to calculate the sensitivity of normal brain to different radiation time–dose-fractionation schemes.[67] These formulas consider total radiation dose, dose per fraction and, to a lesser extent, total treatment time; they indicate that normal brain tissue can tolerate about 60 Gy of radiation delivered in 1.8–2.0 Gy fractions. However, CNS damage from radiation depends not only on total radiation dose, dose per fraction and, to a lesser extent, overall treatment time, but also on additional factors, most of which depend on the host (Table 4.7).

The volume of tissue irradiated is important. Whole-brain radiation is considerably more likely to cause toxicity than partial brain radiation or conformal field radiation. Host factors also play a role. Both the developing (under age 3) and the elderly (over age 60) brain are more susceptible to radiation than the brain of a young adult. For example, in some studies, prophylactic whole-brain RT for leukemia affects the IQ of children under 5, but not those older. Thus, special attempts should be made to avoid RT in infants and children, using chemotherapy to delay radiation as long as possible. Genetic factors may also play a role. Certain familial disorders,

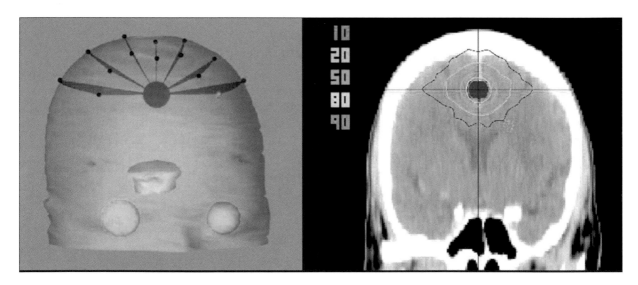

Figure 4.8
Three-dimensionally reconstructed anterior view of a patient showing the placement of seven lateral and superior arcs used for stereotactic radiosurgery of a small midline lesion (left). The brainstem (yellow) and eyes (green) have been delineated for geometrical perspective and to allow the determination of dose to these critical structures. A coronal CT image (right) shows the dose distribution through the center of the target volume for the radiosurgery plan. The prescription level is the 80% isodose line (shown in yellow).

Radiation factors	Host and other factors
Dose per fraction	Age
Total dose	Sex
Total duration of therapy	Genetic predisposition
Volume of tissue irradiated	Pre-existing nervous system disease
Energy of radiation	Infection
	Systemic disease (e.g. hypertension, diabetes, hypoxia)
	Chemotherapy
	Environment (e.g. smoking)

Table 4.7
Risk factors for CNS radiation damage.

particularly those associated with defects in DNA repair, cause marked photosensitivity leading to skin tumors. These and other genetic defects may also cause increased sensitivity to RT. Patients with pre-existing nervous system disease are often more sensitive to radiation. Patients mistakenly given RT for demyelinating lesions appear to be inordinately sensitive.[68] Hypertension and cerebral atherosclerosis may also be risk factors. Hypoxia promotes radiation-induced blood–brain barrier disruption.[69] RT and chemotherapy may be synergistic or at least additive in causing CNS toxicity. This appears to be particularly important in patients treated with chemotherapy and RT for primary CNS lymphoma (Chapter 11). Timing may also be important; some studies suggest that chemotherapy given before RT is safer than that given with or after RT, perhaps because RT disrupts the blood–brain barrier, allowing neurotoxic amounts of chemotherapy to enter.

The mechanism(s) by which the brain is damaged is controversial. Three hypotheses, not necessarily mutually exclusive, have been proposed. The first is that ionizing radiation directly damages nervous system cells. Because RT-induced nervous system damage predominantly affects white matter, glial cells, particularly oligodendroglial, and Schwann cells have been proposed as the most vulnerable. Also, because most neurons are post-mitotic, they are less susceptible to RT damage, although either apoptosis or DNA damage may lead to neuronal dysfunction or death. Radiation damage directed at white matter causes a leukoencephalopathy. Typical is the diffuse white matter destruction seen after whole-brain radiation. Some chemotherapeutic agents appear to exacerbate this type of damage in patients who have received doses of radiation not usually sufficient to cause such damage.

The second mechanism proposed is that RT damages vascular endothelium.[70] Hopewell and Wright[71] postulate that after RT has killed many capillary endothelial cells, a few localized clones survive at irregular locations along the vessel. These clones multiply, leading to focal luminal constrictions and eventually to vascular occlusion. The result is ischemia and necrosis of neural tissue. In this process, luminal occlusion is due to endothelial proliferation; intraluminal clotting plays no role. This hypothesis suffers from the fact that, although vascular occlusions occur in areas of radiation necrosis, the degree of tissue damage is usually greater than can be explained by the degree of vascular insufficiency.

Table 4.8
Cerebral radiation injury.

Designation	Time after RT	Clinical findings	Pathogenesis	Outcome
Acute	Immediate (minutes to hours)	Headache, vomiting, neurologic signs	Increased intracranial pressure	Recovery (usually) with steroids
Early-delayed	4–16 weeks	Somnolence, increased focal signs, worsening MR scan	Demyelination, possibly cerebral edema	Recovery, responds to steroids
Late-delayed	Months to years	Focal signs	Brain necrosis	Responds to steroids
Necrosis	Months to years	MR enhancement, memory loss	Possibly vascular	Surgical removal and steroids
Atrophy, hydrocephalus	Months to years	Dementia, gait ataxia, incontinence, MR atrophy, hydrocephalus, leukoencephalopathy	Cellular loss, demyelination, possibly spongiosis of white matter	Modest response to shunting in some cases
Hemorrhage	Years	Focal signs	Telangiectasia	Partial recovery
Infarction	Years	Focal signs	Cerebral/carotid atherosclerosis	Variable
Encephalopathy	Years	Confusion, disorientation	Hypothyroidism	Recovery with hormone replacement
Neoplasm	Years	Focal signs	RT-induced neoplasm	Usually poor

The third mechanism, proposed by Lampert et al,[72] suggests that damaged glial cells release antigens identified as foreign by the immune system. An immune response leads to both the necrosis and vascular changes of a hypersensitivity reaction. Almost no direct evidence exists for this third hypothesis, although in one patient a focal vasculitis in an irradiated area of brain was associated with circulating immune complexes. Thus, the exact cause of radiation damage to the peripheral and central nervous systems is still unknown, although, at least in experimental animals, lower total RT doses appear to cause neurotoxicity via the endothelial cells, and higher doses via glial cells.

Whatever the mechanism, when radiation injury follows focal radiation for treatment of a brain tumor, the necrosis is focal and the signs and symptoms often mimic those of the original brain tumor. The MR scan may also appear similar, making it difficult to distinguish recurrent tumor from radiation necrosis. The differential diagnosis was discussed in Chapter 3.

Radiation injury can occur at almost any time, from seconds to years after the therapy is delivered. Side-effects can be divided into those that are acute, usually observed within the first few days, early-delayed, seen within 4 weeks to 4 months following RT, or late-delayed, many months to many years after RT is completed. Late-delayed RT-induced brain dysfunction can take several forms (Table 4.8) and is the most important form of RT injury, because it is irreversible and often progressive.

Acute encephalopathy

This disorder usually follows large fractions (more than 300 cGy) delivered to a large volume of brain in patients with increased intracranial pressure from a brain tumor. Because such large doses are rarely used, acute RT toxicity is uncommon; however, absence of corticosteroid treatment increases the risk. Acute effects, usually mild, also follow stereotactic radiotherapy and radiosurgery. Immediately or within a few hours following treatment, susceptible patients develop headache, nausea, vomiting, somnolence, fever, and worsening of pre-existing neurologic symptoms. In rare instances, the disorder culminates in cerebral herniation and death. Acute encephalopathy usually follows the first radiation dose and becomes progressively less severe with each ensuing fraction. A mild form of the disorder is common and consists of headache and nausea immediately following radiation. The pathogenesis of acute encephalopathy is probably disruption of the blood–brain barrier by ionizing radiation, causing increased cerebral edema and a rise in intracranial pressure. Evidence indicates that a single dose of 300 Gy to the brain in an experimental animal causes substantial disruption of the blood–brain barrier if measured 2 h after the radiation. The P-glycoprotein level, a marker of blood–brain barrier function, decreased to 60% of control within 5 days of one dose of 25 Gy to an experimental animal.[73]

These observations carry two clinical messages. First, patients harboring large brain tumors, particularly tumors causing signs of increased intracranial pressure, should probably be treated with fractions no larger than 2.0 Gy. Second, these patients should be protected with corticosteroids such as dexamethasone, 8–16 mg/24 h, or more, if increased intracranial pressure is symptomatic. The drugs should be administered for at least 48–72 h prior to initiating RT. Steroids are not required if the RT portal and the tumor are small.

Early-delayed encephalopathy

This disorder usually begins 4 weeks to 4 months after RT. Early-delayed symptoms do not predict or predispose to later complications. The symptoms of early-delayed encephalopathy simulate tumor progression. The patient develops headache, lethargy, and worsening or reappearance of the original neurologic symptoms. Alternatively, patients may develop memory deficits.[74] The disorder usually peaks 2 months after RT and resolves within 6 months. The symptoms suggest tumor progression but improve spontaneously over the ensuing 4 months. MR or CT scans reveal an increase in the contrast-enhancing area and surrounding edema. In some instances, new areas of contrast enhancement appear. Both clinical and radiologic changes resolve spontaneously over the ensuing months, hastened by corticosteroids. Radiosurgery may also cause an early-delayed encephalopathy, usually characterized by MR scans showing an increased enhancing area, suggesting an increase in tumor volume and more hyperintensity around the tumor, suggesting brain edema. These changes usually appear 3–12 months after treatment and resolve in 5–7 months. They may be accompanied by loss of enhancement in the center of the tumor, suggesting necrosis.

The clinical and scan findings of early-delayed radiation encephalopathy can follow conventional external beam RT or radiosurgery. The clinical implication is that failure of the patient or the scan to improve, or even a worsening within 2 or 3 months of RT, does not mean that the therapy has failed. The usual sequence is that the scan appears somewhat improved immediately at the end of RT and then worsens in the several months following radiation, only to improve once again. The patient should be supported with corticosteroids, with close follow-up examinations and scanning. Because an MRI cannot distinguish either early or late changes due to radiation from those due to residual or recurrent tumor, a number of non-invasive tests have been used in an attempt to make that distinction (Chapter 3). These have included PET and SPECT scanning as well as MRS. However, it is not clear that these tests do make this distinction in early-delayed radiation encephalopathy.

The pathogenesis of early-delayed encephalopathy is believed to be demyelination resulting from transient damage to oligodendroglia with the subsequent breakdown of myelin sheaths. The best evidence supporting this hypothesis comes from pathologic studies in patients with early-delayed brainstem encephalopathy, in whom confluent areas of demyelination with varying degrees of axonal loss were found in areas receiving the radiation. Associated with this is the loss of oligodendrocytes and the occurrence of abnormal, often multinucleated, giant astrocytes. The timing of the appearance and resolution of symptoms tends to parallel the known turnover of myelin. Other pathologic changes include perivenous inflammatory infiltrates. Necrosis and vascular changes are absent.

Late-delayed encephalopathy

Late-delayed radiation damage to the brain can take several forms (Fig. 4.9) (see Table 4.8).

Radiation necrosis

Radiation necrosis usually begins 1–2 years after RT is completed but can start as early as 3 months after treatment or be delayed for several years.[75,76] The symptoms generally recapitulate those of the brain tumor, leading the physician to suspect tumor recurrence. Rarely, new focal signs indicate a lesion distant from the original lesion. The MRI may show increased contrast enhancement at the original tumor site or, less frequently, at a remote site,[77] but within the radiation portal. Neither the clinical symptoms nor CT or MR scans distinguish tumor recurrence from necrosis. PET scan measuring glucose consumption shows hypometabolism in areas of necrosis and hypermetabolism in areas containing tumor, but is not sufficiently sensitive to unequivocally establish a diagnosis.[78] SPECT and MRS may be somewhat better than glucose PET, although they are not infallible. Our experience has been that many patients, particularly those treated for glioma, have a mixture of radiation necrosis and tumor.

Histologically, the typical radiation necrosis lesion consists of coagulative necrosis in the white matter with relative sparing of the overlying cortex and deep gray matter. Microscopically, striking abnormalities are found in blood vessels, with hyalinized thickening and fibrinoid necrosis often associated with vascular thrombosis, hemorrhage, and accumulated perivascular fibrinoid material. In less severely affected areas, demyelination is noted with a loss of oligodendrocytes, variable axonal loss, axonal swellings, dystrophic calcifications, fibrillary gliosis, and scattered perivascular infiltrates and mononuclear cells. Telangiectatic vessels also form there and may be responsible for late hemorrhages.

Radiation necrosis is usually treated by surgical resection. Most patients respond transiently to steroids but relapse when steroids

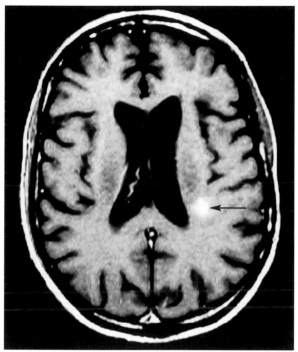

Figure 4.9
A new lesion appearing 14 years post-radiation therapy. This man developed symptoms of a right frontal brain tumor, which was treated surgically and with radiation therapy. The radiation included 40 Gy of whole-brain radiation with a 20 Gy boost to the right frontal area. Sixteen years later, the patient is asymptomatic, working full-time as a physician. Fourteen years after the radiation therapy, a small contrast-enhancing asymptomatic lesion appeared in the posterior frontal area on the left (arrow). This lesion, probably representing a radiation-induced vascular abnormality, is asymptomatic and has not progressed over the ensuing 2 years.

Atrophy, hydrocephalus

A more frequent consequence of brain radiation than radiation necrosis is brain atrophy. If substantial volumes of brain tissue are irradiated, most patients develop MRI-documented evidence of enlarged cerebral sulci and ventriculomegaly. In addition, MR scans may reveal hyperintensity, most marked in cerebral white matter around the ventricles on the T2-weighted or fast fluid-attenuated inversion recovers (FLAIR) images; hypodensity is noted on the CT scan. These changes may worsen over time. Both atrophy and white matter abnormalities are usually clear-cut by 1 year following RT, but occasionally they may become obvious within 2 or 3 months after RT is completed. They can persist or progress thereafter. The symptoms are those of a 'subcortical dementia'[79] with memory loss, apathy and slowed cognitive responses. Some patients also have gait abnormalities suggesting gait apraxia, and urinary urgency followed by incontinence. The triad of gait difficulties, incontinence and dementia suggest the syndrome of normal pressure hydrocephalus.[80] If the scan also suggests hydrocephalus, i.e. if ventricular dilatation is greater than cortical atrophy, the patient may respond at least temporarily to ventricular shunting. The gait disturbance and incontinence respond best to shunting, whereas the memory impairment usually does not respond. Cerebral atrophy is untreatable.

Virtually all patients in whom a substantial portion of the brain is irradiated to treat brain tumors complain of memory loss resembling that experienced by most older people (e.g., forgetting names, telephone numbers, appointments, and recent events but remembering remote events well). The memory loss may even prevent the individual from returning to gainful employment. Recent analysis of long-term survivors of RT

are discontinued, although reports have described prolonged responses after steroid therapy without surgery. Other suggested treatments presupposing a vascular mechanism have included aspirin and anticoagulation, but we have not found them to be effective.

for glioma indicate that 60% were employed at jobs comparable to those they held before receiving RT.[81] In a minority of patients, memory loss progresses and affects other cognitive functions, leading to a more severe dementia.

In our experience, many of our patients complain of two additional symptoms. The first is a feeling of being cold. Characteristically, the patients require more blankets than the spouse, often a reversal of the pre-illness situation. The patients also require more clothing when outdoors than previously. Endocrinological workup does not reveal abnormalities in thyroid function, and the symptoms do not respond to treatment with thyroid hormones. Another frequent symptom is loss of libido or impotence. Patients rarely complain of this symptom but spouses are often quite distressed. Some male patients are not impotent but simply indifferent to sexual activity. It is useful to probe patients and their spouses for the above symptoms, because simply knowing they are common often relieves anxiety. In addition, sildenafil can be useful for some patients with impotence.

Vasculopathy

Radiation therapy decreases microvascular density in tumor and in surrounding normal brain.[82] Telangiectasias sometimes develop that can result in cerebral hemorrhage.[70] Occlusive vasculopathy with subsequent Moya-Moya vessel formation may follow RT to optic gliomas in patients with neurofibromatosis type 1.[80]

Endocrine dysfunction

Hypothyroidism, either primary from cervical irradiation or secondary from cranial irradiation, pituitary failure and retarded bone growth often follow RT, especially when delivered to the entire neuraxis. Growth hormone failure is a particular problem in children with brain tumors.[84]

Principles of chemotherapy

Introduction

Chemotherapeutic agents have been disappointing in the treatment of most brain tumors.[85,86] Exceptions include cerebral germinomas, medulloblastomas, primary lymphomas of the nervous system and some oligodendrogliomas. The role of chemotherapy in the management of astrocytomas is controversial, although most believe it has a small role to play in improving survival in some patients. No adequate chemotherapeutic agents have been developed for meningiomas, acoustic neuromas and most pituitary adenomas.

Certain principles of chemotherapy are believed to apply to all cancers. These are listed in Table 4.9 and discussed in the paragraphs below.

Many of these concepts have been developed by treating tumors in experimental animals and then testing the concepts in humans with systemic cancers, such as carcinoma of the breast. How

Table 4.9
Basic concepts in cancer chemotherapy.

- Chemotherapeutic agents kill only a percentage of cancer cells
- Some drugs kill only dividing cells
- Multiple drugs with differing sites of action are better than a single drug
- High doses are better than low doses

they apply to intracranial tumors is uncertain. The underlying concept is that most tumors are monoclonal, i.e. they arise from a single cell. However, because of genetic instability, as the tumor grows it becomes progressively more heterogeneous, some of the cells having developed intrinsic resistance to some chemotherapeutic agents. Furthermore, although small tumors tend to grow exponentially with virtually all of the cells dividing, as the tumor gets larger, a number of cells enter a quiescent phase, making them less susceptible to many chemotherapeutic agents. In addition, rapidly growing tumors may outstrip their blood supply, leaving cells in relatively ischemic areas less exposed to chemotherapeutic agents and also putting the ischemic cells into a more quiescent phase. When a cancer is exposed to sublethal doses of a chemotherapeutic agent, resistance to further doses of that drug develops. These cells, along with the intrinsically resistant cells, lead to rapid regrowth and restoration of the tumor, now more resistant to treatment than it was initially. Thus, for most cancer therapy, oncologists use the largest possible doses of multiple chemotherapeutic agents. (This is the rationale for high-dose chemotherapy with bone marrow or stem cell rescue, so-called bone marrow transplant protocols.) Each agent should have a different mechanism of action, including cell cycle-specific drugs (drugs which only kill dividing cells) and cell cycle-non-specific (drugs that directly damage DNA and are toxic to resting cells as well as dividing cells). Unfortunately, for most brain tumors, there is no compelling evidence that multiagent chemotherapy is superior to single agent chemotherapy or that dose intensity improves outcome.[87] Controlled trials by the Brain Tumor Study Group (BTSG) failed to demonstrate superiority of multi-agent chemotherapy over 1,3-bischloro-(2-chloroethyl)-7-nitrosourea (BCNU) alone.[88] In the treatment of malignant glioma, one study suggests that multiagent chemotherapy, PCV [procarbazine,

vincristine and 1-(2-chloroethyl)-3-cyclohexyl-1-nitrosourea (CCNU)] may be superior to BCNU for anaplastic astrocytomas but not glioblastoma, but this occurred in a subgroup analysis of an essentially negative study. A recent review of RTOG protocols did not show a survival benefit of PCV over BCNU for patients with anaplastic astrocytoma.[89] A randomized trial from England failed to demonstrate an advantage in survival by using PCV with RT over RT alone,[90] although both randomized trials and a meta-analysis from the US demonstrate that BCNU increases survival in high-grade glioma patients (Chapter 5).[91] Even in chemosensitive tumors such as oligodendroglioma and primary CNS lymphoma, there is no evidence to demonstrate the superiority of multiagent over single agent chemotherapy (BCNU in the former, methotrexate in the latter).[87] Germinomas (Chapter 8) may be an exception, where multiagent therapy does appear to be efficacious.

Table 4.10 classifies antineoplastic drugs and gives some examples of drugs that have been used to treat brain tumors. Individual drugs are considered in the paragraphs below. Recent reviews describe the neurotoxicity of these and a number of other drugs not included in this section.[92]

Problems unique to intracranial tumors

Table 4.11 lists some of the problems specific to the chemotherapy of intracranial tumors.

Many oncologists overrate the blood–brain barrier as a problem for chemotherapy of brain tumors. Many intracranial tumors, including meningiomas, schwannomas, most pineal region tumors and anterior pituitary tumors, do not possess a blood–brain barrier. In other tumors such as metastases and high-grade gliomas, disruption of the blood–brain barrier is often sufficient for water-soluble chemotherapeutic agents to reach tumors in substantial

Table 4.10
Classification of
antineoplastic
drugs.

Class	Examples
• Alkylating agents	Platinum-based, e.g. cisplatin, carboplatin
	Nitrosoureas, e.g. carmustine (BCNU), lomustine (CCNU)
	Temozolomide
• Antibiotics	Doxorubicin
	Bleomycin
	Anthracyclines e.g. doxorubricin
• Antimetabolites	Cytarabine
	5-Fluorouracil
	Methotrexate
• Plant alkaloids	Vincristine
	Epipodophyllotoxins, e.g. etoposide, teniposide
	Taxanes, e.g. paclitaxel
• Miscellaneous	Suramin
	Hydroxyurea
	Procarbazine

Table 4.11
Chemotherapy of intracranial tumors: problems
specific to location.

- Blood–brain barrier
- Paucity of lymphatics
- Heterogeneity of gliomas
- Intrinsic resistance
- Low therapeutic/toxic ratio

concentrations. However, for certain tumors, the blood–brain barrier does prevent entry of water-soluble chemotherapeutic agents. Examples include low-grade gliomas in which the blood–brain barrier is intact, and higher-grade gliomas that disrupt the blood–brain barrier in the bulk of the tumor, but not the edge where tumor infiltrates normal tissue. The blood–brain barrier is relatively or completely intact at the infiltrating margins of the tumor. Perhaps the most striking example is primary lymphoma of the nervous system. The patient usually presents with one or multiple contrast-enhancing lesions, but there is also widespread infiltration of tumor that does not contrast enhance. Standard doses of water-soluble agents may eliminate the area(s) of contrast enhancement, only to have the tumor rapidly appear elsewhere in the brain, where it had been sequestered behind the blood–brain barrier.

A number of attempts have been made to circumvent the blood–brain barrier in the treatment of brain tumors. These have included opening the blood–brain barrier using a hyperosmolar agent such as intra-arterial mannitol or Cereport, a bradykinin analog.[93] The latter is said to open the blood–brain barrier more in tumors than in normal brain. Opening of the blood–brain barrier has been used in the treatment of primary CNS lymphomas (Chapter 11); there is as yet no evidence that barrier opening is superior to chemotherapy without barrier opening. Furthermore, opening the blood–brain barrier, at least with hyperosmolar agents, results in a greater proportionate increase of drug entry into normal brain than into brain tumor. Osmotic blood–brain barrier opening is influenced by the choice of anesthesia; propofol/N_2O with hypercarbia is optimal.[94]

Other approaches have attempted to deliver more chemotherapy to the tumor and less to normal tissue. These include intra-arterial infusions,[95] intratumoral injections using catheters, implanting drug-impregnated wafers[96] or microspheres,[97] and drugs altered to cross the blood–brain barrier.[98,99] None has yet proved more effective or less toxic than conventional routes of administration, and wafer implantation has been reported to result in postoperative complications, including infection and poor wound healing.[100]

The best drugs for the treatment of infiltrating gliomas have proved to be the nitrosoureas (and perhaps temozolomide), which are lipid-soluble and thus not affected by the blood–brain barrier. Nevertheless, despite their ability to reach the entire tumor, they have not proved dramatically effective. On the other hand, methotrexate, which does not easily cross the blood–brain barrier, has been shown, when given in very high doses, to be effective for primary lymphomas of the nervous system, even though it is not a major agent for the treatment of comparable systemic lymphomas.

Major problems with chemotherapy for most brain tumors include: (1) intrinsic resistance to most chemotherapeutic agents,[101,102] probably because of heterogeneity of the higher grade tumors; (2) rapid development of resistance to chemotherapeutic agents; and (3) susceptibility only to doses of chemotherapeutic agents that are unacceptably toxic both to the normal brain and the tissues outside the CNS. Thus, extremely high-dose BCNU with bone marrow rescue given for the treatment of malignant gliomas is successful in eradicating the tumor, but causes severe encephalopathy that eventually kills the patient. Furthermore, there is little evidence that increasing the dose of standard chemotherapeutic agents

within an acceptable range of toxicity is more effective than standard doses.

Other problems unique to intracranial tumors include the fact that a deficient lymphatic system prevents the easy removal of detritus caused by effective chemotherapy from the brain. Necrotic tissue is not cleared easily from the brain and may form a nidus for further edema and worsening of neurologic symptoms. This is one reason why radiation necrosis causes symptoms.

Even the time-honored concept that a small tumor responds better than a big tumor does not appear to apply to many primary brain tumors, perhaps because of their intrinsic resistance. In the treatment of gliomas, current evidence suggests that there is little or no advantage to treating patients in the adjuvant setting with chemotherapy over waiting for a recurrence and then treating. This probably reflects the intrinsic resistance of these tumors to the chemotherapeutic agents that are currently available.

Chemotherapy directed at intracranial tumors can be given by a number of routes of administration. The most common is systemic administration, either oral or intravenous. The advantage of systemic administration is that the agents are easy to administer. The disadvantages include the fact that some drugs are unable to cross the blood–brain barrier easily and that much of the agent reaches and damages tissues other than the tumor. The second route of administration is local. Most intrinsic brain tumors, unlike systemic tumors, do not metastasize, but the vast majority recur at the original site.[42] Accordingly, gliomas should be ideal for focal therapy. Focal therapy has the advantage not only of preventing systemic toxicity, but also of circumventing the blood–brain barrier and getting higher doses of a chemotherapeutic agent to the tumor than one could get by systemic administration. Techniques of local therapy include intra-arterial injection,[103] usually in the carotid artery or one of its branches, intrathecal injection, into the subarachnoid space by lumbar puncture or via an intraventricular cannula, or intratumoral injection. Intra-arterial injection has been compared in a controlled trial with intravenous injection of carmustine and not found to be superior but to increase neurotoxicity.[104] Intrathecal injection may treat leptomeningeal tumor but cannot reach intrinsic tumors of the brain in sufficient concentrations to be effective. Several studies are now investigating the efficacy of intratumoral injection either by the implantation of wafers that slowly release chemotherapeutic agents or by single or repeated injections through an implanted cannula. Wafers impregnated with BCNU implanted in the tumor bed appear to give longer survival than placebo implantation for recurrent gliomas, but the increased survival was only 2 months, so that the advantage, if any, is modest.[96] The advantage of local therapy is that it saves normal tissues from the side-effects of the chemotherapeutic agent. The disadvantage is that it often requires a surgical procedure. Combinations of systemic and local therapy include opening the blood–brain barrier by intra-arterial injection of various substances, followed by either intra-arterial or systemic chemotherapy.

The timing of chemotherapy with respect to radiation is important but controversial. On the one hand, evidence suggests that many chemotherapeutic agents act as radiation sensitizers. Theoretically, if such agents are given along with radiation therapy, the effect will be better than if they are given independently. However, there is no evidence demonstrating enhanced efficacy against brain tumors when chemotherapy and RT are given together than when they are used sequentially. Furthermore, there is some evidence that chemotherapeutic agents such as cisplatin may induce radiation resistance.[105] Chemotherapy given prior to RT

may have an advantage in that the vascular supply to the tumor is better than it is after radiation. In addition, by giving chemotherapy first, one can determine if the agents are effective and, if so, continue using them after RT. If they are ineffective, they can be abandoned. There is also some evidence, at least for methotrexate, that chemotherapy given prior to radiation is less neurotoxic than when it follows radiation. Alternatively, chemotherapy following radiation may encounter a blood–brain barrier that has been partially disrupted by the radiation. This may allow more water-soluble drug to enter both the tumor and, unfortunately, the normal brain. Given all of these considerations, it is not yet clear what the optimal sequence of radiation and chemotherapy should be. We generally prefer to use RT, the more effective modality, first and follow with chemotherapy.

Specific chemotherapeutic agents

Table 4.12 lists some chemotherapeutic agents used for the treatment of brain tumors. Some of these are considered in the paragraphs below.

Alkylating agents

The alkylating agents, including the nitrosoureas, platinum compounds and procarbazine, are among the most widely used drugs for the treatment of brain tumors. Although cell cycle non-specific, they appear to be more active against rapidly dividing cells, probably because of the lesser time these cells have to repair DNA damage. By alkylating DNA bases, they cross-link DNA, resulting in single and double-strand breaks. The most widely used of the alkylating agents for the treatment of brain tumors are the nitrosoureas. Several nitrosoureas treat gliomas, including BCNU (carmustine), CCNU (lomustine), PCNU,

MeCCNU and ACNU [3-((4-amino-2-methyl-5-pyrimidinyl-methyl)-12(2-chloroethyl)-1-nitrosourea] and HeCCNU The drugs have been used in single agent and multiagent chemotherapeutic regimens, either adjuvantly after surgery and radiation, at relapse, or during radiation as radiation sensitizers. The nitrosoureas alkylate O-6-guanine in DNA. Substantial evidence indicates that patients whose tumors intrinsically express the repair enzyme guanine-6-methyltransferase are more resistant to the chemotherapeutic effects of nitrosoureas.[101] Inhibitors of the enzyme are

Table 4.12

Specific chemotherapeutic agents used for intracranial tumors.

Cytosine arabinoside (Ara-C)
Arazidinylbenzoquinone (AZQ)
1,3-bis(2-Chloroethyl)-1-nitrosourea (BCNU)
1-(2-Chloroethyl)-3-cyclohexyl-1-nitrosourea (CCNU)
Cisplatin
Carboplatin
Dianhydrogalacticol
Dibromodulcitol
Dacarbazine (DTIC)
Temozolomide
5-Fluorouracil
Hydroxyurea
Methyl-1-(2-chloroethyl)-3-cyclohexyl-1-nitrosourea (MeCCNU)
Misonidazole
Methotrexate
1-(2-Chloroethyl)-3-(2,6-dioxo-3-piper-idyl)-1-nitrosourea (PCNU)
Procarbazine
Vincristine
Teniposide
Etoposide (VP16)
Paclitaxel (Taxol)
Bromodeoxyuridine (BrdU)
Eflornithine
Irinotecan (CPT-11)

being used experimentally to try to increase tumor sensitivity to nitrosoureas and other chemotherapeutic agents.[106]

The major toxicities of nitrosoureas are bone marrow suppression and pulmonary fibrosis. The drugs are relatively non-neurotoxic. ACNU has been safely given intrathecally. However, high doses of nitrosoureas can cause encephalopathy. Retinal toxicity and encephalopathy were side-effects of an experimental program in which the drug was given intra-arterially to increase the dose delivered to the tumor.

Procarbazine rapidly crosses the blood–brain barrier. Its mechanism of action is not known, although it is believed to interfere with DNA synthesis. The drug has been widely used as part of conventional treatment of malignant gliomas. Encephalopathy and peripheral neuropathy have been reported, but rash and bone marrow suppression are the main side-effects. Because it is a weak monoamine oxidase inhibitor, patients are advised to avoid foods containing tyramine. Although the importance of this precaution is doubtful, monoamine oxidase inhibitors should be discontinued 2 weeks before starting procarbazine.

The platinum compounds, cisplatin and particularly carboplatin, have been used to treat a number of brain tumors. Cisplatin is neurotoxic (Table 4.13), but carboplatin is not. These drugs are efficacious against medulloblastomas and germinomas and although widely used in the treatment of gliomas, their role is not established. A preliminary report suggests that carboplatin in combination with an opening of the blood–brain barrier might be effective in glioma.[107]

Cyclophosphamide is a prodrug that must be metabolized in the liver to 4-hydroxyperoxycyclophosphamide to be active. The active agent has safely been given intrathecally for the treatment

Table 4.13
Neurotoxicity of cisplatin.

- **Common**
  - Peripheral neuropathy (large fiber, sensory)
  - Lhermitte's sign
  - Hearing loss (high frequency)
  - Tinnitus
- **Uncommon**
  - Encephalopathy
  - Visual loss
    Retinal toxicity
    Optic neuropathy
    Cortical blindness
  - Seizures
  - Cerebral herniation (hydration related)
  - Electrolyte imbalance (Ca++, Mg++, Na+, SIADH)
  - Vestibular toxicity
  - Autonomic neuropathy

SIADH = Syndrome of Inappropriate Antidiuretic Hormone Secretion

of leptomeningeal tumor. Cyclophosphamide has been used as part of multiagent chemotherapy for a number of intracranial tumors. It is relatively non-neurotoxic except at high doses, when it can cause lethargy, seizures or both. *Ifosfamide*, a related compound that also requires hydroxylation by liver, more commonly causes encephalopathy.

Thiotepa crosses the blood–brain barrier easily and has been used both intravenously and intrathecally for the treatment of brain tumors. High-dose thiotepa is used in some bone marrow rescue protocols, particularly for the treatment of anaplastic oligodendroglioma. The drug is not neurotoxic, although myelopathy has been reported in a few patients after intrathecal injection.

Dacarbazine (DTIC) and a related compound temozolomide are both cell cycle-non-specific alkylating agents that have been used for the treatment of CNS tumors. DTIC has been used to treat malignant meningiomas. Temozolomide is approved for treatment of malignant gliomas. Early enthusiastic reports suggesting a 50% response rate have not been borne out by more current data. However, temozolomide appears to be active in about 20% of patients with malignant glioma, about the same as the nitrosoureas. The fact that it is administered orally and is relatively nontoxic makes it appealing.[108] These drugs are marrow suppressive and occasionally cause encephalopathy but are basically non-neurotoxic. Hepatic veno-occlusive disease and necrosis have been reported.

Estramustine is an alkylating agent that crosses the blood–brain barrier poorly but has been reported to have some effect on malignant gliomas. It is not neurotoxic.

Diazaquine (AZQ) crosses the blood–brain barrier. The drug has been used to treat malignant gliomas and has been given intrathecally to treat leptomeningeal tumor. Its main toxicities are myelosuppression, nausea, anorexia, and skin discoloration.

Busulfan is a bifunctional alkylating agent that easily crosses the blood–brain barrier. It has been used to treat some malignant brain tumors, but does not appear to be effective. With high-dose therapy used to prepare children for bone marrow transplantation, seizures occur. At standard doses the drug is not neurotoxic.

Plant alkaloids

The plant alkaloids include: the vinca alkaloids, vincristine, vindesine, and vinblastine; podophyllins, including etoposide and teniposide; and the taxanes, paclitaxel and docetaxel. The drugs all bind to tubulin, the microtubular protein, but the antineoplastic mechanism of each is different.

The vinca alkaloids, because of their size, cross the blood–brain barrier poorly. They cause metaphase arrest by binding to tubulin during S-phase and thus are cell cycle specific. Vincristine is part of a common regimen for the treatment of malignant gliomas (PCV). The major side effect is a peripheral neuropathy, but myopathies, autonomic neuropathies, cranial neuropathies and central toxicity, including seizures and inappropriate secretion of antidiuretic hormone with hyponatremia, have been reported (Table 4.14).

The podophyllins are lipid-soluble compounds but do not cross the blood–brain barrier well, because of their size. They bind to tubulin and inhibit microtubular assembly, and thus are cell cycle specific, causing arrest in G_2. Etoposide is widely used for the treatment of gliomas and forms part of multiagent therapy for other brain tumors.[109] It has been given intrathecally without toxicity but can cause mild peripheral neuropathy when given systemically. Teniposide causes peripheral neuropathy less commonly.

The taxanes bind to tubulin, but instead of inhibiting polymerization, as do the vinca alkaloids, they stabilize and promote microtubular assembly. How this interaction causes cytotoxicity is not certain. The drugs have been used for the treatment of a number of brain tumors, particularly malignant gliomas, but their role is not yet established.[110] The taxanes can cause peripheral neuropathy and proximal weakness which is probably neuropathic as well.[111]

Antimetabolites

The antimetabolites are all cell cycle specific and are subdivided into the antifolates, including methotrexate, the cytidine analogs,

Table 4.14
Spectrum of vincristine neurotoxicity.

Toxic effect	Subacute (1 day to 2 weeks)	Intermediate (1 to 4 weeks)	Chronic (> 4 weeks)
Peripheral neuropathy	Depressed Achilles reflex, paresthesias	Other tendon reflexes depressed, paresthesias	Sensory loss, extensor weakness, especially foot-drop
Myopathy	Muscle pain, tenderness (especially quadriceps); jaw pain		
Autonomic neuropathy	Ileus with abdominal cramping, pain	Constipation, urinary hesitancy, impotence, orthostatic hypotension	
Cranial neuropathy (uncommon)			Optic atrophy; ptosis; VIth, VIIth, and VIIIth cranial nerve dysfunction; hoarseness; dysphagia
'Central' toxicity		Seizures, SIADH	

including cytarabine (Ara-C), the fluorinated pyrimidines, including 5-fluorouracil, the purine analogs, including 6-thioguanine, 6-mercaptopurine and cladribine, and a variety of other agents, including hydroxyurea.

Hydroxyurea inhibits ribonucleotide diphosphate reductase, an enzyme required in DNA synthesis. The drug crosses the blood–brain barrier readily and has been used as a radiosensitizer for the treatment of malignant gliomas, without substantial effect. It has also been used as a single agent in the treatment of recurrent meningiomas, also without significant effect. The drug causes mild nausea, anorexia, skin discoloration and myelosuppression but is not neurotoxic.

Methotrexate is a drug widely used in cancer chemotherapy but has limited use in the treatment of brain tumors, with the exception of primary CNS lymphoma. The drug is water-soluble and does not cross the blood–brain barrier well, but intravenous injection of very high doses (with folinic acid rescue) forces enough drug across the blood–brain and blood-CSF barriers to produce therapeutic levels within the CNS (Chapter 11). The drug binds reversibly to dihydrofolate reductase, thus blocking synthesis of tetrahydrofolate, reducing the folate pool and preventing thymidine and purine biosynthesis. The primary side-effects of the drugs are bone marrow suppression and gastrointestinal toxicity, but neurotoxicity is a significant problem (Table 4.15). The drug appears to be synergistic with brain irradiation in producing leukoencephalopathy. High doses of the drug occasionally cause a transient encephalopathy, and intrathecal injection can cause a myelopathy. Gene amplification of dihydrofolate reductase can result in over-production of the enzyme, leading to tumor resistance to methotrexate.

Cytarabine (Ara-C) is an S-phase cell cycle-specific drug that inhibits DNA polymerase-α, is incorporated into DNA and terminates DNA chain elongation. The drug does not cross the blood–brain barrier unless given in very high doses. However, because the enzyme that metabolizes the drug is present at very low levels in the CNS, the drug persists for an extended period. Cytarabine is not widely used for the treatment of brain tumors, with the exception of primary CNS lymphoma (Chapter 11). At very high doses, the drug can cause

Table 4.15
Methotrexate neurotoxicity.

Route of administration	Dose	Toxic effect
Oral or intravenous	Conventional	Leukoencephalopathy (if prior brain irradiation)
Intravenous	High-dose	Acute transient encephalopathy, chronic leukoencephalopathy
Intra-arterial	Conventional or high-dose	Hemorrhagic cerebral infarction, seizures
Intrathecal	Conventional	Acute aseptic meningitis, paraplegia, seizures, chronic leukoencephalopathy, cerebral atrophy, calcification

cerebellar degeneration, a peripheral neuropathy or an encephalopathy. A depo-preparation has been used to treat leptomeningeal tumors (Chapter 11).

5-Fluorouracil is a pyrimidine analog that interferes with DNA synthesis. It is not efficacious in the treatment of brain tumors, even though it crosses the blood–brain barrier well. The drug is generally non-neurotoxic, although high doses can cause encephalopathy or cerebellar degeneration. The major side-effects are stomatitis and diarrhea.

6-Mercaptopurine and 6-thioguanine are purine analogs that inhibit purine biosynthesis. They have been used to treat gliomas but are not widely used anymore. They cause myelosuppression but are not neurotoxic. They do not cross the blood–brain barrier easily.

Antineoplastic antibiotics

The antineoplastic antibiotics consist of the anthracyclines such as doxorubicin, and other agents such as mitomycin and bleomycin. Most are not used for the treatment of brain tumors, although a recent experimental protocol calls for direct injection of bleomycin into the tumor bed. The drugs are generally not neurotoxic, although bleomycin in combination with cisplatin has been reported to cause strokes and myocardial infarction. Doxorubicin is not neurotoxic when given by conventional routes, but accidental injection into the CSF is lethal.

Miscellaneous agents

Camptothecins are topoisomerase inhibitors used experimentally for the treatment of malignant gliomas. Topotecan crosses the blood–brain barrier[112] and encouraging preliminary reports suggest that camptothecins may

have some efficacy in the treatment of intracranial tumors,[113] especially metastases.[114] Camptothecins cause marrow suppression but are not neurotoxic.

Eflornithine (DFMO) inhibits ornithine decarboxylase and depletes cells of putrescine and spermidine. It has been used in brain tumors as a radiation enhancer. The drug does not readily cross the blood–brain barrier. It can cause ototoxicity, but other kinds of neurotoxicity are not reported; its primary toxic effect is on bone marrow.

Tamoxifen is a synthetic anti-estrogen that crosses the blood–brain barrier and appears to concentrate in the brain. It has been reported to have some effect against malignant gliomas[115] and has been used without much effect for the treatment of meningiomas. Its mechanism of action on malignant gliomas, if any, is probably not as an anti-estrogen but as an inhibitor of protein kinase C (PKC); it requires high doses to achieve this effect. The drug at high doses causes dizziness and ataxia,[115] and reversible effects on the retina have been described: the drug may promote thrombophlebitis.

Principles of miscellaneous therapies

Experimental therapies

Table 4.16 lists a number of approaches to therapy now being tried experimentally either in animals or early clinical trials.

Angiogenesis inhibitors

Many brain tumors are highly vascular, and angiogenesis is necessary for their growth. Accordingly, drugs that interfere with angiogenesis might retard the growth of tumors. In

Table 4.16
Experimental therapies.

- Angiogenesis inhibitors[116,117]
- Gene therapy[118]
    Herpes simplex thymidine kinase, p53 gene
- Immunotherapy[119]
    Vaccines
    T-cells
    Tumor cells
    Antibodies
    Dendritic cells
- Growth factor inhibitors
- Toxins[120,121]
- Differentiating agents

experimental animals, anti-angiogenesis factors not only retard the growth of tumor, but have been shown eventually to cure tumors. Furthermore, because blood vessels are not neoplastic, they do not possess the genetic instability of tumor cells and do not develop resistance to the anti-angiogenesis factors. A number of drugs are now in clinical trials, including thalidomide efficacy[122] and analogs of fumagillin. These drugs are being used either alone or in conjunction with chemotherapeutic agents (i.e. thalidomide plus carboplatin). The future roles, if any, of these drugs are unknown.

Gene therapy

Gene therapy is another attractive experimental approach to the treatment of brain tumors. Most studies have focused on the insertion of the herpes simplex thymidine kinase gene into tumor cells; the patient is then treated with ganciclovir, a drug that causes a lethal reaction with the herpes simplex but not the human thymidine kinase gene, killing the tumor cell. Some evidence suggests that not only are tumor cells possessing the gene destroyed, but surrounding tumor cells are also destroyed by a 'bystander' effect.[123] Although clever, this approach has not yet proved efficacious in the treatment of malignant gliomas. The poor outcome may be due to technical limitations that further research may resolve.

An even more attractive therapeutic approach would be to try to normalize mutated genes in tumor cells. Therapeutic attempts using the wild-type p53 gene, which should cause tumor cells that lack this gene to stop reproducing, are underway. Other forms of gene therapy are still in early experimental stages.

Antisense oligonucleotides that probably inhibit the function of the normal messenger RNA are being used in experimental systems. For example, antisense fibroblast growth factor (FGF) and antisense IGF receptors inhibit growth of glioblastoma cells.

Immunotherapy

Immunotherapy has proved a disappointment. A number of human trials involving the injection of T-cells with interleukin-2 (IL-2) into the tumor bed are ongoing, but none have yet proved efficacious. Vaccination of patients with their own radiation-killed tumor cells, or with tumor cells and T-cells incubated with IL-2, has been undergoing therapeutic trials, but, again, efficacy has not been shown.

Growth factor inhibitors

Growth factor inhibitors are also undergoing clinical trials. Most brain tumors are dependent on growth factors such as epidermal growth factor (EGF), platelet-derived growth factor (PDGF) and vascular endothelial growth factor (VEGF), as well as FGF, for both angiogenesis and tumor growth. Monoclonal antibodies against EGF receptor have been used to treat brain tumors but effectiveness has not yet been established. A number of drugs that inhibit growth factors are currently undergoing clinical trials, but again their efficacy is not known.

Supportive therapy

Anticonvulsants

Table 14.17 details the principles of using anticonvulsants.

Seizures comprise one of the common symptoms in patients with intracranial tumors. They usually occur as the presenting symptom but may in some instances be late complications following surgery or radiation therapy. The late onset of seizures does not necessarily presage recurrence of a tumor. It may simply result from damage to surrounding normal brain caused by the tumor or as a result of treatment. All seizures due to intracranial tumor have a focal onset. If the focus of epileptic discharge is in a silent area, the seizure may secondarily generalize without the patient being aware of any initial symptoms. Focal seizures generally resolve spontaneously and do not cause permanent damage. Focal seizures may vary in frequency from rare (a few a month to a few a year) to several times a day. Although occasional focal seizures do not cause significant damage or interfere with activities of daily living, they are distressing and attempts should be made to control them. Generalized seizures, although usually not dangerous, can be lethal if the patient injures himself during the course of a seizure or if repetitive seizures lead to status epilepticus. Thus, as a general principle, attempts should be made to control seizures.

Unfortunately, as Table 4.17 indicates, attempts to control seizures are not without problems. Both focal and generalized seizures may be extremely difficult to control in patients with a brain tumor. In patients with low-grade glioma, there is some evidence that treating the tumor with RT decreases the incidence of intractable seizures. However, there is no good evidence that anticonvulsants themselves are effective in controlling seizures

Table 4.17
Brain tumors: anticonvulsants.

- Prophylaxis
  Does not prevent first seizure
  Probably useful in perioperative period
- Treatment
  Efficacy unclear
  Side-effects more common
  Interactions common
  Hard to control levels
  Best drug unknown

due to brain tumors, either those that occur before or those that occur after treatment. Furthermore, untoward side-effects of anticonvulsants are more common in patients with brain tumors than in the general population. Especially dangerous are skin reactions including the Stevens–Johnson syndrome, which can be fatal[124] (Fig. 4.10). Most (but not all) anticonvulsants have interactions with drugs used to treat patients with brain tumors. The interactions may affect the metabolism of chemotherapeutic agents. Interactions may also affect the metabolism of anticonvulsants, thus making therapeutic levels hard to maintain. Although some of the newer anticonvulsants (e.g. gabapentin) do not have known interactions, presently unknown interactions may eventually surface.

We recommend anticonvulsants for all patients who have either focal or generalized seizures. Table 4.18 lists the anticonvulsants generally used to treat patients with brain tumors. One anticonvulsant does not appear to be superior to the others.[125]

The first-line anticonvulsants include phenytoin, carbamazepine, valproate and phenobarbital. All of these have potentially deleterious effects, including disorders of cognitive function and interactions with

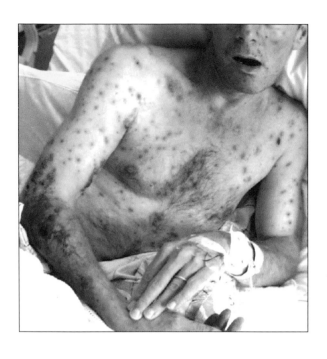

Figure 4.10
Stevens–Johnson syndrome in a man with a brain tumor. Although this patient did not have seizures, he was begun on corticosteroids and phenytoin prior to surgery. The surgery was without incident, and radiation therapy was started about 3 weeks after the operation. A week after radiation was started, he broke out with a total body rash, including involvement of the oral mucosa and the conjunctiva. He was hospitalized for about a week before the rash began to clear. This is a typical Stevens–Johnson syndrome that occurs in patients with a combination of recent onset of anticonvulsant drugs (usually phenytoin or carbamazepine), radiation therapy to the head and tapering of corticosteroids.

Table 4.18
Some antiepileptic drugs for brain tumors.

Drug	Usual daily dose	Dose intervals
Standard agents		
Phenytoin	200–500 mg	Once daily (qd) or twice daily (bid)
Carbamazepine	600–1600 mg	Three times a day (tid) or four times a day (qid) (bid for extended release tablets)
Valproate	15–60 mg/kg	tid or qid
Phenobarbital	1–4 mg/kg	qid
Newer agents		
Gabapentin	900–6000 mg	tid or qid
Lamotrigine	200–800 mg	bid
Topiramate	200–1600 mg	bid
Tiagabine	32–56 mg	bid – qid

chemotherapeutic agents. The newer anticonvulsant drugs appear to have fewer side-effects and many have fewer interactions. In healthy adults, topiramate can cause cognitive dysfunction; gabapentin and lamotrigine rarely do so.[126] However, it is not clear how effective these newer agents are in the treatment of patients with brain tumors, or whether more side-effects will emerge with longer experience. Accordingly, we recommend the following approach. An active seizure should be stopped, first with intravenous lorazepam (0.5–2 mg over 1–2 min), followed by 1000 mg (15 mg/kg) of phenytoin or preferably fosphenytoin by intravenous injection (the latter drug does not cause cardiovascular problems and may be given more rapidly than phenytoin itself). For patients not actively having seizures, we begin either with phenytoin or carbamazepine, increasing the dose until either seizures are stopped or side-effects prevent further increases. Measurement of blood levels will indicate to the physician the likelihood that a further dose increase may be toxic or safe, but it is wise to treat the seizures and not the blood levels. Some patients are well controlled on doses that are considered 'subtherapeutic'. Conversely, many patients tolerate 'supratherapeutic' blood levels without evidence of toxicity. If one drug is ineffective, one can switch to another or add a second drug. We generally add gabapentin to either phenytoin or carbamazepine in an attempt to control seizures. In some patients with non-disabling focal seizures, control with anticonvulsants may not be possible without toxicity and it may be wise to allow the patient to have occasional focal seizures.

There is no evidence that anticonvulsant drugs prevent seizures in patients with brain tumors who have not had prior seizures. Controlled trials indicate that with either metastatic or primary brain tumors, prophylactic anticonvulsants are not helpful.[127] One exception may be in the immediate perioperative period, when the use of prophylactic anticonvulsants for several weeks may be indicated.

Corticosteroids

Table 4.19 lists some of the advantages and disadvantages of using corticosteroids.

Corticosteroids dramatically relieve the symptoms of brain tumors, reducing edema and thus decreasing intracranial pressure. Symptomatic improvement may begin within minutes and patients often become asymptomatic within 24–48 h. The mechanisms by which corticosteroids exert their effects are poorly understood. One mechanism may be a decrease in the flux of water-soluble compounds across the disrupted blood–brain barrier (Chapter 2), thus effectively reconstituting the blood–brain barrier. Unintended effects include reduction of chemotherapeutic drug entry into the tumor. Furthermore, restoring the blood–brain barrier reduces contrast enhancement on MRI, which can sometimes be mistaken for a response to treatment.

Corticosteroids are indicated in all symptomatic patients with intracranial tumors, with the exception of suspected but undiagnosed lymphoma. In a patient with lymphoma, corticosteroids may cause tumor necrosis due to their lympholytic effect, precluding definitive diagnosis (Chapter 11). Corticosteroids are not given to asymptomatic patients, except those undergoing surgery or RT.

Table 4.19
Advantages and disadvantages of corticosteroids.

- Advantages
  Controls neurologic symptoms by
    reducing edema
  Decreases acute RT toxicity
  Relieves emesis from chemotherapy
  Oncolytic (lymphoma)
- Disadvantages
  Side-effects common (see Table 4.20)
  Decreases chemotherapy entry
  Oncolytic (lymphoma)

The corticosteroid usually administered is dexamethasone at 16 mg a day. The drug is long-acting and need not be given more than twice daily, but is often administered more frequently to reduce acute gastrointestinal toxicity and insomnia. We do not routinely use gastric protection for patients receiving corticosteroids. In patients expected to be on corticosteroids for a prolonged period, e.g. more than 6 weeks, prophylactic antibiotics to prevent *Pneumocystis carinii* infection are indicated. Unfortunately, these drugs often cause side-effects, particularly platelet suppression and rash. Once begun, the administration of a corticosteroid is continued until the patient's symptoms are relieved and intracranial pressure is diminished. The drug is then tapered to the lowest dose commensurate with good neurologic function. It can often be completely discontinued after surgery or radiation. There is no upper limit on the use of corticosteroids to control brain edema. If 16 mg a day does not relieve symptoms, it is often wise to double the dose for a few days to see if symptoms improve. Some investigators have indicated that doses of 100 mg a day for several days may be required to fully relieve symptoms of a brain tumor. If one doubles or quadruples the dose of corticosteroids for 48 h and does not see an effect, one can rapidly taper the drug back to baseline. Recent evidence suggests that doses of prednisone less than 5 mg daily can be abruptly withdrawn without causing adrenal suppression.[128]

Despite the necessity for their use, the side-effects of corticosteroids are many (Table 4.20),

Table 4.20
Side effects of corticosteroids.

Common but usually mild	Non-neurologic but serious	Neurologic (common)	Neurologic (uncommon)
Insomnia	Gastrointestinal bleeding	Myopathy[133]	Psychosis
Sensation of	Bowel perforation	Behavioral alterations	Paraparesis
abdominal	Osteoporosis	Hallucinations (high dose)	
bloating	Avascular osteonecrosis	Hiccoughs	
Increased appetite	(usually hip)	Tremor	
Visual blurring	Glaucoma	Visual blurring	
Urinary frequency	Opportunistic infections		
and nocturia	Hyperglycemia		
Acne	Kaposi's sarcoma		
Edema	Pancreatitis		
Lipomatosis			
Genital burning			
(IV push)			
Oral candidiasis			
Memory loss[132]			

IV, intravenous
For further discussion of supportive care of brain tumor patients, see Posner.[67]

and not all are dose-related. Because of the side-effects of steroids, investigators have made efforts to find substitutes with fewer side-effects. These have included 21-amino steroids,[129] corticotropin-releasing factor,[130] and boswellic acid.[131] All of these treatments remain experimental.

Anticoagulants

Deep vein thromboses commonly complicate brain tumors and their therapy. They may be present when the patient is first evaluated or occur after treatment is underway.[134] There are multiple factors which contribute to deep vein thrombosis, including immobility, neurosurgery, the release of thromboplastins from the brain and hypercoagulability related to systemic cancer and/or chemotherapy. Most episodes occur in close proximity to the patient's initial neurosurgical procedure, often beginning during anesthesia. Pneumatic compression boots decrease the incidence of deep vein thrombosis, especially if applied preoperatively and continued in the postoperative period until the patient is fully ambulatory;[135] low molecular weight heparin combined with the boots is even better.[136] However, deep vein thromboses occur even in patients who ambulate the day after craniotomy and are protected by pneumatic boots during and after surgery. A recent study addressed the safety of perioperative subcutaneous heparin for prophylaxis of venous thromboembolism during craniotomy. Treatment was begun at the induction of anesthesia and continued for 7 days. The anticoagulants did not increase intraoperative blood loss, transfusion requirements or postoperative platelet counts. No patient with a brain tumor bled into the tumor bed after surgery. The authors concluded that perioperative heparin at a dose of 5000 units every 12 h is safe.[137,138] Low molecular weight heparin given prophylactically 24 h after surgery also appears to be safe,[136] but one study indicates that, given preoperatively, it

may increase the risk of symptomatic intracranial hemorrhage.[139]

Treatment of an established thrombosis in neurosurgical patients is even more controversial than prophylaxis. Therapeutic options include the placement of a vena cava filter or the use of an anticoagulant such as heparin or low molecular weight heparin. Many neurosurgeons remain reluctant to prescribe anticoagulation during the immediate postoperative period. There is disagreement about when anticoagulation can safely be started after a craniotomy[140] once a clinically apparent thrombosis develops. The brain appears to become less susceptible to hemorrhage after about 48 h. Some neurosurgeons begin heparin treatment at 24 h, while others wait for 5–7 days. When making the decision to begin anticoagulants, the physician must weigh the risk that the patient will suffer a thromboembolic episode against the risk of an intracranial hemorrhage. In patients with thromboembolic disease, anticoagulation, avoiding supratherapeutic levels, is probably safe within 2 or 3 days of surgery. Because the placement of vena cava filters has complications of its own, we prefer anticoagulants to vena cava filters whenever possible;[141] many of our patients who receive filters subsequently require anticoagulation for recurrent thrombosis and chronic venous insufficiency of the legs. We usually start low molecular weight heparin with concurrent coumadin and treat patients for the standard 3–6 months that is recommended for thromboembolism. Occasionally, we have found that daily aspirin can help reduce repeated thromboembolic episodes in patients with chronic venous stasis.

'Alternative therapy'

One study suggests that about one-quarter of brain tumor patients try alternative therapy. Although no major side-effects have been noted, one cannot be sure that the agents did not interfere with conventional therapy. For example, some antioxidants, a favorite alternative therapy, inhibit the cytotoxicity of cisplatin on glioma cells.[142] As in breast cancer patients on alternative therapies, the brain tumor patient using alternative therapies may have a lower quality of life.[143]

Nutrition

Nutrition is often poor in patients with brain tumors. Both the tumor and its treatment may cause nausea or anorexia. Dysphagia and obtundation may also decrease food intake. The physician must be scrupulous in ensuring adequate nutrition. Patients with brain tumors should not suffer the additional and clinically confusing insult of Wernicke's encephalopathy.[144]

Quality of life

The goal of all of the above treatments is not only to promote survival either by curing the tumor or by retarding its growth, but also to ensure that the patient sustains the best quality of life possible. A number of recent studies have addressed quality of life in patients being treated for high-grade brain tumors.[145-147] Patients with brain tumors can suffer other symptoms such as depression or anxiety, which should be vigorously treated and do respond to therapy. Physical therapy can help patients to maximize their functional capacity. Occasionally, stimulants such as methylphenidate can improve a patient's level of alertness and decrease lethargy.[148] Although cognitive dysfunction and mood alterations are common, the quality of life does not appear worse than in patients with other chronic neurologic diseases. Most factors that affect the patient's quality of life are related to the tumor rather than to the treatment.

References

1. Gutin PH, Posner JB. Neuro-oncology: Diagnosis and management of cerebral gliomas – past, present, and future. Neurosurgery 2000; 47: 1–8.
2. Black PM. Surgery for cerebral gliomas: past, present, and future. Clin Neurosurg 2000; 47: 21–45.
3. Kondziolka D, Lunsford LD. The role of stereotactic biopsy in the management of gliomas. J Neurooncol 1999; 42: 205–13.
4. Mohan DS, Suh JH, Phan JL et al. Outcome in elderly patients undergoing definitive surgery and radiation therapy for supratentorial glioblastoma multiforme at a tertiary care institution. Int J Radiat Oncol Biol Phys 1998; 42: 981–7.
5. Simpson JR, Horton J, Scott C et al. Influence of location and extent of surgical resection on survival of patients with glioblastoma multiforme: results of three consecutive Radiation Therapy Oncology Group (RTOG) clinical trials. Int J Radiat Oncol Biol Phys 1993; 26: 239–44.
6. Toms SA, Ferson DZ, Sawaya R. Basic surgical techniques in the resection of malignant gliomas. J Neurooncol 1999; 42: 215–26.
7. Fadul C, Wood J, Thaler H et al. Morbidity and mortality of craniotomy for excision of supratentorial gliomas. Neurology 1988; 38: 1374–9.
8. Sawaya R, Hammoud M, Schoppa D et al. Neurosurgical outcomes in a modern series of 400 craniotomies for treatment of parenchymal tumors. Neurosurgery 1998; 42: 1044–55.
9. Gumprecht HK, Widenka DC, Lumenta CB. BrainLab VectorVision neuronavigation system: technology and clinical experiences in 131 cases. Neurosurgery 1999; 44: 97–104.
10. Pujol J, Conesa G, Deus J et al. Clinical application of functional magnetic resonance imaging in presurgical identification of the central sulcus. J Neurosurg 1998; 88: 863–9.
11. Roux FE, Boulanouar K, Ranjeva JP et al. Cortical intraoperative stimulation in brain tumors as a tool to evaluate spatial data from motor functional MRI. Invest Radiol 1999; 34: 225–9.

12. Schwartz TH, Devinsky O, Doyle W, Perrine K. Preoperative predictors of anterior temporal language areas. J Neurosurg 1998; 89: 962–70.

13. Taylor MD, Bernstein M. Awake craniotomy with brain mapping as the routine surgical approach to treating patients with supratentorial intraaxial tumors: a prospective trial of 200 cases. J Neurosurg 1999; 90: 35–41.

14. North JB, Penhall RK, Hanieh A, Frewin DB, Taylor WB. Phenytoin and postoperative epilepsy. A double-blind study. J Neurosurg 1983; 58: 672–7.

15. Shaw MD, Foy PM. Epilepsy after craniotomy and the place of prophylactic anticonvulsant drugs: discussion paper. J R Soc Med 1991; 84: 221–3.

16. Jansen GFA, Van Praagh BH, Kedaria MB, Odoom JA. Jugular bulb oxygen saturation during propofol and isoflurane/nitrous oxide anesthesia in patients undergoing brain tumor surgery. Anesth Analg 1999; 89: 358–63.

17. Dorward NL, Alberti O, Palmer JD, Kitchen ND, Thomas DGT. Accuracy of true frameless stereotaxy: in vivo measurement and laboratory phantom studies – technical note. J Neurosurg 1999; 90: 160–8.

18. Nimsky C, Ganslandt O, Kober H, Buchfelder M, Fahlbusch R. Intraoperative magnetic resonance imaging combined with neuronavigation: A new concept. Neurosurgery 2001; 48: 1082–9.

19. Matz PG, Cobbs C, Berger MS. Intraoperative cortical mapping as a guide to the surgical resection of gliomas. J Neurooncol 1999; 42: 233–45.

20. Danks RA, Aglio LS, Gugino LD, Black PM. Craniotomy under local anesthesia and monitored conscious sedation for the resection of tumors involving eloquent cortex. J Neurooncol 2000; 49: 131–9.

21. Jennings CR, O'Donoghue GM. Posterior fossa endoscopy. J Laryngol Otol 1998; 112: 227–9.

22. Savargaonkar P, Farmer PM. Utility of intraoperative consultations for the diagnosis of central nervous system lesions. Ann Clin Lab Sci 2001; 31: 133–9.

23. Bowles AP Jr, Perkins E. Long-term remission of malignant brain tumors after intracranial infection: a report of four cases. Neurosurgery 1999; 44: 636–42.

24. Hunter CA, Yu D, Gee M et al. Cutting edge: systemic inhibition of angiogenesis underlies resistance to tumors during acute toxoplasmosis. J Immunol 2001; 166: 5878–81.

25. Hall WA, Martin AJ, Liu HY et al. Brain biopsy using high-field strength interventional magnetic resonance imaging. Neurosurgery 1999; 44: 807–13.

26. King WA, Wackym PA. Endoscope-assisted surgery for acoustic neuromas (vestibular schwannomas): early experience using the rigid Hopkins telescope. Neurosurgery 1999; 44: 1095–100.

27. King WA, Ullman AS, Frazee LG, Post KD, Bergsneider M. Endoscopic resection of colloid cysts: surgical considerations using the rigid endoscope. Neurosurgery 1999; 44: 1103–9.

28. Walker MD, Alexander EJ, Hunt WE et al. Evaluation of BCNU and/or radiotherapy in the treatment of anaplastic gliomas. A cooperative clinical trial. J Neurosurg 1978; 49: 333–43.

29. Walker MD, Strike TA, Sheline GE. An analysis of dose–effect relationship in the radiotherapy of malignant gliomas. Int J Radiat Oncol Biol Phys 1979; 5: 1725–31.

30. Hall EJ. Radiobiology for the radiologist, 3rd edn. Philadelphia: J.B. Lippincott Co., 1988.

31. Withers HR. Radiation biology and treatment options in radiation oncology. Cancer Res 1999; 59: 1676s–84s.

32. Olive PL. DNA organization affects cellular radiosensitivity and detection of initial DNA strand breaks. Int J Radiat Oncol Biol Phys 1992; 62: 389–96.

33. Ang KK. Fractionation effects in clinical practice. In: Leibel SA, Phillips TL, eds. Textbook of radiation oncology. Philadelphia: W.B. Saunders Co., 1998: 26–41.

34. Mandell LR, Kadota R, Freeman C et al. There is no role for hyperfractionated radiotherapy in the management of children with newly diagnosed diffuse intrinsic brainstem tumors: results of a Pediatric Oncology Group phase III trial comparing conventional versus hyperfractionated radiotherapy. Int J Radiat Oncol Biol Phys 1999; 43: 959–64.

35. Haas-Kogan DA, Kogan SS, Yount G et al. p53 function influences the effect of fractionated radiotherapy on glioblastoma tumors. Int J Radiat Oncol Biol Phys 1999; 43: 399–403.

36. Fallai C, Olmi P. Hyperfractionated and accelerated radiation therapy in central nervous system tumors (malignant gliomas, pediatric tumors, and brain metastases). Radiother Oncol 1997; 43: 235–46.

37. Groves MD, Maor MH, Meyers C et al. A phase II trial of high-dose bromodeoxyuridine with accelerated fractionation radiotherapy followed by procarbazine, lomustine, and vincristine for glioblastoma multiforme. Int J Radiat Oncol Biol Phys 1999; 45: 127–35.

38. Tubiana M, Eschwège F. Conformal radiotherapy and intensity-modulated radiotherapy. Clinical data. Acta Oncol 2000; 39: 555–67.

39. Baumert BG, Lomax AJ, Miltchev V, Davis JB. A comparison of dose distributions of proton and photon beams in stereotactic conformal radiotherapy of brain lesions. Int J Radiat Oncol Biol Phys 2001; 49: 1439–49.

40. Barth RF, Yang WL, Rotaru JH et al. Boron neutron capture therapy of brain tumors: Enhanced survival and cure following blood–brain barrier disruption and intracarotid injection of sodium borocaptate and boronophenylalanine. Int J Radiat Oncol Biol Phys 2000; 47: 209–18.

41. Koot RW, Maarouf M, Hulshof MC et al. Brachytherapy: results of two different therapy strategies for patients with primary glioblastoma multiforme. Cancer 2000; 88: 2796–802.

42. Lee SW, Fraass BA, Marsh LH et al. Patterns of failure following high-dose 3-D conformal radiotherapy for high-grade astrocytomas: a quantitative dosimetric study. Int J Radiat Oncol Biol Phys 1999; 43: 79–88.

43. Khoo VS, Oldham M, Adams EJ et al. Comparison of intensity-modulated tomotherapy with stereotactically guided conformal radiotherapy for brain tumors. Int J Radiat Oncol Biol Phys 1999; 45: 415–25.

44. Kortmann RD, Becker G, Perelmouter J et al. Geometric accuracy of field alignment in fractionated stereotactic conformal radiotherapy of brain tumors. Int J Radiat Oncol Biol Phys 1999; 43: 921–6.

45. Shafman TD, Loeffler JS. Novel radiation technologies for malignant gliomas. Curr Opin Oncol 1999; 11: 147–51.

46. Adler JR Jr, Murphy MJ, Chang SD, Hancock SL. Image-guided robotic radiosurgery. Neurosurgery 1999; 44: 1299–306.

47. Pollock BE, Gorman DA, Schomberg PJ, Kline RW. The Mayo Clinic gamma knife experience: indications and initial results. Mayo Clin Proc 1999; 74: 5–13.

48. Foote KD, Friedman WA, Buatti JM, Bova FJ, Meeks SA. Linear accelerator radiosurgery in brain tumor management. Neurosurg Clin N Am 1999; 10: 203–42.

49. Hoban PW, Jones LC, Clark BG. Modeling late effects in hypofractionated stereotactic radiotherapy. Int J Radiat Oncol Biol Phys 1999; 43: 199–210.

50. Tokuuye K, Akine Y, Sumi M et al. Fractionated stereotactic radiotherapy of small intracranial malignancies. Int J Radiat Oncol Biol Phys 1998; 42: 989–94.

51. Loeffler JS, Kooy HM, Tarbell NJ. The emergence of conformal radiotherapy: special implications for pediatric neuro-oncology. Int J Radiat Oncol Biol Phys 1999; 44: 237–8.

52. Suh JH, Barnett GH. Brachytherapy for brain tumor. Hematol Oncol Clin N Am 1999; 13: 635–50.

53. Videtic GMM, Gaspar LE, Zamorano L et al. Use of the RTOG recursive partitioning analysis to validate the benefit of iodine-125 implants in the primary treatment of malignant gliomas. Int J Radiat Oncol Biol Phys 1999; 45: 687–92.

54. Sneed PK, Stauffer PR, McDermott MW et al. Survival benefit of hyperthermia in a prospective randomized trial of brachytherapy boost +/– hyperthermia for glioblastoma multiforme. Int J Radiat Oncol Biol Phys 1998; 40: 287–95.

55. Glimelius B, Isacsson U, Blomquist E et al. Potential gains using high-energy protons for therapy of malignant tumours. Acta Oncol 1999; 38: 137–45.

56. Munzenrider JE, Adams J, Liebsch NJ. Skull base tumors: treatment with three-dimensional planning and fractionated x-ray and

proton radiotherapy. In: Leibel SA, Phillips TL, eds. Textbook of Radiation Oncology. Philadelphia: W.B. Saunders Co., 1998: 347–56.

57. Barth RF, Soloway AH, Goodman JH et al. Boron neutron capture therapy of brain tumors: an emerging therapeutic modality. Neurosurgery 1999; 44: 433–50.

58. Chanana AD, Capala J, Chadha M et al. Boron neutron capture therapy for glioblastoma multiforme: interim results from the phase I/II dose-escalation studies. Neurosurgery 1999; 44: 1182–92.

59. Joel DD, Coderre JA, Micca PL, Nawrocky MM. Effect of dose and infusion time on the delivery of *p*-boronophenylalanine for neutron capture therapy. J Neurooncol 1999; 41: 213–21.

60. Prados MD, Scott CB, Rotman M et al. Influence of bromodeoxyuridine radiosensitization on malignant glioma patient survival: a retrospective comparison of survival data from the Northern California Oncology Group (NCOG) and Radiation Therapy Oncology Group (RTOG) for glioblastoma and anaplastic astrocytoma. Int J Radiat Oncol Biol Phys 1998; 40: 653–9.

61. Carde P, Timmerman R, Mehta MP et al. Multicenter phase Ib/II trial of the radiation enhancer motexafin gadolinium in patients with brain metastases. J Clin Oncol 2000; 19: 2074–83.

62. Lammering G, Valerie K, Lin PS et al. Radiosensitization of malignant glioma cells through overexpression of dominant-negative epidermal growth factor receptor. Clin Cancer Res 2001; 7: 682–90.

63. Valerie K, Hawkins W, Farnsworth J et al. Substantially improved in vivo radiosensitization of rat glioma with mutant HSV-TK and acyclovir. Cancer Gene Ther 2001; 8: 3–8.

64. Gramaglia A, Loi GF, Mongioj V, Baronzio GF. Increased survival in brain metastatic patients treated with stereotactic radiotherapy, omega three fatty acids and bioflavonoids. Anticancer Res 1999; 19: 5583–6.

65. Noel F, Tofilon PJ. Astrocytes protect against X-ray-induced neuronal toxicity in vitro. Neuroreport 1998; 9: 1133–7.

66. Hensley ML, Schuchter LM, Lindley C et al. American Society of Clinical Oncology Clinical Practice Guidelines for the Use of Chemotherapy and Radiotherapy Protectants. J Clin Oncol 1999; 17: 3333–55.

67. Posner JB. Neurologic complications of cancer, 1st Edn. Philadelphia: F.A. Davis, 1995.

68. Peterson K, Rosenblum MK, Powers JM, Alvord EC, Walker RW, Posner JB. Effect of brain irradiation on demyelinating lesions. Neurology 1993; 43: 2105–12.

69. Li YQ, Ballinger JR, Nordal RA, Su ZF, Wong CS. Hypoxia in radiation-induced blood–spinal cord barrier breakdown. Cancer Res 2001; 61: 3348–54.

70. O'Connor MM, Mayberg MR. Effects of radiation on cerebral vasculature: a review. Neurosurgery 2000; 46: 138–49.

71. Hopewell JW, Wright EA. The nature of latent cerebral irradiation damage and its modification by hypertension. Br J Radiol 1970; 43: 161–7.

72. Lampert P, Tom MI, Rider WD. Disseminated demyelination of the brain following Co^{60} (gamma) radiation. Arch Pathol (Chicago) 1959; 68: 322–30.

73. Mima T, Toyonaga S, Mori K, Taniguchi T, Ogawa Y. Early decrease of P-glycoprotein in the endothelium of the rat brain capillaries after moderate dose of irradiation. Neurol Res 1999; 21: 209–15.

74. Armstrong C, Ruffer J, Corn B, DeVries K, Mollman J. Biphasic patterns of memory deficits following moderate-dose partial-brain irradiation: neuropsychologic outcome and proposed mechanisms. J Clin Oncol 1995; 13: 2263–71.

75. Marks JE, Wong J. The risk of cerebral radionecrosis in relation to dose, time and fractionation: a follow-up study. Prog Exp Tumor Res 1985; 29: 210–8.

76. Morris JG, Grattan-Smith P, Panegyres PK et al. Delayed cerebral radiation necrosis. Q J Med 1994; 87: 119–29.

77. Shewmon DA, Masdeu JC. Delayed radiation necrosis of the brain contralateral to original tumor. Arch Neurol 1980; 37: 592–4.

78. Ricci PE, Karis JP, Heiserman JE et al. Differentiating recurrent tumor from radiation necrosis: time for re-evaluation of

positron emission tomography? Am J Neuroradiol 1998; 19: 407–13.

79. Vigliani MC, Duyckaerts C, Hauw JJ et al. Dementia following treatment of brain tumors with radiotherapy administered alone or in combination with nitrosourea-based chemotherapy: a clinical and pathological study. J Neurooncol 1999; 41: 137–49.

80. Thiessen B, DeAngelis LM. Hydrocephalus in radiation leukoencephalopathy – results of ventriculoperitoneal shunting. Arch Neurol 1998; 55: 705–10.

81. Kleinberg L, Wallner K, Malkin MG. Good performance status of long-term disease-free survivors of intracranial gliomas. Int J Radiat Oncol Biol Phys 1993; 26: 129–33.

82. Johansson M, Bergenheim AT, Widmark A, Henriksson R. Effects of radiotherapy and estramustine on the microvasculature in malignant glioma. Br J Cancer 1999; 80: 142–8.

83. Grill J, Couanet D, Cappelli C et al. Radiation-induced cerebral vasculopathy in children with neurofibromatosis and optic pathway glioma. Ann Neurol 1999; 45: 393–6.

84. Brandes AA, Pasetto LM, Lumachi F, Monfardini S. Endocrine dysfunctions in patients treated for brain tumors: incidence and guidelines for management. J Neurooncol 2000; 47: 85–92.

85. Galanis E, Buckner JC. Chemotherapy of brain tumors. Curr Opin Neurol 2001; 13: 619–25.

86. DeAngelis LM. Medical progress: Brain tumors. N Engl J Med 2001; 344: 114–23.

87. Huncharek M, Muscat J, Geschwind JF. Multi-drug versus single agent chemotherapy for high grade astrocytoma; results of a meta-analysis. Anticancer Res 1998; 18: 4693–7.

88. Shapiro WR, Shapiro JR. Biology and treatment of malignant glioma. Oncology 1998; 12: 233–40.

89. Prados MD, Scott C, Curran WJ Jr, Nelson DF, Leibel S, Kramer S. Procarbazine, lomustine, and vincristine (PCV) chemotherapy for anaplastic astrocytoma: a retrospective review of Radiation Therapy Oncology Group Protocols comparing survival with carmustine or PCV adjuvant chemotherapy. J Clin Oncol 1999; 17: 3389–95.

90. Randomized trial of procarbazine, lomustine, and vincristine in the adjuvant treatment of high-grade astrocytoma: a Medical Research Council trial. J Clin Oncol 2001; 19: 509–18.

91. Fine HA, Dear KB, Loeffler JS, Black PM, Canellos GP. Meta-analysis of radiation therapy with and without adjuvant chemotherapy for malignant gliomas in adults. Cancer 1993; 71: 2585–97.

92. Keime-Guibert F, Napolitano M, Delattre J-Y. Neurological complications of radiotherapy and chemotherapy. J Neurol 1998; 245: 695–708.

93. Bartus RT, Snodgrass P, Dean RL, Kordower JH, Emerich DF. Evidence that Cereport's ability to increase permeability of rat gliomas is dependent upon extent of tumor growth: Implications for treating newly emerging tumor colonies. Exp Neurol 2000; 161: 234–44.

94. Remsen LG, Pagel MA, McCormick CI et al. The influence of anesthetic choice, $PaCo_2$, and other factors on osmotic blood–brain barrier disruption in rats with brain tumor xenografts. Anesth Analg 1999; 88: 559–67.

95. Gobin YP, Cloughesy TF, Chow KL et al. Intraarterial chemotherapy for brain tumors by using a spatial dose fractionation algorithm and pulsatile delivery. Radiology 2001; 218: 724–32.

96. Brem H, Piantadosi S, Burger PC et al. Placebo-controlled trial of safety and efficacy of intraoperative controlled delivery by biodegradable polymers of chemotherapy for recurrent gliomas. The Polymer-Brain Tumor Treatment Group. Lancet 1995; 345: 1008–12.

97. Menei P, Venier MC, Gamelin E et al. Local and sustained delivery of 5-fluorouracil from biodegradable microspheres for the radio-sensitization of glioblastoma – a pilot study. Cancer 1999; 86: 325–30.

98. Kreuter J. Nanoparticulate systems for brain delivery of drugs. Adv Drug Deliv Rev 2001; 47: 65–81.

99. Zucchetti M, Boiardi A, Silvani A et al. Distribution of daunorubicin and daunorubicinol in human glioma tumors after administration of liposomal daunorubicin. Cancer Chemother Pharmacol 1999; 44: 173–6.

100. Subach BR, Witham TF, Kondziolka D, Lunsford LD, Bozik M, Schiff D. Morbidity and survival after 1,3-*bis*(2-chloroethyl)-1 nitrosourea wafer implantation for recurrent glioblastoma: a retrospective case matched cohort series. Neurosurgery 1999; 45: 17–22.

101. Esteller M, Garcia-Foncillas J, Andion E et al. Inactivation of the DNA-repair gene MGMT and the clinical response of gliomas to alkylating agents. N Engl J Med 2000; 343: 1350–4.

102. Bredel M. Anticancer drug resistance in primary human brain tumors. Brain Res Brain Res Rev 2001; 35: 161–204.

103. Ashby LS, Shapiro WR. Intra-arterial cisplatin plus oral etoposide for the treatment of recurrent malignant glioma: a phase II study. J Neurooncology 2001; 51: 67–86.

104. Shapiro WR, Green SB, Burger PC et al. A randomized comparison of intra-arterial versus intravenous BCNU, with or without intravenous 5-fluorouracil, for newly diagnosed patients with malignant glioma. J Neurosurg 1992; 76: 772–81.

105. Poppenborg H, Knüpfer MM, Preiss R, Wolff JEA, Galla HJ. Cisplatin (CDDP)-induced radiation resistance is not associated with CDDP resistance in 86HG39 and A172 malignant glioma cells. Eur J Cancer 1999; 35: 1150–4.

106. Friedman HS, McLendon RE, Kerby T et al. DNA mismatch repair and O6–alkylguanine-DNA alkyltransferase analysis and response to Temodal in newly diagnosed malignant glioma. J Clin Oncol 1998; 16: 3851–7.

107. Cloughesy TF, Black KL, Gobin YP et al. Intra-arterial Cereport (RMP-7) and carbo-platin: a dose escalation study for recurrent malignant gliomas. Neurosurgery 1999; 44: 270–8.

108. Dinnes J, Cave C, Huang S, Major K, Milne R. The effectiveness and cost-effectiveness of temozolomide for the treatment of recurrent malignant glioma: a rapid and systematic review. Health Technol Assess 2001; 5: 1–73.

109. Beauchesne P, Soler C, Rusch P et al. Phase II study of a radiotherapy/etoposide combination for patients with newly malignant gliomas. Cancer Chemother Pharmacol 1999; 44: 210–16.

110. Chamberlain MC, Kormanik P. Salvage chemotherapy with taxol for recurrent anaplastic astrocytomas. J Neurooncol 1999; 43: 71–8.

111. Freilich RJ, Balmaceda C, Seidman AD, Rubin M, DeAngelis LM. Motor neuopathy due to docetaxel and paclitaxel. Neurology 1996; 47: 115–8.

112. Stewart CF, Gajjar AJ, Heideman RL, Houghton PJ. Penetration of topotecan into cerebrospinal fluid after intravenous injection. Onkologie 1998; 21: 22–4.

113. Kadota RP, Stewart CF, Horn M et al. Topotecan for the treatment of recurrent or progressive central nervous system tumors – a Pediatric Oncology Group phase II study. J Neurooncol 1999; 43: 43–7.

114. Schütte W, Manegold C, Von Pawel JV. Topotecan in the therapy of brain metastases in lung cancer. Onkologie 1998; 21: 25–7.

115. Chang SM, Barker FG, II, Huhn SL et al. High dose oral tamoxifen and subcutaneous interferon alpha-2a for recurrent glioma. J Neurooncol 1998; 37: 169–76.

116. Miller KD, Sweeney CJ, Sledge GW. Redefining the target: chemotherapeutics as antiangiogenics. J Clin Oncol 2001; 19: 1195–206.

117. Los M, Voest EE. The potential role of antivascular therapy in the adjuvant and neoadjuvant treatment of cancer. Semin Oncol 2001; 28: 93–105.

118. Lam PYP, Breakefield XO. Potential of gene therapy for brain tumors. Hum Mol Genet 2001; 10: 777–87.

119. Parney IF, Hao CH, Petruk KC. Glioma immunology and immunotherapy. Neurosurgery 2000; 46: 778–91.

120. Oldfield EH, Youle RJ. Immunotoxins for brain tumor therapy. Curr Top Microbiol Immunol 1998; 234: 97–114.

121. Arab S, Murakami M, Dirks P et al. Verotoxins inhibit the growth of and induce apoptosis in human astrocytoma cells. J Neurooncol 1998; 40: 137–50.

122. Fine HA, Figg WD, Jaeckle K et al. Phase II trial of the antiangiogenic agent thalidomide in patients with recurrent high-grade gliomas. J Clin Oncol 2000; 18: 708–15.

123. Estin D, Li MW, Spray D, Wu JK. Connexins are expressed in primary brain tumors and

enhance the bystander effect in gene therapy. Neurosurgery 1999; 44: 361–8.

124. Guberman AH, Besag FMC, Brodie MJ et al. Lamotrigine-associated rash: Risk benefit considerations in adults and children. Epilepsia 1999; 40: 985–91.

125. Beenen LFM, Lindeboom J, Trenité DGAK et al. Comparative double blind clinical trial of phenytoin and sodium valproate as anticonvulsant prophylaxis after craniotomy: efficacy, tolerability, and cognitive effects. J Neurol Neurosurg Psychiatry 1999; 67: 474–80.

126. Martin R, Kuzniecky R, Ho S et al. Cognitive effects of topiramate, gabapentin, and lamotrigine in healthy young adults. Neurology 1999; 52: 321–7.

127. Glantz M, Friedberg M, Cole B et al. Double-blind, randomized, placebo-controlled trial of anticonvulsant prophylaxis in adults with newly diagnosed brain metastases. Proc ASCO 1994; 13, 176.

128. Dupond JL, Gil H, De Wazières B, Berthier S, Magy N. Withdrawing corticosteroids: the stress of the last milligrams. Presse Med 1999; 28: 140–2.

129. Kondziolka D, Mori Y, Martinez AJ et al. Beneficial effects of the radioprotectant 21-aminosteroid U-74389G in a radiosurgery rat malignant glioma model. Int J Radiat Oncol Biol Phys 1999; 44: 179–84.

130. Tjuvajev J, Uehara H, Desai R et al. Corticotropin-releasing factor decreases vasogenic brain edema. Cancer Res 1996; 56: 1352–60.

131. Glaser T, Winter S, Groscurth P et al. Boswellic acids and malignant glioma: induction of apoptosis but no modulation of drug sensitivity. Br J Cancer 1999; 80: 756–65.

132. De Kloet ER, Oitzl MS, Joëls M. Stress and cognition: are corticosteroids good or bad guys? Trends Neurosci 1999; 22: 422–6.

133. Gayan-Ramirez G, Vanderhoydonc F, Verhoeven G, Decramer M. Acute treatment with corticosteroids decreases IGF-1 and IGF-2 expression in the rat diaphragm and gastrocnemius. Am J Respir Crit Care Med 1999; 159: 283–9.

134. Marras LC, Geerts WH, Perry JR. The risk of venous thromboembolism is increased throughout the course of malignant glioma – An evidence-based review. Cancer 2000; 89: 640–6.

135. Ruff RL, Posner JB. The incidence of systemic venous thrombosis and the risk of anticoagulation in patients with malignant gliomas. Trans Am Neurol Assoc 1981; 106: 223–6.

136. Agnelli G, Piovella F, Buoncristiani P et al. Enoxaparin plus compression stockings compared with compression stockings alone in the prevention of venous thromboembolism after elective neurosurgery. N Engl J Med 1998; 339: 80–5.

137. Macdonald RL, Amidei C, Lin G et al. Safety of perioperative subcutaneous heparin for prophylaxis of venous thromboembolism in patients undergoing craniotomy. Neurosurgery 1999; 45: 245–51.

138. Constantini S, Kanner A, Friedman A et al. Safety of perioperative minidose heparin in patients undergoing brain tumor surgery: a prospective, randomized, double-blind study. J Neurosurg 2001; 94: 918–21.

139. Dickinson LD, Miller LD, Patel CP, Gupta SK. Enoxaparin increases the incidence of postoperative intracranial hemorrhage when initiated preoperatively for deep venous thrombosis prophylaxis in patients with brain tumors. Neurosurgery 1998; 43: 1074–81.

140. Lazio BE, Simard JM. Anticoagulation in neurosurgical patients. Neurosurgery 1999; 45: 838–47.

141. Levin JM, Schiff D, Loeffler JS et al. Complications of therapy for venous thromboembolic disease in patients with brain tumors. Neurology 1993; 43: 1111–4.

142. Yam D, Peled A, Shinitzky M. Suppression of tumor growth and metastasis by dietary fish oil combined with vitamins E and C and cisplatin. Cancer Chemother Pharmacol 2001; 47: 34–40.

143. Verhoef MJ, Hagen N, Pelletier G, Forsyth P. Alternative therapy use in neurologic diseases – Use in brain tumor patients. Neurology 1999; 52: 617–22.

144. Kuba H, Inamura T, Ikezaki K, Kawashima M, Fukui M. Thiamine-deficient lactic acidosis with brain tumor treatment – report of three cases. J Neurosurg 1998; 89: 1025–8.

145. Giovagnoli AR. Quality of life in patients with stable disease after surgery, radiotherapy, and chemotherapy for malignant brain tumour. J Neurol Neurosurg Psychiatry 1999; 67: 358–63.

146. Weitzner MA. Psychosocial and neuropsychiatric aspects of patients with primary brain tumors. Cancer Invest 1999; 17: 285–91.

147. Whitton AC, Rhydderch H, Furlong W, Feeny D, Barr RD. Self-reported comprehensive health status of adult brain tumor patients using the health utilities index. Cancer 1997; 80: 258–65.

148. Meyers CA, Weitzner MA, Valentine AD, Levin VA. Methylphenidate therapy improves cognition, mood, and function of brain tumor patients. J Clin Oncol 1998; 16: 2522–7.

II

Management of specific tumors

5

Glial tumors

Introduction

Although their exact lineage is unknown, most intrinsic brain tumors are believed to originate from glial cells or their precursors.[1,2] Central nervous system (CNS) glia can be divided into astrocytes, oligodendrocytes, microglia and ependyma. Schwann cells, the peripheral nervous system's oligodendrocytes, are also found within the intracranial cavity, synthesizing myelin in the distal intracranial portions of some cranial nerves (Chapter 9). Microglia are not true glia. Unlike the other glia, which are ectodermal in origin, microglia are mesodermal, probably of hematopoietic origin; they are involved in inflammatory and immune responses in the CNS and will not be discussed in this chapter. Ependymal cells line the cerebral ventricles and form the surface of the choroid plexus, which is why choroid plexus tumors are discussed in this chapter. Although the word glia (from the Greek meaning 'glue')

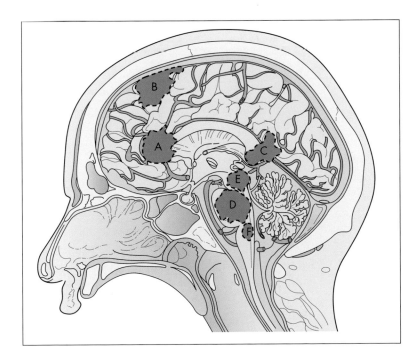

Figure 5.1
A schematic sagittal section showing common locations for diffuse glial tumors. (A) Most arise within the white matter of the hemispheres. The tumors often infiltrate the cortex. (B) The genu of the corpus callosum and (C) the splenium of the corpus callosum are common sites of gliomas. From these sites, the tumor can infiltrate both hemispheres. Gliomas can arise anywhere in the brainstem, usually the pons (D), but occasionally the midbrain (E) or the medulla (F). Low-grade astrocytomas commonly arise within the cerebellum (Fig. 5.10). All are discussed in the text.

implies that these cells just support and hold neurons in place, glia have far more important metabolic functions than just providing structural support,[3] for example, they maintain the blood–brain barrier (Chapter 2).

Tumors of glial origin can be divided into those that infiltrate into normal brain structures (diffuse tumors, Fig. 5.1) and those with more discrete boundaries, i.e. focal tumors (Table 5.1). The division is relative: some diffuse glial tumors have relatively discrete boundaries (e.g. so-called type 1 astrocytomas[4]) and some focal tumors invade surrounding normal brain (e.g. invasive ependymomas).

Diffuse glial tumors

Diffuse glial tumors range from very low grade (astrocytoma, oligodendroglioma) to extremely high grade (glioblastoma multiforme). They are more common in adults than in children and generally arise in the cerebral hemispheres, although they may affect brainstem, optic nerve, cerebellum or spinal cord. Low-grade tumors have a tendency to progress to a high-grade phenotype. High-grade tumors, i.e. glioblastoma, may either arise by progression from a lower grade tumor or may develop de novo.

Astrocytomas

Introduction

Astrocytoma (from the Greek word 'astro' for star) refers to the stellate shape of some astrocytes. Diffuse astrocytic tumors can be divided by histologic characteristics into astrocytoma, a low-grade tumor, and anaplastic astrocytoma and glioblastoma multiforme, both high-grade tumors (Fig. 5.2). Also included in this group are tumors that diffusely infiltrate all or much of the brain without necessarily forming a mass lesion (gliomatosis cerebri) and tumors restricted to the brainstem (brainstem gliomas); both may be of either grade. Because of different age and growth characteristics, and because their location often precludes biopsy, brainstem gliomas are considered separately from supratentorial gliomas. Almost by definition, diffuse astrocytomas, even those that appear to be histologically discrete, are not amenable to surgical cure.

Incidence

As indicated in Chapter 1, diffuse astrocytic tumors represent about 25% of primary intracranial tumors encountered at autopsy, but 35% of **symptomatic** primary intracranial tumors (Table 1.3). Glial tumors affect 5–7 new patients per 100 000 population per year, or about 18 000 new cases in the USA annually. In addition to being the most common symptomatic tumor, diffuse astrocytic

Table 5.1
Glial tumors.

Diffuse glial tumors
• Astrocytic tumors
Astrocytoma
Anaplastic astrocytoma
Glioblastoma multiforme
Gliomatosis cerebri
Brainstem glioma
• Oligodendroglial tumors
Oligodendroglioma
Anaplastic oligodendroglioma
Glioblastoma multiforme
Focal glial tumors
Pilocytic astrocytoma
Pleomorphic xanthoastrocytoma (PXA)
Ependymoma
Subependymoma
Choroid plexus papilloma

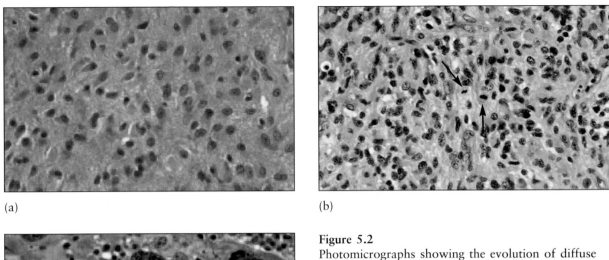

(a)

(b)

(c)

Figure 5.2
Photomicrographs showing the evolution of diffuse astrocytic tumors. A glioblastoma multiforme, the highest grade of diffuse astrocytoma, may arise by progressive evolution of the lesion from astrocytoma (a) showing hypercellular tumor tissue with angulated hyperchromatic atypical astrocytic nuclei; no mitoses are evident. The next stage is anaplastic astrocytoma (b) showing increased nuclear atypia and the presence of mitoses (arrows). The glioblastoma (GBM) (c) shows highly atypical giant tumor cells and mitotic figures (arrow). A GBM may also arise de novo. Genetic pathways of these primary and secondary astrocytomas are outlined in Table 5.2.

Table 5.2
Comparison of World Health Organization (WHO) and St Anne/Mayo classification of astrocytomas.[25]

WHO grade	WHO designation	St Anne/Mayo designation	Histological criteria
I	Pilocytic astrocytoma	Astrocytoma grade 1	Rosenthal fibers, piloid cells (low-grade diffuse) zero criterion
II	Diffuse astrocytoma	Astrocytoma grade 2	One criterion, usually nuclear atypia
III	Anaplastic astrocytoma	Astrocytoma grade 3	Two criteria, usually nuclear atypia and mitosis
IV	Glioblastoma multiforme	Astrocytoma grade 4	Three of four criteria: the two above plus endothelial proliferation and/or necrosis

tumors, unlike some other common brain tumors such as meningiomas and pituitary tumors, are not curable.

Also as discussed in Chapter 1, diffuse astrocytic tumors may be increasing in incidence. The most dramatic data are those of Olney et al,[5] showing the annual incidence of astrocytomas, anaplastic astrocytomas and glioblastomas between 1975 and 1992 increasing from 45 to 53 tumors per million population, with a dramatic increase in the incidence of anaplastic astrocytomas and glioblastomas and a corresponding fall in (low-grade) astrocytomas. The changing incidence of histologic subtypes could be attributed to changes in interpretation of microscopic slides by neuropathologists, although it is not known if there has been a tendency for neuropathologists to 'upgrade' their interpretation of diffuse astrocytic tumors (i.e. call tumors previously read as astrocytoma, anaplastic). If there has been substantial upgrading in histologic interpretation, one would expect to see reported improvement in survival via the 'Will Rogers effect'. (Will Rogers, a humorist, stated that during the depression of the 1930s, the migration of individuals from Oklahoma to California raised the IQ of both states.) If a tumor that was once considered low-grade is now considered high-grade, and if low-grade tumors have longer survival than high-grade tumors, then the change in pathologic reading should lead to longer survival in both patient groups. To date, there has been no evidence of improved survival in populations of patients with high-grade gliomas, so this is an unlikely explanation for any observed changes in epidemiology of gliomas. In addition, changes in pathologic interpretation can also lead to optimistic reports of phase 2 studies done in an institution where the neuropathologist habitually upgrades.

Etiology

Risk factors. With the exception of ionizing radiation (Chapter 1), no risk factors have been established for sporadic diffuse astrocytomas. Even with respect to ionizing radiation, in any given individual, one cannot be certain whether a diffuse astrocytic tumor occurring in a previously irradiated patient is related or coincidental. If the tumor occurs within the radiation portal, then the presumption of radiation as causal is strong. In one of our patients, an anaplastic astrocytoma developed in the radiation portal of a pituitary tumor 4 years after treatment. However, careful examination of previous scans suggested that the tumor had been there shortly following radiation therapy (RT), a latency too short for it to be other than coincidence. On the other hand, we have encountered a glioblastoma in a patient irradiated successfully 20 years earlier for a pineal region germinoma. The glioblastoma was bilateral and symmetrical, effectively outlining the radiation port. The development of a radiation-induced astrocytic tumor does not preclude the re-use of radiation if the patient's normal brain can tolerate it.

As discussed in Chapter 1, two alleged additional risk factors specifically linked to diffuse astrocytic tumors are ingestion of aspartame and electromagnetic (non-ionizing) radiation, particularly that produced by the portable cellular telephone. In portable cellular telephones, the antenna is part of the headset and the user's head is exposed to radiofrequency energy. As discussed in Chapter 1, studies of cellular telephones have failed to show a correlation with brain tumors. Also, as discussed in Chapter 1, the aspartame data are unconvincing. At least one recent study failed to provide evidence of DNA damage after exposure to electromagnetic radiation within the cellular phone communication frequency band. A study from Sweden addressing occupational exposure and glioma suggests an increased risk associated with solvents, pesticides and plastic materials.[6] A study from China suggests that nutritional factors (fresh vegetables, vitamin E and calcium protective; salted vegetables and salted fish deleterious) may play a role.[7]

About 5% of gliomas are familial,[8] most not belonging to the recognized syndromes. A few familial disorders that predispose to astrocytoma are discussed in Chapter 12. Astrocytomas occasionally complicate neurofibromatosis-1 and neurofibromatosis-2, the Li–Fraumeni syndrome and Turcot's syndrome. A specific type of astrocytoma, the subependymal giant cell astrocytoma, complicates tuberous sclerosis.

Genetic alterations

Figure 5.3 illustrates some of the genetic changes encountered in patients with diffuse astrocytomas.

Genetic changes leading to the formation of gliomas affect two major cell functions: signal transduction and the cell cycle.[2] The first is affected by overexpression of growth factors or their receptors (e.g. EGF, PDGF) that through autocrine and paracrine pathways activate signaling pathways such as RAS and AKT.[2] Alternately, mutations of tumor suppressors such as PTEN may fail to inhibit signaling. Either change can lead to uncontrolled growth. The second general mechanism is an alteration of the cell cycle. Loss of inhibitors of the cell cycle such as INK4A, RB,

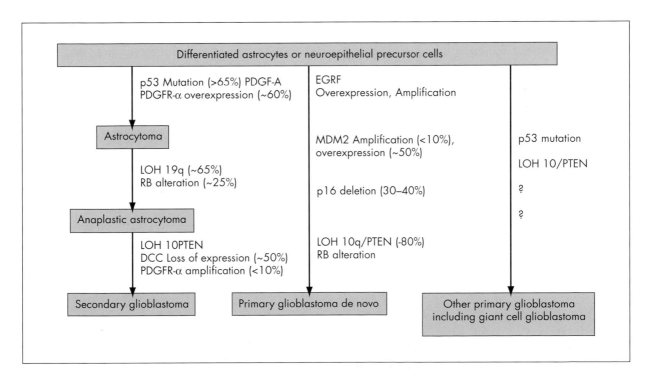

Figure 5.3
Genetic change in diffuse astrocytoma. (Modified from[2,25] with permission.)

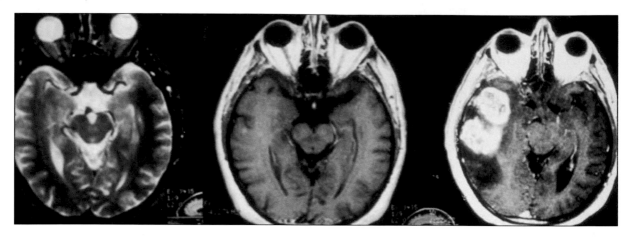

Figure 5.4
A unique patient with a symptomatic diffuse astrocytoma and a negative MR scan. The T2 (left) and T1 contrast-enhanced image (middle) were negative when the patient first presented with a generalized convulsion. Nine months later in the face of progressive symptoms, a repeat scan showed the image on the right, which on resection was a glioblastoma multiforme.

p53 and others can also lead to uncontrolled growth, genetic instability and failure of normal apoptosis (Chapter 1).

Glioblastoma (GBM) can arise de novo (Fig. 5.4, center and right panels) or progress from a low-grade tumor. The de novo pathway usually occurs in older patients in whom there is a short history of symptoms and no known pre-existing low-grade lesion. Alternatively, a GBM can arise through the progressive accumulation of genetic defects (Fig. 5.3, left panel) that lead first to an astrocytoma, then an anaplastic astrocytoma and finally a GBM. This pathway primarily occurs in young adults who often have a 3–10 year history before a GBM develops. The rate of progression to anaplasia correlates directly with age.[10] These alternative pathways indicate that no single genetic change is either essential or sufficient for GBM development.

Two major abnormalities that lead a differentiated astrocyte or neuroepithelial precursor cell to become an astrocytoma are p53 mutations and/or overexpression of platelet-derived growth factor A (PDGF-A) or platelet-derived growth factor receptor alpha (PDGFR-α). Progressive genetic changes in low-grade astrocytomas, including the loss of heterozygosity on 19q or alteration in the retinoblastoma tumor suppressor gene, lead the low-grade tumor to become anaplastic. Other genetic changes, including mutations in the PTEN gene, loss of expression of the DCC gene, or amplification of PDGFR-α, lead to GBM (secondary GBM). De novo or primary GBM arises by amplification or overexpression of epidermal growth factor receptor (EGFR); p53 mutations are rare. In about 40% of GBMs the EGFR is truncated with an in-frame deletion of approximately 30 amino acids. The truncated form is constitutively active, i.e. active without the need for ligand binding. The truncated receptor gene is not found in normal glial cells and thus forms a potential tumor-specific therapeutic target. PTEN inactivation plays an equal role in de novo and secondary glioblastomas.[11]

The differentiation between primary and secondary GBM may be difficult and cannot be made on a molecular basis alone. If a patient has a history of low-grade glioma that becomes a GBM, or if histologic evidence of both low-grade and high-grade astrocytoma is found in the same tumor specimen, the GBM is probably secondary. However, some apparently de novo glioblastomas have areas of low-grade as well as high-grade tumor. The low-grade areas in these primary GBMs have more 10q deletions and fewer p53 mutations than are found in the usual low-grade astrocytoma. These tumors lack EGFR amplification, suggesting that they represent a subset of secondary GBM with unusually rapid progression.[12] An MR scan showing areas of non-enhancing as well as enhancing tumor, or serial MR scans changing from non-enhancing to enhancing, suggest a secondary GBM. The development of an intensely enhancing tumor on the background of a previously normal scan suggests a primary GBM. Primary and secondary GBMs may differ in biology as well as genetics. Primary GBM is associated with a shorter survival than is secondary GBM.

High-grade gliomas often show abnormalities of genes coding for proteins that regulate the cell cycle (see Fig. 1.9). Control of the transition from G_1 to S phase is affected by mutation or deletion of the retinoblastoma gene but also by deletion or alterations of cyclins, including deletion of CDKN2A and CDKN2B, as well as amplification or overexpression of CDK4 and CDK6. D-type cyclin genes that regulate cyclin-dependent kinases are overexpressed in a few high-grade gliomas.[13] In high-grade astrocytoma, CDKN2/p16 is decreased and associated with a poor prognosis.[14] The tumor suppressor genes p53, p16, p14 and PTEN may be co-mutated in high-grade gliomas, each leading to a different alteration in cellular pathways.[15] PTEN mutations are present only in high-grade gliomas and may be associated with the transition to anaplasia.[16] Exogenous PTEN induces G_1 cell cycle arrest in glioma cells in culture.[17] One in vitro study suggests that tumors with mutated p53 are more resistant to fractionated RT than are those with wild-type p53. Those tumors with mutated p53 may respond better to fewer, larger fractions of radiation.[18] Deletions of chromosome 22q occur in about 30% of astrocytic tumors and the frequency of these deletions increases with progressive anaplasia (17% astrocytomas, 38% GBMs).[19] The nature of the suppressor gene on 22q is not known.

The matrix metalloproteinases, gelatinase A and B, are overexpressed in glioma, with expression of the B isoform related to higher tumor grade. These substances are involved in tumor invasion and angiogenesis (Chapter 2).[20,21] The tumor suppression gene DCC (Deleted in Colorectal Cancer) is reduced or absent in most glioblastomas, but is usually normal in low-grade tumors. Its absence predicts a poor prognosis.[22] Other genetic changes include proteosome-induced degradation of p27, a protein that regulates the cell cycle at G_1 to S transition.[23] Whether mutations in p21 contribute to the development of gliomas is uncertain.[24]

Pathology

Most astrocytic tumors are gray or yellow and soft to the touch, but focal calcifications give a gritty feeling to some astrocytomas. Microcyst formation in low-grade tumors may cause a gelatinous appearance. Sometimes a single large cyst filled with clear fluid is present. However, even when the boundaries appear distinct macroscopically, microscopic infiltration of brain is present. Grossly, it is often impossible to distinguish a low-grade from a high-grade diffuse astrocytoma unless necrosis, characteristic of GBM, is present.

Owing to their infiltrative nature, diffuse astrocytomas usually show blurring of gross anatomic boundaries, particularly loss of the gray–white matter border. Edema surrounds the tumor, but where tumor ends and edema begins cannot be identified grossly. GBM is more likely to appear well-demarcated from surrounding normal brain. Hemorrhage and necrosis are generally not found in lower grade tumors but may be grossly visible in GBM.

Microscopically, there may be infiltration of tumor cells several centimeters from the gross bulk of tumor.[4] Nuclear atypia, increased cellularity, endothelial proliferation, mitoses and necrosis are used to grade diffuse astrocytic tumors. Two grading systems for diffuse astrocytomas are widely used (Table 5.2).

The WHO uses a four-tiered system with Grade I reserved for pilocytic astrocytomas, Grade II for astrocytoma (low-grade), Grade III anaplastic astrocytoma, and Grade IV GBM (both high-grade), respectively.[25] The St Anne/Mayo system also uses numerical grades. It is often difficult to distinguish astrocytomas from anaplastic astrocytomas, leading to some disagreement between pathologists about interpreting individual tumors. The difficulty is compounded by the recent use of stereotactic needle biopsy, which gives the neuropathologist a very small sample to examine. Because of the well-known heterogeneity of astrocytic tumors, the smaller the sample, the less likely it is that one can grade the tumor accurately. Intratumoral heterogeneity can be demonstrated not only microscopically but also at the molecular level by comparative genomic hybridization.[26] In controlled trials of the treatment of diffuse astrocytomas, it is important to have one pathologist examining all of the tumors, ensuring consistency if not absolute accuracy.

Figure 5.2 illustrates the several grades of diffuse astrocytomas. In the panel on the left, a diffuse astrocytoma (WHO Grade II) or astrocytoma grade II (St Anne/Mayo designation) shows atypical nuclei, increased cellularity and microcysts. No mitotic activity, endothelial proliferation or necrosis can be identified. In the next panel, an anaplastic astrocytoma (WHO Grade III) or astrocytoma grade 3 (St Anne/Mayo) shows higher cellularity and nuclear atypia as well as mitotic activity. GBM (WHO Grade IV) or astrocytoma Grade 4 (St Anne/Mayo criteria) shows nuclear atypia, mitosis, endothelial proliferation and necrosis. Cellular proliferation evaluated by the MIB-1 labeling index helps distinguish among WHO Grade I (pilocytic) and Grades II and III. In Grades II and III astrocytomas, the MIB-1 index is the single best prognostic factor; however, for an individual patient, the labeling index alone should not determine therapy.[27] Surprisingly, the index does not give prognostic information for recurrent tumors.[28] Gemistocytes (from Latin gemma meaning 'bud') are large eosinophilic cells with spherical, eccentric nuclei. Gemistocytic astrocytomas, especially those with > 20% gemistocytes, indicate a poor prognosis.[29]

Occasionally, glial tumors can acquire histologic features suggestive of other tumor types, such as ependymal differentiation leading to confusion with an ependymoma. An experienced neuropathologist can usually discern the correct nature of the lesion; however, sometimes additional pathologic evaluation is necessary. For example, electron microscopy will identify the cilia characteristic of a true ependymoma, which are absent in an astrocytic tumor with ependymal differentiation.

Two biological characteristics of diffuse astrocytomas are invasion of normal surrounding brain and angiogenesis (Chapter 2). Unlike cancers elsewhere in the body, which usually have the capacity not only to invade surrounding tissue but also to metastasize distantly, astrocytomas usually invade and may spread widely within the CNS but rarely metastasize outside of it. Normal glial cells in vitro, and probably in vivo as well, are motile. This property is enhanced in glioma cells, and the degree of motility appears to be directly related to the grade of the tumor cell. Cell migration appears to follow white matter pathways; the corpus callosum and anterior commissure are among the major pathways for spread of astrocytomas. These two routes allow tumors to spread from one hemisphere to the other.

In patients with brain tumors, Kelly et al have demonstrated by stereotactic needle biopsy of tumor and surrounding brain that tumor cells often invade normal brain to a variable degree.[4] In some tumors, there is little or no invasion and the tumor is grossly as well as microscopically reasonably well circumscribed. In other tumors, cells can be found several centimeters beyond the apparent border of the tumor with normal brain. The series of mutations necessary to allow astrocytoma cells to invade surrounding normal brain are discussed in Chapter 2 (see Table 2.2). Several factors apply primarily to glioma, the major invasive brain tumor: integrins, transmembrane glycoproteins that anchor extracellular matrix components with the intracellular cytoskeleton, and transcriptional machinery are overexpressed in glioma cells. Interactions between integrins and extracellular matrix components, including tenascin, fibronectin and osteopontin, are necessary for invasion to occur. CD44, a glycoprotein receptor for several extracellular matrix components, including hyaluronic acid, is expressed weakly in astrocytomas but more strongly expressed in anaplastic astrocytomas and GBM. This receptor mediates tissue invasion by glioma cells. Adhesion molecules such as neural cell adhesion molecules (N-CAM)[30] promote cell–cell interaction; glioma cells lacking N-CAM loosen that interaction, which facilitates motility. Proteases are expressed by glioma cells and some, particularly metalloproteinases, are probably important for invasion. Growth factors, including transforming growth factor beta-1 (TGF-β_1), contribute to the spread of tumor cells within the CNS.

The capacity to invade not only makes it impossible to completely remove diffuse astrocytic tumors, but also allows them to appear in multiple places in the brain. Somewhere between 5% and 10% of diffuse astrocytomas are said to be 'multicentric'. A multicentric glioma is a clinical challenge because the imaging may resemble that of brain metastasis and lead to an incorrect evaluation or diagnosis. It is possible that so-called multicentric gliomas represent spread from a single focus, with areas of grossly apparent tumor being connected by bridges of microscopic glioma cells. In its most florid form, gliomas can invade the entire brain (gliomatosis cerebri) without any focal regions of obvious tumor apparent on neuroimaging. The second major factor in glioma growth is angiogenesis, discussed in Chapter 2. Angiogenesis supports tumor growth and facilitates clinical diagnosis.

Both the tumor and clinician depend on angiogenesis. The tumor needs new blood vessels to nourish a mass beyond a few millimeters. The clinician relies on the fact that the neovasculature induced by the tumor is leaky, lacking an intact blood–brain barrier and leading to contrast enhancement on the MR scan.

Clinical findings

Symptoms and signs

The symptoms and signs, as well as the diagnostic evaluation of diffuse astrocytomas, are, for the most part, described in Chapter 3.

Some distinctions will be highlighted here. Astrocytomas are more likely than their higher-grade counterparts to present with seizures, either focal or generalized.[31] Occasional seizures over many months or years, without the development of other neurologic symptoms, occur with astrocytomas and even more frequently with oligodendrogliomas (see below). If seizures are the presenting symptom of an anaplastic astrocytoma, they are generally soon followed by other neurologic dysfunction. Higher-grade lesions are more likely to present with focal neurologic symptoms such as memory loss, personality change, contralateral motor or sensory symptoms, and visual field deficits.

Imaging

In general, an infiltrative non-enhancing lesion, hyperintense on T2, connotes a low-grade glioma, whereas an enhancing lesion connotes a high-grade lesion. A large enhancing lesion that shifts the midline indicates a poor prognosis.[32] A normal MR scan usually excludes a diffuse astrocytoma as the cause of a patient's symptoms, and no further workup for brain tumor is required. However, we have encountered one exception to the above rule – a patient who had an entirely normal MR scan after a generalized convulsion, but several months later, after another seizure, was found to have a glioblastoma multiforme (Fig. 5.4). Others have encountered similar situations.[33] In all other instances where reportedly normal scans were found in patients with neurologic symptoms due to diffuse astrocytoma, a careful review of the scans identified either an inadequate study or hyperintensity on the T2-weighted image that eventually became an obvious tumor. To complicate the situation, transient MRI abnormalities occasionally are caused by long-lasting seizures in the absence of a structural defect.[34] Difficulties in inter-preting the MR scan in diffuse astrocytomas may arise in older patients who have multiple areas of white matter hyperintensity related to vascular disease. One additional area of hyper-intensity might be disregarded unless contrast is given to reveal enhancement. However, the hyperintensity from tumor is usually immediately subcortical and more diffuse than most periventricular white matter hyperintense foci seen with vascular disease.

Positron emission tomography

PET scans are helpful in some patients with putative low-grade diffuse astrocytomas prior to biopsy. The PET scan is done with fluorodeoxyglucose to determine glucose metabolic rate. If the PET scan is hypometabolic in a patient with a non-enhancing lesion who suffers only seizures controllable by anticonvulsants, and has no other neurologic symptoms or signs, we may elect to follow that patient rather than biopsy or treat immediately (see below). If a generally hypometabolic PET scan shows an area of hypermetabolism suggesting a focus of high-grade tumor, the neurosurgeon can direct his stereotactic needle biopsy to that area, because treatment is determined by the highest grade in a heterogeneous tumor. Amino acid PET imaging, usually with methionine, can characterize low vs. high grade glioma with greater accuracy than fluorodeoxyglucose PET, but it is currently limited to a research setting. PET scanning has also been used to distinguish tumor recurrence from radiation necrosis,[35] as have SPECT scans. Thallium SPECT scanning has been reported to demonstrate response to chemotherapy better than does MRI.[36]

Magnetic resonance spectroscopy

Recent evidence suggests that this technique may have the capacity to distinguish diffuse astrocytomas from other intrinsic tumors of the brain and may play a role in establishing astro-cytoma grade non-invasively.[37] The data are still preliminary and the technique should be considered experimental.

Functional magnetic resonance imaging and cortical mapping

As indicated in Chapter 3, fMRI prior to surgery and cortical mapping during surgery have important roles to play in the treatment of diffuse astrocytomas. Functional magnetic imaging can identify not only sensory and motor areas, but also language areas of brain that cannot be identified at neurosurgery unless the patient is operated on under local anesthesia. Mapping during the course of surgery can identify sensory and motor areas, even under general anesthesia. These tests are particularly important in patients with diffuse astrocytomas because of their infiltrative nature. By delineating the exact location of these critical areas, these tests enable the surgeon to plan his approach appropriately. Many patients with diffuse astrocytomas suffering from focal neurologic symptoms improve after compression of an eloquent area is relieved without the area itself being violated.

Biopsy

In most instances, if a suspected diffuse astro-cytoma is encountered on MR scan, craniotomy and removal of as much tumor as is technically feasible is the best diagnostic and therapeutic approach. In some instances, usually because the tumor is located in a criti-cal area, surgical resection is not feasible. In that case, a stereotactic needle biopsy should be performed to establish the diagnosis before beginning definitive treatment. It is important not only to establish that the abnormality on the MR scan is indeed a diffuse astrocytoma, but also to grade the tumor, because grading determines treatment. The limitations and complications of stereotactic biopsy were discussed in Chapter 3.

Differential diagnosis

Table 5.3 lists some neoplastic and non-neoplastic lesions that are sometimes mistaken for astrocytic tumors by MRI and occasionally even by biopsy. The neoplasms include glial and non-glial tumors. For most glial tumors, the exact histologic diagnosis is less important than the tumor grade; however, distinguishing

Neoplastic lesions	Non-neoplastic lesions
Other glial tumors	Cerebral infarction
Oligodendrogliomas	Cerebral hemorrhage
Ependymoma	Multiple sclerosis/Demyelinating pseudotumor
Focal astrocytic tumor	Herpes simplex encephalitis
	Brain abscess
Non-glial tumors	
Lymphoma	
Metastases	
Neuronal tumors	
Others	

Table 5.3
Differential diagnosis of diffuse astrocytoma.

astrocytic from oligodendroglial tumors can affect treatment (see below).

Other glial tumors are discussed later in this chapter. Non-glial tumors may be difficult or impossible to distinguish from glial tumors on imaging study. Biopsy is essential to establish the correct diagnosis and treatment.

A major problem is distinguishing cerebrovascular disease, either infarction or hemorrhage, from tumor. When an older patient presents with a seizure or sudden neurologic defect, the physician usually suspects vascular disease, particularly if the patient recovers rapidly. Patients with diffuse astrocytomas often present with transient symptoms, and when they are elderly, cerebrovascular disease must be a leading diagnostic consideration. A CT scan without contrast may show an area of hypodensity that is interpreted as cerebral infarction. Cerebral infarcts give their abnormal signal in a vascular distribution and often are triangular, with the base in the cortical gray matter and the apex deep. Tumors are rounder, primarily involve white matter and do not necessarily respect a vascular territory. When the cortex is involved, the gyri are expanded. On diffusion MR scan, an infarct is hyperintense and a tumor usually hypo- or isointense. A contrast-enhanced MR scan often establishes the diagnosis but, too often, the patient is assumed to have vascular disease and no further work-up is initiated beyond the initial CT scan.

Cerebral hemorrhage may announce the presence of a tumor. Unlike other hemorrhages, those into tumor often show enhancement of the underlying tumor immediately after the ictus; enhancement of a hematoma can take days to weeks to develop. Even without enhancement, tumors will demonstrate T2 hyperintensity around the hemorrhage, often outlining peritumoral edema that was present before hemorrhage occurred. This is apparent on the initial imaging procedure whereas edema usually takes several days to develop around a primary intracerebral hemorrhage. Thus, imaging can often suggest the presence of an underlying tumor even when hemorrhage is the presentation.

Focal seizures can have many causes other than brain tumor. However, unlike short-lived focal seizures occurring with other epileptic lesions, the episodes may last many minutes to hours and are often associated with abnormalities of cognition and behavior. Focal seizures themselves can alter brain images. One report describes enhancement and hypermetabolism on PET scan following multiple focal seizures in a patient in clinical remission from a brain tumor. The image normalized after the seizures were controlled.[38]

A non-neoplastic lesion that can mimic tumor is demyelination (Fig. 5.5). Masdeu and colleagues have pointed out that one radiographic distinction between demyelinating pseudotumor and GBM is that the contrast-enhancing ring is incomplete in demyelinating disease, frequently where the lesion is adjacent to the ventricle, but complete in GBM.[39] MRS may also aid in the distinction,[40] but the reliability of this technique is unknown. Generally, the lesions are not easily distinguished on scan, and biopsy is usually necessary to establish the correct diagnosis. It is the obligation of the neurologist and neurosurgeon to call the neuropathologist's attention to the possibility of demyelinating disease, because the macrophages in a demyelinating lesion may be interpreted as tumor cells, with the patient unnecessarily subjected to major resection and RT. RT appears to be particularly damaging in these patients[41] and the distinction, therefore, is vital. Usually demyelinating pseudotumor is an isolated event and a minority of

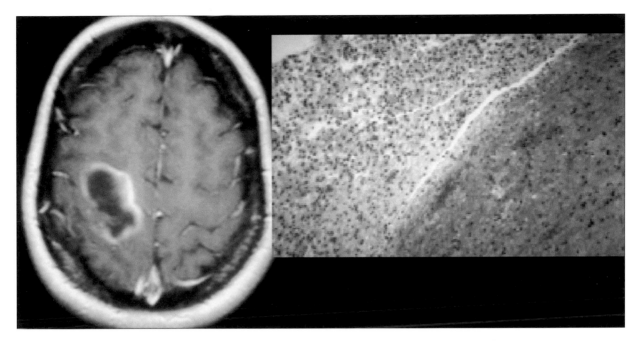

Figure 5.5
Differential diagnosis of glioblastoma multiforme. The axial scan shows a ring-enhancing mass surrounded by edema, suggesting a neoplasm. Note that the ring is incomplete, which might give a clue to a demyelinating lesion (Chapter 3). A myelin stain of the lesion reveals a sharp border between the demyelinated lesion (left half) containing many macrophages, and the adjacent brain with preserved myelin (right half).

patients go on to develop multiple sclerosis. Most patients recover and do well. Other inflammatory lesions (e.g. sarcoid) may also mimic tumor and require biopsy.

Herpes simplex encephalitis usually presents acutely with headache, seizures and neurologic dysfunction suggesting a temporal lobe lesion. Brain tumors may present in the same way. Each year we encounter at least 2 patients who 'recover' from encephalitis but then relapse and are discovered to have a diffuse astrocytoma.

Treatment

The treatment of diffuse astrocytomas depends on the grade, and in the paragraphs below is divided by both grade and specific tumor type.

Astrocytoma

The best treatment for astrocytomas has not been established.[42] Surgery establishes the diagnosis and often relieves neurologic symptoms but whether it prolongs survival is controversial.[43] Older patients (> 40 years) with tumors >3 cm and with mass effect do appear to benefit from resection. Surgery seems to improve both quality and duration of life in children with astrocytomas, both low- and high-grade[44] and we believe that it also does so in adults. However, surgery does not cure (pilocytic astrocytoma is an exception – see below); surgery conventionally has been followed by RT. This approach remains valid for patients with progressive neurologic signs or intractable seizures. However, for asymptomatic patients, including those with controlled seizures, immediate postoperative radiation therapy improves progression-free survival but not overall duration of survival when compared with radiation therapy delivered after the patient has developed clinical or radiographic progression.[45] Furthermore, radiation causes dose-related cognitive abnormalities and diminishes quality of life.[42,46] A PET study indicated that RT has no effect on either methionine or glucose uptake in the tumor area compared to patients not irradiated.[47] However, although the 'normal brain' areas of patients with astrocytomas who did not receive radiotherapy have lower glucose uptake than normal individuals, the glucose uptake in normal brain areas was even lower in patients who received radiation therapy,[48] indicating radiation damage to normal brain.

When used, the best dose of radiation has not been established. An EORTC study comparing 45 Gy in 5 weeks with 59.4 Gy in 6.5 weeks revealed no difference in survival, but patients who received the higher dose radiation tended to report lower levels of function and more symptom burden following completion of radiotherapy. The group differences were statistically significant for fatigue/malaise and insomnia immediately after RT, and emotional functioning at 7–15 months after treatment.[49] Low-grade gliomas do respond to RT with a greater than 50% decrease in tumor area on scan, but there is no statistically significant association between response as measured on scan, symptomatology and progression-free survival.[50]

Each patient's treatment must be individualized but we adhere to the following general rules and recommendations:

- If the tumor is in a relatively silent area of brain (e.g. right frontal lobe), whether or not it is causing neurologic symptoms and signs other than controllable seizures, an attempt should be made to remove the tumor. Patients who undergo a gross total resection of a low-grade tumor are not cured, but survival appears to be longer and quality of life better than in those who do not have resection.

- Patients whose tumors involve critical brain structures, e.g. language cortex, and who are asymptomatic save for focal seizures, particularly if the PET scan is hypometabolic, can be followed without treatment (an area of hypermetabolism on the PET scan is an indication for biopsy and perhaps treatment as indicated below for anaplastic tumors). Some patients can be followed for many years without substantial growth of the lesion. At the time of clinical or radiographic progression, biopsy should be performed to ascertain whether the tumor is an astrocytoma, oligodendroglioma or something else, and to determine grade. Treatment would then be dictated by histology.

- Symptomatic patients should undergo resection to the maximum extent feasible, or a stereotactic needle biopsy should be performed when resection cannot be done. After a diagnosis is established, RT should be delivered to a limited field encompassing the visible tumor on MR scan and a 2 cm margin. Conventional treatment is delivered in fractions no larger than 1.8 Gy to a total dose of 54 Gy. Lower doses might be equally effective (or ineffective).[49] There is no evidence at the present time that radiosurgery, brachytherapy or radiation sensitizers have any role to play.

Anaplastic astrocytomas and glioblastoma multiforme

In most treatment series, anaplastic astrocytomas (anaplasia comes from the Greek words *plasso*, meaning 'to form', and *ana*, meaning 'repeat or again'; anaplasia is generally taken to mean growth without appropriate form or structure) and GBMs (glioblastoma from the Greek *glia* for 'glue', *blastos* for 'germ or sprout' and *oma* for 'tumor'; *multiforme* from the Latin for 'polymorphic'), also called astrocytomas grade III and IV by WHO and St. Anne-Mayo criteria, are usually lumped together under the term 'malignant glioma' or 'malignant astrocytoma'. However, these two tumors have different prognoses (see below), and if a clinical trial is heavily weighted with one or the other, one may observe different survival rates that are not due to treatment.

The conventional treatment of anaplastic astrocytoma is removal of as much of the tumor as is surgically feasible, delivery of RT to a limited field encompassing the tumor and a 2.5–3 cm margin to a dose of 59.4 Gy in 1.8-Gy fractions, and chemotherapy following the irradiation. Most studies suggest that extensive surgery increases both duration and quality of survival. RT also improves quality and duration of life. There is a correlation between the amount of radiation and the duration of survival. However, the maximum feasible dose appears to be the equivalent of 60 Gy given in 1.8–2.0 Gy fractions to a limited field. After three-dimensional conformal radiotherapy to a dose of 70–80 Gy, recurrences still occur primarily within the irradiated field,[51] and the increased dose does not improve survival. Although a few

reports describe benefit, there is at the present time no firm evidence that hyperfractionation, radiosurgery[52] or brachytherapy[53] are better than standard RT, even when the total dose has been escalated as high as 120 Gy with brachytherapy. Accelerated hyperfractionation radiotherapy (70 Gy in 44 fractions given twice daily) is reported to be comparable to but not better than standard RT.[54] Re-irradiation with lower doses (34.5 Gy in 23 fractions), to treat recurrences that occur after initial RT and chemotherapy, may improve survival with little toxicity.[55]

Elderly patients (> 70 years) treated with surgery and radiation therapy survive longer than those treated with less aggressive regimes,[56] but the prognosis is still poor. Some recommend reducing the dose and duration of radiation therapy to those over 70 (45 Gy/25 fractions).[57] Some older patients in poor neurological condition, who have extensive GBM achieve maximum palliation with a short course of RT, so that the decision to use a short course of RT is based on the clinical situation.

Two conventional **chemotherapeutic** regimens are carmustine (BCNU) at a dose of 200 mg/m^2 every 8 weeks to a total dose of 1500 mg/m^2, and procarbazine, vincristine and lomustine (PCV), as indicated in Table 5.4. The two are equally effective,[58] but and because PCV is more

Table 5.4
Chemotherapy of anaplastic gliomas* and oligodendrogliomas.

Drug	Dose		Route	Schedule
	Intensive[a]	*Standard[b]*		
Carmustine (BCNU)	130 mg/m^2	110 mg/m^2	PO	Day 1
Vincristine[a]	1.4 mg/m^2[b]	1.4 mg/m^2[b]	IV	Days 8 and 28
Procarbazine	75 mg/m^2/day	60 mg/m^2/day	PO	Days 8–21

*Standard dose chemotherapy is used for anaplastic gliomas
[a]Intensive cycle is 6 weeks, standard is 8 weeks
[b]2 mg limit in standard dose, no limit in intensive dose

toxic, we generally prefer BCNU as a single agent. Although a number of phase II trials have shown that other chemotherapeutic agents are modestly effective,[59] none are superior to BCNU or PCV. Increasing the dose of PCV with stem cell support increases toxicity but not efficacy.[60] BCNU does not substantially increase the median survival, but in 20–30% of patients it prolongs survival. Good prognostic factors (e.g. favorable histology) do not predict benefit from adjuvant chemotherapy and benefit has been demonstrated for patients up to age 65.[61]

There is no evidence to indicate that chemotherapy given prior to RT or concomitant with RT promotes either quality or duration of survival. There are some data to demonstrate that pre-RT chemotherapy may be harmful, with a high rate of rapid tumor regrowth frequently necessitating reoperation before RT can be administered, and occasionally early death. We have also had the occasional experience of profound unexpected myelosuppression when BCNU was administered concurrently with RT. Therefore, we usually start chemotherapy after completion of RT.

Inevitably, patients with anaplastic astrocytoma and glioblastoma multiforme relapse after treatment (Fig. 5.6). In many circumstances, a second surgical procedure will improve symptoms and increase survival for about 6

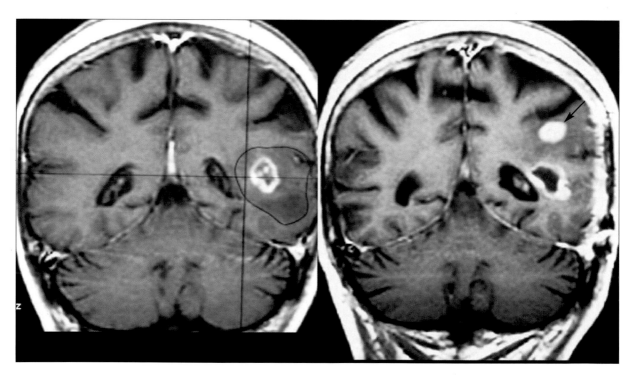

Figure 5.6
Response of a glioblastoma to radiation therapy but with recurrence outside the radiation portal. An elderly patient presented with language difficulty and at surgery was found to have a glioblastoma multiforme. The lesion was partially resected. The patient then received 60 Gy to the area outlined in black on the left panel. One year later, the patient began to complain of right-sided weakness and a repeat scan revealed that the tumor in the irradiated area had not grown but that a new lesion had appeared outside of the radiation portal (arrow).

months. As indicated above, re-irradiation at relapse is feasible and stereotactic RT, brachytherapy, other chemotherapeutic agents and experimental therapeutic techniques can also be considered at that point. One study indicated that BCNU wafers implanted into the tumor bed at relapse may increase survival, but the study compared placebo wafers with a BCNU wafer, not with intravenous BCNU.[62] Implantation of wafers may be associated with a higher risk of postoperative complications, particularly infection and poor wound healing.[63] One study suggests that a combination of interstitial and systemic chemotherapy may promote survival.[64]

Temozolomide (200 mg/m[2] daily for 5 days followed by 23 days rest) is now the most used second-line agent if the patient has originally been treated with a nitrosourea or PCV. Temozolomide is given orally and has few side-effects, so that many physicians use it in preference to BCNU as initial chemotherapy although data regarding its use in the adjuvant setting is not yet available. A number of other chemotherapeutic agents have been reported in phase II trials to have moderate activity, including topotecan, carboplatin and cisplatin (Table 4.12), but none induce prolonged remission. Intrathecal thiotepa may help some patients with ependymal or leptomeningeal spread of tumor.[65]

Tamoxifen in high doses (80 mg/m[2] or more) inhibits protein kinase C (PKC). It has little neurotoxicity, although dizziness and ataxia may occur, but the drug has little or no efficacy.[66] At the present time, newer forms of treatment, including immunotherapy, radio-active antibodies,[67] gene therapy,[68] antiangiogenesis therapy, and antisense therapy, have not been shown to be efficacious.

Prognosis

Table 1.11 lists the prognosis in diffuse astrocytoma. The median survival for glioblastoma multiforme (Grade IV) is approximately one year, with 15–20% of patients surviving more than 2 years but fewer than 5% more than 3 years.[69] There are rare long-term survivors, particularly among the young. Gliosarcomas have a prognosis similar to GBM.[70] Young age is the most important favorable prognostic factor.[71] Other favorable factors include performance status, histology (anaplastic astrocytoma vs GBM), extent of surgery and adjuvant chemotherapy.[69] A serum albumin level < 3.4 mg/dl predicts a poor prognosis;[72] the low levels are probably part of an acute-phase response regulated by cytokines that also induce angiogenesis.[72] In anaplastic astrocytomas (Grade III), the median survival is approximately 3 years, with 10–15% surviving beyond 5 years. Diffuse astrocytomas have a wide range of behavior, but the median survival is 5–8 years, with 15–20% surviving 10 years. Good prognostic factors include young age, good performance status and no enhancement on MRI.[73] Prognosis for these tumors has not changed substantially for the past 20–30 years; clearly, new therapies are required.

Gliomatosis cerebri

Diffuse astrocytomas sometimes infiltrate the brain so widely that they involve the entire brain with or without an identifiable focal lesion. Such diffuse infiltration is called gliomatosis cerebri (Fig. 2.2). Pathologically, the disorder is an astrocytoma that may vary from low to high grade and may differ in grade from area to area. Rarely, an oligodendroglioma may present as gliomatosis cerebri.[74] The symptoms may be either generalized (i.e. headaches, papilledema, cognitive changes) or focal, including corticospinal tract abnormalities and seizures. Some patients present with brainstem or even spinal cord signs, as the entire neuraxis may be infiltrated occasionally.

The MR scan is usually characterized by hyper-intensity on the T2 image, either diffusely or multifocally. On some occasions, one or more areas of contrast enhancement are present within the diffuse or multifocal non-enhancing areas. On rare occasions, there is no abnormality of signal intensity but simply diffuse enlargement of the brain leading to smaller ventricles and sulci than would be expected for the patient's age. When gliomatosis cerebri is suspected, a stereotactic needle biopsy will establish the diagnosis. The needle biopsy should be directed toward the most abnormal area of the brain. The prognosis is poor; more than half the patients die within a year of symptom onset and less than a quarter survive more than 3 years.

Patients with gliomatosis cerebri are treated with RT.[75] Unlike focal anaplastic astrocytomas or glioblastoma, the radiation is delivered to the whole brain to a total dose of 60 Gy. In patients with biopsy or scan evidence of anaplasia, adjuvant chemotherapy with BCNU can be given after the radiation, although its efficacy is not known.

Brainstem glioma

Gliomas arising in the brainstem are heterogeneous[76] (Fig. 5.7). They have been categorized in three ways: diffuse and focal, by location, i.e. pontine, midbrain and medullary, and subdivided into cystic or exophytic lesions. Each has a different biology and prognosis. The most common of the brainstem gliomas is the diffuse pontine astrocytoma that usually occurs in childhood. These tumors are astrocytic and may be low or high grade. Tumors that occur in adulthood differ little in signs or symptoms from those in children, usually beginning with cranial nerve palsies, especially diplopia, and subsequently evolving to cause long tract signs. Hydrocephalus is uncommon. The diagnosis is made by MR scan. The tumors look histologically identical to astrocytomas in other areas of the brain. Focal brainstem lesions, less than 2 cm and often dorsally exophytic, are more likely to be pilocytic astrocytomas or gangliogliomas, and open biopsy is safe. Some neurosurgeons recommend stereotactic needle biopsy even when the tumor remains within the confines of the brainstem, but others believe that the complication rate is too high and that MR scan is sufficiently characteristic to establish the diagnosis. Some neurosurgeons recommend partial excision if tumors are exophytic, but the diffuse lesions widely infiltrate the brainstem and cannot be approached surgically. For most brainstem gliomas, focal RT is the treatment of choice. Hyperfractionated radiotherapy is not more effective than conventional radiotherapy.[77] Adjuvant chemotherapy, even when given in high doses, has not been effective, although studies to find effective agents continue.[78] The prognosis is better in adults than it is for children, with 45% of adults living longer than 5 years in our experience.[79] Tumors that arise in the midbrain or medulla, focal or exophytic tumors of the pons and tumors that are amenable to subtotal resection have a better prognosis than the usual diffuse pontine tumor.[76] Brainstem gliomas associated with neurofibromatosis type 1 usually have a good prognosis and often do not require treatment[80] (see Chapter 12).

A peculiarly low-grade tumor sometimes affects the midbrain. These tumors have variously been called tectal gliomas or pencil gliomas of the aqueduct, depending on their appearance on MR scan. They present in adolescence or early adulthood with hydrocephalus caused by compression of the aqueduct, the symptoms of which can be relieved by shunting of the cerebral ventricles.

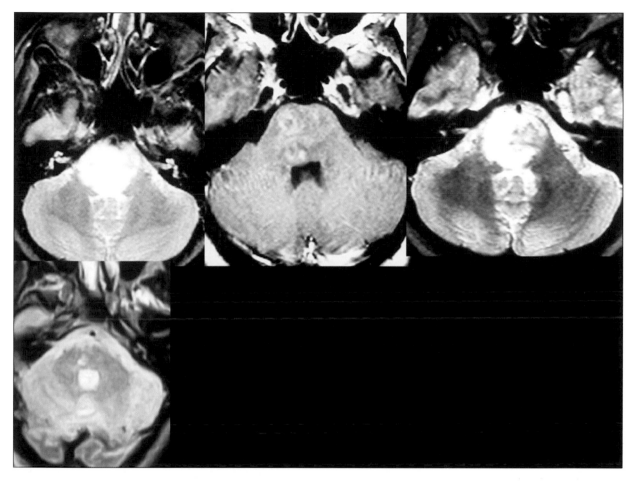

Figure 5.7
A brainstem glioma in a young woman. This patient originally presented with facial myokymia and mild facial weakness. The MRI revealed an infiltrating tumor in the brainstem (see also Fig. 3.1C). She was lost to follow-up for approximately a year. She returned with increasing facial weakness. The scan at that time showed diffuse hyperintensity on the T2-weighted image of the entire pons (left upper) with some contrast enhancement (left middle). Six months after radiation, she was clinically stable and the scan showed some decrease in the size of the T2-weighted lesion (upper right). Four years later she continued to have mild facial weakness but the tumor on scan had largely resolved. No biopsy was performed.

Many such tumors appear to require no additional treatment, as they do not grow, and as long as the hydrocephalus is relieved, the patient remains asymptomatic, often for many years. If there is evidence of tumor growth on scan or if symptoms of brainstem dysfunction develop, RT is the treatment.

Subependymal giant cell astrocytoma

This low-grade tumor typically arises as a single or multiple lesions lining the wall(s) of the lateral ventricles.[81] The tumor is believed to arise from subependymal stem cells, giving it a mixed neuronal and glial phenotype. The tumor usually occurs in patients suffering from tuberous sclerosis and generally affects children, although infants and adults have also been reported. Interestingly, although tuberin, the protein product of the tuberous sclerosis gene, is expressed in tubers, it is not expressed in these tumors.[82] Their characteristic site within the walls of the ventricle, the calcification seen on CT scan and the stigmata of tuberous sclerosis (see Chapter 12) help establish the diagnosis. Surgical treatment is necessary only in the rare instance when the tumor obstructs the ventricular system, causing hydrocephalus. Malignant degeneration is extremely rare.

Oligodendroglial tumors

Introduction

Oligodendroglial tumors (from the Greek words *oligo* meaning 'few', *dendro* meaning 'tree' and *glia* meaning 'glue', meaning few dendritic processes when compared with astrocyts) are believed to arise from the oligodendrocyte by dedifferentiation or from neoplastic transformation of a progenitor such as the O-2A cell,[83] a precursor of oligodendrocytes and type II astrocytes. The tumors occur both in pure form and mixed with neoplastic cells that appear astrocytic (oligoastrocytoma). Like diffuse astrocytomas, many tumors progress from low grade to a higher grade (Fig. 5.8).

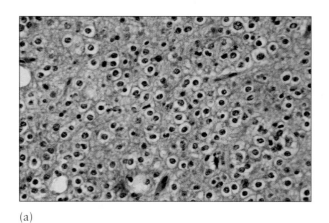

(a)

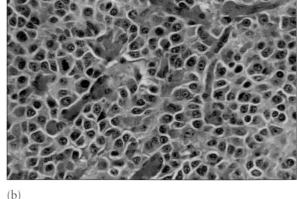

(b)

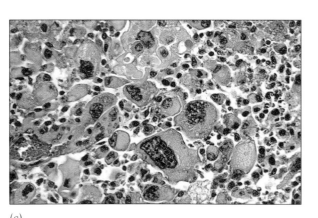

(c)

Figure 5.8
The evolution of oligodendrogliomas as indicated in Table 5.5. Oligodendrogliomas can evolve from non-neoplastic precursors and low-grade tumors, anaplastic oligodendrogliomas to glioblastomas multiforme. This figure illustrates the changes in that sequence. (a) Uniform round nuclei with surrounding clear halo, the so-called 'fried egg' appearance of a typical low-grade oligodendroglioma. (b) More cellular tumor with brisk mitoses and atypical cells with eosinophilic cytoplasm. (c) The oligodendrocytic phenotype is lost and anaplastic glial forms, including giant cells, appear.

Because they are less common than astrocytomas, and because of the difficulty of definitive diagnosis, many aspects of the tumor are poorly understood. For example, no unequivocal marker identifies a tumor as being oligodendroglial in origin. About 50% of oligos that are otherwise typical express glial fibrillary acidic proteins (GFAP), usually considered an astrocytic marker. In many tumors, microgemistocytes are prominent, often leading to an incorrect diagnosis of a gemistocytic astrocytoma (an astrocytoma variant, believed to have a worse prognosis than other astrocytomas of the same grade). In addition, the relationship between histopathology and prognosis is less clear when oligodendrogliomas are compared with astrocytomas. In past years, differentiating between an oligodendroglioma and an astrocytoma was unimportant therapeutically, and many pathologists paid little attention to distinguishing these tumors. Because of the recent evidence that oligodendrogliomas are much more chemosensitive than astrocytomas (see below), more attention has been paid to the histologic differentiation; consequently, the apparent frequency of diffuse oligodendrogliomas has risen. In one series they represented slightly under 5% of all primary brain tumors. A recent study attempting to define the histologic criteria indicated that about 25% of gliomas are of oligodendroglial origin.[84] Genetic studies (see below) may settle the issue. Furthermore, the majority of oligos (approximately 90%) are low-grade at diagnosis, in contrast to the astrocytic tumors that are more frequently malignant.

Oligodendrogliomas usually occur in young individuals with a peak incidence at about age 30. The tumors are uncommon in childhood. Unlike astrocytomas that are more common in men; oligodendrogliomas occur equally in men and women.

Etiology

Risk factors. There are no established risk factors for the development of oligodendrogliomas. Similar tumors can be produced in experimental animals by ethylnitrosourea and methylnitrosourea, but chemical carcinogenesis is not established in humans. Occasional families have oligodendrogliomas in more than one member, but this finding could be a coincidence and its meaning is unclear.

Genetics

Table 5.5 outlines the genetic changes thought to be associated with oligodendrogliomas. The most important alteration is loss of heterozygosity on the long arm of chromosome 19 and the short arm of chromosome 1. Up to 80% of patients with oligodendrogliomas have the 19q deletion, representing an as yet unidentified tumor suppressor gene that resides between 19q 13.2 and 19q 13.4. The deletion

Table 5.5
Genetic alteration in oligodendroglial tumors.

Oligodendroglial cells or precursor (? 0–2A)
19q LOH
1p LOH
4q LOH
EGFR overexpression
PDGF/PDGFR overexpression
Oligodendroglioma
9p LOH
10p LOH
CDCKN2A deletion
CDKN2C mutation/deletion
VEGF overexpression
TP53 mutation
P53 mutation (~10%)
Anaplastic oligodendroglioma
?
Glioblastoma multiforme
Modified from Kleihues and Cavenee.[25]

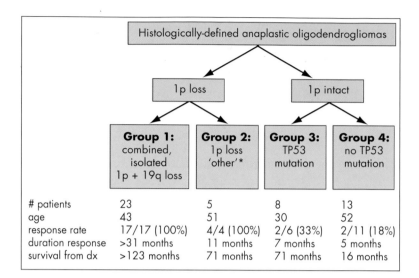

Figure 5.9
Response of anaplastic
oligodendrogliomas to chemotherapy
by genetic makeup. From [88] with
permission.

The figure contains:

Histologically-defined anaplastic oligodendrogliomas

→ 1p loss → 1p intact

	Group 1: combined, isolated 1p + 19q loss	Group 2: 1p loss 'other'*	Group 3: TP53 mutation	Group 4: no TP53 mutation
# patients	23	5	8	13
age	43	51	30	52
response rate	17/17 (100%)	4/4 (100%)	2/6 (33%)	2/11 (18%)
duration response	>31 months	11 months	7 months	5 months
survival from dx	>123 months	71 months	71 months	16 months

on the short arm of chromosome 1 has been reported in up to 90% of oligodendrogliomas.[85] Candidate genes on 1p include the cell cycle regulator gene CDKN2C.[86,87] Ino and colleagues[88] have identified 4 molecular subtypes of anaplastic oligodendrogliomas. Those with isolated losses of 1p and 19q have a dramatic and prolonged (years) response to chemotherapy; those with 1p but not 19q deletions respond but with shorter duration (1 year); those without 1p deletions but with p53 mutations may respond for a short time (7 months); those with neither 1p nor p53 alterations do not respond (Fig. 5.9).[88]

Pathology

Oligodendrogliomas are usually supratentorial, often arising in the frontal lobe and involving the corpus callosum. Their gross appearance does not differ from that of astrocytomas, except that calcifications can occasionally be identified in the gross specimen, a rarity in astrocytomas. Microscopically, low-grade oligodendrogliomas appear as a moderately cellular tumor with spherical hyperchromatic nuclei surrounded by swollen clear cytoplasm.

The swollen clear cytoplasm, surrounded by a well-defined plasma membrane, has given the cells a so-called 'fried egg' appearance, actually an artifact of fixation. Mitoses are rare. In the background are delicate blood vessels, often arranged in a 'chicken wire pattern'. This delicate vasculature may account for the relatively high rate of hemorrhage even in low-grade oligodendrogliomas. Endothelial proliferation is absent in the low-grade tumors. In anaplastic oligodendrogliomas, vascular proliferation, mitotic activity and necrosis may be seen. Calcifications are prominent. Table 5.6 details the histologic changes in oligodendrogliomas and their high-grade counterparts. Although this four-tiered grading system has been developed, the only clinically useful classification of oligodendrogliomas is low-grade versus anaplastic. Thus, functionally, a two-tiered system is used by most neuropathologists. The close relationship of cellularity, nuclear atypia and even mitotic figures to prognosis is less certain in oligodendroglial tumors than in astrocytic tumors, but endothelial proliferation appears predictive of poor prognosis.[89]

Table 5.6
Classification and grading of oligodendroglioma.

Grade	Grades based on progressive development
1	Hypercellularity, cellular anaplasia, and mitotic activity No pleomorphism Mild hypercellularity Neuropil persists between cells
2	Moderate hypercellularity with loss of neuropil between cells Mild pleomorphism
3	Moderate hypercellularity and pleomorphism Mitoses present and usually frequent
4	Moderate hypercellularity with increasing pleomorphism and mitoses Microvascular proliferation

Modified from Kleihuer and Cavenee.[25]

Clinical features

Symptoms and signs. Oligodendrogliomas grow more slowly than their astrocytic counterparts and thus are likely to cause symptoms, particularly focal seizures, for a longer period of time before the diagnosis is made. Before the advent of MRI, many patients suffered focal seizures for years before a diagnosis was finally established. One of our patients had a 20-year history of focal seizures beginning in the left foot prior to the establishment of the diagnosis of what was still a low-grade oligodendroglioma. The tumor subsequently became biologically more aggressive and was responsible for his death. The seizures are likely to be either focal motor or have partial complex emotional or intellectual components. One of our patients was treated for many months at a university center for 'panic attacks' that were episodes of sudden, overwhelming fear lasting 20–30 seconds and not relieved by psychotropic medication. When she had a generalized convulsion, a scan revealed a frontal tumor that proved to be an oligodendroglioma. Because the tumor was not resectable and the seizures were well controlled, she was followed for several years without significant change in tumor size.

Headaches are uncommon, because of the slow-growing infiltrative nature of the tumor. Because most of the tumors are in the frontal lobe, hemiparesis is relatively common and focal parietal or occipital signs are less common. The anaplastic oligodendroglioma tends to manifest more lateralizing symptoms than the low-grade oligodendroglioma. Seizures may be the presenting symptom, but they are often accompanied by hemiparesis, cognitive changes and hemisensory loss.

Imaging. Oligodendrogliomas cannot be distinguished from diffuse astrocytomas on routine MR imaging. Characteristically, the low-grade tumor is hypointense on the T1-weighted image and hyperintense on the T2-weighted image. Most oligodendrogliomas do not contrast enhance, and most anaplastic oligodendrogliomas do. Thus, the presence of contrast enhancement is a poor prognostic sign. If the tumor is heavily calcified, the calcium can sometimes be identified on the MR scan as either hyper- or hypointensity; however, calcium is better seen on a CT scan. Our policy in patients with infiltrating gliomas identified on MR scan who are not symptomatic, save for seizures that are controlled with anticonvulsants, is to perform a CT scan to look for calcification, a fluorodeoxyglucose PET (recent evidence suggests that methionine PET scans differentiate low-grade and high-grade tumors better than glucose[90]) and an MRS. Low-grade tumors are usually hypometabolic on PET scan and higher grade tumors are hypermetabolic. MRS may help distinguish astrocytic tumors from oligodendroglial lesions as preliminary data suggest different patterns. However, these data are still early and their meaning is not yet clear.

Treatment. The same treatment considerations that apply in low-grade astrocytomas also apply to oligodendrogliomas. There is even less reason for treating asymptomatic oligodendrogliomas than for treating asymptomatic astrocytomas, because the course is so much longer and the patients usually present with seizures but without other neurologic disability. If a substantial resection can be safely done, that is the treatment of choice for low-grade tumors. It ensures that the tumor is low-grade and probably delays the onset of symptoms. The following represents our therapeutic approach:

1. If the tumor is resectable, it should be resected. If the patient is asymptomatic save for controllable seizures, no further therapy should be administered and the patient should be carefully followed. All tumors resected or biopsied should undergo chromosomal analysis.[91]
2. If the tumor is not resectable and the patient is asymptomatic save for controllable seizures, a PET scan, an MRS and a CT scan should be done. If these all indicate a low-grade tumor, and particularly if the tumor is calcified, no further therapy is carried out. If the tumor is symptomatic, a biopsy, preferably with debulking, is performed and the patient is treated with chemotherapy[92] (see below). Some, but not all, patients with low-grade oligodendrogliomas respond to chemotherapy with shrinkage of the tumor and resolution of symptoms.[93] One of our patients remains well 7 years post-treatment. Her hemiparesis resolved over

several months and, although the tumor is still present, it is substantially smaller than when first treated and she is asymptomatic. Four to six cycles of chemotherapy are given, usually with an MRI every other cycle to evaluate tumor size, and then the treatment is stopped. If successful, i.e. the tumor decreases in size and/or the patient becomes asymptomatic; we then follow without further therapy until relapse.
3. If chemotherapy fails, limited-field radiation to a dose of 54 Gy is delivered.
4. Late recurrences are treated with surgery where feasible, followed by RT if not previously administered and/or chemotherapy.

For anaplastic oligodendrogliomas, the only chemotherapy regimen that has been extensively tested is PCV[94] (many physicians use temozolomide up-front, but the only published data concern its use at recurrence[95]). The tumors are treated with up-front chemotherapy as outlined in Table 5.4. Four to six cycles of chemotherapy, depending on the patient's tolerance, are delivered followed by limited-field radiation. One chemotherapy regimen is an intensive version of PCV (I-PCV) with both an increase in dose of all three drugs and a shortened time between cycles from 8 to 6 weeks. One cycle is defined as the period of therapy (i.e. 28 days) plus 2 weeks of observation for a total of 42 days. It is unknown whether I-PCV is better than standard PCV for malignant oligodendrogliomas, but it is more toxic and most patients have trouble tolerating it. We prefer the standard-dose regimen.

An experimental protocol is testing the role of high-dose chemotherapy with stem cell rescue without RT for newly diagnosed anaplastic oligodendrogliomas. This study will explore the limits of chemosensitivity for anaplastic oligodendrogliomas and defer RT to try and limit neurotoxicity. Recurrences after

Survival (%)	Low-grade		High-grade	
	Oligo	Oligo-Astro	Oligo	Oligo-Astro
Median (year)	9.8	7.1	4.5	4.3
2-year	93	89	67	82
5-year	73	63	45	45
10-year	49	33	26	23
15-year	49	17	13	17

Table 5.7
Survival of oligodendrogliomas by grade and histologic type. From Shaw et al.[97]

aggressive treatment of anaplastic oligodendrogliomas are treated similarly to astrocytomas. However, chemotherapeutic options at recurrence include melphalan, carboplatin, cisplatin and etoposide and temozolomide.[95]

Prognosis. The prognosis of oligodendrogliomas is much better than that of their astrocytic counterparts, with a median survival of 16 years in our series;[96] however, because of the difficulty in accurate identification of these tumors, their exact prognosis is not well established (Table 5.7, see also Table 1.11). Furthermore, genetic evidence suggests that only some tumors are chemosensitive and prognosis varies accordingly (Fig. 5.9).

Data from two randomized prospective Brain Tumor Study Group (BTSG) protocols were combined to analyze the effects of prognostic factors on survival by treatment group. These studies assessed all 'malignant' gliomas without differentiation of astrocytomas from oligodendrogliomas. Adjuvant chemotherapy increased long-term survival regardless of prognostic factors. Oligodendrogliomas were overrepresented among long-term survivors, whether or not they were treated with chemotherapy, but the benefits of adjuvant chemotherapy were not restricted to pathologically defined oligodendrogliomas.[61] Thus, prognostic factors did not predict benefit from adjuvant nitrosourea in malignant gliomas, and all of the long-term survival with chemotherapy was not explained by oligodendroglial tumors.

Oligoastrocytoma

Tumors that contain significant elements of both astrocytic and oligodendroglial tumor may account for 10% of diffuse gliomas. Unfortunately, no histologic markers unequivocally distinguish tumor cells of astrocytic origin from those of oligodendroglial origin, making the diagnosis a subjective one about which pathologists often disagree. However, a recent report suggests that a specific marker may have been identified.[98] Current evidence suggests that these mixed tumors, when low grade, respond to chemotherapy and RT but have a higher recurrence rate and shorter time to progression than do pure oligodendrogliomas. Current evidence suggests that 1p and 19q deletions do not predict response in these mixed tumors.[99]

Focal glial tumors

Introduction

These tumors affect predominantly children and young adults and, taken together, represent no more than a few per cent of adult brain

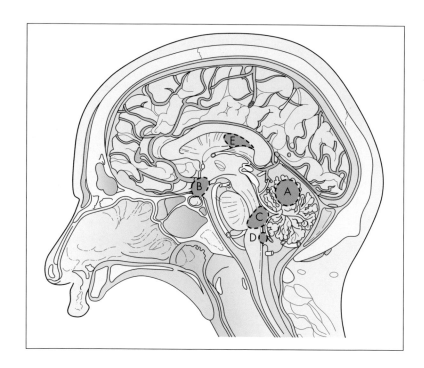

Figure 5.10
A schematic sagittal section illustrating the common location of focal glial tumors. Focal glial tumors include the pilocytic astrocytoma commonly found in the cerebellum (A), optic nerve, chiasm or hypothalamus (B). Brainstem gliomas are occasionally focal and exophytic (C). Other focal gliomas include ependymoma that often arise within the 4th ventricle (D) and choroid plexus papillomas (E).

tumors, although they represent a more substantial percentage of childhood brain tumors. They differ from diffuse astrocytomas in that they tend to be well-circumscribed and, if accessible, may be cured surgically (Fig. 5.10). Even though they are low-grade, contrast enhancement tends to be the rule rather than the exception. These tumors may have a pleomorphic appearance histologically, with mitoses and vascular proliferation which, when combined with contrast enhancement, often leads the physician to believe that one is dealing with a high-grade neoplasm. A careful review by an expert neuropathologist is essential to establish the correct diagnosis. Most patients with focal gliomas should not be treated with RT or chemotherapy immediately after surgery, but should be followed clinically. Patients are often cured or have long remissions after surgery alone. Uncommonly, these generally low-grade tumors may recur aggressively and even seed the leptomeninges.

Pilocytic astrocytoma

Pilocytic astrocytomas are low-grade tumors of astrocytic origin, corresponding to a WHO grade I astrocytoma (see Table 5.2). The tumor is named for its bipolar fusiform cell processes ('piloid' is from the Greek for 'hair'). Pilocytic astrocytoma is the most common glioma of children but also occurs in young adults; over 75% occur in those under age 20. These tumors are found in the cerebellum (Fig. 5.11),[100] optic nerve or optic chiasm[101] and hypothalamus of children. They are sometimes found in the basal ganglia and in the brainstem as a dorsally exophytic brainstem glioma. In young adults, they are usually in the cerebral hemispheres and cerebellum (Fig. 5.11). They constitute more than half of spinal astrocytomas, where they displace rather than invade tissue. About 15% of optic nerve pilocytic astrocytomas are associated with neurofibromatosis-1 (NF-1).

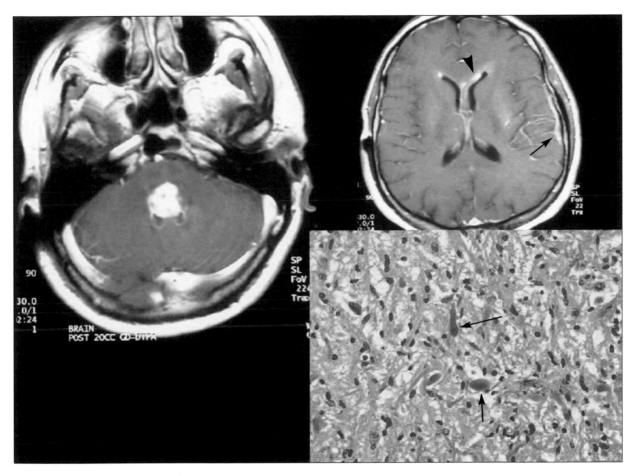

Figure 5.11
A pilocytic astrocytoma of the brainstem (left) in an adult that has seeded the leptomeninges (right arrow) and the ventricular ependymomas (right, arrowhead). The histology of leptomeningeal infiltration often remains low-grade, as does the histology of the tumor. The photomicrograph shows hyperchromatic, pleomorphic glial nuclei. Many Rosenthal fibers (arrows) are present.

Etiology

Pilocytic astrocytomas do not have a distinct cytogenetic pattern. Unlike diffuse astrocytomas, p53 mutations are not common in pilocytic astrocytomas. One study of 18 pilocytic astrocytomas (including one anaplastic tumor), 3 of which were NF-1 related, showed no p53 gene mutations,[102] but a more recent study demonstrated p53 mutations in 7 of 20 pilocytic astrocytomas.[103] A few sporadic pilocytic astrocytomas show loss of chromosome 17q, including the region encoding the NF-1 gene, but this is not the case in most instances. In a cytogenetic study of 24 pilocytic astrocytomas, 12 had normal karyotypes. In the other 12, there were structural and/or numerical abnormalities most frequently in chromosomes 7, 8 and 11; these genetic abnormalities may indicate tumor progression.[104] Telomerase activity, believed to occur early in glial tumorigenesis, is absent in pilocytic astrocytomas, dysembryoplastic neuroepithelial tumors (see below) and pleomorphic xanthoastrocytomas (see below). With the exception of NF-1, there are no known risk factors for pilocytic astrocytomas.

Pathology

Grossly, the tumors are usually well demarcated from surrounding normal tissue and are often cystic. The typical tumor cell has long bipolar hair-like extensions that, taken together, form a dense fibrillar background. The cells often contain Rosenthal fibers, a brightly eosinophilic intracytoplasmic mass, that helps establish the diagnosis. Microcysts are common. The tumor may show hyperchromatism, pleomorphism and microvascular proliferation. In the absence of significant mitotic activity these findings do not portend a poor prognosis. The MIB-1 labeling index ranges from 0% to 19% in pilocytic astrocytomas.[105] Pilocytic astrocytomas with low labeling indices do not appear to show progression after partial resection, whereas those with higher indices are more likely to progress.[105] Some tumors appear to be mixed with non-pilocytic components. Tumors with a monomorphous pilomyxoid pattern are more likely to recur than are more typical tumors.[106] Although the vast majority of pilocytic astrocytomas are benign, some may seed the leptomeninges[107] or even spread distantly within the CNS. Biopsy of a metastasis usually reveals the same histology as the primary tumor, indicating that the biological behavior cannot always be predicted by the histologic appearance; the metastases may also behave in a relatively indolent fashion, like the primary. Smear preparations may help in establishing the diagnosis during surgery.[108]

Clinical findings

The symptoms and signs of pilocytic astrocytoma depend on both the tumor's location and rate of growth. The typical cerebellar pilocytic astrocytoma is in the cerebellar hemisphere (in contradistinction to medulloblastomas, which are usually in the vermis) and usually presents with gait and ipsilateral limb ataxia. Later, patients develop headache, nausea and vomiting, diplopia from VI nerve palsy and often papilledema. Hypothalamic pilocytic astrocytomas may present with cognitive and behavioral abnormalities or with endocrine dysfunction, especially diabetes insipidus, and occasionally precocious puberty. Optic nerve tumors present with visual field defects or occasionally blindness. As with most brain tumors, symptoms are progressive, with one exception: a number of patients with optic gliomas develop some visual loss and then stabilize or improve without treatment for many years.[101]

Imaging. MR scans often show a combination of solid and cystic mass. Sometimes the solid tumor, which usually contrast enhances, is small and presents as a mural nodule in a large cyst, a finding characteristic of the cerebellar pilocytic astrocytoma. The tumor appears well demarcated and often lacks the surrounding edema of other neoplasms. When pilocytic astrocytomas occur in the brainstem they tend to be exophytic and also contrast enhancing, distinguishing them from the more common diffuse astrocytomas that affect the brainstem of children. The presence, absence, or degree of enhancement has no prognostic significance.

PET scanning with glucose or methionine tends to show more uptake in pilocytic astrocytomas than the low-grade nature of the tumor would suggest.[109] Thus, PET scans must be interpreted carefully in children and young adults with cystic tumors, recognizing that hypermetabolic lesions may be biologically benign. MRS has shown a choline/*N*-acetyl aspartate ratio of 3.4, a lipid/choline ratio below 1, and a lactate peak.[110]

Differential diagnosis. Although imaging characteristics, especially a cystic tumor with an enhancing nodule, and location can suggest the diagnosis, only biopsy will unequivocally establish it. Pilocytic astrocytomas must be distinguished from other neoplasms that arise in the same area, e.g. medulloblastoma in the cerebellum, astrocytoma in the brainstem, craniopharyngioma in the suprasellar area and other glial tumors in the hemisphere. Pilocytic astrocytomas must also be distinguished from non-neoplastic lesions such as eosinophilic granuloma in the suprasellar area (Chapter 10).

Treatment. Whenever possible, the treatment is surgical.[44] Most pilocytic astrocytomas involving the cerebellum, and a few involving the brainstem, can be successfully removed without the necessity for further treatment. Reports suggest that even partial removal of cerebellar astrocytomas may yield prolonged remissions. Optic gliomas and hypothalamic pilocytic astrocytomas can sometimes be successfully debulked using microsurgical techniques, but total removal is rarely possible, even though the tumors are well circumscribed. Nevertheless, after partial removal, symptoms improve in many patients and some have a prolonged remission. Accordingly, if one can remove much or all of the tumor surgically, no further therapy should be instituted until there is evidence of progression. In some patients, only a biopsy can be performed to establish the diagnosis. If symptoms can be relieved by an alternative procedure, such as ventriculoperitoneal (VP) shunt, then definitive anti-tumor therapy is withheld until the patient develops progressive symptoms. RT and fractionated stereotactic radiotherapy[111] have been reported to have some effect. However, since many of the patients are young, a number of investigators have attempted chemotherapy with a variety of agents[112] to delay RT. The usual chemotherapeutic regimen is carboplatin and vincristine,[113] which appears to have some efficacy, particularly in optic pathway and hypothalamic tumors.

Prognosis. Overall, the prognosis is usually excellent, with a 15-year survival of about 80%.[114] For cerebellar pilocytic astrocytomas, the overall 5-year survival rate is 93%, but is 100% after complete resection. Younger age (< 14 years) and classic histology are good prognostic factors.[115] Those with complete surgical resection do better than those with partial resection, who in turn do better than those with biopsy. Brainstem involvement is a negative prognostic factor.[116] However, recurrences do affect some patients, even after long quiescent intervals. One of our patients treated in childhood for a cerebellar astrocytoma relapsed after 33 years. The tumor at second surgery appeared identical to the initial tumor but kept recurring over several years and was ultimately responsible for the patient's death, although the histology remained low-grade. A low MIB-1 labeling index is associated with a reduced risk of recurrence, but a high labeling index, e.g. > 5%, does not necessarily predict recurrence.[105] Leptomeningeal dissemination has been reported and usually indicates aggressive biological behavior with poor outcome even if the histology remains low-grade.[107]

Pleomorphic xanthoastrocytomas

This tumor is so named because it consists of a mixture of pleomorphic tumor cells, ranging from normal astrocytes to giant multinucleated

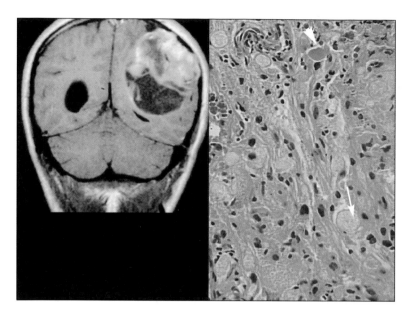

Figure 5.12
A pleomorphic xanthoastrocytoma in an 18-year-old man. This man presented with increasing headache and was found to have a large contrast-enhancing cystic tumor. At surgery, the tumor was originally interpreted as glioblastoma multiforme, but further review suggested a pleomorphic xanthoastrocytoma. He received no further treatment and is free from recurrence 5 years later. The tumor cells exhibit pleomorphism with scattered lipidized forms (arrow), and a granular body (arrowhead).

cells.[117] The latter contain lipid and they also express GFAP. The tumor occurs in children and young adults and usually arises superficially in the temporal lobes, often extensively involving the meninges.[118] No specific cytogenetic or molecular genetic abnormalities characterize this tumor. p53 missense mutations have been described in some patients, and EGFR amplification has also been described.

Because of cortical involvement, patients usually present with seizures that may be present for many years before the diagnosis is made. On MR scan, the tumor appears as an inhomogeneous mixed signal intensity mass that is well-circumscribed, often contrast enhances and may be cystic (Fig. 5.12). Surrounding edema is usually modest, as would befit a very slow-growing tumor.

The treatment is surgical. Patients with complete resections recur less often than those with partial resections. The pleomorphic appearance of the tumor and its invasion of the leptomeninges often suggest to the physician that he is dealing with a malignant tumor.

Expert neurologic and neuropathologic examination usually establishes the diagnosis, and no further treatment after surgery is indicated, other than careful follow-up. The tumors occasionally recur and sometimes seed the leptomeninges, but these are the exceptions. A high mitotic index and atypical mitoses may suggest recurrence.[117] Recurrence-free survival rates are 72% at 5 years and 61% at 10 years. Overall survival is 70% at 10 years.[117]

Ependymomas

Ependymomas are tumors that arise from the ependymal cells that line the ventricular system (Fig. 5.13) and the central canal of the spinal cord.[119,120] They account for about 10% of childhood intracranial tumors (30% of those arising in children younger than 3 years old) and 5% of adult intracranial tumors. They are the most frequent neuroepithelial tumor of the spinal cord, accounting for over 50% of spinal gliomas in children and adults. A slight preponderance of males is affected. The incidence is

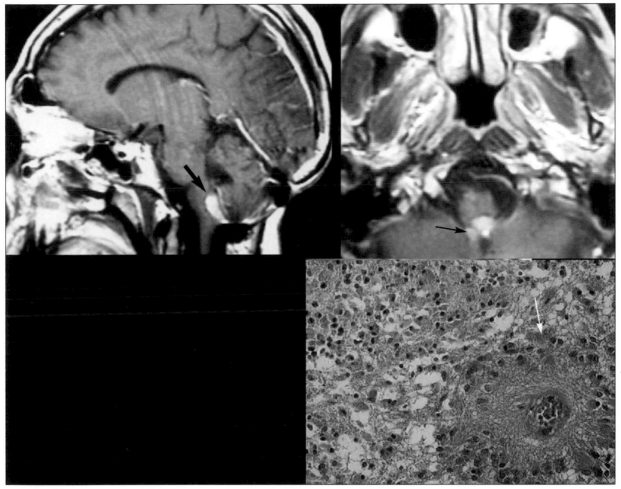

Figure 5.13
An ependymoma of the fourth ventricle. This man presented with hydrocephalus, headache and ataxia in 1981. A 4th ventricular mass (black arrow) was discovered and resected. Because resection was incomplete, he received radiation therapy. In 1992, a surveillance scan indicated recurrence of the tumor in the 5th ventricle. He received 2 years of carboplatin chemotherapy without a change in size of the tumor. It has remained unchanged for the ensuing 3 years. Uniform tumor cells with round/oval nuclei and delicate processes form a perivascular pseudorosette (white arrow).

bimodal, with the major peak at 5 years and a smaller peak at about 35 years.

Ependymomas can arise anywhere ependymal cells are present. A particular site of predilection is the IVth ventricle, where they grow within the ventricular system (Fig. 5.13). Supratentorial ependymomas also arise from ependymal structures but grow into the parenchyma of the hemisphere and may have no obvious intraventricular component. Myxopapillary ependymomas are tumors of the filum terminale of the spinal canal and are not discussed in this book.

A number of cytogenetic abnormalities have been described in ependymomas, none characteristic.[121] Loss of chromosome 22 is the most common. One report describes a 50% incidence of allelic loss on the short arm of chromosome 17 in pediatric ependymomas. p53 mutations are rare. p73 mRNA, which shares functional and structural homology with p53, is overexpressed in ependymomas.[122]

Histologically,[123] ependymomas are characterized by perivascular pseudorosettes, i.e. tumor cells arranged radially around blood vessels, and ependymal or Homer–Wright rosettes, i.e. columnar cells, which arrange themselves around a central lumen. The tumors are GFAP positive. Histologic subtypes of intracranial ependymoma include clear cell, cellular and papillary. The latter may be mistaken for a choroid plexus papilloma (see below). The diagnosis can be established unequivocally in problematic cases by electron microscopy, where tumor cells show the elaborate cilia and microvilli of normal ependyma. The tumors are generally low-grade but may be aggressive and spread via the cerebrospinal fluid (CSF) to seed the meninges and even rarely metastasize to extraneural structures, primarily the lungs. Many, but not all, studies have found histology to be an unreliable prognostic factor, independent of tumor location, extent of resection and age at diagnosis. However, as with many other glial tumors, mitotic figures, vascular proliferation and a high (> 4%) MIB-1 labeling index are encountered more often in those tumors destined to recur or kill.[124]

Clinical findings depend on the site of the tumor. Unlike brainstem gliomas, IVth ventricular ependymomas cause hydrocephalus early along with headache, dizziness or vertigo and, especially in children, nausea and vomiting as presenting complaints; ataxia and diplopia are also common. Spinal ependymomas may present in a similar fashion because otherwise asymptomatic tumors can cause hydro-

cephalus, probably by obstruction of CSF absorptive pathways due to a high CSF protein concentration.[125] Supratentorial tumors cause progressive focal neurologic symptoms, depending on their location.

MR scan demonstrates a mass lesion that is heterogeneously hypo- and isointense on T1 and hyperintense on T2 and may or may not contrast enhance; edema may be prominent. Hemorrhage may be present. Calcification, seen best on CT scan, is present in about 15% of ependymomas. The differential diagnosis includes other tumors that can occur in the same area, e.g. medulloblastoma and brainstem glioma.

The initial treatment of ependymomas is surgical.[44] A gross total resection prolongs survival, but the location of the tumor, particularly when it involves structures at the floor of the 4th ventricle, frequently makes that impossible. Surgical resection should be followed by RT.[126] Despite the fact that about 10% of posterior fossa tumors eventually seed the leptomeninges, they usually do so in the setting of local recurrence, so that RT is delivered to the site of the tumor and not to the whole neuraxis.[127] If symptomatic leptomeningeal seeding develops later, one can prescribe additional RT. There is no role for adjuvant chemotherapy at this time. Isolated reports describe recurrent ependymomas responding to chemotherapy, particularly carboplatin, and also several other chemotherapeutic agents. These reports make chemotherapy worth trying in patients who have failed surgery and radiation therapy, but response is usually poor.[128] Young children have been treated with chemotherapy initially in order to delay RT[129] and minimize neurotoxicity.

Unlike most glial tumors, the prognosis is worse in children than in adults, probably because posterior fossa ependymomas are more common in children and their IVth ventricular location makes them difficult to resect; these tumors often cause severe neurologic disability leading to early death. However, the overall prognosis of intracranial ependymomas is better than that for most other glial tumors. Five-year survival rates are about 80%, and 10-year survival rates about 50%.[119] Anaplastic ependymomas may be invasive and more likely to spread by CSF pathways than their lower-grade counterpart; however, it is not clear whether anaplastic features reliably confer a worse prognosis. Treatment does not differ for an anaplastic ependymoma and for all patients, most eventually succumb to local recurrence rather than metastatic disease.

Subependymoma

Subependymomas are low-grade intraventricular tumors, usually found in the IVth ventricle and, less frequently, in the lateral ventricle. They may be multiple. Their cell of origin is unknown. They were named because of their histologic resemblance to areas of tumor sometimes found in ependymomas. However, cytogenetic studies of subependymoma give a normal karyotype.[130] When they cause symptoms, they usually do so by ventricular obstruction, but many are asymptomatic, encountered incidentally at autopsy, or when a scan is done. The tumors are iso- to hypointense on T1 and may be heterogeneous due to calcification and/or hemorrhage. Some contrast enhance. Histologically, clusters of GFAP- and S100-positive monomorphic cells are found in a fibrillary background; sclerotic vessels and nuclear pleomorphism may be found, but mitotic figures, vascular proliferation and necrosis are absent and the MIB-1 labeling index is lower than that of other ependymal tumors.[131] If symptomatic, surgery is curative.

Choroid plexus tumors

Choroid plexus papillomas and choroid plexus carcinomas are rare, accounting for less than 1% of all intracranial tumors.[132,133] The tumors originate from the epithelium of the choroid plexus of the cerebral ventricles (Fig. 5.14) and typically occur in children. Choroid plexus papilloma is the most common intracranial tumor in the first year of life. However, these tumors also occur in adults. The most common site in children is the lateral ventricle. In adults, IVth ventricular tumors are more common. Some evidence suggests a possible role for simian virus-40 (SV-40) or a related DNA virus in pathogenesis.[134] p53 mutations have been reported in a few tumors. The tumors are well-demarcated intraventricular masses that may be cystic and/or hemorrhagic. Microscopically, they resemble normal choroid plexus, but with more crowded and elongated cells. Most choroid plexus tumors cause symptoms by hydrocephalus.

The hydrocephalus usually results from obstruction of CSF pathways by the tumor mass, but in children there may be an excessive production of CSF that overwhelms spinal fluid absorptive pathways, leading to enlargement of the ventricular system. Occasionally, choroid plexus tumors present with an intraventricular hemorrhage.

The MR or CT scan shows an intensely contrast-enhancing lobulated intraventricular mass which may be calcified. The majority of these tumors are histologically benign, although even benign tumors may occasionally seed the subarachnoid space. About 20% of tumors are malignant (choroid plexus carcinoma); they seed the leptomeninges along CSF pathways. Choroid plexus tumors must be distinguished from other intraventricular tumors and cysts; they must also be distinguished from metastatic papillary carcinomas.

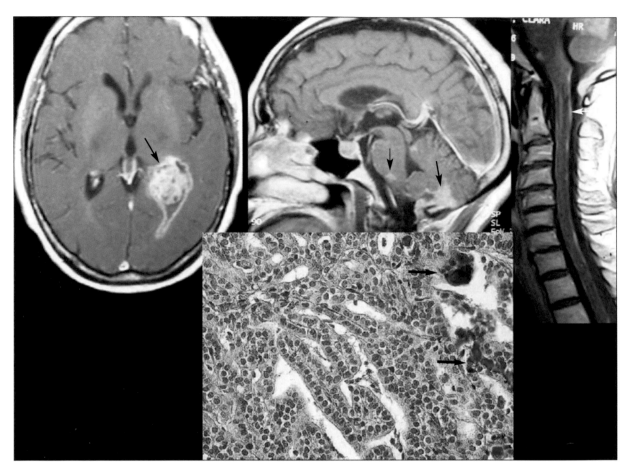

Figure 5.14
A choroid plexus papilloma has seeded the leptomeninges. The scan on the left shows the contrast-enhancing lesion involving the choroid plexus (arrow). The (middle) and (right) scans show infiltration of the leptomeninges in the brainstem, cerebellum and cervical cord (arrows). Ribbons of regimented tumor cells with uniform round nuclei and a cuboidal cytoplasm surround fibrovascular cores forming papillary structures. Stromal concretions can be encountered (arrow).

The treatment of choroid plexus tumors is surgical. The 5-year survival rate after gross total removal is about 80%. Choroid plexus carcinomas should receive RT in the postoperative period even if there has been a gross total resection.[135] If there is cytologic or clinical evidence of subarachnoid seeding, whole neuraxial radiation is required.[133] Chemotherapy, either postoperatively[133] or preoperatively to reduce tumor volume and vascularity[136,137] may be helpful.

References

1. Linskey ME. Glial ontogeny and glial neoplasia: the search for closure. J Neurooncol 1997; 34: 5–22.
2. Holland EC. Gliomagenesis: genetic alterations and mouse models. Nat Rev Genet 2001; 2: 120–9.
3. Kettenmann H, Ransom BR. Neuroglia. New York: OUP, 1999.
4. Kelly PJ, Daumas-Duport C, Scheithauer BW. Stereotactic histologic correlations of computed

tomography and magnetic resonance imaging-defined abnormalities in patients with glial neoplasms. Mayo Clin Proc 1987; 62: 450–9.

5. Olney JW, Farber NB, Spitznagel E, Robins LN. Increasing brain tumor rates: is there a link to aspartame? J Neuropathol Exp Neurol 1996; 55: 1115–23.

6. Rodvall Y, Ahlbom A, Spannare B, Nise G. Glioma and occupational exposure in Sweden, a case–control study. Occup Environ Med 1996; 53: 526–37.

7. Hu J, La Vecchia C, Negri E et al. Diet and brain cancer in adults: a case-control study in northeast China. Int J Cancer 1999; 81: 20–3.

8. Malmer B, Iselius L, Holmberg E et al. Genetic epidemiology of glioma. Br J Cancer 2001; 84: 429–34.

9. Kleihues P, Ohgaki H. Genetics of glioma progression and the definition of primary and secondary glioblastoma. Brain Pathol 1997; 7: 1131–6.

10. Shafqat S, Hedley-Whyte ET, Henson JW. Age-dependent rate of anaplastic transformation in low-grade astrocytoma. Neurology 1999; 52: 867–9.

11. Zhou XP, Li YJ, Hoang-Xuan K et al. Mutational analysis of the *PTEN* gene in gliomas: molecular and pathological correlations. Int J Cancer 1999; 84: 150–4.

12. Cheng Y, Ng HK, Ding M et al. Molecular analysis of microdissected de novo glioblastomas and paired astrocytic tumors. J Neuropathol Exp Neurol 1999; 58: 120–8.

13. Büschges R, Weber RG, Actor B et al. Amplification and expression of cyclin D genes (*CCND1*, *CCND2* and *CCND3*) in human malignant gliomas. Brain Pathol 1999; 9: 435–42.

14. Miettinen H, Kononen J, Sallinen P et al. *CDKN2/p16* predicts survival in oligodendrogliomas: comparison with astrocytomas. J Neurooncol 1999; 41: 205–11.

15. Ishii N, Maier D, Merlo A et al. Frequent co-alterations of *TP53*, *p16/CDKN2A*, *p14ARF*, *PTEN* tumor suppressor genes in human glioma cell lines. Brain Pathol 1999; 9: 469–79.

16. Duerr EM, Rollbrocker B, Hayashi Y et al. PTEN mutations in gliomas and glioneuronal tumors. Oncogene 1998; 16: 2259–64.

17. Adachi J, Ohbayashi K, Suzuki T, Sasaki T. Cell cycle arrest and astrocytic differentiation resulting from PTEN expression in glioma cells. J Neurosurg 1999; 91: 822–30.

18. Haas-Kogan DA, Kogan SS, Yount G et al. p53 function influences the effect of fractionated radiotherapy on glioblastoma tumors. Int J Radiat Oncol Biol Phys 1999; 43: 399–403.

19. Ino Y, Silver JS, Blazejewski L et al. Common regions of deletion on chromosome 22q12.3–q13.1 and 22q13.2 in human astrocytomas appear related to malignancy grade. J Neuropathol Exp Neurol 1999; 58: 881–5.

20. Forsyth PA, Wong H, Laing TD et al. Gelatinase-A (MMP-2), gelatinase-B (MMP-9) and membrane type matrix metalloproteinase-1 (MT1-MMP) are involved in different aspects of the pathophysiology of malignant gliomas. Br J Cancer 1999; 79: 1828–35.

21. Nakada M, Kita D, Futami K et al. Roles of membrane type 1 matrix metalloproteinase and tissue inhibitor of metalloproteinases 2 in invasion and dissemination of human malignant glioma. J Neurosurg 2001; 94: 464–73.

22. Nakatani K, Yoshimi N, Mori H et al. The significance of the expression of tumor suppressor gene DCC in human gliomas. J Neurooncol 1998; 40: 237–42.

23. Piva R, Cancelli I, Cavalla P et al. Proteasome-dependent degradation of p27/kip1 in gliomas. J Neuropathol Exp Neurol 1999; 58: 691–6.

24. Gran S, Tali T. p53 and p16INK4A mutations during the progression of glomus tumor. Pathol Oncol Res 1999; 5: 41–5.

25. Kleihues P, Cavenee WK. World Health Organization Classification of Tumours: Tumours of the Nervous System – Pathology and Genetics. Lyon: IRAC Press, 2000.

26. Jung V, Romeike BFM, Henn W, Feiden W et al. Evidence of focal genetic microheterogeneity in glioblastoma multiforme by area-specific CGH on microdissected tumor cells. J Neuropathol Exp Neurol 1999; 58: 993–9.

27. Giannini C, Scheithauer BW, Burger et al. Cellular proliferation in pilocytic and diffuse astrocytomas. J Neuropathol Exp Neurol 1999; 58: 46–53.

28. Litofsky NS, Mix TC, Baker SP et al. Ki-67 (clone MIB-1) proliferation index in recurrent glial neoplasms: no prognostic significance. Surg Neurol 1998; 50: 579–85.

29. Kosel S, Scheithauer BW, Graeber MB. Genotype-phenotype correlation in gemistocytic astrocytomas. Neurosurgery 2001; 48: 187–93.

30. Maidment SL, Rucklidge GJ, Rooprai HK, Pilkington GJ. An inverse correlation between expression of NCAM-A and the matrix-metalloproteinases gelatinase-A and gelatinase-B in human glioma cells in vitro. Cancer Lett 1997; 116: 71–7.

31. Liigant A, Haldre S, Oun A et al. Seizure disorders in patients with brain tumors. Eur Neurol 2001; 45: 46–51.

32. Gamburg ES, Regine WF, Patchell RA et al. The prognostic significance of midline shift at presentation on survival in patients with glioblastoma multiforme. Int J Radiat Oncol Biol Phys 2000; 48: 1359–62.

33. Landy HJ, Lee TT, Potter P et al. Early MRI findings in high grade glioma. J Neurooncol 2000; 47: 65–72.

34. Amato C, Elia M, Musumeci SA et al. Transient MRI abnormalities associated with partial status epilepticus: a case report. Eur J Radiol 2001; 38: 50–4.

35. Langleben DD, Segall GM. PET in differentiation of recurrent brain tumor from radiation injury. J Nucl Med 2000; 41: 1861–7.

36. Roesdi MF, Postma TJ, Hoekstra OS, Van Groeningen CJ, Wolbers JG, Heimans JJ. Thallium-201 SPECT as response parameter for PCV chemotherapy in recurrent glioma. J Neurooncol 1998; 40: 251–5.

37. Vigneron D, Bollen A, McDermott M et al. Three-dimensional magnetic resonance spectroscopic imaging of histologically confirmed brain tumors. Magn Reson Imaging 2001; 19: 89–101.

38. Quan D, Hackney DB, Pruitt AA, Lenkinski RE, Cecil KM. Transient MRI enhancement in a patient with seizures and previously resected glioma: use of MRS. Neurology 1999; 53: 211–3.

39. Masdeu JC, Quinto C, Olivera C et al. Open-ring imaging sign – highly specific for atypical brain demyelination. Neurology 2000; 54: 1427–33.

40. De Stefano N, Caramanos Z, Preul MC et al. In vivo differentiation of astrocytic brain tumors and isolated demyelinating lesions of the type seen in multiple sclerosis using ^{1}H magnetic resonance spectroscopic imaging. Ann Neurol 1998; 44: 273–8.

41. Peterson K, Rosenblum MK, Powers JM et al. Effect of brain irradiation on demyelinating lesions. Neurology 1993; 43: 2105–12.

42. Peterson K, DeAngelis LM. Weighing the benefits and risks of radiation therapy for low-grade glioma. Neurology 2001; 56: 1255–6.

43. Bampoe J, Bernstein M. The role of surgery in low grade gliomas. J Neurooncol 1999; 42: 259–69.

44. Pollack IF. The role of surgery in pediatric gliomas. J Neurooncol 1999; 42: 271–88.

45. Karim AB, Cornu P, Bleehen N. Immediate postoperative radiotherapy in low grade glioma improves progression free survival but not overall survival: preliminary results of an EROTC/MRC randomized phase III study. Proc Am Soc Clin Oncol. 17, 400a. 1998.

46. Surma-Aho O, Niemela M, Vilkki J et al. Adverse long-term effects of brain radiotherapy in adult low-grade glioma patients. Neurology 2001; 56: 1285–90.

47. Roelcke U, von Ammon K, Hausmann O et al. Operated low grade astrocytomas: a long term PET study on the effect of radiotherapy. J Neurol Neurosurg Psychiatry 1999; 66: 644–7.

48. Bruehlmeier M, Roelcke U, Amsler B et al. Effect of radiotherapy on brain glucose metabolism in patients operated on for low grade astrocytoma. J Neurol Neurosurg Psychiatry 1999; 66: 648–53.

49. Kiebert GM, Curran D, Aaronson NK et al. Quality of life after radiation therapy of cerebral low-grade gliomas of the adult: results of a randomised phase III trial on dose response (EORTC trial 22844). EORTC Radiotherapy Co-operative Group. Eur J Cancer 1998; 34: 1902–9.

50. Bauman G, Pahapill P, Macdonald D et al. Low grade glioma: measuring radiographic response to radiotherapy. Can J Neurol Sci 1999; 26: 18–22.

51. Lee SW, Fraass BA, Marsh LH et al. Patterns of failure following high-dose 3-D conformal

radiotherapy for high-grade astrocytomas: a quantitative dosimetric study. Int J Radiat Oncol Biol Phys 1999; 43: 79–88.

52. Shrieve DC, Alexander E III, Black PM et al. Treatment of patients with primary glioblastoma multiforme with standard postoperative radiotherapy and radiosurgical boost: prognostic factors and long-term outcome. J Neurosurg 1999; 90: 72–7.

53. Gaspar LE, Zamorano LJ, Shamsa F et al. Permanent ^{125}iodine implants for recurrent malignant gliomas. Int J Radiat Oncol Biol Phys 1999; 43: 977–82.

54. Prados MD, Wara WM, Sneed PK et al. Phase III trial of accelerated hyperfractionation with or without difluromethylornithine (DFMO) versus standard fractionated radiotherapy with or without DFMO for newly diagnosed patients with glioblastoma multiforme. Int J Radiat Oncol Biol Phys 2001; 49: 71–7.

55. Arcicasa M, Roncadin M, Bidoli E et al. Reirradiation and lomustine in patients with relapsed high-grade gliomas. Int J Radiat Oncol Biol Phys 1999; 43: 789–93.

56. Mohan DS, Suh JH, Phan JL et al. Outcome in elderly patients undergoing definitive surgery and radiation therapy for supratentorial glioblastoma multiforme at a tertiary care institution. Int J Radiat Oncol Biol Phys 1998; 42: 981–7.

57. Pierga JY, Hoang-Xuan K, Feuvret L et al. Treatment of malignant gliomas in the elderly. J Neurooncol 1999; 43: 187–93.

58. Prados MD, Scott C, Curran WJ Jr et al. Procarbazine, lomustine, and vincristine (PCV) chemotherapy for anaplastic astrocytoma: a retrospective review of Radiation Therapy Oncology Group protocols comparing survival with carmustine or PCV adjuvant chemotherapy. J Clin Oncol 1999; 17: 3389–95.

59. Nieder C, Grosu AL, Molls M. A comparison of treatment results for recurrent malignant gliomas. Cancer Treat Rev 2000; 26: 397–409.

60. Jakacki RI, Siffert J, Jamison C, Velasquez L, Allen JC. Dose-intensive, time-compressed procarbazine, CCNU, vincristine (PCV) with peripheral blood stem cell support and concurrent radiation in patients with newly diagnosed high-grade gliomas. J Neurooncol 1999; 44: 77–83.

61. DeAngelis LM, Burger PC, Green SB, Cairncross JG. Malignant glioma: who benefits from adjuvant chemotherapy? Ann Neurol 1998; 44: 691–5.

62. Brem H, Piantadosi S, Burger et al. Placebo-controlled trial of safety and efficacy of intraoperative controlled delivery by biodegradable polymers of chemotherapy for recurrent gliomas. The Polymer-Brain Tumor Treatment Group. Lancet 1995; 345: 1008–12.

63. Subach BR, Witham TF, Kondziolka D et al. Morbidity and survival after 1,3-*bis*(2-chloroethyl)-1 nitrosourea wafer implantation for recurrent glioblastoma: a retrospective case matched cohort series. Neurosurgery 1999; 45: 17–22.

64. Boiardi A, Silvani A, Pozzi A et al. Interstitial chemotherapy plus systemic chemotherapy for glioblastoma patients: improved survival in sequential studies. J Neurooncol 1999; 41: 151–7.

65. Witham TF, Fukui MB, Meltzer CC et al. Survival of patients with high grade glioma treated with intrathecal thiotriethylenephosphoramide for ependymal or leptomeningeal gliomatosis. Cancer 1999; 86: 1347–53.

66. Chamberlain MC, Kormanik PA. Salvage chemotherapy with tamoxifen for recurrent anaplastic astrocytomas. Arch Neurol 1999; 56: 703–8.

67. Akabani G, Reist CJ, Cokgor I et al. Dosimetry of ^{131}I-labeled 81C6 monoclonal antibody administered into surgically created resection cavities in patients with malignant brain tumors. J Nucl Med 1999; 40: 631–8.

68. Spear MA. Gene therapy of gliomas: receptor and transcriptional targeting. Anticancer Res 1998; 18: 3223–31.

69. Scott JN, Rewcastle NB, Brasher PMA et al. Which glioblastoma multiforme patient will become a long-term survivor? A population-based study. Ann Neurol 1999; 46: 183–8.

70. Galanis E, Buckner JC, DiNapoli RP et al. Clinical outcome of gliosarcoma compared with glioblastoma multiforme: North Central Cancer Treatment Group results. J Neurosurg 1998; 89: 425–30.

71. Perry A, Jenkins RB, O'Fallon JR et al. Clinicopathologic study of 85 similarly treated patients with anaplastic astrocytic tumors – an analysis of DNA content (ploidy), cellular proliferation, and p53 expression. Cancer 1999; 86: 672–83.

72. Schwartzbaum JA, Lal P, Evanoff W et al. Presurgical serum albumin levels predict survival time from glioblastoma multiforme. J Neurooncol 1999; 43: 35–41.

73. Bauman G, Lote K, Larson D et al. Pretreatment factors predict overall survival for patients with low-grade glioma: a recursive partitioning analysis. Int J Radiat Oncol Biol Phys 1999; 45: 923–9.

74. Tancredi A, Mangiola A, Guiducci A, Peciarolo A, Ottaviano P. Oligodendrocytic gliomatosis cerebri. Acta Neurochir (Wien) 2000; 142: 469–72.

75. Horst E, Micke O, Romppainen ML et al. Radiation therapy approach in gliomatosis cerebri – case reports and literature review. Acta Oncologica 2000; 39: 747–51.

76. Farmer JP, Montes JL, Freeman CR et al. Brainstem gliomas: a 10-year institutional review. Pediatr Neurosurg 2001; 34: 206–14.

77. Mandell LR, Kadota R, Freeman C et al. There is no role for hyperfractionated radiotherapy in the management of children with newly diagnosed diffuse intrinsic brainstem tumors: results of a Pediatric Oncology Group phase III trial comparing conventional versus hyperfractionated radiotherapy. Int J Radiat Oncol Biol Phys 1999; 43: 959–64.

78. Allen J, Siffert J, Donahue B et al. A phase I/II study of carboplatin combined with hyperfractionated radiotherapy for brainstem gliomas. Cancer 1999; 86: 1064–9.

79. Landolfi JC, Thaler HT, DeAngelis LM. Adult brainstem gliomas. Neurology 1998; 51: 1136–9.

80. Pollack IF, Shultz B, Mulvihill JJ. The management of brainstem gliomas in patients with neurofibromatosis 1. Neurology 1996; 46: 1652–60.

81. Shepherd CW, Scheithauer BW, Gomez MR, Altermatt HJ, Katzmann JA. Subependymal giant cell astrocytoma: a clinical, pathological, and flow cytometric study. Neurosurgery 1991; 28: 864–8.

82. Arai Y, Ackerley CA, Becker LE. Loss of the TSC2 product tuberin in subependymal giant-cell tumors. Acta Neuropathol (Berl) 1999; 98: 233–9.

83. Mao X, Jones TA, Tomlinson I et al. Genetic aberrations in glioblastoma multiforme: translocation of chromosome 10 in an O-2A-like cell line. Br J Cancer 1999; 79: 724–31.

84. Coons SW, Johnson PC, Scheithauer BW, Yates AJ, Pearl DK. Improving diagnostic accuracy and interobserver concordance in the classification and grading of primary gliomas. Cancer 1997; 79: 1381–93.

85. Bigner SH, Rasheed K, Wiltshire RN, McLendon R. Morphologic and molecular genetic aspects of oligodendroglial neoplasms. Neurooncology 1999; 1: 52–60.

86. Pohl U, Cairncross JG, Louis DN. Homozygous deletions of the CDKN2C/p18[INK4C] gene on the short arm of chromosome 1 in anaplastic oligodendrogliomas. Brain Pathol 1999; 9: 639–43.

87. Husemann K, Wolter M, Büschges R et al. Identification of two distinct deleted regions on the short arm of chromosome 1 and rare mutation of the CDKN2C gene from 1p32 in oligodendroglial tumors. J Neuropathol Exp Neurol 1999; 58: 1041–50.

88. Ino Y, Betensky RA, Zlatescu MC et al. Molecular subtypes of anaplastic oligodendroglioma: implications for patient management at diagnosis. Clin Cancer Res 2001; 7: 839–45.

89. Giannini C, Scheithauer BW, Weaver AL et al. Oligodendrogliomas: Reproducibility and prognostic value of histologic diagnosis and grading. J Neuropathol Exp Neurol 2001; 60: 248–62.

90. Derlon JM, Chapon F, Noël MH et al. Non-invasive grading of oligodendrogliomas: correlations between in vivo metabolic pattern and histopathology. Eur J Nucl Med 2000; 27: 778–87.

91. Cairncross JG, Ueki K, Zlatescu MC et al. Specific genetic predictors of chemotherapeutic response and survival in patients with anaplastic oligodendrogliomas. J Natl Cancer Inst 1998; 90: 1473–9.

92. Soffietti R, Rudà R, Bradac GB, Schiffer D. PCV chemotherapy for recurrent oligodendrogliomas and oligoastrocytomas. Neurosurgery 1998; 43: 1066–73.

93. Mason WP, Krol GS, DeAngelis LM. Low-grade oligodendroglioma responds to chemotherapy. Neurology 1996; 46: 203–7.

94. Paleologos N, Cairncross JG. Treatment of oligodendroglioma: an update. J Neurooncol 1999; 1: 61–8.

95. Chinot OL, Honore S, Dufour H et al. Safety and efficacy of temozolomide in patients with recurrent anaplastic oligodendrogliomas after standard radiotherapy and chemotherapy. J Clin Oncol 2001; 19: 2449–55.

96. Olson JD, Riedel E, DeAngelis LM. Long-term outcome of low-grade oligodendroglioma and mixed glioma. Neurology 2000; 54: 1442–8.

97. Shaw EG, Scheithauer BW, O'Fallon JR. Supratentorial gliomas: A comparative study by grade and histologic type. J Neurooncol 1997; 31: 273–8.

98. Marie Y, Sanson M, Mokhtari K et al. OLIG2 as a specific marker of oligoden-droglial tumour cells. Lancet 2001; 358: 298–300.

99. Smith JS, Perry A, Borell TJ et al. Alterations of chromosome arms 1p and 19q as predic-tors of survival in oligodendrogliomas, astro-cytomas, and mixed oligoastrocytomas. J Clin Oncol 2000; 18: 636–45.

100. Morreale VM, Ebersold MJ, Quast LM, Parisi JE. Cerebellar astrocytoma: experience with 54 cases surgically treated at the Mayo Clinic, Rochester, Minnesota, from 1978 to 1990. J Neurosurg 1997; 87: 257–61.

101. Parsa CF, Hoyt CS, Lesser RL et al. Spontaneous regression of optic gliomas: thirteen cases documented by serial neuroimaging. Arch Ophthalmol 2001; 119: 516–29.

102. Ishii N, Sawamura Y, Tada M et al. Absence of p53 gene mutations in a tumor panel representative of pilocytic astrocytoma diver-sity using a p53 functional assay. Int J Cancer 1998; 76: 797–800.

103. Hayes VM, Dirven CMF, Dam A et al. High frequency of *TP53* mutations in juvenile pilocytic astrocytomas indicates role of *TP53* in the development of these tumors. Brain Pathol 1999; 9: 463–7.

104. Zattara-Cannoni H, Gambarelli D, Lena G et al. Are juvenile pilocytic astrocytomas benign tumors? A cytogenetic study in 24 cases. Cancer Genet Cytogenet 1998; 104: 157–60.

105. Dirven CM, Koudstaal J, Mooij JJ, Molenaar WM. The proliferative potential of the pilocytic astrocytoma: the relation between MIB-1 labeling and clinical and neuro-radio-logical follow-up. J Neurooncol 1998; 37: 9–16.

106. Tihan T, Fisher PG, Kepner JL et al. Pediatric astrocytomas with monomorphous pilomyx-oid features and a less favorable outcome. J Neuropathol Exp Neurol 1999; 58: 1061–8.

107. Tamura M, Zama A, Kurihara H et al. Management of recurrent pilocytic astro-cytoma with leptomeningeal dissemination in childhood. Childs Nerv Syst 1998; 14: 617–22.

108. Teo JG, Ng HK. Cytodiagnosis of pilocytic astrocytoma in smear preparations. Acta Cytol 1998; 42: 673–8.

109. Kaschten B, Stevenaert A, Sadzot B et al. Preoperative evaluation of 54 gliomas by PET with fluorine-18-fluorodeoxyglucose and/or carbon-11-methionine. J Nucl Med 1998; 39: 778–85.

110. Hwang JH, Egnaczyk GF, Ballard E et al. Proton MR spectroscopic characteristics of pediatric pilocytic astrocytomas. Am J Neuroradiol 1998; 19: 535–40.

111. Debus J, Kocagöncü KO, Höss A, Wenz F, Wannenmacher M. Fractionated stereotactic radiotherapy (FSRT) for optic glioma. Int J Radiat Oncol Biol Phys 1999; 44: 243–8.

112. Kato T, Sawamura Y, Tada M et al. Cisplatin/vincristine chemotherapy for hypothalamic/visual pathway astrocytomas in young children. J Neurooncol 1998; 37: 263–70.

113. Gropman AL, Packer RJ, Nicholson HS et al. Treatment of diencephalic syndrome with chemotherapy: growth, tumor response, and long term control. Cancer 1998; 83: 166–72.

114. Shaw EG, Scheithauer BW, O'Fallon JR. Supratentorial gliomas: A comparative study by grade and histologic type. J Neurooncol 1997; 31: 273–8.

115. Haapasalo H, Sallinen SL, Sallinen P et al. Clinicopathological correlation of cell prolif-eration, apoptosis and p53 in cerebellar pilocytic astrocytomas. Neuropathol Appl Neurobiol 1999; 25: 134–42.

116. Pencalet P, Maixner W, Sainte-Rose C et al. Benign cerebellar astrocytomas in children. J Neurosurg 1999; 90: 265–73.

117. Giannini C, Scheithauer BW, Burger PC et al. Pleomorphic xanthoastrocytoma: what do we really know about it? Cancer 1999; 85: 2033–45.

118. Tonn JC, Paulus W, Warmuth-Metz M et al. Pleomorphic xanthoastrocytoma: report of six cases with special consideration of diagnostic and therapeutic pitfalls. Surg Neurol 1997; 47: 162–9.

119. Schwartz TH, Kim S, Glick RS et al. Supratentorial ependymomas in adult patients. Neurosurgery 1999; 44: 721–31.

120. Applegate GL, Marymont MH. Intracranial ependymomas: a review. Cancer Invest 1998; 16: 588–93.

121. Hamilton RL, Pollack IF. The molecular biology of ependymomas. Brain Pathol 1997; 7: 807–22.

122. Loiseau H, Arsaut J, Demotes-Mainard J. *p73* gene transcripts in human brain tumors: overexpression and altered splicing in ependymomas. Neurosci Lett 1999; 263: 173–6.

123. Rosenblum MK. Ependymal tumors: A review of their diagnostic surgical pathology. Pediatr Neurosurg 1998; 28: 160–5.

124. Prayson RA. Clinicopathologic study of 61 patients with ependymoma including MIB-1 immunohistochemistry. Ann Diagn Pathol 1999; 3: 11–18.

125. Kordas M, Czirjak S, Doczi T. The spinal tumour related hydrocephalus. Acta Neurochir (Wien) 1997; 139: 1049–54.

126. Schild SE, Nisi K, Scheithauer BW et al. The results of radiotherapy for ependymomas: The Mayo Clinic Experience. Int J Radiat Oncol Biol Phys 1998; 42: 953–8.

127. Paulino AC. The local field in infratentorial ependymoma: Does the entire posterior fossa need to be treated? Int J Radiat Oncol Biol Phys 2001; 49: 757–61.

128. Mason WP, Goldman S, Yates AJ et al. Survival following intensive chemotherapy with bone marrow reconstitution for children with recurrent intracranial ependymoma – a report of the Children's Cancer Group. J Neurooncol 1998; 37: 135–43.

129. Horn B, Heideman R, Geyer R et al. A multi-institutional retrospective study of intracranial ependymoma in children: identification of risk factors. J Pediatr Hematol Oncol 1999; 21: 203–11.

130. Dal Cin P, Van den Berghe H, Buonamici L et al. Cytogenetic investigation in subependymoma. Cancer Genet Cytogenet 1999; 108: 84.

131. Prayson RA, Suh JH. Subependymomas: clinicopathologic study of 14 tumors, including comparative MIB-1 immunohistochemical analysis with other ependymal neoplasms. Arch Pathol Lab Med 1999; 123: 306–9.

132. Schiff D, Wen PY. Uncommon brain tumors. Neurol Clin 1995; 13: 953–74.

133. Chow E, Reardon DA, Shah AB et al. Pediatric choroid plexus neoplasms. Int J Radiat Oncol Biol Phys 1999; 44: 249–54.

134. Gallia GL, Gordon J, Khalili K. Tumor pathogenesis of human neurotropic JC virus in the CNS. J Neurovirol 1998; 4: 175–81.

135. Wolff JE, Sajedi M, Coppes MJ, Anderson RA, Egeler RM. Radiation therapy and survival in choroid plexus carcinoma. Lancet 1999; 353: 2126.

136. St Clair SK, Humphreys RP, Pillay PK et al. Current management of choroid plexus carcinoma in children. Pediatr Neurosurg 1991; 17: 225–33.

137. Souweidane MM, Johnson JH Jr, Lis E. Volumetric reduction of a choroid plexus carcinoma using preoperative chemotherapy. J Neurooncol 1999; 43: 167–71.

6

Meningeal tumors

Introduction

The meninges (from the Greek for 'membrane') consist of three layers. The dura mater (from the Latin for 'hard mother') is a tough, fibrous membrane with a consistency of canvas that forms the outer covering of the brain and spinal cord. The arachnoid (from the Greek for 'spider web'[1]) is a delicate fibrous membrane that is apposed to the dura mater and forms the outer layer of the subarachnoid space. The pia mater (from the Latin for 'tender mother') is adherent to the glial capsule of the brain and spinal cord (pial–glial membrane) and surrounds arterial blood vessels as they enter the substance of the brain, leaving a potential space between the blood vessel and the brain. The spaces are sometimes true spaces, large enough to be identified on MRI and occasionally mistaken for a cyst, tumor or infarct.[2] These Virchow–Robin spaces are potential sites of brain invasion from meningeal tumors. The arachnoid membrane forms granulations that protrude into dural veins, particularly the sagittal sinus, and are a site of cerebrospinal fluid (CSF) absorption.

Tumors may arise from any cells found in the meninges. These include not only meningeal cells, but also melanocytes and connective tissue cells. Furthermore, non-meningeal tumors originating in or outside of the intracranial cavity may spread to and invade the leptomeninges either focally or diffusely.

Most primary meningeal tumors are focal. A few, such as meningeal melanoma, may infiltrate the meninges diffusely. Meningeal tumors are classified by the World Health Organization[3] as listed in Table 6.1, with modifications. Those meningiomas generally considered to be more aggressive in behavior are indicated by italics.

Meningioma is a common tumor; all of the others are rare. Hemangiopericytomas were once considered a subtype of meningioma (angioblastic meningioma) but are now recognized as a separate and malignant tumor. Hemangioblastoma is a tumor of uncertain cell origin usually found in the cerebellum and often involving the leptomeninges. The WHO classifies it with meningeal tumors because of its meningeal location, recognizing that its cellular origin is unknown. Sarcomas of mesenchymal but non-meningothelial origin, especially chondrosarcomas, may rarely arise in the leptomeninges. The meninges also contain melanocytes that may give rise to either relatively indolent melanocytomas or frankly malignant melanomas. Primary melanocytic intracranial and intraspinal tumors are less common than malignant melanomas that originate in the skin and metastasize to the leptomeninges.

Table 6.1
Tumors of meninges.

Tumors of meningothelial origin
- Meningioma
  - Variants

Meningothelial	WHO grade 1
Fibrous (fibroblastic)	WHO grade 1
Transitional (mixed)	WHO grade 1
Psammomatous	WHO grade 1
Angiomatous	WHO grade 1
Microcystic	WHO grade 1
Secretory	WHO grade 1
Clear cell	WHO grade 2
Choroid	WHO grade 2
Lymphoplasmacyte-rich	WHO grade 1
Rhabdoid	WHO grade 3
Papillary	WHO grade 3
Atypical	WHO grade 2
Anaplastic (malignant)	WHO grade 3

Mesenchymal, non-meningeal tumors
- Benign neoplasms
  - Osteocartilaginous tumors
  - Lipoma
  - Fibrous histiocytoma
  - Others
- Malignant neoplasms
  - Hemangiopericytoma
  - Chondrosarcoma
  - Variant mesenchymal chondrosarcoma
  - Malignant fibrous histiocytoma
  - Rhabdomyosarcoma
  - Meningeal sarcomatosis
  - Others

Primary melanocytic lesions
- Diffuse melanosis
- Melanocytoma
- Malignant melanoma
- Meningeal melanomatosis

Tumors of uncertain histogenesis
- Hemangioblastoma
  (Capillary hemangioblastoma)

Meningioma

Introduction

The term 'meningioma' was coined by Cushing in 1922 to give a non-specific name to a tumor that was almost always found in proximity to the meninges. Fig. 6.1 illustrates the common location of intracranial meningiomas. Meningeal cells, actually meningothelial arachnoid cap cells, are also found in choroid plexus, tela choroidea, and the arachnoid villi at the spinal nerve exit, explaining why tumors are common in the spinal canal and can also occur intraventricularly and in the pineal region (Table 6.2).

Meningiomas are benign, slowly growing tumors that compress the brain but rarely invade it (Fig. 6.2). When they compress brain substance, they usually cause seizures initially, followed by focal neurologic signs. When they compress cranial nerves in the cavernous sinus or the optic nerve, they cause diplopia or visual loss respectively. They also frequently evoke an

Table 6.2
Sites of intracranial meningiomas.

Site	Relative incidence (%)
Parasagittal/falcine	25
Convexity	19
Sphenoid ridge	17
Suprasellar (tuberculum)	9
Posterior fossa	8
Olfactory groove	8
Middle fossa/Meckel's cave	4
Tentorial	3
Peritorcular (sagittal sinus)	3
Lateral ventricle	1–2
Foramen magnum	1–2
Orbit/optic nerve sheath – spinal	1–2

Modfied from DeMonte et al.[4]

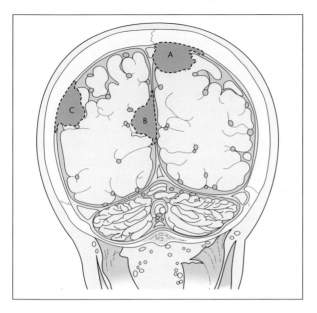
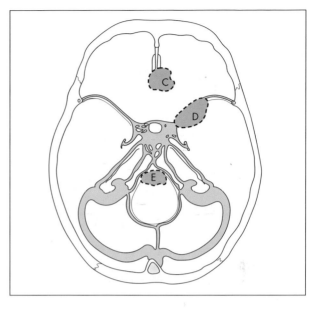

Figure 6.1
Typical location of meningiomas. (A) Parasagittal meningiomas may compress the sagittal sinus, causing a pseudotumor-like syndrome without focal findings. (B) Convexity meningiomas not close to the sensorimotor strip may grow to substantial size without causing symptoms, as may olfactory groove meningiomas (C). (D) Meningiomas involving the sphenoid ridge may compress or enter the cavernous sinus to surround the carotid artery and involve nerves to the ocular muscles. Meningiomas also occur in the posterior fossa, particularly in the cerebello-pontine angle and around the foramen magnum (E).

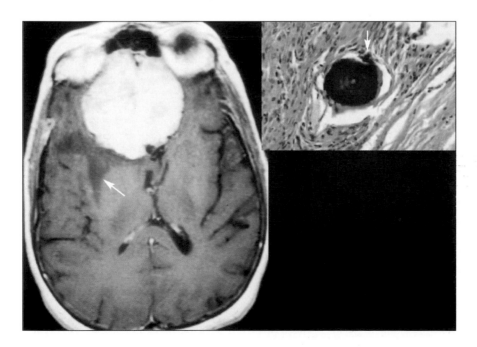

Figure 6.2
A large olfactory groove meningioma in a patient who presented with a slowly developing history of memory loss and some headache. (A) Note the modest amount of edema within the brain substance (arrow). (B) Meningioma showing the benign morphology and a typical psammoma (Greek for sand) body (arrow) with its concentric layers of calcification.

osteoblastic response in the surrounding bone called 'hyperostosis' that can be identified on plain skull films. Hyperostosis may cause symptoms by compressing cranial nerves at the skull base. Meningiomas may spread along the dura (en plaque meningioma), impairing multiple cranial nerves.

As indicated in Table 6.1, the usually benign meningioma has a large number of variants. These are primarily of neuropathologic interest and do not, for the most part, affect the clinical course, treatment or prognosis. There are exceptions. The **secretory meningioma**,[5] a tumor which often secretes vascular endothelial growth factor (VEGF),[6] may, unlike most other meningiomas, cause edema in the underlying brain, leading the clinician to believe that he is dealing with a malignant tumor such as a metastasis. The course of secretory meningiomas is, however, quite benign. The **angiomatous meningioma** has prominent vascular channels between rather inconspicuous nests of meningothelial cells. The tumor, particularly when capillary-size vessels are numerous, may mimic hemangioblastoma. The **clear cell meningioma** may be mistaken for other clear cell tumors, e.g. hemangioblastoma, metastatic renal cell carcinoma or neurocytoma.[7] Immunohistochemistry and electron microscopy can establish the diagnosis. Clear cell meningiomas often appear at an earlier age than other meningiomas and may behave more aggressively than other benign variants.[8]

Incidence

In population-based studies, intracranial meningiomas represent more than 20% of primary intracranial neoplasms.[9] When autopsy data are considered, meningiomas represent over 40% of intracranial neoplasms. In the Mayo Clinic series, 75% of meningiomas were asymptomatic, found either incidentally at autopsy or on a brain CT/MR scan performed for an unrelated problem.[10] In a Japanese incidence study, 32% of primary intracranial tumours were meningiomas: 39% were asymptomatic, dicovered incidentally on scan, and only 1/3 of these grew on follow-up.

Although the tumors can occur at any age, they are more common in late middle age. Symptomatic tumors are less common in the very elderly, but asymptomatic tumors found by scan or at autopsy indicate an increasing incidence with increasing age.

Meningiomas are substantially more common in women than in men, with female/male ratios varying from 3:2 to 2:1. Africans and African-Americans show equal male/female ratios and may actually have higher rates of meningiomas than their Caucasian counterparts. Multiple meningiomas are characteristic of NF-2 and other familial meningioma syndromes. Multiple tumors also occur sporadically but at an incidence of less than 10%. Atypical meningiomas represent about 5% of meningiomas, and frankly malignant meningiomas about 3%.[11] Meningiomas are also the most common intradural but extramedullary tumors of the spinal canal. Spinal meningiomas of the thoracic spinal cord virtually always occur in women.

Etiology

Genetics

The genetic progression of meningiomas is depicted in Table 6.3.

As the table indicates, multiple cytogenetic changes have been noted in meningiomas.[12,13] The most consistent is deletion of chromosome 22, which occurs in approximately 50% of meningiomas and probably involves the NF-2 tumor suppressor gene and its protein product, merlin (see Chapter 12). The NF-2 gene does not appear to be involved in meningothelial meningiomas,[14]

Table 6.3
Genetic changes in meningiomas.

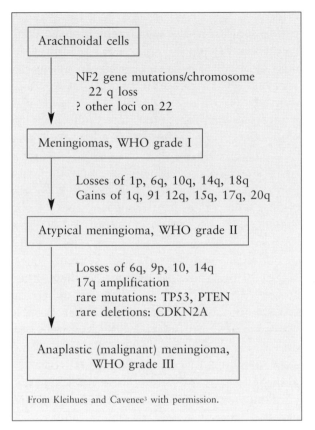

From Kleihues and Cavenee[3] with permission.

or in radiation-induced meningiomas.[15] In a few studies, abnormalities of chromosome 22 have been detected outside the NF-2 region, perhaps involving the INI1 tumor suppressor gene.[16]

Chromosomal changes are more extensive in atypical and anaplastic tumors than in the more benign variety. Allelic losses are found at 1p, 3p, 6q, 9q, 10q, 14q and 17p,[12] as well as other sites. These genes may be responsible for progression of the tumor from a benign to a malignant form. Complex karyotypes and abnormalities of chromosomes 1, 3 and 6 are present in aggressive tumors.[17] Losses on chromosome 10 are not due to deletions or

mutations of PTEN, as they are in glioblastoma.[18] Loss of heterozygosity on 17p and 22q is associated with aggressive tumors.[19] Studies of X-chromosome inactivation have suggested that meningiomas are monoclonal tumors when single, and when they are multiple, about half appear to be monoclonal.[20,21] However, other studies conclude that meningiomas are heterogeneous in clonal composition.[22] Recurrent meningiomas, whether near or distant from the original lesions, are clonal, suggesting that the meninges were seeded at the time of surgery.[23]

Of some interest is the role of sex hormones.[13] Meningiomas rarely express estrogen receptors or, if they do, they do so at very low levels,[24] but more than half express estrogen receptor mRNA.[25] Approximately two-thirds of meningiomas express progesterone receptors, more often in female than in male patients. The role of these receptors in the pathogenesis of the tumor remains unknown, but their presence has been an impetus for hormonal therapy, particularly progesterone receptor blockers, so far without success.[26] Some have suggested that sex hormone receptors account for the reportedly more rapid growth of meningiomas during pregnancy, but there is little scientific evidence that sex hormones function as growth factors for meningiomas.[27] One population-based study showed no relationship between number of pregnancies or age at first pregnancy and the development of meningiomas.[28]

Absence of progesterone receptors is associated with anaplastic tumors[13] and a shorter time to recurrence after surgery. Estramustine-binding protein, believed to correlate with sensitivity to the chemotherapeutic agent estramustine (a combination of estradiol and a nitrogen mustard), has been found in some meningiomas.[29] Other abnormalities that have been described in meningiomas include co-expression of platelet-derived growth factor (PDGF) and PDGF receptor genes and their protein products and perhaps EGF and IGF as well. Some meningiomas, especially secretory and microcystic types, express VEGF.[30] Neurotensin receptors have also been described in meningiomas. Growth hormone receptor mRNA is expressed in most meningiomas; blockade of the receptor retards meningioma growth in culture.[31] Proteins of the JAK and STAT superfamilies, which mediate signals from prolactin and PDGF, are expressed in meningiomas; these proteins may be the mechanism by which interferon-alpha (IFN-α) inhibits meningioma cell growth.[32] Some meningiomas also express somatostatin receptors and telomerase.[13]

Risk factors

Both familial and environmental risk factors have been implicated in the pathogenesis of meningiomas.[33] As mentioned above, NF-2 is a common cause of meningiomas, but there is also an increased incidence of meningiomas in families without NF-2 abnormalities. Meningiomas may be increased in Gorlin and Cowden syndromes (Chapter 12). Meningiomas

of all grades are over-represented in Africans, Asians and particularly Asians of Chinese origin.[34]

Ionizing radiation is the only established risk factor for meningioma (Fig. 6.3). Both low-dose radiation for the treatment of tinea capitis and high-dose radiation for the treatment of other brain tumors[35] cause meningiomas,[36] many of which are atypical or frankly malignant. Ron et al[37] identified a 10-fold increase in meningiomas in patients who had been treated as children with low-dose radiation to the scalp for tinea capitis. Meningiomas also occur after high-dose radiation for brain tumors such as germinomas or medulloblastomas or after prophylactic cranial RT for childhood leukemia.

One of our patients was operated on at age 14 in 1945 for what was originally believed to be an anaplastic astrocytoma (probably a more benign focal astrocytoma) and received postoperative RT. Over 30 years later, she developed a meningioma within the radiation portal. The tumor was at first slow growing, but eventually became more aggressive, leading to her death.

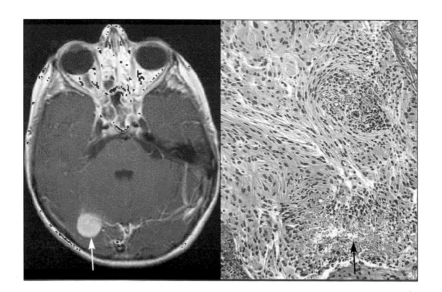

Figure 6.3
Radiation-induced atypical meningioma. A 30-year-old man who had received prophylactic cranial irradiation for leukemia 26 years previously had a CT scan following a fall. The scan revealed a tentorial lesion. An MRI, left, showed the lesion (arrow) to be uniformly contrast enhancing. He was asymptomatic but craniotomy revealed an atypical meningioma with mitosis and areas of necrosis (arrow). Atypical meningiomas require resection and postoperative radiation therapy (see text).

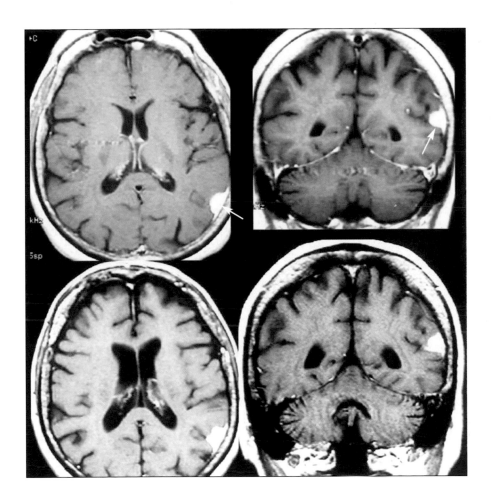

Figure 6.4
Multiple meningiomas in a patient with breast cancer. This neurologically asymptomatic patient was scanned in 1995 (top) as part of a screening workup for metastatic breast cancer (not conventional screening for breast cancer). Two small contrast-enhancing meningiomas were identified (arrows). A diagnosis of meningioma was made tentatively because of the absence of other metastatic lesions. Four years later (bottom), the tumors had not changed in size.

Trauma was suggested by Cushing as a significant etiologic factor; he had successfully removed a meningioma from the army chief-of-staff, who had suffered an injury at the same site years previously.[38] A number of epidemiologic studies have investigated this risk factor. Most have been negative, but a recent study reported a head injury odds ratio of 1.5 for men with meningiomas; the ratio was lower for serious injury, raising a question as to relevance.[39] Head injury causing meningioma still arises as a source of lawsuits. Others have implicated viral infections, particularly SV-40 virus, as a potential pathogenic cause but the evidence is unconvincing.

Meningiomas are probably more common in women with a history of breast cancer than in women without such a history[40] (Fig. 6.4). Meningiomas may be difficult to distinguish from dural metastases from breast cancer, particularly when there is prominent edema surrounding the lesion. Furthermore, breast cancer may metastasize to a meningioma.[41] However, in the majority of patients, the diagnosis can be established on MRI and the meningioma treated accordingly.

Pathology

Grossly, meningiomas are smooth lobulated tumors with a fine vascular pattern on their surface. When benign, they separate easily from underlying brain tissue, which they compress but do not invade. They may, however, invade venous structures, particularly the sagittal sinus, making surgery difficult unless the sinus has been occluded by tumor, in which case the occluded sinus can sometimes be removed with the tumor. Acute occlusion of the posterior portion of the superior sagittal sinus, as might occur during surgery, causes infarction of the brain,[42] and, therefore, a surgeon may need to leave a small amount of disease behind to avoid this complication. Meningiomas may encase cerebral arteries, particularly the carotid artery at the base of the brain. They may infiltrate the arterial wall, making arterial reconstruction necessary if the tumor is to be resected, but this is rarely advisable. Occasionally, meningiomas may penetrate bone and present as a scalp mass. Some meningiomas grow as a flat en plaque mass infiltrating substantial portions of the meninges, often making resection impossible.

The histologic appearance varies with the type of meningioma.[11] Certain features are common to all subtypes. They include a lobular structure, the presence of psammoma bodies and calcification. Microcystic and lymphoplasmacytic-rich variants contain the structures that their names imply. Most meningiomas, particularly benign meningiomas, react with epithelial membrane antigen (EMA) and vimentin on immunohistochemical studies. EMA immunoreactivity is less apparent in atypical and malignant tumors. S-100 protein is usually absent. Estrogen receptors are rarely found in meningiomas but there is an inverse correlation between tumor grading and the intensity of reaction with progesterone receptors.[13] Secretory meningiomas are carcinoembryonic antigen (CEA) and cytokeratin positive, and may elevate serum CEA. One of our patients, after successful treatment for

colon cancer, was found to have a persistently elevated CEA. A search of the body revealed only an enhancing dural-based lesion which was interpreted as metastatic colon cancer. Surgical excision revealed a secretory meningioma, and the serum CEA level fell after resection. The MIB-1 labeling index correlates well with the likelihood of recurrence after resection,[43] although mitoses are uncommon in the usual benign variants. DNA ploidy and p53 immunohistochemistry do not provide useful prognostic information.

Although most histologic subtypes do not have clinical significance, some subtypes behave in a more aggressive fashion than others. The aggressive subtypes include rhabdoid[44] and clear cell meningiomas. Lymphoplasmacytic-rich meningiomas may be associated with polyclonal gammopathy or anemia.

Atypical meningiomas are characterized by increased mitotic activity (4 or more/10 high power fields) and at least 3 of the following histologic features: increased cellularity, high nucleus/cytoplasm ratio, prominent nucleoli, necrosis, and patternless or sheet-like growth. Invasion of the brain warrants a diagnosis of atypical meningioma, but it alone does not indicate an **anaplastic (malignant) meningioma**, whereas 20 mitoses per 10 high power fields, or histology resembling carcinoma, sarcoma or melanoma does[3] (Fig. 6.5). Occasional pleomorphic nuclei and mitoses are noted in benign meningiomas and do not connote aggressive behavior. Although less than 1% of meningiomas metastasize, about half of malignant meningiomas metastasize, usually to liver or bone.[45] One patient presented with severe hypoglycemia from liver metastases 2 years after removal of a frontal anaplastic meningioma. It is particularly important to identify atypical and frankly malignant meningiomas, as their treatment

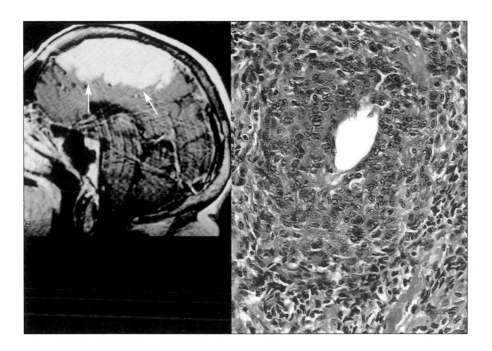

Figure 6.5
Left frontal malignant meningioma showing an irregular margin invading the brain (arrows), typical of a malignant meningioma. Histologically, it was a highly cellular tumor with complete loss of meningothelial differentiation and many mitoses.

differs from that of the benign meningioma (see below).

Clinical findings

Symptoms and signs

Meningiomas usually grow slowly and many appear not to grow even when followed for several years.[46,47] The vast majority of meningiomas do not invade the brain but cause symptoms by: (1) compression of central nervous system (CNS) structures, (2) shift of CNS structures with or without increased intracranial pressure, (3) hydrocephalus, and (4) brain edema (Table 6.4).

The symptoms of compression of CNS tissue depend on the site of the tumor. Tumors over the convexity, particularly when they are near the sensorimotor cortex, usually present with focal seizures. Simple partial or complex partial seizures, including many with behavioral and intellectual features, may mark the presence of

a meningioma. As the tumor grows, it may further compress areas of the brain, leading to sensory and motor changes, visual field defects or other focal symptoms (see Table 3.5). Meningiomas involving the orbit, optic nerve

Table 6.4
Meningioma pathophysiology of signs and symptoms.

- Compression of CNS tissue
  Seizures
  Cranial nerve palsies
  Focal sensory and motor signs
- Shift of CNS structures
  Cognitive and behavioral changes
  False localizing signs (see Table 3.6)
- Hydrocephalus
  Cognitive failure
  Gait ataxia
  Urinary incontinence
- Brain edema (Fig. 6.6)
  Focal sensory and motor signs
  Seizures

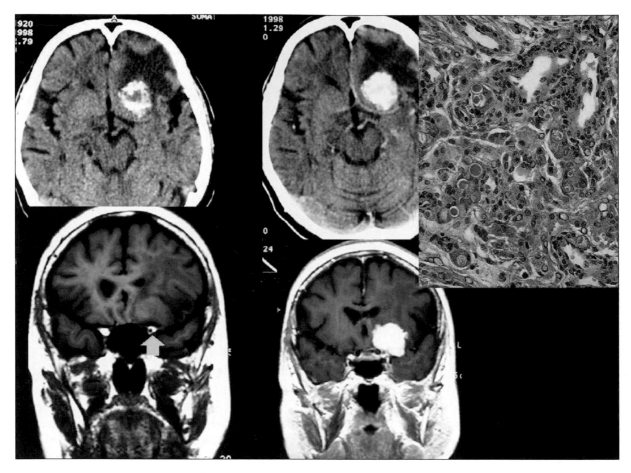

Figure 6.6
A meningioma with extensive surrounding edema. The CT and MR scan show a lesion that is hyperdense before contrast on the CT scan, suggesting calcification, and which uniformly contrast enhances. The MR scan does not show the lesion well without contrast (arrow), but the tumor intensely contrast enhances. The tumor proved to be a secretory meningioma with hyalin inclusion bodies 'pseudopsammoma bodies' in an otherwise typical meningioma.

or cavernous sinus present with visual loss, ophthalmoplegia or proptosis (Fig. 6.7). Tumors at the foramen magnum may mimic amyotrophic lateral sclerosis. In one unselected series of 59 patients examined in the modern era, headache was the most common symptom, followed by visual loss and cognitive changes (Table 6.5).

Because meningiomas are so slow-growing, they may reach a gigantic size before symptoms are recognized, particularly if they involve relatively silent areas of brain such as the non-dominant frontal lobe. This is because the compressed but usually non-edematous brain adapts to the lesion and no significant shift of intracranial structures occurs.

Headache is a common symptom in patients with all brain tumors, including meningiomas. In many patients with meningiomas, the headaches are not related to the tumor, the

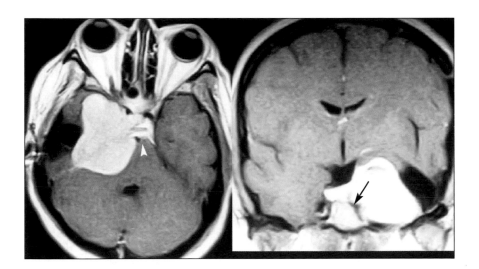

Figure 6.7
A large cavernous sinus meningioma causing a partial non-progressive third nerve palsy. Except for diplopia, the patient was well for many years until she developed signs of hydrocephalus requiring a shunt. This is the same patient illustrated in Fig. 3.5. Note that the tumor surrounds the carotid artery (arrow) and partially surrounds the basilar artery (arrowhead).

tumor being found incidentally when an imaging study is performed for evaluation of the headache. One study[49] suggests that typical migraine or cluster headaches may be related to meningiomas. The authors reviewed 514 meningiomas, selecting patients with headache but without papilledema, vomiting or mass effect on the scan. Four patients met the clinical criteria for cluster headaches, and three

patients met the clinical criteria for migraine headache. In all seven patients, the headache ceased after surgery. As indicated in Chapter 3 these patients all had a recent change in the pattern of their long-standing headache that prompted further evaluation; either the frequency of the attacks increased or the pain became persistent and more intense. Patients with brain tumors and a pre-existing headache problem are more likely to have headache associated with their brain tumor than patients without an underlying headache problem. This emphasizes the importance of evaluating changing headaches even when they seem typically vascular or benign.

As indicated above, many meningiomas are discovered incidentally, usually when the patient presents with headache or another neurologic problem that leads to a scan. Thus, one must be extremely careful in attributing coincidental symptoms to the tumor. One of our patients presented with sudden onset of painless ptosis and diplopia. Examination revealed paralysis of the oculomotor nerve without pupillary involvement. An MR scan revealed a meningioma on the appropriate side not involving the oculomotor nerve. After a

Table 6.5
Presenting symptoms of 59 meningiomas by side of lesion.

	Left	Right	Bilateral	% of total
Headache	9	12	1	37.3
Visual	3	7	5	25.4
Cognitive	6	3	5	23.7
LOC	8	2	3	22.0
Weakness	6	5		18.6
Seizure	6	3	1	16.9
Dizziness	4	3	1	11.9
Nausea	1	1		3.3

LOC, loss of consciousness.
From Bornstein and Witt.[48]

glucose tolerance test, a diagnosis of diabetic ophthalmoplegia was made. The patient made a full recovery, and the meningioma was just followed.

Patients, particularly those with large frontal lobe tumors, may present with cognitive and personality changes, usually apathy and depression. The patient may undergo psychiatric evaluation and prolonged psychiatric treatment before a tumor is suspected. A sudden personality change should lead one to suspect a structural lesion and evaluation by brain imaging.

Slow-growing meningiomas may also be responsible for false localizing signs. Some of these signs are listed in Table 3.6. A particularly vexing problem before the age of neuroimaging was gait ataxia from a frontal meningioma. Neurosurgeons would operate on the posterior fossa, expecting to find the tumor there rather than in the frontal lobe.

Although most meningiomas do not cause brain edema, some, particularly secretory meningiomas, can cause substantial edema leading to clinical symptoms. The cause of the edema is not entirely established and may be multifactorial. Substantial evidence implicates VEGF, and perhaps other chemical substances, as important factors.[50] VEGF is secreted by some meningiomas, particularly those that receive vascular supply from the brain (most meningiomas are supplied by vessels such as the external carotid artery that do not supply the brain itself). The role of VEGF in angiogenesis is described in Chapter 2, but, in addition, if VEGF diffuses from the tumor into surrounding normal brain, it causes increased vascular permeability and edema as well as promoting angiogenesis.[51] Other chemical factors that may play a role include platelet-activating factor produced by leukocyte infiltration into meningiomas[52] and prostaglandins.[53] A non-chemical factor that may play a role is compression by the tumor

of cortical veins, leading to venous hypertension and edema. The severity of peritumoral edema is closely related to the labeling index, suggesting a relationship between tumor aggressiveness and edema.[54] Tumor recurrence also correlates with the degree of edema.[55]

Meningiomas may also cause symptoms by hydrocephalus. Some meningiomas at the base of the brain or in the posterior fossa cause hydrocephalus by compressing and thus obstructing the ventricular system. Others exude proteinaceous material(s) that interferes with normal CSF absorption, causing communicating hydrocephalus (i.e. hydrocephalus without ventricular obstruction). The hydrocephalus is characterized by ataxia, urgency incontinence, and short-term memory loss. It usually responds to shunting of the cerebral ventricles, without necessarily treating the underlying meningioma. We have encountered a number of patients with large, quiescent or slowly-growing meningiomas at the base of the brain that cause symptoms of hydrocephalus. Characteristically, the tumors were in the cerebellopontine angle or the cavernous sinus and caused cranial nerve palsies that were relatively static. After many years, the patient would complain of gait unsteadiness and urgency incontinence sometimes associated with poor short-term memory. MR scan might reveal no change in the meningioma (Fig. 6.5) but a progressive increase in the size of the ventricles. The symptoms are characteristic of hydrocephalus, and even though the ventricles are dilated, the pressure is usually normal (normal-pressure hydrocephalus). Symptoms are relieved by ventricular shunting. One of our patients went from being unable to walk and incontinent to full normality after the shunt. Communicating hydrocephalus can also develop or be the presenting symptom of a spinal meningioma. In this situation, cranial imaging only reveals dilated ventricles. A careful neurologic history and examination often reveals a myelopathy in addition to the symptoms and signs of hydrocephalus. Spinal imaging will reveal the meningioma or other spinal tumor.

Another unusual symptom of meningioma is the mimicking of pseudotumor cerebri (benign intracranial hypertension); the meningioma typically compresses or invades the posterior portion of the superior sagittal sinus,[56,57] increasing venous, and thus CSF, pressure. The patient develops headache and papilledema, usually without change in ventricular size. The syndrome is indistinguishable from that of pseudotumor cerebri, except that MR venogram reveals obstruction of the sagittal sinus. The same syndrome can result from compression of the dominant transverse sinus by a posterior fossa meningioma.

Imaging

The diagnosis of meningioma is often established by neuroimaging,[58] particularly MRI. A typical meningioma is hypointense or isointense with brain on T1, usually hypointense on T2, and intensely and uniformly contrast enhances (98%). Hyperintense T2 images correlate with tumor invasion of cerebral cortex.[59] In heavily calcified meningiomas (67%), contrast enhancement may sometimes be minimal and CT scan may be more useful for identifying the tumor. Many meningiomas either erode bone or cause hyperostosis (27%). When hyperostosis of the base of skull is associated with a meningioma, there is usually invasion of that bone by tumor.[60] However, some meningiomas cause hyperostosis without invasion, probably by secretion of products such as alkaline phosphatase; that enzyme may also play a role in the calcifications found in most meningiomas. Both hyperostosis and bone erosion are better identified on CT than on MR scan. Meningiomas typically have an enhancing 'dural tail' that spreads out from the body of the tumor along the dura, a less common finding in other dural tumors, including metastasis. The dural tail is often not tumor, but a hypervascular response of the dura to the tumor. Thus, it is not specific for meningioma and may occur with an extra- or intra-axial tumor[61] and even with an aneurysm, confusing the diagnosis. A large tumor compressing brain but not causing edema is probably a meningioma, although one report describes edema in 66% of meningiomas seen on MR scan.[62] Sometimes meningiomas have unusual imaging features caused by hemorrhage, cystic degeneration or necrosis.[58]

Magnetic resonance spectroscopy (MRS) shows well-defined peaks for choline (CHO), a low phosphocreatine (PCr)/creatine (Cr) ratio and a decrease of n-acetyl aspartate (NAA). The reduction in PCr/Cr is greater than that seen in astrocytomas. An alanine peak is characteristic of meningiomas, and is usually much larger than the creatine peak.[58] Nuclear scanning is sometimes useful in the diagnosis of meningioma. The somatostatin analog, octreotide is taken up by meningiomas but not most other skull-based tumors.[63] PET findings of skull-based tumors have shown a much higher accumulation of the amino acid methionine in meningiomas compared with surrounding cerebellar tissue, making the tumor easy to identify and demarcate. Methionine uptake correlates better with proliferative potential than does F[18] flourodeoxyglucose (FDG) PET.[64] Neuromas show a lower uptake compared to cerebellum,[65] making a clear distinction between these two common tumors.

Differential diagnosis

The differential diagnosis of meningioma is indicated in Table 6.6. It includes dural metastasis, the other primary meningeal tumors

Table 6.6
Differential diagnosis of meningioma.

Dural metastasis
Other primary meningeal tumors (Table 6.1)
Metastasis to leptomeninges
Meningeal lymphoma/plasmacytoma
Inflammatory pseudotumor
Granulomas (e.g. sarcoid, foreign body)
Aneurysm

listed in Table 6.1, metastasis to leptomeninges and primary meningeal lymphomas, plasmacytomas or melanomas as well as inflammatory lesions that can mimic tumors.[66] Because systemic cancer can metastasize to a meningioma, both may be present in the same patient. The diagnosis can be suspected by the more rapid development of symptoms than one would expect from a meningioma and by neuroimaging where edema and central necrosis suggest a more aggressive process.

Sometimes only a biopsy will settle the diagnosis. However, most meningiomas are so characteristic on MRI that the diagnosis is 'established' on the basis of neuroimaging alone. This is particularly true when resection or biopsy would be hazardous.

Treatment

The diagnosis of meningioma is usually made by the combination of symptoms and imaging. The first step in management is to determine whether the patient requires treatment. Many meningiomas are either discovered incidentally or cause focal seizures or cranial nerve palsies and appear not to grow when followed over several years[47] (Fig. 6.8). Calcified tumors are less likely to grow.[46] If they do not grow, surgical intervention may not be necessary if the patient is asymptomatic, if symptoms are due to another cause, or if seizures are the only symptom and are easily controlled with

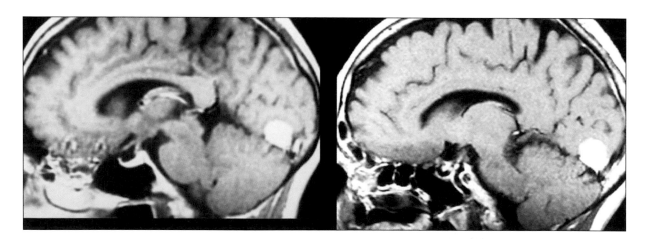

Figure 6.8
No growth in a meningioma over ten years. This woman presented with focal visual seizures. A scan done in 1989 (left panel) revealed a contrast-enhancing lesion arising from the tentorium without surrounding edema. It was presumptively diagnosed as a meningioma. She elected for no therapy other than anticonvulsants, which have controlled her seizures for the past 10 years. A repeat scan in 1999 (right panel) shows that the tumor has not changed over the 10-year period.

anticonvulsants. We have followed one such patient for over 10 years after she presented with a seizure and was found to have a meningioma involving the occipital area. Surgery was recommended when she was first seen, but she refused. The seizures have been completely controlled with anticonvulsants and no new symptoms have developed. The tumor has not altered in size over the last decade.

Other meningiomas are not treated because removal would be difficult and dangerous, out of proportion to the symptoms from which the patient suffers. Typically, these are large meningiomas at the base of the brain, often invading the cavernous sinus, that present with cranial nerve palsies without evidence of increased intracranial pressure. At least two of our patients with oculomotor palsies have been followed for more than two decades with stable neurologic symptoms and no change in the meningioma. An additional patient developed, after several years, a visual field abnormality which improved after microsurgery with subtotal resection.

Surgery
The treatment of most symptomatic meningiomas is by surgery. In many instances, the entire tumor can be removed surgically and the patient cured. Thus, if complete surgical removal can be achieved, no further therapy is indicated. However, in about 15–20% of patients, even when the tumor has been 'completely' removed, there is recurrence. Tumors that are 'mushroom'-shaped or lobulated are more likely to recur than those that are round. Wide dural resection decreases the likelihood of recurrence.[67] Thus, after successful surgery, patients should be followed closely with MR scans beginning at about 6-month intervals and gradually increasing to 24-month intervals.

Because meningiomas can occur virtually anywhere in or around the brain or spinal cord, the surgery to remove them involves many different approaches, ranging from the relatively simple (convexity tumors) to the very complex (skull base tumors[68,69]). The guiding principle in all cases is removal of as much tumor as possible without causing or adding to neurologic injury. Because of the relatively slow growth rate of these tumors, a subtotal resection is often enough, particularly in elderly patients. Obviously, a complete resection for cure should be contemplated in every case.

Postoperative cerebral edema is a particular problem in meningioma patients. This should be anticipated, particularly in patients with larger tumors. Patients should receive steroids and be fluid-restricted in the immediate postoperative period. The peak edema period can be delayed, often 24–48 hours after surgery. Edema may compress cerebral vessels, leading to delayed ischemia and even infarction in the days following surgery.

If the tumor recurs, a second surgical procedure should be carried out, if feasible, again with the intent of removing all or as much of the tumor as possible. This should be followed by focal RT (see below). A small percentage of tumors are atypical or frankly anaplastic, either initially or at recurrence. All of these should be treated with radiation therapy after surgery. Patients with anaplastic tumors should receive periodic bone and body scans to detect asymptomatic metastases that can be treated either surgically or by irradiation.

Modern surgical techniques have made meningioma surgery much more successful and less dangerous. Preoperative embolization can reduce the size and vascularity[58] of the tumor, making resection easier; viable tumor in the perinecrotic areas may show an increased labeling index, but this is transient and does not indicate an increased proliferative potential of the tumor.[70] Techniques to preserve the carotid artery and to remove tumor from around cranial nerves in the cavernous sinus have considerably increased the safety of operations in that area. Reconstruction of the carotid artery can often be carried out now as part of a procedure to remove tumor from the cavernous sinus.

Despite these advances, there is still a small mortality and significant morbidity associated with surgical treatment of meningiomas. In part, this is because many of the patients are elderly and the tumors have grown to a large size prior to diagnosis, and in part because the tumor often directly involves important nerve and vascular structures. Thus, in the absence of feasible surgery and if the tumor is growing, RT should be considered.

In those patients in whom only partial resection or no resection is possible, RT may either prevent further growth or cause some shrinkage but rarely, if ever, eradicates the tumor. Unlike the case with every other type of primary brain tumor, biopsy is not necessary for tissue diagnosis in unresectable meningioma prior to the administration of RT. The clinical and radiographic appearance are usually so characteristic, and the differential diagnosis so clear, that surgery is performed only if it can be helpful therapeutically, and a diagnostic biopsy is limited to the unusual patient who requires tissue confirmation before treatment can start.

Radiation therapy

RT is applied as primary treatment to inoperable tumors and as secondary treatment after partial surgery in some patients, after recurrence, after surgery and in all instances of atypical or malignant meningioma even if completely excised.[71] In patients whose tumor is benign and totally resected, postoperative RT is unnecessary. If the tumor recurs, it is resected again and postoperative RT given.

Atypical and malignant meningiomas are treated with 59.4 Gy.[72] Conformal radiation giving a tumor dose of 54 Gy has been the standard treatment of 'benign' meningiomas. Evidence from uncontrolled retrospective studies indicates that recurrence is less frequent and survival is longer in those patients who receive postoperative therapy.[73] Thus, postoperative irradiation should be considered after subtotal resection. The size of the residual tumor predicts response to RT. Progression-free survival was significantly poorer for those tumors > 5 cm than for those < 5 cm (40% versus 93%).[74] However, even after partial resection, we may elect to follow the patient by MRI, and if the tumor grows, re-resect and then radiate (see prognosis below). Skull-based meningiomas often can only be subtotally resected. Radiation therapy can produce long-term control of unresected or partially resected meningiomas with few side-effects.[75]

Radiosurgery is another option which has received increasing attention.[76,77] The role of radiosurgery in the treatment of meningiomas is still not established, but many radiation oncologists are enthusiastic about the ability to treat meningiomas with high doses of radiation while sparing surrounding brain. Radiosurgery is limited to tumors 3 cm in size or less and may be particularly useful in elderly or infirm patients who cannot easily tolerate surgery. In one series 93% of patients followed for 5–10 years required no other therapy.[76] Radiosurgery is being increasingly advocated for small tumors in surgically difficult areas such as near a patent sagittal sinus[78] or at the base of the brain.[79] The benefit of radiosurgery may be delayed, and improvement may take months to years. Thus, radiosurgery is not a good option for patients with rapidly progressive symptoms. Side effects of radiosurgery both acute[80] (brain edema) and delayed[81] (cranial nerve palsy,

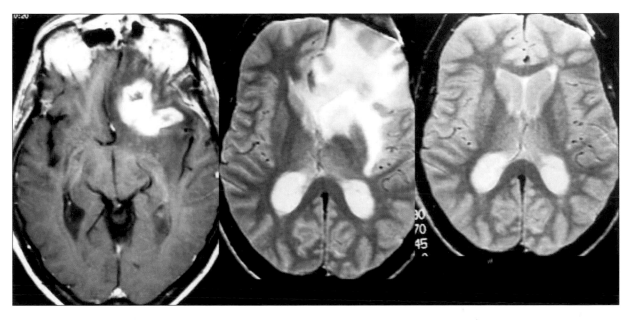

Figure 6.9
Side effects of radiosurgery. This patient received radiosurgery for treatment of a meningioma at the base of the brain. The meningioma decreased somewhat in size but she developed severe headache. The MR scan revealed a contrast-enhancing area in the frontal lobe (the meningioma had not directly involved the frontal lobe) surrounded by edema (left). The T2-weighted image (middle) revealed marked edema with mass effect. She was treated with steroids with amelioration of symptoms. When a routine scan was done 2 years later (right), the radiation toxicity had resolved.

visual loss, radiation necrosis), are uncommon but do occur (Fig. 6.9).

Chemotherapy

The role of chemotherapy for meningiomas is not established.[82] Isolated reports have suggested that octreotide, hydroxyurea,[83] tamoxifen, doxorubicin-based regimens, IFN-α[84] and mifepristone (RU486) have controlled the growth of some meningiomas. Hydroxyurea has not produced responses in our experience. A number of investigative protocols for the treatment of meningioma are underway, including growth factor and angiogenesis inhibitors and gene therapy, but none has proved efficacious as yet. Retinoic acid is reported to stimulate meningioma cell adhesion and inhibit invasion in vitro.[85]

Prognosis

The prognosis after treatment of meningiomas depends on the histology of the tumor and on the adequacy of resection. Age at diagnosis, tumor size and postoperative RT may also play a role.[86] A low-grade meningioma that is totally resected has recurrence rates of about 20% in 5 years[86] and 25% in 10 years.[87] Tumors with less than gross total resection have about a 60% chance of progressing without postoperative RT. Overall, younger patients do better than the elderly. The 5-year survival rate of patients aged 21–64 is 81%, whereas it is 56% for patients 65 and older. The 5-year survival rate for benign tumors overall is 70%, whereas it is 55% with malignant tumors, even with aggressive surgery and adjuvant radiation.[88] The higher the MIB-1 labeling index at initial surgery, the shorter the time to recurrence.[89] In general quality of life remains good after treatment of either young or elderly patients.[90,91]

Hemangiopericytoma

Introduction

Originally called hemangioblastic meningioma (as were hemangioblastomas – see below), or angioblastic meningioma, this tumor is now recognized as a distinct tumor of uncertain cellular origin that behaves much more aggressively than meningiomas. The dural-based highly vascular tumor is indistinguishable histologically from hemangiopericytomas arising in soft tissues elsewhere in the body. Hemangiopericytomas represent less than 1% of primary CNS tumors and are about 2% as common as meningiomas.[92] About 8% of all hemangiopericytomas are meningeal, and about two-thirds of intracranial hemangiopericytomas are supratentorial. Their peak incidence is between 30 and 50 years of age and they are slightly more common in men than in women. Like meningiomas, they are often found in the parasagittal area, particularly around and attached to the torcular herophili (from Latin for 'wine press' – the confluence of dural venous sinuses), and, very rarely, in the ventricle.[93]

Etiology

Several cytogenetic abnormalities have been found in hemangiopericytomas. The most common is the rearrangement of chromosome 12q13. Cytogenetic alterations have also been found in 19q, 6p and 7p. Approximately 25% of meningeal hemangiopericytomas have homologous deletions of CDKN2/p16[94] on chromosome 9p, suggesting that the p16-mediated cell cycle regulatory pathway may be involved in transformation or progression of these tumors. Unlike meningiomas, there is no alteration in the NF2 gene. Somatostatin receptors are expressed by some tumors.[95] There are no known risk factors for the development of meningeal hemangiopericytomas.

Pathology

Hemangiopericytomas are highly vascular but look no different grossly from meningiomas.[96] Microscopically, the tumor consists of uniformly plump or polygonal cells with oval nuclei and scant ill-defined cytoplasm. There is often a dense intercellular pattern of reticular staining surrounding vascular spaces that are lined by normal endothelium. The wide and branching vascular spaces that distinguish this tumor from meningiomas have been called 'stag horn sinusoids'. They separate the tumor into small nodules. Unlike meningiomas, there is no calcification, and no psammoma bodies. Occasionally, the tumor invades the brain. Hemangiopericytomas do not react with epithelial membrane antigen, but are immunoreactive for vimentin and CD34. VEGF is produced by some tumors, probably causing brain edema by a paracrine mechanism. Mitotic activity is usually prominent, with MIB-1 labeling indices varying from 0.6% to 36%.

Clinical findings

The signs and symptoms of meningeal hemangiopericytomas are similar to those of the more common meningiomas (Table 6.7).

The common occurrence of these tumors compressing the torcula may lead to intracranial hypertension with headache and papilledema but no other neurologic signs.

Table 6.7
Presenting signs and symptoms in 44 patients with intracranial hemangiopericytoma.

Location	%
Supratentorial	
Headache	68
Papilledema	50
Hemiparesis	40
Visual field defect	20
Seizure	16
Altered sensorium	15
Infratentorial	
Gait disturbance	56
Ataxia	44
Headache, papilledema	44
Hypacusis	33
Vertigo, dizziness	33
Neck pain	33

From Guthrie et al.[96]

Hemangiopericytomas are occasionally associated with two different paraneoplastic syndromes. One is hypoglycemia, probably a result of tumor production of insulin-like growth factor.[97] The second is osteomalacia.[95] Patients may present with fractures, and are found to have hypophosphatemia and low 1,25-dihydroxy vitamin D_3 with normocalcemia and normal levels of alkaline phosphatase. The tumor is believed to produce some humoral factor inhibiting 25-hydroxy vitamin D-1 α-hydroxylase activity and phosphorus reabsorption in the kidney. The factor may act via parathyroid hormone-related protein receptors,[98] but is unrelated to cyclic AMP production in the proximal renal tubules. One of our patients had symptoms of osteomalacia for over a decade before headache led to cranial imaging and the discovery of the indolent meningeal tumor.

Except for the fact that meningeal hemangiopericytomas are rarely calcified, their CT and MR appearance is identical to that of meningiomas. However, MRS yields a myoinositol peak that distinguishes them from meningiomas. Hemangiopericytomas are dural-based, isodense before contrast, and uniformly and sharply contrast enhance. The tumors may also differ slightly from meningiomas in that they tend to cause lytic destruction of adjacent bone rather than hyperostosis. The presence of hyperostosis probably excludes hemangiopericytoma. PET scans are characterized by low glucose utilization but increased methionine uptake, similar to meningiomas.[99] Octreotide scans (for somatostatin receptors) may be positive.

Treatment

Whenever possible, the treatment is surgical.[100] However, despite apparent complete removal of tumor, local recurrence occurs in the majority of patients.[101] Approximately a quarter of patients suffer recurrence after 5 years and two-thirds after 10 years. Metastases are also common, usually to bones, lungs and liver. Because of the likelihood of local recurrence, and later distant metastases, all patients, even those with apparently complete surgical removal, should be irradiated in the postoperative period.[102] RT to a dose of 59.4 Gy appears to reduce the local recurrence rate, prolonging disease-free and overall survival from 65 months with surgery alone to 96 months with surgery plus RT.[103] Adjuvant chemotherapy has no role.

When tumor recurs, it should be reoperated if feasible.[92] This should be followed by external beam radiation, if not previously given. For patients with small tumors at recurrence, radiosurgery may give a complete response in 30%.[92,104] In previously irradiated patients, radiosurgery produced partial responses in 70%, with 15% remaining stable. Doxorubicin-based chemotherapy regimens were not particularly effective.[92] In general, chemotherapy is believed be ineffective in the treatment of recurrent or metastatic hemangiopericytomas.[105]

Prognosis

Unlike meningioma, where the prognosis is excellent, the prognosis of hemangiopericytoma is poor, albeit 'prolonged'. In several series, the recurrence rate after 15 years is about 90% for local recurrence and about 70% for metastases, usually to bones, lung or liver. Once metastases occur, survival is about 2 years. RT probably delays recurrence about two-fold. Recurrent hemangiopericytomas can sometimes be treated by reoperation. The median survival after first recurrence is about 5 years.[92] There is some, but not total, correlation between markers of cell proliferation and likelihood of recurrence.[106]

Hemangioblastoma
Introduction

Hemangioblastoma,[107] a tumor that typically involves the leptomeninges, was once classified as a hemangioblastic meningioma. Hemangioblastomas are benign tumors of uncertain origin that usually occur in the cerebellum but may appear anywhere in the nervous system, including the cerebral hemispheres, spinal cord, optic nerve[108] and peripheral nerves. In about 25% of patients, hemangioblastomas occur as part of the Von Hippel–Lindau (VHL) syndrome, an autosomal dominant disorder characterized by hemangioblastomas in the CNS and retina,

renal cell carcinoma, pheochromocytoma, endolymphatic sac tumors[109] and cysts in various visceral organs (Chapter 12). Hemangioblastomas are the most common primary tumor of the cerebellum in adults; however, they are much less common than metastases to the cerebellum. Sporadic hemangioblastomas usually appear in adulthood, primarily between the ages of 30 and 60. Hemangioblastomas associated with VHL disease occur at an earlier age, the mean being 29 years. The mean age for sporadic retinal hemangioblastomas is 48, whereas that associated with VHL is 24. The age difference fits a formula that requires only a single somatic mutation for the tumor to develop in VHL disease (the first mutation having been inherited in the germline), but two independent mutations for the sporadic form, thus supporting Knudson's two-hit hypothesis[110] (Chapter 1). Sporadic hemangioblastomas, which can occur anywhere in the nervous system, are usually single, whereas patients with VHL disease usually have multiple hemangioblastomas along the neuraxis.

Etiology

The VHL gene is located on chromosome 3q 25.[111] It is a tumor suppressor gene with three exons. The gene is widely expressed in normal adult tissues. The protein product consists of 213 amino acids and binds to the catalytic subunit of elongin, thus interfering with the activity of RNA polymerase. The protein also regulates the expression of VEGF, platelet-derived growth factor beta (PDGF-β) and Glut-1. The tumor cells synthesize VEGF, leading to the exuberant growth of endothelial cells associated with the tumor. VEGF expression is low in solid tumors, moderate in microcystic tumors and high in macrocystic tumors.[112] Because mutations may occur in any one of the exons, the clinical manifestations vary from affected family to affected family; they may also vary within affected members of a given family. Allelic loss, or mutations of the VHL gene, is found in stromal cells of most sporadic cerebellar hemangioblastomas.[113] One series suggests that more than 10% of patients with 'sporadic' hemangioblastoma show germline mutations of VHL,[114] suggesting that the range of VHL disease may be wider than previously recognized. There are no known environmental risk factors for the development of sporadic hemangioblastomas.

Pathology

Grossly, the tumor is seen as a well-circumscribed, highly vascularized red nodule, usually in the wall of a cyst. The tumor consists of two cell types, the stromal cells and vascular cells. The stromal cells are believed to be the neoplastic cells. The vascular cells are believed to represent a non-neoplastic proliferation of capillary endothelial cells as the result of VEGF production by the stromal cells. Stromal cell nuclei vary in size and have inconspicuous nucleoli. The nuclei may occasionally be atypical and hyperchromatic. The cytoplasm is eosinophilic and lipid-rich, with lipid-containing vacuoles giving the tumor a clear cell appearance,[7] similar to metastatic renal cell carcinoma (Table 6.8), an important distinction in VHL patients.

The stromal cells are vimentin and neuron-specific enolase positive; they may show glial fibrillary acidic protein (GFAP) expression but

Table 6.8
Clear cell lesions of the CNS: differential diagnosis.

General list of lesions	Differential diagnosis
Hemangioblastoma	Metastatic renal cell carcinoma
	Microcystic meningioma
Meningioma variants	Meningeal hemangioblastoma
	Metastatic carcinoma
	Chordoma
	Clear cell pituitary adenoma
Germinoma	Metastatic carcinoma
	Clear cell pituitary adenoma
	Large cell lymphoma
Oligodendroglioma	Mixed glial neoplasms
	Dysembryoplastic neuroepithelial tumor infarct
	Demyelinating disorder
	Neoplasms with clear cell foci (central neurocytoma, medulloblastoma, ependymoma, choroid plexus carcinoma, pilocytic astrocytoma)
	Clear cell carcinoma
Xanthomatous lesions	Pleomorphic xanthoastrocytoma
	Lipid-rich glioblastoma multiforme
	Malakoplakia
	Xanthomatous reactions to Langerhan's cell histiocytosis and colloid cyst
	Xanthomatous changes in Schwannoma, choroid plexus, meningioma

From Gokden et al[7] with permission.

are negative for EMA. The stromal cells are distributed within an intricate network of capillaries. The tumor is low-grade with mitoses absent or infrequent; labeling indices are usually less than 1%. In keeping with their low-grade nature, the tumors may show Rosenthal fibers.

Clinical findings

Tumors in the cerebellar hemisphere usually cause ipsilateral cerebellar signs, including gait and unilateral appendicular ataxia.[107] By compression of the 4th ventricle, they can cause hydrocephalus with attendant symptoms of headache, nausea and vomiting, cognitive change, ataxia and urgency incontinence. Because the tumors synthesize erythropoietin in about 20% of patients, erythrocytosis, an elevated hemoglobin without a change in the white cell or platelet count, may be the presenting manifestation, often identified on a blood count done for other reasons. When tumors are in the spinal cord or optic nerve, they cause slowly progressive symptoms appropriate to their location.

The MR scan of hemangioblastoma is characteristic (Fig. 6.10). The tumor is an intensely contrast-enhancing nodule, usually surrounded by a large cyst. The cyst fluid is hyperintense on the T2 image. The tumor often contains hypointense flow voids as a result of its hypervascularity. When more than one tumor is seen on cranial imaging, the patient probably has VHL disease, and a complete workup should include an enhanced spine MRI, complete ophthalmologic examination and body CT scan. Renal cell carcinoma, pheochromocytoma and multiple cysts of other organs are found in patients with VHL disease; renal cell cancer is the primary cause of death in these patients. Furthermore, renal cell carcinoma metastatic to the cerebellum can have an identical MR appearance to a hemangioblastoma and has a predilection to metastasize to the posterior fossa as opposed

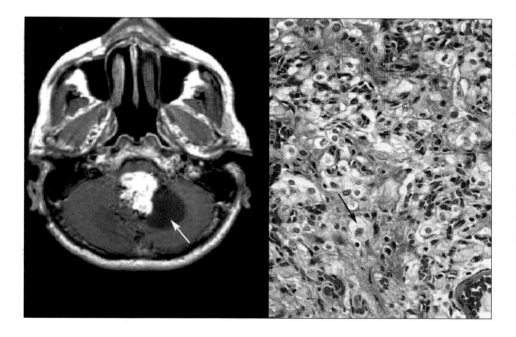

Figure 6.10
A hemangioblastoma of the cerebellum. The lesion is cystic (arrow) and intensely contrast enhances. Headache and cerebellar symptoms resolved after surgery. Histologically, one can identify foamy stromal cells (arrow) embedded in a rich capillary network.

to supratentorial structures. We encountered one patient with hemangioblastoma of one cerebellar hemisphere and a renal cell metastasis in the other cerebellar hemisphere. The two looked alike on neuroimaging.

Treatment

The treatment is surgical.[107] Complete excision results in cure in most instances; recurrence after total excision is less than 10%. Tumors in the spinal cord can often be completely excised. Some brainstem tumors can also be excised, but the morbidity is high. For tumors that cannot be completely excised, RT should follow subtotal resection. Radiosurgery may give better results than standard RT.[115] Those patients with VHL disease should have imaging of the entire nervous system, because tumors are often multiple. Small, asymptomatic tumors might warrant treatment before symptoms develop, but tumors are frequently so numerous that many are followed and not treated until symptoms develop. Early detection of tumors is crucial to ensure a good prognosis, and periodic screening of patients with VHL disease is indicated to look for recurrence and to detect new tumors.[107] Once-yearly should suffice. Screening should include first-degree relatives.

Prognosis

The prognosis of hemangioblastomas of the cerebellum depends in part on the effectiveness of surgery and in part on whether the lesion is sporadic or associated with VHL disease. Complete surgical removal ensures cure. Partial surgical removals are often well controlled with either RT or radiosurgery. Sporadic tumors do not become malignant or metastasize. However, in VHL disease, other tumors may appear either within or outside the CNS and may adversely effect prognosis. The overall 5-year survival is over 80%.

Melanocytic tumors

Introduction

Melanocytes normally found in the leptomeninges can give rise to either benign or malignant tumors.[117] The tumors may either form mass lesions or diffusely involve the leptomeninges. The lesions are divided into three groups: diffuse melanosis, a cytologically benign, diffuse proliferation of melanocytes involving the leptomeninges;[117] melanocytoma, a low-grade but ultimately fatal tumor of the leptomeninges (Table 6.9); and primary melanoma, a malignant meningeal tumor.

Combined, these lesions account for less than 0.1% of primary CNS tumors. When they occur as mass lesions, they involve the posterior fossa and the spinal canal more frequently than supratentorial areas. Primary melanoma of the leptomeninges is far less common than metastatic melanoma and is usually easily distinguished clinically.

Melanocytomas and primary meningeal melanomas are believed to arise from

Table 6.9
Clinical findings in 16 patients with intracranial meningeal melanocytomas.[119]

Median age at diagnosis	38
Female/Male ratio	2.2:1
Age at presentation (years)	9–71
Duration of symptoms (years)	0.1–14
Location of tumor	Posterior fossa
Postoperative survival (years)	0.04–35

Modified from Clarke et al.[118]

melanocytes that are derived from the neural crest. In the normal CNS, melanocytes are localized around the base of the brain, the ventral medulla oblongata, and along the upper cervical spinal cord, which may explain the predilection for tumors to occur in these areas. There are no known risk factors, and genetic abnormalities have not been established.

Pathology

Grossly, the lesions may appear as black tumors involving the subarachnoid space or may give the entire subarachnoid space a dark appearance. The tumors may also appear as non-pigmented, fleshy masses. Histologically, melanocytomas consist of monomorphic cells with low mitotic activity. Small amounts of necrosis or hemorrhage may be present. They occur mostly in the spinal cord but occasionally in the posterior fossa.[119] In melanomas, the cells are pleomorphic with multinucleated giant cells. Many mitoses, necroses and hemorrhages are found. The tumors do not express GFAP, neurofilament, cytokeratins or EMA, but most express HMB 45. About 25% of patients with diffuse meningeal melanocytosis have concomitant cutaneous lesions (neurocutaneous melanosis),[120,121] and approximately 10% of patients with large melanocytic nevi of the skin have CNS melanocytosis. Occasionally, melanosis may be associated with a melanoma.[122]

Clinical findings

The signs and symptoms depend on the location of greatest growth. The tumors begin as leptomeningeal involvement but may involve the brain either by invasion down Virchow–Robin spaces or by compression. Thus, patients may present with seizures, ataxia or spinal cord signs suggesting a focal mass lesion. Alternatively, diffuse invasion of the leptomeninges may interfere with normal CSF absorption, leading to hydrocephalus and signs of generalized brain dysfunction, including headache, mental status changes and ataxia. Symptoms of hydrocephalus may also develop later in the course of these tumors.

MR scan aids in the diagnosis when the leptomeninges are diffusely involved.[117] The meninges appear thickened and contrast enhance. Mass lesions are either isointense or hyperintense on the T1-weighted image with intense enhancement, and hypointense on the T2-weighted image. Melanin is paramagnetic and may yield hyperintensity on short echo time MR sequences. Because the tumors are highly vascular, they may hemorrhage, leading to hyperintensity on the T1-weighted image.

Lumbar puncture may establish the diagnosis by revealing abnormal melanin-containing cells on cytologic examination.[121] The cells may show immunoreactivity for S100 protein, HMB 45 and vimentin. HMB 45 positivity establishes the diagnosis but does not distinguish melanocytomas from malignant melanomas, either primary or metastatic. If there is sufficient melanin in the CSF, it may appear black. More commonly, the CSF is xanthochromic, a result of multiple small hemorrhages. Red cells may or may not be present at the time of the examination.

When the patient presents with mass lesions, the diagnosis is usually not made until surgery, when the surgeon, expecting to encounter an intrinsic brain tumor, instead finds a black tumor that involves the leptomeninges[123] with secondary brain invasion. Biopsy then establishes the diagnosis. Microscopically, melanocytomas and melanomas must be distinguished from other pigmented lesions of the meninges, including melanotic meningiomas and melanotic schwannomas.

Two important problems in differential diagnosis are to distinguish the more benign melanocytomas from melanomas, and to distinguish primary melanomas of the leptomeninges from metastatic melanomas. The former can be done by careful pathologic evaluation, and the latter by a search for a primary tumor of the skin, either by history or examination at the time of diagnosis. Accordingly, all patients with melanotic tumors of the leptomeninges should be examined both for congenital melanotic lesions of the skin (neurocutaneous melanosis) or for malignant melanomas that have not been detected previously.

Treatment

If a mass lesion is present, it should be removed to the maximum extent possible. Patients with melanomas should receive RT to the involved area in the postoperative period. It is not clear whether melanocytomas are best treated with radiation or simply followed until recurrence. However, the tumors are highly radioresistant, and it is questionable whether RT has any substantial effect. Radiosurgery has been reported to be highly effective in the treatment of brain metastases from melanoma and might be considered if only a few small areas of the nervous system are involved in primary melanocytoma or malignant melanoma.[124] Chemotherapy has largely been restricted to the use of chemotherapeutic agents for metastatic melanoma and most are ineffective. Individual reports of dacarbazine, given intrathecally for the treatment of meningeal melanoma, and immunotherapeutic agents such as Interleukin-2 (IL-2), are limited to a few case reports.[125] Some case reports are suspect because of the failure to distinguish between melanocytoma and malignant melanoma. Symptomatic hydrocephalus can be relieved by ventriculoperitoneal (VP) shunt even if the underlying tumor cannot be treated effectively.

The prognosis in all of these tumors is poor. Although long survival in patients with melanocytoma is possible, including one patient alive 35 years after total excision and RT of an intracranial melanocytoma, most patients with melanocytomas succumb within several years and most patients with melanoma within several months. Even diffuse melanosis has a poor prognosis.

Miscellaneous tumors

Several other tumors can occasionally arise from the meninges. These include both benign and malignant tumors. The benign tumors include chondromas, osteomas, lipomas, fibrous histiocytomas, solitary plasmacytomas[126] (Chapter 11) and myxomas.[127] Malignant tumors include chondrosarcomas,[128] Ewing's sarcoma, rhabdomyosarcoma,[129] leiomyosarcoma[130] and fibrosarcoma.[131] Both high- and low-grade gliomas can either arise in or metastasize to the leptomeninges.[132] The low-grade gliomas include pilocytic astrocytomas[133] (Chapter 5). All of these tumors can present with meningeal mass lesions that, when malignant, grow more rapidly than most meningiomas. Primary CNS lymphomas characteristically involve the leptomeninges but rarely as mass lesions (Chapter 11).

Sometimes, the diagnosis may be suspected by MR or CT scan. For example, lipomas have a characteristic hyperintensity on both T1- and T2-weighted images and do not contrast enhance. Lipomas characteristically involve the corpus callosum or the cerebellopontine angle. In the latter case, they present with hearing loss, dizziness and tinnitus. Surgical resection may not remove the entire tumor and may lead to postoperative deficits. Observation may be the best approach[134] until either the patient becomes symptomatic, or the tumor is seen to be growing on serial scans.

Intracranial chondromas are usually found at the base of the skull, most commonly in the sella and parasellar regions with varying degrees of involvement of the cavernous sinus.[135] Rarely, they are confined to the cavernous sinus. The tumors are slowly growing and are best treated surgically. Fibrous histiocytomas may be either benign or malignant.[136] Malignant rhabdoid tumors are a rare, but extremely aggressive, tumor of childhood of unclear histogenesis but characteristic histology.[137] These lesions are usually approached surgically and, if malignant, followed by RT. Despite treatment, outcome is poor due to rapid relapse.

References

1. Sanan A, van Loveren HR. The arachnoid and the myth of Arachne. Neurosurgery 1999; 45: 152–5.
2. Bastos AC, Andermann F, Melancon D et al. Late-onset temporal lobe epilepsy and dilatation of the hippocampal sulcus by an enlarged Virchow–Robin space. Neurology 1998; 50: 784–7.
3. Kleihues P, Cavenee WK. World Health Organization Classification of Tumours: Tumours of the Nervous System – Pathology and Genetics. Lyon: IRAC Press, 2000.
4. DeMonte F, Marmon E, Al-Mefty O. Meningiomas. In: Kaye AH, Laws ERJ, eds. Brain tumors. 2nd edn New York: Churchill Livingstone, 2001: 719–54.
5. Buhl R, Hugo HH, Mihajlovic Z, Mehdorn HM. Secretory meningiomas: clinical and immunohistochemical observations. Neurosurgery 2001; 48: 297–301.
6. Lamszus K, Lengler U, Schmidt NO et al. Vascular endothelial growth factor, hepatocyte growth factor/scatter factor, basic fibroblast growth factor, and placenta growth factor in human meningiomas and their relation to angiogenesis and malignancy. Neurosurgery 2000; 46: 938–47.
7. Gokden M, Roth KA, Carroll SL et al. Clear cell neoplasms and pseudoneoplastic lesions of the central nervous system. Semin Diagn Pathol 1997; 14: 253–69.
8. Pimentel J, Fernandes A, Pinto AE et al. Clear cell meningioma variant and clinical aggressiveness. Clin Neuropathol 1998; 17: 141–6.
9. CBTRUS (2000). Statistical Report: Primary Brain Tumors in the United States, 1992–1997. 2000. Central Brain Tumor Registry of the United States.
10. Radhakrishnan K, Mokri B, Parisi JE et al. The trends in incidence of primary brain tumors in the population of Rochester, Minnesota. Ann Neurol 1995; 37: 67–73.
11. Perry A, Scheithauer BW, Stafford SL et al. Malignancy in meningiomas – a clinicopathologic study of 116 patients, with grading implications. Cancer 1999; 85: 2046–56.
12. Cerdá-Nicolás M, López-Gines C, Pérez-Bacete M et al. Histopathological and cytogenetic findings in benign, atypical and anaplastic human meningiomas: a study of 60 tumors. J Neurooncol 2000; 47: 99–108.
13. Sanson M, Cornu P. Biology of meningiomas. Acta Neurochir (Wien) 2000; 142: 493–505.
14. Evans JJ, Jeun SS, Lee JH et al. Molecular alterations in the *neurofibromatosis Type 2* gene and its protein rarely occurring in meningothelial meningiomas. J Neurosurg 2001; 94: 111–7.
15. Shoshan Y, Chernova O, Jeun SS et al. Radiation-induced meningioma: a distinct molecular genetic pattern? J Neuropathol Exp Neurol 2000; 59: 614–20.
16. Schmitz U, Mueller W, Weber M et al. INI1 mutations in meningiomas at a potential hotspot in exon 9. Br J Cancer 2001; 84: 199–201.
17. Perry A, Jenkins RB, Dahl RJ et al. Cytogenetic analysis of aggressive meningiomas: possible diagnostic and prognostic implications. Cancer 1996; 77: 2567–73.
18. Bostrom J, Cobbers JM, Wolter M et al. Mutation of the PTEN (MMAC1) tumor suppressor gene in a subset of glioblastomas but not in meningiomas with loss of chromosome arm 10q. Cancer Res 1998; 58: 29–33.
19. Kim JH, Lee SH, Rhee CH et al. Loss of heterozygosity on chromosome 22q and 17p correlates with aggressiveness of meningiomas. J Neurooncol 1998; 40: 101–6.

20. Zhu J, Frosch MP, Busque L et al. Analysis of meningiomas by methylation- and transcription-based clonality assays. Cancer Res 1995; 55: 3865–72.

21. Zhu JJG, Maruyama T, Jacoby LB et al. Clonal analysis of a case of multiple meningiomas using multiple molecular genetic approaches: pathology case report. Neurosurgery 1999; 45: 409–16.

22. Wu JK, MacGillavry M, Kessaris C et al. Clonal analysis of meningiomas. Neurosurgery 1996; 38: 1196–200.

23. von Deimling A, Larson J, Wellenreuther R et al. Clonal origin of recurrent meningiomas. Brain Pathology 1999; 9: 645–50.

24. Moresco RM, Scheithauer BW, Lucignani G et al. Oestrogen receptors in meningiomas: a correlative PET and immunohistochemical study. Nucl Med Commun 1997; 18: 606–15.

25. Carroll RS, Zhang J, Black PM. Expression of estrogen receptors alpha and beta in human meningiomas. J Neurooncol 1999; 42: 109–16.

26. Koide SS. Mifepristone. Auxiliary therapeutic use in cancer and related disorders. J Reprod Med 1998; 43: 551–60.

27. Roelvink NC, Kamphorst W, August H, van Alphen M, Rao BR. Literature statistics do not support a growth stimulating role for female sex steroid hormones in haemangiomas and meningiomas. J Neurooncol 1991; 11: 243–53.

28. Lambe M, Coogan P, Baron J. Reproductive factors and the risk of brain tumors: a population-based study in Sweden. Int J Cancer 1997; 72: 389–93.

29. Karlsson AE, Bergenheim AT, Björk P, Henriksson R. Estramustine-binding protein in meningioma. Acta Neuropathol (Berl) 1999; 98: 135–40.

30. Christov C, Lechapt-Zalcman E, Adle-Biassette H, Nachev S, Gherardi RK. Vascular permeability factor/vascular endothelial growth factor (VPF/VEGF) and its receptor flt-1 in microcystic meningiomas. Acta Neuropathol (Berl) 1999; 98: 414–20.

31. Friend KE, Radinsky R, McCutcheon IE. Growth hormone receptor expression and function in meningiomas: effect of a specific receptor antagonist. J Neurosurg 1999; 91: 93–9.

32. Magrassi L, De Fraja C, Conti L et al. Expression of the JAK and STAT superfamilies in human meningiomas. J Neurosurg 1999; 91: 440–6.

33. Bondy M, Ligon BL. Epidemiology and etiology of intracranial meningiomas: a review. J Neurooncol 1996; 29: 197–205.

34. Das A, Tang WY, Smith DR. Meningiomas in Singapore: demographic and biological characteristics. J Neurooncol 2000; 47: 153–60.

35. Nishio S, Morioka T, Inamura T et al. Radiation-induced brain tumours: potential late complications of radiation therapy for brain tumours. Acta Neurochir (Wien) 1998; 140: 763–70.

36. Pollak L, Walach N, Gur R, Schiffer J. Meningiomas after radiotherapy for tinea capitis – still no history. Tumori 1998; 84: 65–8.

37. Ron E, Modan B, Boice JD Jr et al. Tumors of the brain and nervous system after radiotherapy in childhood. N Engl J Med 1988; 319: 1033–9.

38. Kotzen RM, Swanson RM, Milhorat TH, Boockvar JA. Post-traumatic meningioma: case report and historical perspective. J Neurol Neurosurg Psychiatry 1999; 66: 796.

39. Preston-Martin S, Pogoda JM, Schlehofer B et al. An international case–control study of adult glioma and meningioma: the role of head trauma. Int J Epidemiol 1998; 27: 579-86.

40. Markopoulos C, Sampalis F, Givalos N, Gogas H. Association of breast cancer with meningioma. Eur J Surg Oncol 1998; 24: 332–4.

41. Lee A, Wallace C, Rewcastle B, Sutherland G. Metastases to meningioma. Am J Neuroradiol 1998; 19: 1120–2.

42. Kondziolka D, Flickinger JC, Perez B. Judicious resection and/or radiosurgery for parasagittal meningiomas: outcomes from a multicenter review. Gamma Knife Meningioma Study Group. Neurosurgery 1998; 43: 405–13.

43. Perry A, Stafford SL, Scheithauer BW, Suman VJ, Lohse CM. The prognostic significance of MIB-1, p53, and DNA flow cytometry in

completely resected primary meningiomas. Cancer 1998; 82: 2262–9.

44. Perry A, Scheithauer BW, Stafford SL, Abell-Aleff PC, Meyer FB. 'Rhabdoid' meningioma: an aggressive variant. Am J Surg Pathol 1998; 22: 1482–90.

45. Enam SA, Abdulrauf S, Mehta B, Malik GM, Mahmood A. Metastasis in meningioma. Acta Neurochir (Wien) 1996; 138: 1172–7.

46. Go RS, Taylor BV, Kimmel DW. The natural history of asymptomatic meningiomas in Olmsted County, Minnesota. Neurology 1998; 51: 1718–20.

47. Braunstein JB, Vick NA. Meningiomas: the decision not to operate. Neurology 1997; 48: 1459–62.

48. Bornstein RA, Witt NJ. Are right-hemisphere lesions really larger? Lesion size and laterality in meningioma patients. Acta Neurol Scand 1984; 69: 176–81.

49. Talacchi A, Lombardo C, Bricolo A. Vascular headache due to intracranial meningioma: a curable form of headache. Lancet 1997; 350: 1004–5.

50. Bitzer M, Opitz H, Popp J et al. Angiogenesis and brain oedema in intracranial meningiomas: influence of vascular endothelial growth factor. Acta Neurochir (Wien) 1998; 140: 333–40.

51. Bitzer M, Opitz H, Popp J, Morgalla M, Gruber A, Heiss E, Voigt K. Angiogenesis and brain oedema in intracranial meningiomas: influence of vascular endothelial growth factor. Acta Neurochir (Wein) 1998; 140: 333–40.

52. Hirashima Y, Hayashi N, Fukuda O et al. Platelet-activating factor and edema surrounding meningiomas. J Neurosurg 1998; 88: 304–7.

53. Constantini S, Tamir J, Gomori MJ, Shohami E. Tumor prostaglandin levels correlate with edema around supratentorial meningiomas. Neurosurgery 1993; 33: 204–10.

54. Ide M, Jimbo M, Yamamoto M et al. MIB-1 staining index and peritumoral brain edema of meningiomas. Cancer 1996; 78: 133–43.

55. Mantle RE, Lach B, Delgado MR, Baeesa S, Bélanger G. Predicting the probability of meningioma recurrence based on the quantity of peritumoral brain edema on computerized tomography scanning. J Neurosurg 1999; 91: 375–83.

56. Oka K, Go Y, Kimura H, Tomonaga M. Obstruction of the superior sagittal sinus caused by parasagittal meningiomas: the role of collateral venous pathways. J Neurosurg 1994; 81: 520–4.

57. Anegawa S, Hayashi T, Torigoe R, Furukawa Y. Diffuse calvarial meningioma – case report and review of the literature. J Neurosurg 1999; 90: 970–3.

58. Engelhard HH. Progress in the diagnosis and treatment of patients with meningiomas. Part I: diagnostic imaging, preoperative embolization. Surg Neurol 2001; 55: 89–101.

59. Ildan F, Tuna A, Göçer AI et al. Correlation of the relationships of brain–tumor interfaces, magnetic resonance imaging, and angiographic findings to predict cleavage of meningiomas. J Neurosurg 1999; 91: 384–90.

60. Pieper DR, Al-Mefty O, Hanada Y, Buechner D. Hyperostosis associated with meningioma of the cranial base: secondary changes or tumor invasion. Neurosurgery 1999; 44: 742–6.

61. Pierallini A, Bonamini M, Di Stefano D, Siciliano P, Bozzao L. Pleomorphic xantho-astrocytoma with CT and MRI appearance of meningioma. Neuroradiology 1999; 41: 30–4.

62. Kizana E, Lee R, Young N, Dorsch NW, Soo YS. A review of the radiological features of intracranial meningiomas. Australas Radiol 1996; 40: 454–62.

63. Hildebrandt G, Scheidhauer K, Luyken C et al. High sensitivity of the in vivo detection of somatostatin receptors by 111indium (DTPA-octreotide)-scintigraphy in meningioma patients. Acta Neurochir (Wien) 1994; 126: 63–71.

64. Iuchi T, Iwadate Y, Namba H et al. Glucose and methionine uptake and proliferative activity in meningiomas. Neurol Res 1999; 21: 640–4.

65. Nyberg G, Bergstrom M, Enblad P, Lilja A, Muhr C, Langstrom B. PET-methionine of skull base neuromas and meningiomas. Acta Otolaryngol (Stockh) 1997; 117: 482–9.

66. Yamaki T, Ikeda T, Sakamoto Y, Ohtaki M, Hashi K. Lymphoplasmacyte-rich meningioma with clinical resemblance to inflammatory pseudotumor. Report of two cases. J Neurosurg 1997; 86: 898–904.

67. Nakasu S, Nakasu Y, Nakajima M, Matsuda M, Handa J. Preoperative identification of meningiomas that are highly likely to recur. J Neurosurg 1999; 90: 455–62.

68. Lee JH, Jeun SS, Evans J, Kosmorsky G. Surgical management of clinoidal meningiomas. Neurosurgery 2001; 48: 1012–9.

69. Selesnick SH, Nguyen TD, Gutin PH, Lavyne MH. Posterior petrous face meningiomas. Otolaryngol Head Neck Surg 2001; 124: 408–13.

70. Patsouris E, Laas R, Hagel C, Stavrou D. Increased proliferative activity due to necroses induced by pre-operative embolization in benign meningiomas. J Neurooncol 1998; 40: 257–64.

71. Hug EB, DeVries A, Thornton AF et al. Management of atypical and malignant meningiomas: role of high-dose, 3D-conformal radiation therapy. J Neurooncol 2000; 48: 151–60.

72. Milosevic MF, Frost PJ, Laperriere NJ, Wong CS, Simpson WJ. Radiotherapy for atypical or malignant intracranial meningioma. Int J Radiat Oncol Biol Phys 1996; 34: 817–22.

73. Maire JP, Caudry M, Guerin J et al. Fractionated radiation therapy in the treatment of intracranial meningiomas: local control, functional efficacy, and tolerance in 91 patients. Int J Radiat Oncol Biol Phys 1995; 33: 315–21.

74. Connell PP, Macdonald RL, Mansur DB, Nicholas MK, Mundt AJ. Tumor size predicts control of benign meningiomas treated with radiotherapy. Neurosurgery 1999; 44: 1194–9.

75. Dufour H, Muracciole X, Métellus P et al. Long-term tumor control and functional outcome in patients with cavernous sinus meningiomas treated by radiotherapy with or without previous surgery: is there an alternative to aggressive tumor removal? Neurosurgery 2001; 48: 285–94.

76. Kondziolka D, Levy EI, Niranjan A, Flickinger JC, Lunsford LD. Long-term outcomes after meningioma radiosurgery: physician and patient perspectives. J Neurosurg 1999; 91: 44–50.

77. Roche PH, Regis J, Dufour H et al. Gamma knife radiosurgery in the management of cavernous sinus meningiomas. J Neurosurg 2000; 93 Suppl 3: 68–73.

78. Kondziolka D, Flickinger JC, Perez B, Gamma Knife Meningioma Study Group. Judicious resection and/or radiosurgery for parasagittal meningiomas: outcomes from a multicenter review. Neurosurgery 1998; 43: 405–13.

79. Roche PH, Regis J, Dufour H et al. Gamma knife radiosurgery in the management of cavernous sinus meningiomas. J Neurosurg 2000; 93 Suppl 3: 68–73.

80. Singh VP, Kansal S, Vaishya S, Julka PK, Mehta VS. Early complications following gamma knife radiosurgery for intracranial meningiomas. J Neurosurg 2000; 93: 57–61.

81. Stelzer KJ. Acute and long-term complications of therapeutic radiation for skull base tumors. Neurosurg Clin N Am 2000; 11: 597–604.

82. Kyritsis AP. Chemotherapy for meningiomas. J Neurooncol 1996; 29: 269–72.

83. Schrell UMH, Rittig MG, Anders M et al. Hydroxyurea for treatment of unresectable and recurrent meningiomas. II. Decrease in size of meningiomas in patients treated with hydroxyurea. J Neuro Surg 1997; 86: 840–4.

84. Kaba SE, DeMonte F, Bruner JM et al. The treatment of recurrent unresectable and malignant meningiomas with interferon alpha-2B. Neurosurgery 1997; 40: 271–5.

85. Pereda MP, Hopfner U, Pagotto U et al. Retinoic acid stimulates meningioma cell adhesion to the extracellular matrix and inhibits invasion. Br J Cancer 1999; 81: 381–6.

86. McCarthy BJ, Davis FG, Freels S et al. Factors associated with survival in patients with meningioma. J Neurosurg 1998; 88: 831–9.

87. Stafford SL, Perry A, Suman VJ et al. Primarily resected meningiomas: outcome and prognostic factors in 581 Mayo Clinic patients, 1978 through 1988. Mayo Clin Proc 1998; 73: 936–42.

88. Dziuk TW, Woo S, Butler EB et al. Malignant meningioma: an indication for initial aggressive surgery and adjuvant radiotherapy. J Neurooncol 1998; 37: 177–88.

89. Nakaguchi H, Fujimaki T, Matsuno A et al. Postoperative residual tumor growth of

meningioma can be predicted by MIB-1 immunohistochemistry. Cancer 1999; 85: 2249–54.

90. Kalkanis SN, Quiñones-Hinojosa A, Buzney E, Ribaudo HJ, Black PM. Quality of life following surgery for intracranial meningiomas at Brigham and Women's Hospital: a study of 164 patients using a modification of the functional assessment of cancer therapy–brain questionnaire. J Neurooncol 2000; 48: 233–41.

91. Tucha O, Smely C, Lange KW. Effects of surgery on cognitive functioning of elderly patients with intracranial meningioma. Br J Neurosurg 2001; 15: 184–8.

92. Galanis E, Buckner JC, Scheithauer BW, Kimmel DW, Schomberg PJ, Piepgras DG. Management of recurrent meningeal hemangiopericytoma. Cancer 1998; 82: 1915–20.

93. Abrahams JM, Forman MS, Lavi E, Goldberg H, Flamm ES. Hemangiopericytoma of the third ventricle. Case report. J Neurosurg 1999; 90: 359–62.

94. Ono Y, Ueki K, Joseph JT, Louis DN. Homozygous deletions of the *CDKN2/p16* gene in dural hemangiopericytomas. Acta Neuropathol (Berl) 1996; 91: 221–5.

95. Sandhu FA, Martuza RL. Craniofacial hemangiopericytoma associated with oncogenic osteomalacia: case report. J Neurooncol 2000; 46: 241–7.

96. Guthrie BL, Ebersold MJ, Scheithauer BW, Shaw EG. Meningeal hemangiopericytoma: histopathological features, treatment, and long-term follow-up of 44 cases. Neurosurgery 1989; 25: 514–22.

97. Hoekman K, van Doorn J, Gloudemans T, Maassen JA, Schuller AG, Pinedo HM. Hypoglycaemia associated with the production of insulin-like growth factor II and insulin-like growth factor binding protein 6 by a haemangiopericytoma. Clin Endocrinol (Oxf) 1999; 51: 247–53.

98. Nelson AE, Namkung HJ, Patava J et al. Characteristics of tumor cell bioactivity in oncogenic osteomalacia. Mol Cell Endocrinol 1996; 124: 17–23.

99. Kracht LW, Bauer A, Herholz K et al. Positron emission tomography in a case of intracranial hemangiopericytoma. J Comput Assist Tomogr 1999; 23: 365–8.

100. Brunori A, Delitala A, Oddi G, Chiappetta F. Recent experience in the management of meningeal hemangiopericytomas. Tumori 1997; 83: 856–61.

101. Spitz FR, Bouvet M, Pisters PW, Pollock RE, Feig BW. Hemangiopericytoma: a 20-year single-institution experience. Ann Surg Oncol 1998; 5: 350–5.

102. Dufour H, Métellus P, Fuentes S et al. Meningeal hemangiopericytoma: A retrospective study of 21 patients with special review of postoperative external radiotherapy. Neurosurgery 2001; 48: 756–63.

103. Bastin KT, Mehta MP. Meningeal hemangiopericytoma: defining the role for radiation therapy. J Neuro oncology 1992; 14: 277–87.

104. Kocher M, Voges J, Staar S et al. Linear accelerator radiosurgery for recurrent malignant tumors of the skull base. Am J Clin Oncol 1998; 21: 18–22.

105. Younis GA, Sawaya R, DeMonte F, Hess KR, Albrecht S, Bruner JM. Aggressive meningeal tumors: review of a series. J Neurosurg 1995; 82: 17–27.

106. Nakaguchi H, Fujimaki T, Matsuno A, Matsuura R, Asai A, Suzuki I, Sasaki T, Kirino T. Postoperative residual tumor growth of meningioma can be predicted by MIB-1 immunohistochemistry. Cancer 1999; 85: 2249–54.

107. Conway JE, Chou D, Clatterbuck RE et al. Hemangioblastomas of the central nervous system in von Hippel–Lindau syndrome and sporadic disease. Neurosurgery 2001; 48: 55–62.

108. Richard S, Campello C, Taillandier L, Parker F, Resche F. Haemangioblastoma of the central nervous system in von Hippel–Lindau disease. French VHL Study Group. J Intern Med 1998; 243: 547–53.

109. Kawahara N, Kume H, Ueki K et al. VHL gene inactivation in an endolymphatic sac tumor associated with von Hippel–Lindau disease. Neurology 1999; 53: 208–10.

110. Chang JH, Spraul CW, Lynn ML, Drack A, Grossniklaus HE. The two-stage mutation model in retinal hemangioblastoma. Ophthalmic Genet 1998; 19: 123–30.

111. Kondo K, Kaelin WG, Jr. The von Hippel–Lindau tumor suppressor gene. Exp Cell Res 2001; 264: 117–25.

112. Vaquero J, Zurita M, Oya S, Coca S, Salas C. Vascular permeability factor expression in cerebellar hemangioblastomas: correlation with tumor-associated cysts. J Neurooncol 1999; 41: 3–7.

113. Lee JY, Dong SM, Park WS et al. Loss of heterozygosity and somatic mutations of the VHL tumor suppressor gene in sporadic cerebellar hemangioblastomas. Cancer Res 1998; 58: 504–8.

114. Olschwang S, Richard S, Boisson C et al. Germline mutation profile of the VHL gene in von Hippel–Lindau disease and in sporadic hemangioblastoma. Hum Mutat 1998; 12: 424–30.

115. Jawahar A, Kondziolka D, Garces YI et al. Stereotactic radiosurgery for hemangioblastomas of the brain. Acta Neurochir (Wien) 2000; 142: 641–4.

116. Brat DJ, Giannini C, Scheithauer BW, Burger PC. Primary melanocytic neoplasms of the central nervous system. Am J Surg Pathol 1999; 23: 745–54.

117. Byrd SE, Darling CF, Tomita T et al. MR imaging of symptomatic neurocutaneous melanosis in children. Pediatr Radiol 1997; 27: 39–44.

118. Clarke DB, Leblanc R, Bertrand G, Quartey GR, Snipes GJ. Meningeal melanocytoma. Report of a case and a historical comparison. J Neurosurg 1998; 88: 116–21.

119. Prabhu SS, Lynch PG, Keogh AJ, Parekh HC. Intracranial meningeal melanocytoma: a report of two cases and a review of the literature. Surg Neurol 1993; 40: 516–21.

120. DeDavid M, Orlow SJ, Provost N et al. Neurocutaneous melanosis: clinical features of large congenital melanocytic nevi in patients with manifest central nervous system melanosis. J Am Acad Dermatol 1996; 35: 529–38.

121. Alameda F, Lloreta J, Galito E, Roquer J, Serrano S. Meningeal melanocytoma: a case report and literature review. Ultrastruct Pathol 1998; 22: 349–56.

122. Murray C, D'Intino Y, MacCormick R, Nassar B, Walsh N. Melanosis in association with metastatic malignant melanoma: report of a case and a unifying concept of pathogenesis. Am J Dermatopathol 1999; 21: 28–30.

123. Barut S. Primary leptomeningeal melanoma simulating a meningioma. Neurosurg Rev 1995; 18: 143–7.

124. Lavine SD, Petrovich Z, Cohen-Gadol AA et al. Gamma knife radiosurgery for metastatic melanoma: an analysis of survival, outcome, and complications. Neurosurgery 1999; 44: 59–64.

125. Fathallah-Shaykh HM, Zimmerman C, Morgan H et al. Response of primary leptomeningeal melanoma to intrathecal recombinant interleukin-2 – a case report. Cancer 1996; 77: 1544–50.

126. Vaicys C, Schulder M, Wolansky LJ, Fromowitz FB. Falcotentorial plasmacytoma – case report. J Neurosurg 1999; 91: 132–5.

127. Graham JF, Loo SYT, Matoba A. Primary brain myxoma, an unusual tumor of meningeal origin: case report. Neurosurgery 1999; 45: 166–9.

128. Forbes RB, Eljamel MS. Meningeal chondrosarcomas, a review of 31 patients. Br J Neurosurg 1998; 12: 461–4.

129. Kobayashi S, Hirakawa E, Sasaki M, Ishikawa M, Haba R. Meningeal rhabdomyosarcoma. Report of a case with cytologic, immunohistologic and ultrastructural studies. Acta Cytol 1995; 39: 428–34.

130. Bejjani GK, Stopak B, Schwartz A, Santi R. Primary dural leiomyosarcoma in a patient infected with human immunodeficiency virus: case report. Neurosurgery 1999; 44: 199–202.

131. Donnet A, Figarella-Branger D, Grisoli F. Primary meningeal fibrosarcoma: a particular neuroradiological presentation. J Neurooncol 1999; 42: 79–83.

132. Ng HK, Poon WS. Primary leptomeningeal astrocytoma. Case report. J Neurosurg 1998; 88: 586–9.

133. Tamura M, Zama A, Kurihara H et al. Management of recurrent pilocytic astrocytoma with leptomeningeal dissemination in childhood. Childs Nerv Syst 1998; 14: 617–22.

134. Bigelow DC, Eisen MD, Smith PG et al. Lipomas of the internal auditory canal and cerebellopontine angle. Laryngoscope 1998; 108: 1459–69.

135. Brownlee RD, Sevick RJ, Rewcastle NB, Tranmer BI. Intracranial chondroma. Am J Neuroradiol 1997; 18: 889–93.

136. Martinez-Salazar A, Supler M, Rojiani AM. Primary intracerebral malignant fibrous histiocytoma: immunohistochemical findings and etiopathogenetic considerations. Mod Pathol 1997; 10: 149–54.

137. Yachnis AT, Neubauer D, Muir D. Characterization of a primary central nervous system atypical teratoid/rhabdoid tumor and derivative cell line: immunophenotype and neoplastic properties. J Neuropathol Exp Neurol 1998; 57: 961–71.

7

Neuronal, mixed neuronal–glial and embryonal tumors

Introduction

Since Lhermitte and Duclos first described a neuronal tumor of the cerebellum in 1920, the field of neuronal and mixed neuronal–glial neoplasms has been fraught with controversy. One reason is that until recently neurologists and neuropathologists have had a strong bias against the diagnosis of neuronal neoplasm because of the view that all neurons were postmitotic and neuronal precursors did not exist in the adult brain. Current evidence indicates that this is untrue and may lead neuropathologists to reconsider this preconception. A second reason has been that glial tumors may infiltrate cerebral cortex widely, and it often becomes difficult to distinguish neurons that are trapped within a glial tumor from neurons that are themselves neoplastic.

Nevertheless, a number of advances in neurology, neuroimaging and neuropathology have led neuropathologists to diagnose these rare neuronal tumors more frequently (Fig. 7.1). Those advances include non-invasive imaging techniques that allow diagnosis of neoplasms in patients who are asymptomatic save for seizures. A second advance has been the surgical treatment of epilepsy. Early on it was discovered that resections for temporal lobe epilepsy often identified cortically based, otherwise asymptomatic tumors, most of which were probably dysembryoplastic neuroepithelial tumors (DNT) (see below). The recent

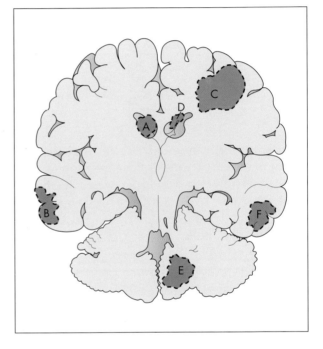

Figure 7.1
Location of neuronal, mixed neuronal–glial and embryonal tumors. Central neurocytomas are found in or close to the lateral ventricle (A). DNTs are found in the cortex of the temporal lobe (B). Gangliogliomas and ganglioneurocytomas are found in the frontal lobe, involving both cortex and subcortex (C). Subependymal giant cell astrocytomas arise from the wall of the lateral ventricles (D). Medulloblastomas are found in the inferior vermis of the cerebellum (E). Other primitive neuroectodermal tumors can arise anywhere in the central nervous system, particularly in the cerebral hemispheres (F).

Gangliocytoma
Dysplastic gangliocytoma of cerebellum (Lhermitte–Duclos) (Chapter 12)
Desmoplastic infantile astrocytoma/ganglioglioma
Dysembryoplastic neuroepithelial tumor
Ganglioglioma
Anaplastic (malignant) ganglioglioma
Central neurocytoma
Paraganglioma of the filum terminale
Olfactory neuroblastoma (esthesioneuroblastoma) (Chapter 9)
    Variant: olfactory neuroepithelioma

Table 7.1
Neuronal, mixed neuronal–glial and neuroblastic tumors.

more aggressive surgical approach to epilepsy is identifying more such tumors. A third advance has been in neuropathology and immunohistochemistry. The identification of synaptic vesicles in neoplastic cells by electron microscopy allows the neuropathologist to distinguish the rare central neurocytoma from the more common similarly appearing oligodendroglioma. The immunohistochemical stain for synaptophysin also reveals synaptic activity in neuronal tumors. Absence of glial fibrillary acidic proteins (GFAP) supports the diagnosis. Perhaps more important has been the discovery of two neuronal nuclear markers, Neu-N[1] and anti-Hu,[2] which appear, when positive, to unequivocally identify neoplastic cells as neuronal in origin. The lack of a reaction with these neuronal markers, however, does not exclude the possibility that the tumor arose from a neuronal precursor.

Table 7.1 shows the World Health Organization (WHO) classification of tumors believed to be of neuronal or mixed neuronal and glial origin. These tumors usually affect children or young adults and, if in the cerebral hemisphere, usually present as epilepsy. The neuropathologic classification has undergone a dramatic change between the first WHO edition in 1979 and the current edition in 2000[3] for some of the reasons indicated above.

This chapter also considers tumors classified by the WHO as embryonal in origin because some evidence suggests these tumors may be neuronal or neuronal precursor in origin. Unlike the other neuronal tumors, they are not rare, but they also primarily affect the young.

The neuronal and embryonal tumors discussed in this chapter generally affect children and young adults, with no particular sex or ethnic predilection. Their exact incidence is unknown, but they may constitute as many as 5% of primary brain tumors and, in selected populations such as children and adults with pharmaco-resistant epilepsy, the incidence may be much higher.

Unlike gliomas, neuronal and neuronal–glial tumors are usually low-grade and have a relatively benign prognosis. They often present with seizures and, before modern imaging techniques, patients could suffer seizures for many years (as long as 39 years in one report) before a diagnosis was made. Embryonal tumors, although probably neuronal in origin (at least, often expressing neuronal markers),[2] differ from the relatively benign neuronal and neuronal–glial tumors in that they are much more aggressive and do not respond well to current therapeutic endeavors. The characteristics of neuronal and neuronal–glial tumors are shown in Table 7.2.

Table 7.2
Characteristics of neuronal and neuronal–glial tumors.

	Age (years) at presentation	Preferential/ pathognomonic site	Imaging characteristics – pathognomonic
Ganglioglioma/gangliocytoma	< 30	Temporal lobe	Cystic, calcified, sharply demarcated, frequently enhancing
Dysplastic Ganz gliocytoma of the cerebellum (Lhermitte–Duclos)	20–40	Cerebellum	Striated pattern, not enhancing
Desmoplastic infantile ganglioglioma	< 2	Hemispheric	Massive, multicystic, multidensity/intensity, solid portion enhancing meningeal attachment
Central neurocytoma	20–40	Intraventricular	Multicystic, attached to septum pellucidum/lateral ventricle wall Prominent enhancement
Dysembryoplastic neuroepithelial tumor	< 30	Temporal lobe	Cystic with ½ of tumors enhancing Cortical Multinodular

From Krouwer[18] with permission.

Neuronal and neuronal–glial tumors

Central neurocytoma

This tumor was identified as a separate histopathological entity in 1982. Central neurocytomas arise from subependymal matrix cells close to a lateral ventricle and usually present as an intraventricular mass within the frontal horn of one or both lateral ventricles[4] (Fig. 7.2) or, rarely, the 4th ventricle[5] or elsewhere.[6] They represent less than 1% of intracranial tumors and have a peak incidence between 20 and 40 years of age. They affect both sexes equally. There are no known environmental risk factors for neurocytoma and, with the exception of one tumor associated with von Hippel–Lindau (VHL) disease, no familial incidence. The genetics of central neurocytomas are not established but chromosomal imbalances have been found on 2p, 10q, 18q.[7] Gain of chromosome 7 has been observed in a few patients but epidermal growth factor receptor located on chromosome 7, is not amplified.[8] p53 mutations have not been detected.[9]

Pathology

Central neurocytomas look like oligodendrogliomas, including the presence of gross calcification and occasionally hemorrhage. The tumors consist of round cells with round or oval nuclei and finely speckled chromatin. There is a promi-

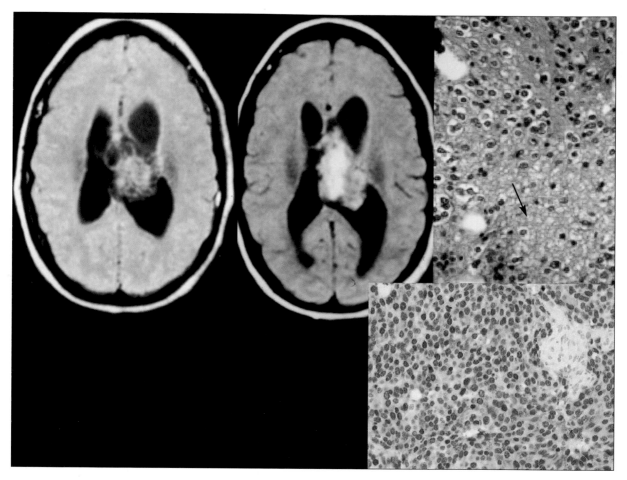

Figure 7.2

A central neurocytoma. An unenhanced (left) and enhanced (right) MRI showing the typical honeycombed appearance of a central neurocytoma obstructing the ventricular system and causing hydrocephalus. The upper photomicrograph shows the typical H&E histology of a central neurocytoma. The cellular elements are bland round cells with clear halos mimicking oligodendroglioma cells, neuropil and a hypocellular zone (arrow). The intense neuronal nuclear staining with the anti-Hu antibody (lower photomicrograph) indicates that this is a neuronal tumor, not an oligodendroglioma.

nent nucleus and scanty cytoplasm. The correct diagnosis is made by either immunohisto-chemistry or electron microscopy.[10] Synapto-physin stains reveal the tumor to be of neuronal origin, as do the more recently used markers, Neu-N[1] and anti-Hu.[2] GFAP is usually absent, but occasional tumor cells and reactive astrocytes may be GFAP and vimentin positive.[10] Neuro-

filaments are not seen, but vascular endothelial growth factor (VEGF) and the neurotrophin receptor protein, Trk[11] immunoreactivity may be present, as may photoreceptors.[12] Electron microscopy identifies features typical of neurons, including synapses in some instances.[10]

Mitoses and necrosis are uncommon. The MIB-1 labeling index ranges from 0.1 to 6.0, with little correlation between histologic atypia and the labeling index. Whether histologic atypia (i.e. cellular pleomorphism, endothelial proliferation and necrosis) or the labeling index predicts outcome is controversial.[13–15]

Clinical findings

Because the tumor arises in the ventricular system, it usually presents with hydrocephalus due to blockage of the foramen of Monro. Headache, nausea, vomiting, diplopia and visual field defects secondary to compression of the optic chiasm are common. Some patients develop pituitary insufficiency as a result of compression of the pituitary stalk. Other hormonal dysfunctions, including gigantism in children and inappropriate secretion of antidiuretic hormone, have been associated with neurocytomas involving the septum, 3rd ventricle and hypothalamus. The tumor does have the capacity to invade the parenchyma and cause focal neurologic deficits, including seizures and hemiparesis. Although benign in their behavior and histologic characteristics, central neurocytomas occasionally seed the leptomeninges.[16] Because of the generalized symptoms of hydrocephalus, the history is usually of short duration before the diagnosis is established.

The MRI of neurocytomas is characteristic. T1-weighted images demonstrate an intraventricular mass which is usually isointense or hyperintense compared to surrounding brain. Speckled areas of hypointensity represent calcifications that occur in 50–60% of tumors. These are better seen on CT scan. Microcystic regions may also appear as hypointense areas, giving the tumor a honeycombed appearance. The tumors sometimes hemorrhage, although usually not symptomatically, and evidence of blood may be found on

MR scan. T2-weighted images are usually hyperintense but may have areas of hypointensity representing hemosiderin. The tumors intensely contrast enhance, revealing a sharply demarcated mass within the ventricle. SPECT scan has been reported to demonstrate significant uptake of technetium-99-labeled hexamethylpropyleneamine oxine (HMPAO) and thallium-201 chloride.[17]

Because of their pathological appearance, central neurocytomas were once thought to be intraventricular oligodendrogliomas or ependymomas. Also included in the differential diagnosis are subependymomas, giant cell astrocytomas, choroid plexus papillomas, meningiomas and other clear cell lesions.

Treatment

The treatment of neurocytoma and other neuronal or mixed neuronal–glial tumors is outlined in Fig. 7.3. Surgery is the treatment of choice. The surgeon should aim for a complete resection, after which no further therapy is indicated. Even partial resections may be associated with prolonged survival. Accordingly, we recommend follow-up with careful monitoring for patients with both complete and partial resections who are otherwise asymptomatic. Follow-up should be especially scrupulous in patients whose tumor shows an elevated labeling index.[13] Recurrence can be treated by further surgery followed by RT or by RT without re-resection.[19] Radiosurgery has also been reported to be effective.[20] If the patient is symptomatic after surgery from residual tumor, external beam radiation therapy to a dose of 54 Gy is probably the best approach. Responses to chemotherapy have been reported, but chemotherapy should probably be reserved for recurrence after surgery and RT or leptomeningeal dissemination.[21]

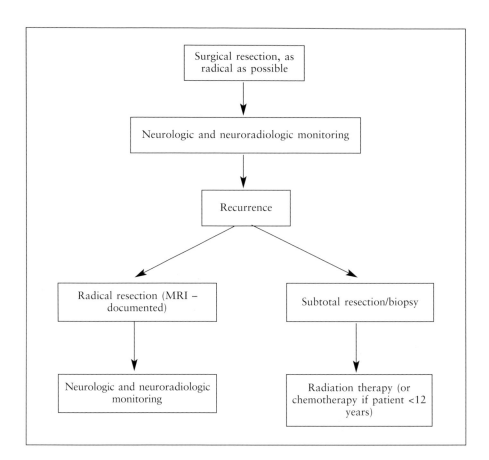

Figure 7.3
Algorithm for treatment of neuronal and mixed neuronal–glial tumors. Patients with a recurrent central neurocytoma should have an MR scan of the spine without and with contrast. (From Krouwer[18] with permission.)

Prognosis

The tumor is relatively benign, with a 5-year actuarial survival rate of 81% and a 5-year local control rate of 100% after gross total resection,[22] but recurrences and meningeal dissemination may occur.[23] The tumor may become more aggressive in pathologic appearance with each recurrence.

Dysembryoplastic neuroepithelial tumor (DNT)

This low-grade cortical-based tumor[24,25] was originally identified in patients undergoing epilepsy surgery for the treatment of long-standing partial, usually temporal lobe, seizures (Fig. 7.4). These tumors represent only a fraction of 1% of intracranial tumors. DNTs are of mixed glial and neuronal origin but, unlike most other neuroepithelial tumors, predominantly involve the temporal lobe cerebral cortex rather than the white matter. Occasionally, the tumors are found elsewhere, including the septum pellucidum[26] and posterior fossa. DNTs usually occur in infants and children but have been reported in young and occasionally elderly adults. Among patients undergoing epilepsy surgery in whom a tumor is encountered, DNTs are relatively common.[25]

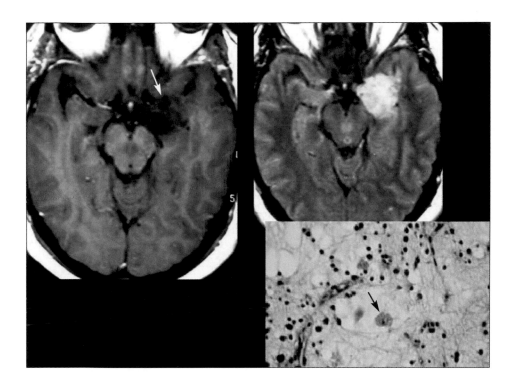

Figure 7.4
A DNT in a young adult with seizures. The panel on the left is a T1-weighted MRI demonstrating the typical cortical involvement and temporal lobe location of this lesion (arrow). Contrast enhancement may be present. The panel on the right is a T2-weighted image. The photomicrograph shows sparse collections of oligodendroglia-like cells and neurons (arrow) 'floating' in a myxoid matrix. The neural elements stain with neuronal markers such as anti-Hu.

Etiology

The only established risk factor for DNT is its occasional occurrence in patients with neuro-fibromatosis type-1. Genetic abnormalities have not been identified. Telomerase expression[27] and PTEN mutations[28] are not present. The apoptosis associated proteins, bcl and bax, are expressed in tumor cells, suggesting that they may play a role in pathogenesis.[29] Brain neurotrophic factor (BNDF) and its receptor (TrkB) are overexpressed in DNTs.[30] These agents promote neuronal survival and may increase neuronal excitability, perhaps playing a role in both tumorigenesis and in the seizures that so commonly characterize these tumors.

Pathology

Grossly, the tumor expands the cortex and appears as multiple firm nodules within the cortex. Three histologic types – simple, complex and non-specific – have been described. In the simple form, glioneuronal elements oriented perpendicular to the cortical surface are present, and columns are formed by bundles of axons lined by small oligodendrocyte-like cells. Between the neoplastic columns, neurons appear to float within an interstitial fluid.[31] The complex form, in addition to these changes, has a micronodular architecture consisting of neoplastic oligodendrocytes and astrocytes with foci of cortical dysplasia. The third form, said to be without specific morphologic features, cannot be distinguished on histologic criteria alone from astrocytomas or other gliomas.[25] Here the diagnosis is made based on clinical history, location and MR findings. It is not clear that the non-specific form is indeed a DNT. In one such patient, a mixed DNT and ganglioglioma was identified.[32] The MIB-1 labeling index is usually quite low, although figures up to 8% have been reported. The tumors react with the neuronal markers, anti-Hu and Neu-N, differentiating even the non-specific type from pure glioma. Hemorrhage is occasionally present histologically.[33]

Clinical findings

As indicated above, most patients present with long-standing, usually drug-resistant, partial seizures with or without secondary generalization.[34] The seizures usually begin in childhood, although they have been reported to begin in adulthood. Seizures are usually unassociated with other neurologic symptoms or signs, although, rarely, hemorrhage may cause acute neurologic dysfunction.[33]

On MR scan, the lesions are located cortically and usually subcortically as well.[35] About half the tumors are poorly demarcated, while the others are sharply demarcated. Tumors are cystic, with most having multiple cysts. There may be a mass effect but surrounding edema is usually absent. Calcification and occasionally hemorrhage may be present.[33] On T1 images, the lesion usually appears as a well-defined, sharply marginated, hypointense mass; on T2 it is hyperintense. About half the tumors contrast enhance, either in a nodular or ring-like pattern. In long-standing tumors of childhood, deformity of the skull overlying the mass may be identified on CT scan or even plain skull films. The deformity results from chronic pressure of the tumor molding the child's pliable skull. The tumors are metabolically inactive on PET scans, either with glucose or methionine,[36] differentiating them from other childhood low-grade tumors.

Treatment

The treatment is surgical.[35] A total resection is indicated if possible, but even partial resection may control seizures and tumor growth. No additional therapy is required. The tumor usually does not recur unless the initial resection is incomplete.[37] At 5 years about 60% of DNT patients are seizure-free[38] Rarely, patients develop psychotic symptoms with paranoid and depressive features,[39] postoperatively after resection of DNT or temporal lobe ganglioglioma.

Gangliogliomas and gangliocytomas

These low-grade tumors are composed either of neoplastic neurons (gangliocytoma) or a combination of neoplastic neurons and glial cells (ganglioglioma)[40] (Fig. 7.5). A rare variant, called ganglioglioneurocytoma, has also been described.[41] Although almost always low-grade, the glial component has the capacity to become anaplastic and behave aggressively, even disseminating throughout the leptomeninges. Together, the tumors are believed to represent about 1% of primary intracranial tumors, but up to 4% of pediatric tumors.[42] However, in one institution[43] the incidence of these tumors was 5% of intrinsic brain tumors. In selected populations of resistant focal epilepsy, the incidence may be even higher. The tumor occurs mostly in children and young adults,[44] but the age range is from 3 days to 80 years and there is an equal sex distribution. The tumors may be found anywhere in the central nervous system (CNS) but the majority are found superficially in the temporal lobe. In one series, 84% of tumors were in the temporal lobe, 10% in the frontal lobe and 4% in the brainstem.[43] Tumors located in the hemisphere are generally diagnosed at an older age than those located in midline structures such as the optic chiasm, hypothalamus, brainstem and spinal cord.

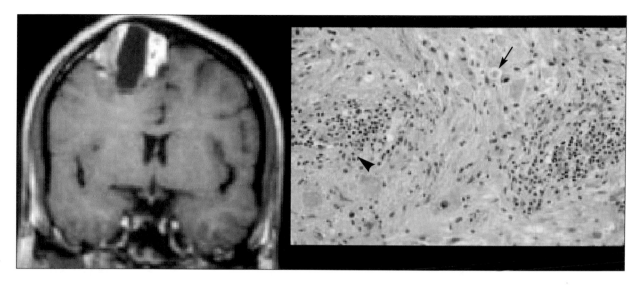

Figure 7.5
A ganglioglioma in a young woman with complex partial seizures. At the original resection this tumor was believed to be an anaplastic astrocytoma, and radiation therapy and chemotherapy were recommended. Careful histologic review (right) revealed a mixture of neoplastic ganglion cells (arrow) and glial cells embedded in a collagen-rich matrix with foci of lymphocytic infiltrates (arrowhead). The patient has been followed for several years without recurrence.

Etiology

There are no known environmental risk factors. Gangliocytomas and gangliogliomas are usually sporadic, but have been reported in association with NF-1.[45] Gangliogliomas are usually karyotypically (from Greek for 'nucleus', thus the chromosomal pattern) normal,[46] but abnormal karyotypes, including ring chromosome 1, trisomy of chromosomes 5, 6 and 7, and deletion of chromosome 6, have been reported. One report describes aberrant p53 protein expression in 20 of 21 specimens.[47] Deletions of portions of chromosome 17p, where p53 resides, have been observed in an anaplastic ganglioglioma with leptomeningeal spread.[48] No PTEN mutations were detected in 16 gangliogliomas.[49] As in DNTs (see above) BNDF and TrkB are overexpressed.[30] Immunoreactivity of the stem cell marker CD34 is present in most gangliogliomas.[50]

Pathology

Gangliocytomas are composed of large pleomorphic neurons within a network of collagen fibers. Perivascular lymphocytic infiltration is common, and a few mitotic figures are sometimes present. The lymphocytic infiltrates may be so prominent as to suggest the diagnosis of encephalitis. Eosinophilic granular bodies, which are liposomes filled with cellular debris, are a characteristic feature. Their presence suggests the diagnosis of a low-grade ganglion cell tumor, even when other elements look aggressive and suggest a diagnosis such as fibrosarcoma. In gangliogliomas, the neural elements may be abundant or sparse. The glial elements may contain eosinophilic granular or hyaline bodies, and the tumor often contains microcysts, calcification and an occasional desmoplastic focus. The glial component is often GFAP positive. The neuronal component is anti-

Hu positive. No cells with intermediate histologic features were identified in one series,[47] but we have seen cells that are both GFAP and anti-Hu reactive.[2] Electron microscopy identifies dense core granules and sometimes synaptic junctions, indicating the neuronal component. Labeling indices are usually low, with MIB-1 varying from 1% to 3%. Malignant ganglion cells are rare. Extreme care should be taken in evaluating these tumors neuropathologically. Inexperienced neuropathologists may interpret the mildly pleomorphic cells as representing an anaplastic astrocytoma rather than a ganglioglioma. Careful review, considering the clinical symptomatology, the pre- and postoperative MR scans, and the immunohistochemistry, will usually reveal the correct diagnosis.[47]

Clinical findings

The symptoms and signs depend on the tumor's location. The vast majority of patients present with seizures, either focal or generalized (Table 7.3).

In various series, seizures occurred in 45–100% of patients. Because of the tumor's usual location in the temporal lobe, partial–complex seizures are the most common

seizure type. In the days before MR scanning, the seizures were often present for many years, in one case up to 45 years prior to diagnosis. Electroencephalograms are often performed to evaluate the seizure disorder; most are abnormal but may misidentify tumor location.[51] Those tumors that present in the midline often present with hydrocephalus and signs of increased intracranial pressure, including headache, nausea and vomiting. Brainstem tumors present with cranial nerve dysfunction and ataxia. When the lesion is in the midline, symptoms are only present for a short time before diagnosis is made.

On MR scan, most tumors are hypointense on the T1-weighted image and hyperintense on the T2-weighted image. About half of the tumors have a cystic component. The tumors usually contrast enhance but not all do. The most characteristic finding is a cystic tumor without much mass effect or surrounding edema, with an area of contrast enhancement near the margin of the cyst. Calcification may be present either on scan or microscopically. Hemorrhage and necrosis are rare. Interestingly, both thallium SPECT and PET scans (high uptake) and MRS (high choline peak relative to creatine and N-acetyl aspartate) may suggest high-grade tumor despite a very low labeling index.[52]

Treatment

The treatment is surgical. A total resection can be achieved in most cases and is usually curative.[40] Even if total resection is not possible, intractable seizures may improve, especially if the epileptogenic focus is identified by corticography and resected. The best outcome with respect to seizure control is associated with younger age, shorter duration of epilepsy, absence of generalized seizures and no epileptiform discharge on postoperative EEG.[51] Often, particularly when the tumor is

Table 7.3
Signs and symptoms in 51 patients with gangliogliomas.

Signs/symptoms	Patients	
	No.	%
Epilepsy	47	92
Cranial nerve deficit	1	2
Hemiparesis	1	2
Quadriparesis	2	4
Increased intracranial pressure	2	4

From Zentner et al,[43] with permission.

located in a midline structure, substantial resection is not possible. If the patient is asymptomatic apart from seizures, careful follow-up without further treatment is recommended even after partial resection. If the tumor recurs after complete or partial resection, a second operation should be considered, followed by conformal RT to 54 Gy.

Gangliogliomas with an anaplastic-appearing glial element should be treated in the same way, without adjuvant RT. Survival of 34 years has been reported with one such tumor.[53] Some authors recommend a more aggressive approach to these tumors when they occur in midline structures such as hypothalamus or brainstem, when the glial component has an anaplastic component.[54] Patients have a higher recurrence rate and a shorter median survival; thus, some investigators recommend adjuvant RT in this 'high-risk' group. However, a recent report suggests that RT of low-grade gangliogliomas may promote malignant degeneration.[55] The concept is interesting but the issue is unsettled. Recurrence of anaplastic gangliogliomas may also be associated with histologic degeneration to a glioblastoma multiforme. This is another reason to consider re-resection at recurrence; subsequent postoperative treatment is determined by histology.

The role of chemotherapy in anaplastic or recurrent low-grade tumor is unknown. One might also consider it in rapidly progressive recurrent tumors in very young children to avoid RT, or in older patients in whom RT has failed. Nitrosoureas, retinoic acid[56] and cisplatinum have all been reported to have some effect. Occasionally, gangliogliomas seed the leptomeninges, in which case chemotherapy should be considered.

Prognosis

The prognosis of low-grade gangliocytomas and gangliogliomas is excellent. Sixty to 80% of patients become seizure-free after surgery.[38,51] Four-year progression-free survival rates after gross total resection of low- and high-grade tumors were 78% and 75%, respectively. After subtotal resection, the figures were 63% and 25%.[40]

Embryonal tumors

Introduction

The WHO lists several tumors as being of embryonal origin. Table 7.4 represents a slight modification. Many of these tumors, including medulloblastoma, neuroblastoma and primitive neuroectodermal tumors, probably originate from neurons or neuronal precursors and thus are considered in this chapter. Ependymoblastomas are rare primitive neuroectodermal tumors of young children that are considered to be embryonal tumors by the WHO. They differ from anaplastic ependymomas (Chapter 5). Because they are so rare and so little is known about them, they are not discussed further. The classification of medulloblastomas is controversial. Because the tumors appear histologically identical to both peripheral and central nervous system

Table 7.4
Embryonal tumors.

Medulloepithelioma
Ependymoblastoma
Medulloblastoma
    Variants: desmoplastic medulloblastoma
    Medullomyoblastoma
    Melanotic medulloblastoma
Supratentorial primitive neuroectodermal
    tumors (PNET)
        Neuroblastoma
        Ganglioneuroblastoma
Atypical teratoid/rhabdoid tumor

tumors called primitive neuroectodermal tumors, as well as pineal region tumors, and central and peripheral neuroblastomas, some pathologists consider all of these tumors together as primitive neuroectodermal tumors. The WHO has chosen not to do so. One reason for keeping these tumors separate is that the prognosis for medulloblastoma is relatively good, whereas similar appearing tumors occurring elsewhere in the brain usually have a dismal prognosis (see below). Another reason is that medulloblastomas differ genetically from other primitive neuroectodermal tumors (see below).

Taken together, embryonal tumors constitute an important fraction of pediatric brain tumors. Most appear similar, with a background of undifferentiated round cells showing a variety of divergent patterns of differentiation, including glial and neuronal. Genetic markers may eventually reveal their origin and lead to reclassification.

Medulloblastoma

The medulloblastoma is a malignant childhood tumor located in the vermis of the cerebellum but with a tendency to seed the leptomeninges and cause widespread metastases within the CNS and occasionally extraneural metastases, especially to bone.[57] Medulloblastoma is the most common intracranial tumor of children, accounting for about 25% of childhood brain tumors.[58] The incidence of medulloblastoma is 0.5–0.6/100 000 children[59] per year, peaking at the age of 7. Seventy percent of medulloblastomas occur before age 16. In one epidemiologic series, 34% of medulloblastomas occurred in patients over age 15, but the highest incidence in adults 15–19 years old was only 0.23/100 000/year.[60] Males outnumber females by about 2:1. These childhood tumors almost always arise in the cerebellar vermis (often inferior vermis) and may compress or invade

the 4th ventricle, causing hydrocephalus. In adults, the tumor can arise in the cerebellar hemisphere (Fig. 7.6), resulting in a somewhat different clinical picture than in children.

Etiology

The disorder is usually sporadic but a number of cases of medulloblastoma in monozygotic and dizygotic twins and siblings have been reported.[61] Medulloblastomas have also been reported in several familial cancer syndromes, including Li–Fraumeni syndrome, the nevoid basal cell carcinoma syndrome, and Turcot's syndrome (Chapter 12). Some patients with extraneural malignancies, including Wilm's tumor and malignant renal rhabdoid tumors, have also been observed to develop medulloblastomas. Conversely, some studies suggest that relatives of patients with medulloblastoma are at increased risk of developing childhood leukemia or lymphoma. No environmental risks have been identified. One study suggested that exposure to SV40, which contaminated the polio vaccine in the 1950s, might be a risk factor, but a more recent study refutes that finding.[62]

A number of chromosomal abnormalities have been identified;[63] the most common is isochromosome 17q.[64] (An isochromosome is a chromosome that has split transversely and fused so that one arm, in this case the long arm of chromosome 17, is doubled.) This abnormality can be found in as many as 60% of medulloblastomas, but not in most other pediatric tumors.[65,66] Abnormalities in several other chromosomes have also been reported.[67] Loss of 9q and loss of 22 occur in a minority of tumors,[64] and PTEN mutations are rare in this disorder. A recent study implicates the DMBT1 tumor suppressor gene in almost 50% of medulloblastomas.[67] Mutations of the PTCH gene, the causal mutation in medulloblastomas associated with the nevoid basal cell carcinoma syndrome (Chapter 12), are found in only about 10% of sporadic medulloblastomas.[68]

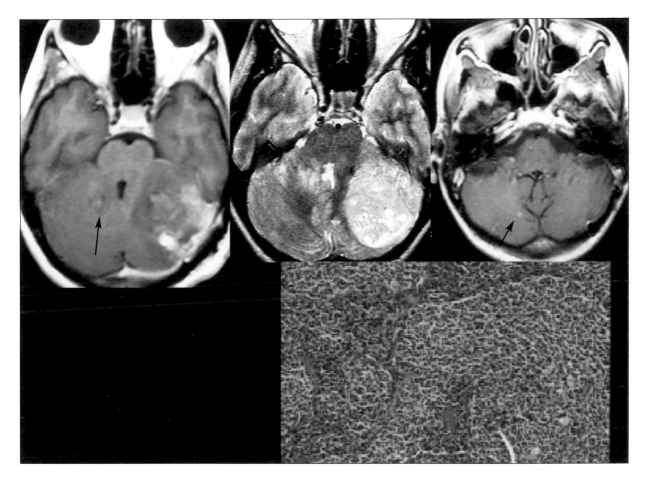

Figure 7.6
A medulloblastoma. This young woman presented with headache and ataxia and was found to have two lesions, one in the left and one in the right cerebellar hemisphere. The larger lesion enhanced with contrast (left panel). The smaller lesion enhanced poorly (arrow). Both are apparent on the T2-weighted image. She was treated with the protocol outlined in Figure 7.2. Three years later, a small enhancing lesion appeared in the right cerebellum away from the original tumor (right panel, arrow). Although initially a recurrence was feared, follow-up has shown no change in the lesion over 2 years, suggesting that it represents a vascular anomaly caused by the radiation. The photomicrograph shows dense collections of undifferentiated neuroepithelial cells forming nodules. Almost 90% of the tumors show neuronal differentiation as indicated by anti-Hu staining. Some others show glial differentiation. These differentiations have no prognostic significance.

Pathology

Medulloblastomas vary in their gross appearance. Some, particularly in adults, are hemorrhagic and necrotic; others appear discrete and relatively firm. The histologic variants of medulloblastoma include classic desmoplastic tumor (desmoplastic tumors are infiltrated by hyperplastic fibroblasts and collagen; the term is from the Greek '*desmo*' meaning 'band' and '*plastikos*' related to 'molding'), medullomyoblastoma, melanotic medulloblastoma and cerebellar neuroblastoma. These variants may lead to some histologic confusion but they have little bearing on the clinical signs, treatment or prognosis.

The typical medulloblastoma is composed of densely packed cells with round, oval or carrot-shaped hyperchromatic nuclei surrounded by scanty cytoplasm (Fig. 7.6). Homer Wright rosettes are found in about 40% of patients; mitoses are frequent and areas of necrosis with pseudopalisading can sometimes be found. The desmoplastic variety is more common in adults than in children. The term 'cerebellar neuro-blastoma' is used to describe the desmoplastic variety with extreme lobularity. In large cell medulloblastoma, the tumor is composed of cells with large round nuclei and prominent nucleoli; it contains large areas of necrosis and resembles atypical rhabdoid teratoid tumors of the cerebellar region.

Medulloblastomas can show differentiation along several lines, including neural, glial and ependymal. The labeling indices are usually high, MIB-1 often being higher than 20%. The anti-Hu antibody is positive in almost 90% of cases,[2] indicating that some degree of neuronal differentiation is found in most medulloblastomas, prompting us to classify them under neuronal or mixed neuronal glial tumors.

Clinical findings

Symptoms and signs. In children, headache and vomiting are the most common presenting symptoms. The headache may be frontal or occipital, and unilateral or bilateral. When unilateral and occipital, it defines the site of the lesion. When unilateral but not occipital, it defines the side of the lesion. Early in the evolution of the tumor, headache is often present in the morning upon waking, only to disappear for the rest of the day. Disappearance of the headache may be associated with vomiting, particularly in children.

Because the patient is too ill to go to school, but seems fine later in the day, a diagnosis of 'school phobia' may delay the appropriate evaluation. When the tumor pushes the cerebellar tonsils through the foramen magnum (tonsillar herniation), patients may complain of neck pain. Nausea may or may not precede the vomiting. Some patients receive extensive gastrointestinal evaluation before a correct diagnosis is made. However, the delay in diagnosis does not seem to affect the prognosis.[69] In infants, medulloblastoma may present simply as failure to thrive associated with vomiting and irritability.

Gait ataxia is usually the first sign. Because the posterior vermis controls balance, children either complain of trouble walking or seem to be unsteady on their feet, staggering as if drunk when they walk. Early in the evolution of symptoms, point-to-point testing in the extremities, including the finger-to-nose and the heel-to-knee-to-shin tests, may be normal and lead the physician to believe that there is no cerebellar dysfunction and that the reeling gait has a psychogenic basis. Additional signs include diplopia from unilateral or bilateral abducens paralysis, transient loss of vision (visual obscurations) related to papilledema and head tilt. 'Cerebellar fits', episodic extensor spasms of trunk and extremities, also called decerebrate rigidity, are an ominous sign, suggesting tonsillar herniation.

Because leptomeningeal dissemination may occur early in the course of the disease, patients may present with more widespread symptoms, including seizures in 5–10% of children. Cranial nerve palsies, with the exception of the abducens nerve, back pain, absent deep tendon reflexes in the legs, and radicular sensory or motor changes suggest leptomeningeal dissemination, the symptoms resulting from direct infiltration of cranial nerves or spinal roots.

Hydrocephalus from compression or invasion by tumor of the 4th ventricle is usually present at diagnosis. Hydrocephalus may evolve quite rapidly, in some patients requiring emergency decompression of the ventricular system before definitive therapy. In some patients the ataxia is relieved by treating hydrocephalus with a shunt, suggesting that frontal lobe dysfunction may play a role in the gait disorder. Rarely, medulloblastoma may invade the leptomeninges without causing a mass lesion. We have encountered a few patients with hydrocephalus associated with cerebrospinal fluid (CSF) pleocytosis but without abnormalities on MR scan. Because the cells in the spinal fluid were interpreted cytologically as lymphocytes and the patients had hydrocephalus, they were shunted. In one instance, the diagnosis was not made until the patient, whose symptoms had been relieved by a ventriculoperitoneal (VP) shunt, developed a pelvic mass that on biopsy proved to be a metastatic medulloblastoma that had spread via the shunt.

Imaging

The diagnosis is strongly suspected on neuroimaging. In children, the tumor is usually in the vermis of the cerebellum and appears hyperdense on CT scan, hypointense on T1 and hyperintense on T2-weighted MR sequences. The tumor enhances intensely and homogeneously, with no evidence of cyst formation or necrosis;[70] rarely, the tumor is non-enhancing. Hydrocephalus is quite common.

In adults, the tumor is usually in the cerebellar hemisphere rather than the vermis, and hydrocephalus occurs in less than half of the patients.[71] The CT scan shows a hyperdense tumor, often with low-density areas suggesting cysts or necrosis. The same cysts or necrosis can be seen on MR scan, where the tumor is hypointense on T1 and hyperintense on T2. Enhancement is variable but usually less than that seen in children.

All patients in whom a diagnosis of medulloblastoma is suspected on imaging should be evaluated for metastatic disease. This can be done by gadolinium-enhanced MR scan of the entire CNS.[72] Areas of contrast enhancement, either nodular or linear in the cerebral hemispheres or spinal cord, suggest metastatic disease. In the absence of symptoms, systemic staging with a bone scan or bone marrow biopsy is probably unnecessary.[73]

The CSF should be examined for malignant cells, but because of the dangers of herniation from a posterior fossa mass, this procedure is not indicated until the patient's tumor has been resected surgically. Preoperative imaging of the spine is important for the surgeon, because radical resection of the focal tumor, with its attendant risk, does not confer survival advantage in a patient who already has disseminated CNS disease. CSF examination should probably be carried out 2–3 weeks after resection, allowing time for a few cells that may have floated into the CSF at surgery to either seed, giving a positive cytology, or disappear, indicating that the neuraxis is free of metastasis. Sampling of ventricular fluid via a shunt is inadequate. Ventricular CSF may not contain malignant cells even when they are abundant in the lumbar CSF.[74] Both imaging and CSF examination are required; some leptomeningeal metastases will be missed with either alone.[75]

Treatment

Treatment is determined in part by preoperative staging (Table 7.5) and in part by the completeness of surgical resection of the tumor.[76,77] If the patient presents with marked hydrocephalus and plateau waves suggesting imminent herniation, a ventriculostomy or ventriculoperitoneal (VP) shunt should be placed prior to definitive surgery. If the patient has leptomeningeal disease, shunting for hydrocephalus may lead to systemic dissemination of the tumor. A number of devices have been designed to reduce the incidence of ventricular shunt metastases; how well these work is unclear.[57]

In all patients, a maximally feasible resection of the tumor should be carried out. If the tumor presents as a single focus without MR evidence of dissemination, a radical resection is indicated. If there is evidence of widespread dissemination, a debulking operation attempting to decrease tumor volume to < 1.5 cm, without attempt at radical resection, is the preferred choice.

After the surgical procedure, the patient is defined as being either average or high risk. An average-risk patient is a patient: (1) who is > 3 and ≤21 years old at diagnosis; (2) whose postoperative MR scan is either free of tumor or has residual tumor < 1.5 cm in largest dimension (the MR should be a contrast-enhanced image performed within 72 h of surgery); (3) with no evidence of metastatic disease in the neuraxis, as defined by absence of masses on total neuraxial MR scan and negative cytologic examination of lumbar CSF performed 2–3 weeks after surgery. Patients with brainstem involvement are still considered to be at average risk. High risk includes patients with residual tumor > 1.5 cm or staged as M1–M4 (Table 7.5). Most investigators believe that staging after surgery, as indicated above, is more important than staging before surgery for determining further therapy and for predicting prognosis.

Figure 7.7 outlines a standard treatment scheme.[79] All patients require whole-neuraxial radiation.[80] The procedure should be performed by a skilled and experienced radiation oncologist; the quality of the radiation targeting correlates with outcome.[81] A standard dose is 36 Gy to the entire nervous system, with a boost to the tumor site of approximately 18 Gy (total to tumor – 54 Gy). Some physicians do not reduce the craniospinal axis dose of RT for average-risk patients (Fig. 7.7), but

Table 7.5
Staging of medulloblastoma.[78]

T_1	Tumor < 3 cm in diameter
T_2	Tumor ≥ 3 cm in diameter
T_{3a}	Tumor > 3 cm in diameter with extension into the aqueduct of Sylvius and/or into foramen of Luschka
T_{3b}	Tumor > 3 cm in diameter with unequivocal extension into the brainstem. T_{3b} can be defined by intraoperative demonstration of tumor extension into the brainstem in the absence of radiographic evidence.
$T_4{}^a$	Tumor > 3 cm in diameter with extension up past the aqueduct of Sylvius and/or down past the foramen magnum. No consideration is given to the number of structures invaded or the presence of hydrocephalus.
M_0	No evidence of subarachnoid cells found in CSF
$M_1{}^a$	Microscopic tumor cells found in CSF
$M_2{}^a$	Gross nodular seeding in the cerebellar, cerebral subarachnoid space, or the 3rd or lateral ventricles
$M_3{}^a$	Gross nodular seeding in spinal subarachnoid space
$M_4{}^a$	Metastasis outside the cerebrospinal axis. Residual tumor > 1.5 cm postoperatively*

*High risk.

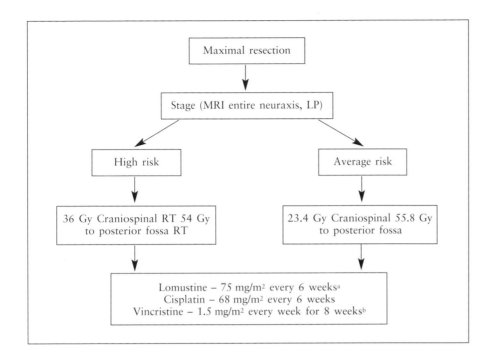

Figure 7.7
Treatment of patients with medulloblastoma.[a] Cisplatin begins 6 weeks post-RT.[b] Vincristine begins during RT[b], maximum dose 2 mg/m[2].

most do when RT is combined with chemotherapy, as there appears to be no difference in progression-free survival at 5–6 years and cognitive deficits are less pronounced.[82,83] One study suggests 55.8 Gy to the tumor and 23.4 Gy to the remainder of the nervous system in children with localized tumors.[83] Hyperfractionationed radiation does not appear to lengthen survival, at least in good-risk patients.[84] Patients at high risk (see Table 7.5) should be treated with adjuvant chemotherapy. Several chemotherapeutic protocols have been suggested,[73] but none has proved superior to the protocol outlined in Fig. 7.7. This chemotherapy regimen is usually well tolerated by children, but the cumulative amount of vincristine (VCR) is not tolerated by most adults. Consequently, we usually administer the VCR only once every other week during RT to adults, and even that dose may have to be modified because of peripheral nerve toxicity. A controlled trial comparing carmustine with cyclophosphamide is underway. To date, the addition of adjuvant chemotherapy for average-risk patients has not improved survival. However, many pediatric neuro-oncologists are treating all patients with adjuvant therapy, given the sensitivity of medulloblastomas to these agents, the 40% incidence of relapse over 5 years with RT alone, and the opportunity to reduce the dose of neuraxis RT.

In infants, some investigators have suggested that RT be deferred if chemotherapy can control the growth of the tumor after surgery. Several such protocols exist. Busulphan is effective for treating medulloblastoma and/or primitive neuroectodermal tumor implanted into athymic mice,[85] but its utility in patients has not been tested.

Surveillance MRI scans after therapy detect asymptomatic recurrences, and may make subsequent therapy easier, but whether they increase survival is controversial.[86] We have encountered patients whose surveillance scans revealed contrast enhancement not caused by tumor.[87]

Treatment complications

The successful treatment of medulloblastoma comes at a price.[88] (See Fig. 7.8.) Several significant complications of treatment, both acute and delayed, are relatively common. Among the acute complications are postoperative aseptic meningitis (hemogenic meningitis) and the cerebellar mutism syndrome. Hemogenic meningitis follows some posterior fossa operations, when blood is spilled into the cisterna magna.[89,90] Elements in the blood (probably red cell membranes) irritate the leptomeninges and initiate an inflammatory response. The patient

develops fever, headache and sometimes hydrocephalus. The CSF shows a pleocytosis with an elevated protein. Cultures are negative. An increased dose of corticosteroids usually suppresses the inflammation and patients then recover spontaneously. Antibiotics are not required. Bacterial meningitis is an extremely rare complication of 'clean' (i.e. surgery through an uncontaminated field) posterior fossa surgery. A CSF lactate level, which is high in bacterial but not elevated hemogenic meningitis, may assist in the diagnosis.[91] On rare occasions, particularly in patients on high doses of steroids, the symptoms of hemogenic meningitis do not develop until the patient has been discharged and the steroids tapered to low doses. We have seen a few patients in whom

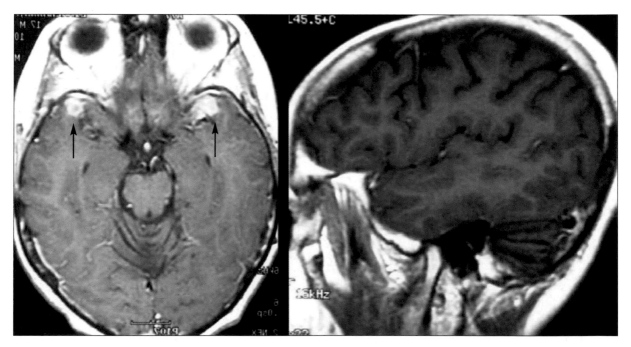

Figure 7.8
Failure of radiation therapy in a patient with a medulloblastoma. The patient's cerebellum was successfully treated, but a routine surveillance scan 18 months after treatment showed contrast-enhancing masses at the inferior tips of the temporal lobes (arrows). On biopsy, this proved to be metastatic medulloblastoma. Evidently, the radiation portals had been poorly drawn and did not include the inferior temporal lobes.

the symptoms of hemogenic meningitis persisted for many weeks, requiring a very gradual tapering of the steroids. The same syndrome sometimes follows spinal surgery and supratentorial surgery when the lateral ventricle has been entered. Rarely, chronic subclinical bleeding after surgery for cerebellar tumors may lead to siderosis of the meninges, with hearing loss, ataxia and cognitive dysfunction appearing years after surgery. The diagnosis is established by the hypointense coating of the brainstem and cerebellum on the MRI.[92]

The cerebellar mutism syndrome is virtually always restricted to children who undergo cerebellar surgery.[93] In the postoperative period, after a latent period of a few days, during which time the child speaks normally, the child becomes mute, often refuses to swallow and may have other behavioral abnormalities resembling autism (e.g. irritability and lack of social interaction). Visual impairment, probably cortical blindness, may also be present. Most patients recover speech spontaneously after days to weeks. The pathogenesis of this syndrome is unknown, and postoperative MR scans fail to demonstrate brainstem or hemispheric abnormalities. However, the cerebellum contributes to cognitive functions, and, therefore, intellectual, language and behavorial disturbances affect many children after posterior fossa surgery.[94,95]

Delayed manifestations of treatment toxicity after medulloblastoma include growth failure, endocrine disturbances, cognitive dysfunction, vasculopathy and secondary tumors. Growth failure results in part from radiation to the spinal column, which inhibits vertebral growth, and in part from radiation to the hypothalamus and pituitary gland, which causes growth hormone deficiency.[96] As a result, most children treated for medulloblastoma remain small. Growth hormone will restore long bone growth, but spinal growth remains impaired.

Thyroid dysfunction, resulting from radiation to the thyroid gland within the spinal cord radiation portal, can occur at any time, even many years after radiation has been completed. Accordingly, patients should be followed with thyroid stimulating hormone (TSH) and T4 levels for the rest of their lives. In some children, T4 remains normal and patients are clinically euthyroid but TSH is high. Some have suggested that such patients should be treated with thyroid hormone to diminish the possibility that high TSH levels may drive their irradiated thyroid to become neoplastic.

Many but not all children treated for medulloblastoma demonstrate a decreased IQ.[82] Cognitive dysfunction is probably related to both the posterior fossa RT[97,98] and the total dose to the brain.[82,83] Some have difficulty at school. Several risk factors increase the likelihood of such patients developing cognitive dysfunction:

1. The presence of hydrocephalus in either the pre- or postoperative period. Accordingly, patients should be followed and hydrocephalus corrected as soon as detected.
2. Postoperative infectious meningitis, probably because it increases intracranial pressure and the likelihood of developing hydrocephalus. It is not known if hemogenic meningitis is a risk factor.
3. RT. One study found a full-scale IQ drop of 14 points 2 years after treatment for medulloblastoma. Patients with posterior fossa tumors who were not irradiated (e.g. cerebellar astrocytoma) had no significant decline in IQ, but most did not suffer from hydrocephalus in the preoperative period, as do children with medulloblastoma. Both the dose of radiation and the age of the patient (young age) are risk factors for chronic radiation encephalopathy.

4. The posterior fossa surgery itself. As indicated above, some patients who undergo operations on the cerebellum for tumors develop mutism, pseudobulbar symptoms and behavioral changes after surgery. Although the mutism and swallowing difficulty always improve, behavioral symptoms may persist and interfere with cognitive function later in life.[99]

Late post-irradiation occlusive vasculopathy is a rare complication of childhood medulloblastoma.[100] Vessels in the posterior fossa become stenotic and may occlude, leading to occipital lobe and posterior fossa infarction. Hyperfractionated radiotherapy is associated with MR evidence of necrosis, telangiectasia and white matter changes.[101] Finally, RT to the CNS may lead to secondary tumors. Children treated for brain tumors have a nine-fold higher risk for developing a second cancer. In one series of 187 children treated for medulloblastoma, the actuarial incidence of death due to a second malignant tumor was 13% at 30 years. The tumors may occur either in the radiation field, e.g. sarcoma of the occipital bone, be part of a familial tumor syndrome such as neurofibromatosis, occur as a result of alkylating chemotherapeutic agents, e.g. leukemia, or occur from radiation of the neck, e.g. thyroid cancer, as indicated above. Children cured of medulloblastoma must be followed life-long for these potential complications.

Prognosis
Medulloblastoma is one of the intracranial tumors in which there has been a substantial improvement in survival as a direct result of therapy. The 5-year survival rate in the 1960s was about 30%, and was as low as 8% in one series.[102] It is now closer to about 70% using modern protocols combining surgery and radiation along with chemotherapy for high-risk patients. For average-risk patients, progression-free survival in one series was 86% at 3 years and 79% at 7 years. Sex is an important predictor for survival, with girls having a much better outcome than boys.[103] Very young children have a worse prognosis, perhaps due to the lower radiation doses often given.[104] Interestingly, the duration of symptoms is inversely related to disease stage and, thus, survival.[105] Among adults late relapse is common and systemic failure occurs even in low-risk patients: both problems require prolonged and careful surveillance.[106]

Children should be followed with a uniform surveillance program which includes repeat lumbar punctures and MR scans. In 25–30% of patients, surveillance scans will reveal asymptomatic relapse, but current evidence suggests that these patients do not benefit from salvage therapy more than those with symptomatic relapses.[86] The outlook following recurrence of medulloblastoma is poor. Salvage chemotherapy produces some response in about half of the patients, and a complete response in about a fourth. In one series, the median survival was only several months and only a few patients lived longer than 2 years. High-dose chemotherapy with autologous stem cell rescue for relapse yields a 30% progression-free survival at a median of 54 months.[107] Early detection of relapse and aggressive treatment seem to be warranted to prevent the development of neurologic symptoms.

How long it is necessary to follow patients who are free from recurrence is unclear. Collins' law states that for embryonal tumors of childhood the risk of recurrence ends when the child is free of disease for years equal to his age when the tumor appeared plus 9 months. The law, with some exceptions, seems to apply to childhood medulloblastomas[108] and other brain tumors of young children, although rare late relapses have been observed.[109]

Other tumors of 'embryonal' origin

Not all cerebellar lesions are medulloblastomas, or even tumors (Fig. 7.9). Other tumors in this category, including CNS neuroblastoma and ganglioneuroblastoma, primitive neuroectodermal tumors (PNET) and rhabdoid tumors, are all quite rare. Collectively, these tumors represent less than 1% of childhood brain tumors and usually occur before 2 years of age. The tumors are similar in neuroimaging and histologic appearance to cerebellar medulloblastomas. The treatment is the same but the prognosis is much worse. Children with non-pineal supratentorial PNETs have an overall 5-year survival rate of 34%.

Atypical teratoid/rhabdoid tumors are uncommon tumors of childhood found in the cerebral hemispheres, cerebellum or cerebellopontine angle.[110] They all contain rhabdoid cells (a cell with an apparent autoplasmic inclusion consisting of bundles of intermediate filaments) and represent about 2% of childhood neuroepithelial tumors. They usually occur in young children; the median age is 20 months but a few adults have been reported. They differ from other embryonal tumors in

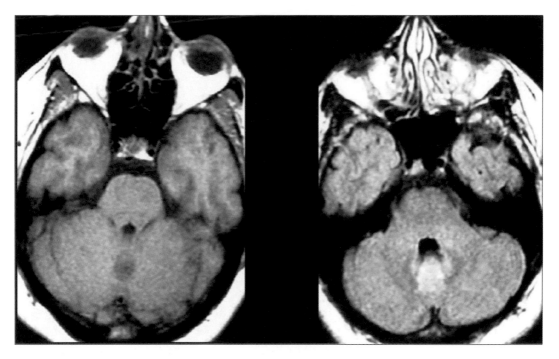

Figure 7.9
Pitfalls in the diagnosis of neuronal tumors. This young woman presented to medical attention with a two week history of ataxia and mild vertigo. Her examination was normal save for a slightly unsteady gait and a vertiginous sensation when she moved suddenly. An MR scan showed a non-contrast enhancing mass in the vermis of the cerebellum. The mass was hypointense on the T1 (left) and hypointense on the T2 (right) image. Medulloblastoma was considered but because she was so mildly symptomatic it was decided to follow her. Two months later the lesion completely disappeared. Its nature remains a mystery.

their histopathology. Some consist only of rhabdoid cells, while others consist of a combination of rhabdoid and PNET-appearing cells. The tumor may be vimentin, GFAP, epithelial membrane agonist (EMA) and smooth muscle actin positive. They are sometimes mistaken for medulloblastoma when they occur in the posterior fossa. Unlike other embryonal tumors, most show abnormalities of chromosome 22, either monosomy or deletion of 22q.[111] The tumors are highly malignant, and with treatment similar to that of medulloblastoma, median survival is about 6 months. About 30% show leptomeningeal spread at diagnosis. High-dose chemotherapy with autologous bone marrow or stem cell support, and RT have yielded improved survival in some children;[112,113] however, vigorous treatment,

particularly RT, is likely to produce significant neurologic sequelae in these young survivors.

Neuroblastoma, a childhood tumor of the adrenal gland and sympathetic nervous system, is the third most common childhood tumor after leukemia and brain tumors. This tumor may occasionally arise within the intracranial cavity, usually deep in the cerebral hemisphere. The tumors have a histologic appearance identical to their peripheral counterparts, with Homer Wright rosettes and expression of neurofilament protein and synaptophysin. The tumor must be differentiated from metastatic neuroblastoma, which usually spreads to the dura rather than the parenchyma of the brain, and must be differentiated histologically from other PNETs and

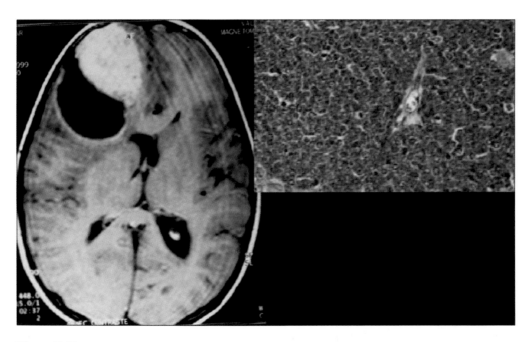

Figure 7.10
The MRI of a young child presenting with headache. A dural-based tumor with a large cyst was identified on the MR scan. At surgery, the tumor appeared to be a primitive neuroectodermal tumor with sheets of uniform round cells with small amounts of cytoplasm. Genetic evaluation revealed it to be a Ewing's sarcoma. Extraskeletal Ewing's sarcomas are uncommon. Those arising in the meninges are extremely rare.

medulloblastoma, which the neuroblastoma resembles histologically.

Primitive neuroectodermal tumor (Fig. 7.10) is a term that some apply to a number of histologically identical tumors that in the brain include cerebral neuroblastoma, medulloblastoma and pinealoblastoma (see Chapter 8). PNETs above the tentorium cerebelli are different from medulloblastoma of the cerebellum both in their genetic composition and in their clinical course. Isochromosome 17q observed in medulloblastoma is not found in supratentorial PNETs. Loss of chromosome 14q, detected in about 40% of supratentorial PNETs, is not detected in medulloblastoma.[114] Loss of chromosome 3p is common in supratentorial PNETs but not in medulloblastoma.[64] The clinical symptoms obviously differ, because PNETs arise in the cerebral hemisphere, whereas medulloblastomas arise in the cerebellum. PNETs disseminate throughout the neuraxis, and whole-neuraxial radiation is recommended for all. However, the 5-year recurrence-free survival is much lower in patients with supratentorial PNETs[115,116] than in those with medulloblastoma.

References

1. Wolf HK, Buslei R, Schmidt-Kastner R et al. NeuN: a useful neuronal marker for diagnostic histopathology. J Histochem Cytochem 1996; 44: 1167–71.
2. Gultekin SH, Dalmau J, Graus Y, Posner JB, Rosenblum MK. Anti-Hu immunolabeling as an index of neuronal differentiation in human brain tumors – a study of 112 central neuroepithelial neoplasms. Am J Surg Pathol 1998; 22: 195–200.
3. Kleihues P, Cavenee WK. World Health Organization Classification of Tumours: Tumours of the nervous system – pathology and genetics. Lyon: IRAC Press, 2000.
4. Maiuri F, Spaziante R, De Caro ML et al. Central neurocytoma: clinico-pathological study of 5 cases and review of the literature. Clin Neurol Neurosurg 1995; 97: 219–28.
5. Warmuth-Metz M, Klein R, Sörensen N, Solymosi L. Central neurocytoma of the fourth ventricle – case report. J Neurosurg 1999; 91: 506–9.
6. Ashkan K, Casey ATH, D'Arrigo C, Harkness WF, Thomas DGT. Benign central neurocytoma – a double misnomer? Cancer 2000; 89: 1111–20.
7. Yin XL, Pang JCS, Hui ABY, Ng H. Detection of chromosomal imbalances in central neurocytomas by using comparative genomic hybridization. J Neurosurg 2000; 93: 77–81.
8. Tong CY, Ng IIK, Pang JC et al. Central neurocytomas are genetically distinct from oligodendrogliomas and neuroblastomas. Histopathology 2000; 37: 160–5.
9. Nozaki M, Tada M, Matsumoto R, Sawamura Y, Abe H, Iggo RD. Rare occurrence of inactivating p53 gene mutations in primary nonastrocytic tumors of the central nervous system: reappraisal by yeast functional assay. Acta Neuropathol (Berl) 1998; 95: 291–6.
10. Ishiuchi S, Tamura M. Central neurocytoma: an immunohistochemical, ultrastructural and cell culture study. Acta Neuropathol (Berl) 1997; 94: 425–35.
11. Nishio S, Morioka T, Hamada Y, Fukui M, Nakagawara A. Immunohistochemical expression of tyrosine kinase (Trk) receptor proteins in mature neuronal cell tumors of the central nervous system. Clin Neuropathol 1998; 17: 123–30.
12. Mena H, Morrison AL, Jones RV, Gyure KA. Central neurocytomas express photoreceptor differentiation. Cancer 2001; 91: 136–43.
13. Favereaux A, Vital A, Loiseau H et al. Histopathological variants of central neurocytoma: Report of 10 cases. Ann Pathol 2000; 20: 558–63.
14. Mackay IR. Central neurocytoma: histologic atypia, proliferation potential, and clinical outcome. Cancer 1999; 85: 1606–10.
15. Mackenzie IRA. Central neurocytoma – histologic atypia, proliferation potential, and clinical outcome. Cancer 1999; 85: 1606–10.

16. Eng DY, DeMonte F, Ginsberg L, Fuller GN, Jaeckle K. Craniospinal dissemination of central neurocytoma. Report of two cases. J Neurosurg 1997; 86: 547–52.

17. Oguchi M, Higashi K, Taniguchi M et al. Single photon emission CT images in a case of intraventricular neurocytoma. Ann Nucl Med 1998; 12: 161–4.

18. Krouwer HGJ. Neuronal and mixed neuronal–glial tumors. In: Vecht C, ed. Neurooncology, part 2. Amsterdam: Elsevier, 1997: 137–57.

19. Wharton SB, Antoun NM, Macfarlane R, Anderson JR. The natural history of a recurrent central neurocytoma-like tumor Clin Neuropathol 1998; 17: 136–40.

20. Anderson RC, Elder JB, Parsa AT, Issacson SR, Sisti MB. Radiosurgery for the treatment of recurrent central neurocytomas. Neurosurgery 2001; 48: 1231–7.

21. Brandes AA, Amistà P, Gardiman M et al. Chemotherapy in patients with recurrent and progressive central neurocytoma. Cancer 2000; 88: 169–74.

22. Schild SE, Scheithauer BW, Haddock MG et al. Central neurocytomas. Cancer 1997; 79: 790–5.

23. Sgouros S, Carey M, Aluwihare N, Barber P, Jackowski A. Central neurocytoma: a correlative clinicopathologic and radiologic analysis. Surg Neurol 1998; 49: 197–204.

24. Cabiol J, Acebes JJ, Isamat F. Dysembryoplastic neuroepithelial tumor. Crit Rev Neurosurg 1999; 9: 116–25.

25. Daumas-Duport C, Varlet P, Bacha S et al. Dysembryoplastic neuroepithelial tumors: nonspecific histological forms – a study of 40 cases. J Neurooncol 1999; 41: 267–80.

26. Baisden BL, Brat DJ, Melhem ER et al. Dysembryoplastic neuroepithelial tumor-like neoplasm of the septum pellucidum: a lesion often misdiagnosed as glioma: report of 10 cases. Am J Surg Pathol 2001; 25: 494–9.

27. Chong EY, Lam PY, Poon WS, Ng HK. Telomerase expression in gliomas including the nonastrocytic tumors. Hum Pathol 1998; 29: 599–603.

28. Duerr EM, Rollbrocker B, Hayashi Y et al. PTEN mutations in gliomas and glioneuronal tumors. Oncogene 1998; 16: 2259–64.

29. Prayson RA. Bcl-2, bcl-x, and bax expression in dysembryoplastic neuroepithelial tumors. Clin Neuropathol 2000; 19: 57–62.

30. Aronica E, Leenstra S, Jansen GH et al. Expression of brain-derived neurotrophic factor and tyrosine kinase B receptor proteins in glioneuronal tumors from patients with intractable epilepsy: colocalization with N-methyl-D-aspartic acid receptor. Acta Neuropathol (Berl) 2001; 101: 383–92.

31. Kleihues P, Cavenee WK. Pathology and genetics of tumours of the nervous system. Lyons: International Agency for Research on Cancer, 1997.

32. Hirose T, Scheithauer BW. Mixed dysembryoplastic neuroepithelial tumor and ganglioglioma. Acta Neuropathol (Berl) 1998; 95: 649–54.

33. Thom M, Gomez-Anson B, Revesz T et al. Spontaneous intralesional haemorrhage in dysembryoplastic neuroepithelial tumours: a series of five cases. J Neurol Neurosurg Psychiatry 1999; 67: 97–101.

34. Schiff D, Wen PY. Uncommon brain tumors. Neurol Clin 1995; 13: 953–74.

35. Lee DY, Chung CK, Hwang YS et al. Dysembryoplastic neuroepithelial tumor: radiological findings (including PET, SPECT, and MRS) and surgical strategy. J Neurooncol 2000; 47: 167–74.

36. Kaplan AM, Lawson MA, Spataro J et al. Positron emission tomography using [18F] fluorodeoxyglucose and [11C] L-methionine to metabolically characterize dysembryoplastic neuroepithelial tumors. J Child Neurol 1999; 14: 673–7.

37. Prayson RA, Morris HH, Estes ML, Comair YG. Dysembryoplastic neuroepithelial tumor: a clinicopathologic and immunohistochemical study of 11 tumors including MIB1 immunoreactivity. Clin Neuropathol 1996; 15: 47–53.

38. Aronica E, Leenstra S, Van Veelen CWM et al. Glioneuronal tumors and medically intractable epilepsy: a clinical study with long-term follow-up of seizure outcome after surgery. Epilepsy Res 2001; 43: 179–91.

39. Andermann LF, Savard G, Meencke HJ et al. Psychosis after resection of ganglioglioma or DNET: evidence for an association. Epilepsia 1999; 40: 83–7.

40. Selch MT, Goy BW, Lee SP et al. Gangliogliomas: experience with 34 patients and review of the literature. Am J Clin Oncol 1998; 21: 557–64.

41. Alkhani AM, Bilbao JM, Medline P, Ogundimu FA. Ganglioglioneurocytoma of the posterior fossa. Can J Neurol Sci 1999; 26: 207–10.

42. Johnson JH Jr, Hariharan S, Berman J et al. Clinical outcome of pediatric gangliogliomas: ninety-nine cases over 20 years. Pediatr Neurosurg 1997; 27: 203–7.

43. Zentner J, Wolf HK, Ostertun B et al. Gangliogliomas: clinical, radiological, and histopathological findings in 51 patients. J Neurol Neurosurg Psychiatry 1994; 57: 1497–502.

44. Hakim R, Loeffler JS, Anthony DC, Black PM. Gangliogliomas in adults. Cancer 1997; 79: 127–31.

45. Geraci AP, de Csepel J, Shlasko E, Wallace SA. Ganglioneuroblastoma and ganglioneuroma in association with neurofibromatosis type I: report of three cases. J Child Neurol 1998; 13: 356–8.

46. Bhattacharjee MB, Armstrong DD, Vogel H, Cooley LD. Cytogenetic analysis of 120 primary pediatric brain tumors and literature review. Cancer Genet Cytogenet 1997; 97: 39–53.

47. Hirose T, Scheithauer BW, Lopes MBS et al. Ganglioglioma. An ultrastructural and immunohistochemical study. Cancer 1997; 79: 989–1003.

48. Wacker MR, Cogen PH, Etzell JE et al. Diffuse leptomeningeal involvement by a ganglioglioma in a child. Case report. J Neurosurg 1992; 77: 302–6.

49. Duerr EM, Rollbrocker B, Hayashi Y, et al. PTEN mutations in gliomas and glioneuronal tumors. Oncogene 1998; 16: 259–64.

50. Blumcke I, Lobach M, Wolf HK, Wiestler OD. Evidence for developmental precursor lesions in epilepsy-associated glioneuronal tumors. Microsc Res Tech 1999; 46: 53–8.

51. Morris HH, Matkovic Z, Estes ML et al. Ganglioglioma and intractable epilepsy: clinical and neurophysiologic features and predictors of outcome after surgery. Epilepsia 1998; 39: 307–13.

52. Kumabe T, Shimizu H, Sonoda Y, Shirane R. Thallium-201 single-photon emission computed tomographic and proton magnetic resonance spectroscopic characteristics of intracranial ganglioglioma: three technical case reports. Neurosurgery 1999; 45: 183–7.

53. Celli P, Scarpinati M, Nardacci B, Cervoni L, Cantore GP. Gangliogliomas of the cerebral hemispheres. Report of 14 cases with long-term follow-up and review of the literature. Acta Neurochir (Wien) 1993; 125: 52–7.

54. Haddad SF, Moore SA, Menezes AH, VanGilder JC. Ganglioglioma: 13 years of experience. Neurosurgery 1992; 31: 171–8.

55. Rumana CS, Valadka AB. Radiation therapy and malignant degeneration of benign supratentorial gangliogliomas. Neurosurgery 1998; 42: 1038–43.

56. Kaba SF, Langford LA, Yung WK, Kyritsis AP. Resolution of recurrent malignant ganglioglioma after treatment with cis-retinoic acid. J Neurooncol 1996; 30: 55–60.

57. Halperin EC, Samulski T, Oakes WJ, Friedman HS. Fabrication and testing of a device capable of reducing the incidence of ventricular shunt promoted metastasis. J Neurooncol 1996; 27: 39–46.

58. Packer RJ. Childhood medulloblastoma: progress and future challenges. Brain Dev 1999; 21: 75–81.

59. Agerlin N, Gjerris F, Brincker H et al. Childhood medulloblastoma in Denmark 1960–1984. A population-based retrospective study. Childs Nerv Syst 1999; 15: 29–36.

60. Giordana MT, Schiffer P, Lanotte M, Girardi P, Chio A. Epidemiology of adult medulloblastoma. Int J Cancer 1999; 80: 689–92.

61. Bayani J, Zielenska M, Marrano P et al. Molecular cytogenetic analysis of medulloblastomas and supratentorial primitive neuroectodermal tumors by using conventional banding, comparative genomic hybridization, and spectral karyotyping. J Neurosurg 2000; 93: 437–48.

62. Strickler HD, Rosenberg PS, Devesa SS, Fraumeni JFJ, Goedert JJ. Contamination of poliovirus vaccine with SV40 and the incidence of medulloblastoma. Med Pediatr Oncol 1999; 32: 77–8.

63. Reardon DA, Michalkiewicz E, Boyett JM et al. Extensive genomic abnormalities in childhood medulloblastoma by comparative genomic hybridization. Cancer Res 1997; 57: 4042–7.

64. Nicholson JC, Ross FM, Kohler JA, Ellison DW. Comparative genomic hybridization and histological variation in primitive neuroectodermal tumours. Br J Cancer 1999; 80: 1322–31.

65. Giordana MT, Migheli A, Pavanelli E. Isochromosome 17q is a constant finding in medulloblastoma. An interphase cytogenetic study on tissue sections. Neuropathol Appl Neurobiol 1998; 24: 233–8.

66. Avet-Loiseau H, Vénuat AM, Terrier-Lacombe MJ et al. Comparative genome hybridization detects many recurrent imbalances in central nervous system primitive neuroectodermal tumours in children. Br J Cancer 1999; 79: 1843–7.

67. Yin XL, Pang JC, Liu YH et al. Analysis of loss of heterozygosity on chromosomes 10q, 11, and 16 in medulloblastomas. J Neurosurg 2001; 94: 799–805.

68. Dong J, Gailani MR, Pomeroy SL, Reardon D, Bale AE. Identification of PATCHED mutations in medulloblastomas by direct sequencing. Hum Mutat 2000; 16: 89–90.

69. Halperin EC, Friedman HS. Is there a correlation between duration of presenting symptoms and stage of medulloblastoma at the time of diagnosis? Cancer 1996; 78: 874–80.

70. Tortori-Donati P, Fondelli MP, Rossi A et al. Medulloblastoma in children: CT and MRI findings. Neuroradiology 1996; 38: 352–9.

71. Becker RL, Becker AD, Sobel DF. Adult medulloblastoma: review of 13 cases with emphasis on MRI. Neuroradiology 1995; 37: 104–8.

72. Harrison SK, Ditchfield MR, Waters K. Correlation of MRI and CSF cytology in the diagnosis of medulloblastoma spinal metastases. Pediatr Radiol 1998; 28: 571–4.

73. Zeltzer PM, Boyett JM, Finlay JL et al. Metastasis stage, adjuvant treatment, and residual tumor are prognostic factors for medulloblastoma in children: conclusions from the Children's Cancer Group 921 randomized phase III study. J Clin Oncol 1999; 17: 832–45.

74. Gajjar A, Fouladi M, Walter AW et al. Comparison of lumbar and shunt cerebrospinal fluid specimens for cytologic detection of leptomeningeal disease in pediatric patients with brain tumors. J Clin Oncol 1999; 17: 1825–8.

75. Fouladi M, Gajjar A, Boyett JM et al. Comparison of CSF cytology and spinal magnetic resonance imaging in the detection of leptomeningeal disease in pediatric medulloblastoma or primitive neuroectodermal tumor. J Clin Oncol 1999; 17: 3234–7.

76. Chintagumpala M, Berg S, Blaney SM. Treatment controversies in medulloblastoma. Curr Opin Oncol 2001; 13: 154–9.

77. Greenberg HS, Chamberlain MC, Glantz MJ, Wang S. Adult medulloblastoma: multiagent chemotherapy. Neurooncol 2001; 3: 29–34.

78. Packer RJ, Sutton LN, Elterman R et al. Outcome for children with medulloblastoma treated with radiation and cisplatin, CCNU, and vincristine chemotherapy. J Neurosurg 1994; 81: 690–8.

79. Packer RJ, Sutton LN, Goldwein JW et al. Improved survival with the use of adjuvant chemotherapy in the treatment of medulloblastoma. J Neurosurg 1991; 74: 433–40.

80. Paulino AC. Radiotherapeutic management of medulloblastoma. Oncology (Huntingt) 1997; 11: 813–23.

81. Carrie C, Hoffstetter S, Gomez F et al. Impact of targeting deviations on outcome in medulloblastoma: Study of the French Society of Pediatric Oncology (SFOP). Int J Radiat Oncol Biol Phys 1999; 45: 435–9.

82. Mulhern RK, Kepner JL, Thomas PR et al. Neuropsychologic functioning of survivors of childhood medulloblastoma randomized to receive conventional or reduced-dose craniospinal irradiation: a pediatric oncology group study. J Clin Oncol 1998; 16: 1723–8.

83. Packer RJ, Goldwein J, Nicholson HS et al. Treatment of children with medulloblastomas with reduced-dose craniospinal radiation therapy and adjuvant chemotherapy: A children's cancer group study. J Clin Oncol 1999; 17: 2127–36.

84. Prados MD, Edwards MSB, Chang SM et al. Hyperfractionated craniospinal radiation therapy for primitive neuroectodermal tumors: results of a phase II study. Int J Radiat Oncol Biol Phys 1999; 43: 279–85.

85. Boland I, Vassal G, Morizet J et al. Busulphan is active against neuroblastoma and medulloblastoma xenografts in athymic mice at clinically achievable plasma drug concentrations. Br J Cancer 1999; 79: 787–92.

86. Bouffet E, Doz F, Demaille MC et al. Improving survival in recurrent medulloblastoma: earlier detection, better treatment or still an impasse? Br J Cancer 1998; 77: 1321–6.

87. Fouladi M, Heideman R, Langston JW et al. Infectious meningitis mimicking recurrent medulloblastoma on magnetic resonance imaging – case report. J Neurosurg 1999; 91: 499–502.

88. Sutton LN, Phillips PC, Molloy PT. Surgical management of medulloblastoma. J Neuro-oncol 1996; 29: 9–21.

89. Forgacs P, Geyer CA, Freidberg SR. Characterization of chemical meningitis after neurological surgery. Clin Infect Dis 2001: 32: 179–85.

90. Carmel PW, Greif LK. The aseptic meningitis syndrome: A complication of posterior fossa surgery. Pediatr Neurosurg 1993; 19: 276–80.

91. Leib SL, Boscacci R, Gratzl O, Zimmerli W. Predictive value of cerebrospinal fluid (CSF) lactate level versus CSF/blood glucose ratio for the diagnosis of bacterial meningitis following neurosurgery. Clin Infect Dis 1999; 29: 69–74.

92. Anderson NE, Sheffield S, Hope JKA. Superficial siderosis of the central nervous system – a late complication of cerebellar tumors. Neurology 1999; 52: 163–9.

93. Liu GT, Phillips PC, Molloy PT et al. Visual impairment associated with mutism after posterior fossa surgery in children. Neurosurgery 1998; 42: 253–6.

94. Riva D, Giorgi C. The cerebellum contributes to higher functions during development: evidence from a series of children surgically treated for posterior fossa tumours. Brain 2000; 123: 1051–61.

95. Levisohn L, Cronin-Golomb A, Schmahmann JD. Neuropsychological consequences of cerebellar tumour resection in children: cerebellar cognitive affective syndrome in a paediatric population. Brain 2000; 123 (Pt 5): 1041–50.

96. Clarson CL, Del Maestro RF. Growth failure after treatment of pediatric brain tumors. Pediatrics 1999; 103: E371–6.

97. Grill J, Renaux VK, Bulteau C et al. Long-term intellectual outcome in children with posterior fossa tumors according to radiation doses and volumes. Int J Radiat Oncol Biol Phys 1999; 45: 137–45.

98. Copeland DR, DeMoor C, Moore BD III, Ater JL. Neurocognitive development of children after a cerebellar tumor in infancy: a longitudinal study. J Clin Oncol 1999; 17: 3476–86.

99. Ersahin Y, Mutluer S, Çagli S, Duman Y. Cerebellar mutism: report of seven cases and review of the literature. Neurosurgery 1996; 38: 60–6.

100. Grenier Y, Tomita T, Marymont MH, Byrd S, Burrowes DM. Late postirradiation occlusive vasculopathy in childhood medulloblastoma. Report of two cases. J Neurosurg 1998; 89: 460–4.

101. Russo C, Fischbein N, Grant E, Prados MD. Late radiation injury following hyperfractionated craniospinal radiotherapy for primitive neuroectodermal tumor. Int J Radiat Oncol Biol Phys 1999; 44: 85–90.

102. Agerlin N, Gjerris F, Brincker H et al. Childhood medulloblastoma in Denmark 1960–1984. A population-based retrospective study. Child Nerv Syst 1999; 15: 29–36.

103. Weil MD, Lamborn K, Edwards MS, Wara WM. Influence of a child's sex on medulloblastoma outcome. JAMA 1998; 279: 1474–6.

104. Saran FH, Driever PH, Thilmann C et al. Survival of very young children with medulloblastoma (primitive neuroectodermal tumor of the posterior fossa) treated with craniospinal irradiation. In J Radiat Oncol Biol Phys 1998; 42: 959–67.

105. Halperin EC, Watson DM, George SL. Duration of symptoms prior to diagnosis is related inversely to presenting disease stage in children with medulloblastoma. Cancer 2001; 91: 1444–50.

106. Chan AW, Tarbell NJ, Black PM et al. Adult medulloblastoma: Prognostic factors and patterns of relapse. Neurosurgery 2000; 47: 623–31.

107. Dunkel IJ, Boyett JM, Yates A et al. High-dose carboplatin, thiotepa, and etoposide with autologous stem-cell rescue for patients with recurrent medulloblastoma. J Clin Oncol 1998; 16: 222–8.

108. Brown WD, Tavare CJ, Sobel EL, Gilles FH. The applicability of Collins' Law to childhood brain tumors and its usefulness as a predictor of survival. Neurosurgery 1995; 36: 1093–6.

109. Sala F, Colarusso E, Mazza C, Talacchi A, Bricolo A. Brain tumors in children under 3 years of age – recent experience (1987–1997) in 39 patients. Pediatr Neurosurg 1999; 31: 16–26.

110. Ho DMT, Hsu CY, Wong TT, Ting LT, Chiang H. Atypical teratoid/rhabdoid tumor of the central nervous system: a comparative study with primitive neuroectodermal tumor/medulloblastoma. Acta Neuropathol (Berl) 2000; 99: 482–8.

111. Bruch LA, Hill DA, Cai DX et al. A role for fluorescence in situ hybridization detection of chromosome 22q dosage in distinguishing atypical teratoid/rhabdoid tumors from medulloblastoma/central primitive neuroectodermal tumors. Hum Pathol 2001; 32: 156–62.

112. Hilden JM, Watterson J, Longee DC et al. Central nervous system atypical teratoid tumor rhabdoid tumor: response to intensive therapy and review of the literature. J Neurooncol 1998; 40: 265–75.

113. Olson TA, Bayar E, Kosnik E et al. Successful treatment of disseminated central nervous system malignant rhabdoid tumor. J Pediatr Hematol Oncol 1995; 17: 71–5.

114. Russo C, Pellarin M, Tingby O et al. Comparative genomic hybridization in patients with supratentorial and infratentorial primitive neuroectodermal tumors. Cancer 1999; 86: 331–9.

115. Paulino AC, Melian E. Medulloblastoma and supratentorial primitive neuroectodermal tumors – an institutional experience. Cancer 1999; 86: 142–8.

116. Reddy AT, Janss AJ, Phillips PC, Weiss HL, Packer RJ. Outcome for children with supratentorial primitive neuroectodermal tumors treated with surgery, radiation, and chemotherapy. Cancer 2000; 88: 2189–93.

8

Pineal region tumors

Introduction

The pineal gland (from the Latin for 'pine') is a pine-cone-shaped structure measuring about 8 × 4 mm in the adult and weighing about 200 mg. It is located in the midline of the brain, just above the tectum of the midbrain. It is tethered to the posterior portion of the 3rd ventricle by a neuroepithelial stalk that is partially ependymal-lined. The pineal gland is a neuroendocrine gland that is solid in childhood and has a tendency to calcify later in life. Sometimes cysts form; these are usually but not always asymptomatic.[1] The pineal gland, often referred to as a third eye, recognizes light and darkness via the sympathetic nervous system. Retinal fibers project indirectly to the pineal gland; retinal photoreceptors project to the suprachiasmatic nucleus of the hypothalamus, and then via the median forebrain bundle to the brainstem, the spinal cord and the superior cervical ganglion. Sympathetic fibers from the superior cervical ganglion innervate the pineal gland. In amphibians, there are photoreceptors within the pineal gland, making it truly a 'third eye'. The pineal gland produces the hormone melatonin, which appears to play an important role in the sleep–wake cycle.[2] The pineal gland is enlarged in some patients with systemic cancer but the cause of that enlargement is not known.[3]

Tumors of the pineal gland and pineal region are often detected when they are very small, because of their tendency to compress the underlying brainstem tectum and obstruct the aqueduct of Sylvius, causing hydrocephalus (Fig. 8.1). Many different tumors, some benign and some malignant, arise in or near the pineal gland (Fig. 8.1),[4] including germ cell tumors (GCTs), pineal parenchymal tumors,[5] glial tumors, and meningiomas. In addition, several non-neoplastic mass lesions, including cysts[6] and vascular malformations, may mimic pineal region tumors (Table 8.1). The most common pineal region tumor, the GCT, can also occur in the suprasellar area. All together, tumors of the pineal region represent about 1% of intracranial tumors in adults and about 8% in children (Table 8.2).

Several non-neoplastic lesions found in the pineal region include epidermoid[8] and dermoid cysts (see Chapter 12) and vascular anomalies, in particular aneurysms of the vein of Galen. About one-third of all pineal region masses are benign. The other two-thirds are malignant tumors, but the single most common tumor type, the germinoma, is curable. Pineal parenchymal tumors, GCTs and cysts are discussed in this chapter. Gliomas arising in the pineal region, usually from the tectum of the midbrain, were discussed in Chapter 5.

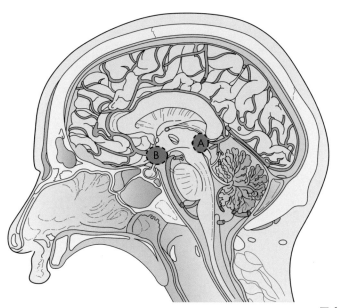

Figure 8.1
Distribution of tumors that commonly arise in the pineal region. The tumors discussed in this chapter mostly arise in or around the pineal gland (A), compressing the aqueduct and causing hydrocephalus. A few, especially germinomas in females, arise in the suprasellar area (B) and cause visual and endocrinologic disturbances. Occasional tumors invade the hypothalamus.

Table 8.2
Relative frequency of pineal region tumors in US series.

Tumor	% of total	
	US Series*	European Series**
Germ-cell	37	35
Germinomas	17	
Teratomas	6	
NGGCT[a]	14	
Pinealoma	22	28
Pineocytoma	12	7
Pineoblastoma or mixed	10	21
Glial	28	27
Astrocytoma	19	
Oligodendroglioma and mixed glioma	3	
Ependymoma	5	
Other	13	10
Cyst	3	
Meningioma	6	7
Melanoma	1	
Metastasis	1	
Other	4	

[a]Non-germinomatous germ cell tumors.
*Data in US series from Paker and Cohen[7]
**Data from European patients, from Fauchon et al.[5]

Table 8.1
Pineal region tumors.

Pineal parenchymal tumors
    Pineocytoma
    Pineoblastoma
    Intermediate differentiation (see text)
Germ cell tumors
    Germinoma
    Non-germinomatous germ cell tumors:
        Embryonal carcinoma
        Yolk sac tumor (endodermal sinus tumor)
        Choriocarcinoma
        Teratoma
        Mature or immature mixed tumors
Others
    Meningioma
    Tectal astrocytoma
    Vein of Galen aneurysms
    Dermoid and epidermoid cysts
    Pineal cysts

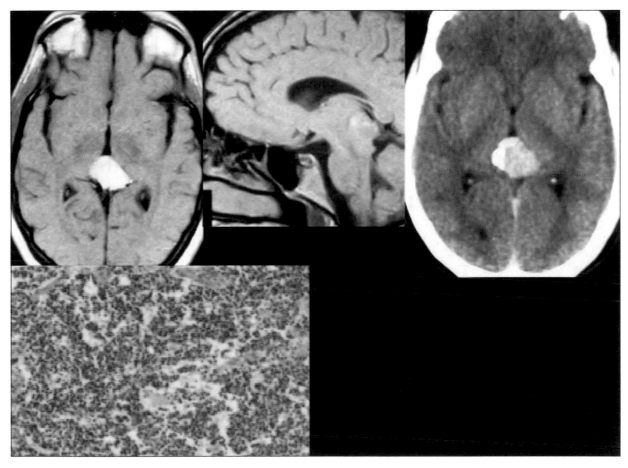

Figure 8.2
A pineocytoma in an adult. The panel on the top left shows an enhancing tumor of the pineal compressing the tectum. The lesion cannot be distinguished from other pineal region tumors by its MR characteristics alone. Sometimes, if the tumor is surrounded by normal pineal calcification, one can infer that the tumor arose within the pineal gland and is either a pineocytoma or a pineoblastoma. Histologically, one sees solid sheets of moderately-sized cells with fibrillar processes occasionally forming pineocytomatous rosettes. No mitoses are identified.

Pineal parenchymal tumors

Introduction

There are three types of pineal parenchymal tumors (Table 8.1), the relatively low-grade pineocytoma, the high-grade pineoblastoma (Fig. 8.2) and pineal parenchymal tumors of interme- diate differentiation[9] with an unpredictable growth rate and clinical behavior. In addition, cysts of the pineal gland can occasionally be large enough to become symptomatic.[6] Pineal parenchymal tumors occasionally complicate inherited retinoblastoma in children,[10] the so- called trilateral retinoblastoma. The higher-grade tumors account for approximately one-third of parenchymal pineal tumors, have a slight male preponderance, and are usually found in children and young adults but occasionally occur in older individuals.[11] The lower-grade tumors tend to occur in adults and account for about 40% of pineal parenchymal tumors. The remaining 25–30% are intermediate or mixed tumors. Both pineocytomas and pineoblastomas can behave aggressively, and either can seed the leptomeninges at diagnosis or at relapse, although pineocytomas do so rarely.[12] Both pineal parenchymal tumors are derived from pineocytes and neuroepithelial cells that have both photosensory and neuroendocrine functions. Pineocytoma cells label with synaptophysin and for neurofilaments, demonstrating neuronal differentiation. Pineal parenchymal tumors cannot be distinguished from each other clinically or by imaging.

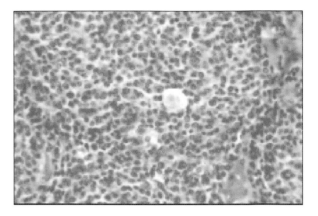

Figure 8.3
The histology of a pineoblastoma. The tumor is typically more cellular with small hyperchromatic nuclei, and has many mitoses and areas of necrosis. An MRI of a pineoblastoma cannot be distinguished from that of a pineocytoma.

Etiology

Aside from hereditary retinoblastoma, no other environmental risk factors for pineal parenchymal tumors have been unequivocally identified. Experiments in mice have implicated SV-40 virus in the development of trilateral retinoblastoma.[13] Multiple chromosomal abnormalities have been described in pineal tumors with higher grade tumors, showing gains of 12q and loss of 22.[14]

Pathology

Grossly, **pineocytomas** tend to be well-circumscribed. They may show hemorrhage or cystic change but usually no necrosis. **Pineoblastomas** are usually larger, and hemorrhage and necrosis are more common. Neither tumor calcifies. Pineocytomas are moderately cellular with delicate connective tissue stroma and Homer–Wright rosettes[15] (Fig. 8.3). Pineocytoma cells label with synaptophysin

and for neurofilaments, evidence of neuronal differentiation. These neoplastic cells may be capable of synthesizing serotonin and melatonin, the neurotransmitters secreted by the normal pineal gland, although this does not cause clinical syndromes of hypersecretion. The pineocytoma is a slowly growing tumor that can demonstrate neuronal, glial, melanocytic, photoreceptor and mesenchymal differentiation.

Pineoblastomas are much more cellular, are more primitive appearing, and have increased mitotic activity and sometimes necrosis; they tend to resemble cerebellar medulloblastomas and may have Homer–Wright rosettes. Some consider them a supratentorial primitive neuroectodermal tumor (Chapter 7). They are often included in that category in clinical trials.

Fauchon et al[5] recognize four grades of pineal parenchymal tumors that correlate with prognosis: grade 1a pineocytoma, without mitosis and positive immunostaining for neuron-specific enolase, synaptophysin, chromogranin A and neurofilaments; grade 2, a transitional tumor with fewer than 6 mitoses/10 high power fields (HPF) and positive immunostaining; grade 3, either fewer than 6 mitoses/10 HPF but negative or weak immunostaining or more than 6 mitoses/HPF with immunostaining; grade 4 pineoblastoma, with many mitoses and weak or absent immunostaining.

Clinical findings

Patients with pineal tumors usually present with hydrocephalus (63/76 patients[5]) caused by the mass compressing the Sylvian aqueduct. Because the superior and inferior colliculi immediately underlie the pineal gland, the compressing mass also causes eye movement abnormalities, specifically Parinaud's syndrome (paralysis of upward gaze, pupils that fail to respond to light but constrict when the patient accommodates, i.e. light/near pupillary dissociation and convergence–retraction nystagmus). Rarely, the tumor causes hearing loss from compression of auditory fibers in the inferior colliculus (Fig. 8.1).

In one series of 30 patients,[16] headaches were present in 73%, impaired vision in 47%, nausea and vomiting in 40%, impaired ambulation (ataxia) in 37%, cognitive dysfunction in 27%, vertigo and dizziness in 23%, fatigue in 17%, dysarthria in 13%, tinnitus in 13% and changes in consciousness in 13%. Signs included papilledema (60%), ataxia (50%), and Parinaud's syndrome (30%) (Table 8.3).

Other signs sometimes result from brainstem or cerebellar compression. Insomnia is a rare symptom of a pineal region tumor[2] or its treatment;[17] melatonin relieves this symptom. Like pituitary tumors (Chapter 10), pineal tumors may bleed, although they do so rarely. A sudden hemorrhage, called pineal apoplexy,

Table 8.3
Symptoms and signs of pineal parenchymal tumors.

Generalized
    Headache
    Nausea/vomiting
    Visual obscurations
    Papilledema
    Tinnitus
    Confusion
    Vertigo/dizziness
    Cognitive dysfunction
Endocrine
    Insomnia
    Precocious puberty
Focal
    Ataxia
    Parinaud's syndrome
    Hearing loss

can cause visual loss, diplopia or abrupt loss of consciousness, mimicking a subarachnoid hemorrhage.

Pineocytomas are usually relatively small when they present (less than 3 cm in diameter). On MR scan, obstructive hydrocephalus is almost always present; and the lesion can be seen compressing the Sylvian aqueduct. The tumors are hypointense on the T1-weighted image and hyperintense on the T2-weighted image with homogeneous enhancement after contrast. Pineoblastomas may be larger and appear more heterogeneous after contrast enhancement but otherwise cannot be distinguished radiographically. Leptomeningeal dissemination can often be identified by enhancement of the cerebral or spinal meninges. Because these tumors cannot be distinguished from GCTs of the region, if hydrocephalus or increased intracranial pressure do not contraindicate, a lumbar puncture to measure cerebrospinal fluid (CSF) markers for GCT should be performed in the preoperative period. Usually, it is not safe to perform a lumbar puncture, and diagnosis is made by biopsy. If hydrocephalus is a major problem threatening herniation, and a shunting procedure is required, ventricular CSF should be assessed for the presence of both tumor cells and CSF markers.

Treatment

Because of the potential danger of surgery in and around the pineal region, some investigators have recommended radiation therapy (RT) without biopsy. Others have suggested stereotactic needle biopsy,[18] but sampling error can occur. Because of the dangers of incorrect histologic diagnosis using either CSF cytology or small samples achieved by stereotactic needle biopsy, and because of the relative safety of modern neurosurgery, we recommend that all lesions be biopsied and, if possible, resected by an open surgical approach. In hydrocephalic patients, ventriculoperitoneal shunts may be placed prior to biopsy.[19] Frameless stereotactic surgical techniques and endoscopic approaches have rendered surgery much safer.[20]

Several different surgical approaches are available.[21,22] One is a combined supra-infratentorial trans-sinus approach.[23] Alternatively, a supracerebellar, infratentorial approach can facilitate tumor resection. For pineocytomas, the treatment following surgery is not established. These are almost always benign tumors that rarely metastasize and have 1-, 3- and 5-year survival rates of 100%, 100% and 67% respectively, after complete resection alone.[16] RT should be delivered to tumors that are incompletely resected. Radiosurgery has been reported to be useful for the treatment of pineocytomas as well as some other tumors within the pineal region.[18]

Pineoblastomas are highly malignant. They infiltrate surrounding structures and often seed the leptomeninges, but usually in the setting of persistent or recurrent primary tumor.[16] Following surgical diagnosis, the entire neuraxis is irradiated with a focal boost to the pineal region. Chemotherapy, either preceding or following RT, using drugs such as etoposide, cisplatin or carboplatin, vincristine and cyclophosphamide, improves prognosis.[24] The 1-, 3- and 5-year survival rates for pineoblastoma are 88%, 78% and 58%.

Pineocytomas and pineoblastomas are most likely to recur locally. Spinal dissemination occurs, but usually when there is also residual or recurrent local tumor. Chemotherapy, either conventional or experimental, is the first treatment modality used at relapse. Recurrent disease is treated with radiotherapy if it was not administered at diagnosis.

Pineal cysts are usually asymptomatic and have a high incidence in young women.[25] Most are identified inadvertently when an MR scan is performed for another reason or the patient has non-specific headache which is unrelated to the cyst. However, pineal cysts can reach a large size and occasionally become symptomatic.[6] Symptomatic cysts average over 15 mm in diameter, whereas asymptomatic cysts are usually less than 10 mm. The symptoms are similar to those of a pineal region tumor, including hydrocephalus and Parinaud's syndrome. A sudden increase in cyst size from hemorrhage may lead to acute hydrocephalus with loss of consciousness and, rarely, sudden death. The cysts differ from pineal parenchymal tumors on MR scan in that they are hypointense on T1 and hyperintense on T2, have a fluid-filled appearance and usually a thin rim of contrast enhancement defining the cyst wall. They are restricted to the pineal gland and, if symptomatic, can be treated by ventricular shunt, 3rd ventriculostomy alone, surgical removal or drainage;[26] however, simple cyst drainage risks recurrence.[1]

Germ cell tumors

Introduction

GCTs mainly occur in children and adolescents[27] and are identical in appearance to GCTs elsewhere, e.g. the ovary and testes. Their biological behavior is also similar but treatment differs.[28] Most GCTs, except for mature teratomas, are highly malignant but do respond to therapy. Cure is usual in germinomas but rare in the other malignant tumors. Therefore, GCTs are divided into germinomas and non-germinomatous germ cell tumors (NGGCTs).

GCTs arise in midline structures, mostly in the pineal region and the suprasellar cistern, and sometimes in both areas simultaneously. Less common sites of GCTs include the cerebral ventricle, basal ganglia, thalamus and cerebellar hemisphere (Fig. 8.4). Germinomas represent about 50% of intracranial GCTs (Table 8.4). Teratomas are the next most common tumor (20%), with mature (relatively benign) teratoma being slightly more common than the more aggressive immature teratoma[29] or teratoma with malignant transformation. Mixed GCTs, yolk sac tumor (endodermal sinus tumor),[30] embryonal carcinoma and

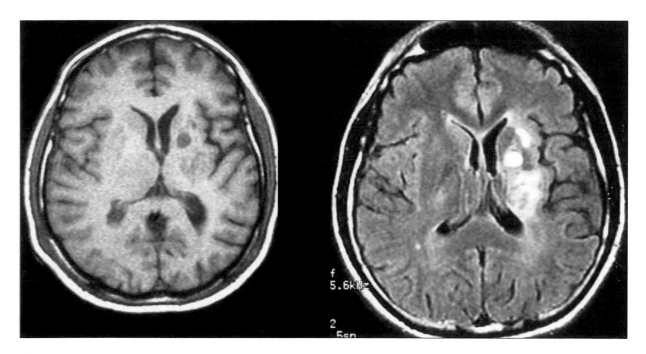

Figure 8.4
A germinoma of the basal ganglia. This patient was 35 in 1990 when he noted that his vision was not right. About a year later he first noticed diplopia on upward gaze (while playing tennis). His pupils were noted to be poorly reactive to light. When he attempted to gaze upward, there was less than 5° of movement and there was retractory nystagmus. Convergence was poor. An MR of the brain showed a lesion in the tectum and right thalamus. A lumbar puncture showed nine white cells with normal biochemical markers and a negative cytologic examination. A stereotactic needle biopsy revealed the lesion to be a granulomatous germinoma (see Fig. 8.8). He was treated with chemotherapy. The tumor and symptoms disappeared and have not recurred.

Table 8.4

Histologic subtypes of central nervous system germ cell tumors.

Type	Approximate percentage
Germinoma	43
Teratoma	20
Mixed tumors	20
Yolk sac tumors	2
Embryonal carcinoma	4
Choriocarcinoma	2

From Campos et al,[29] with permission.

choriocarcinomas together represent about 25% of tumors.

GCTs, rare in Caucasians, are more common in Asians. Taken together, GCTs represent only about 0.5–1% of all primary intracranial neoplasms encountered in the USA, and only 3% of such neoplasms in children and adolescents. In Japan and Taiwan, however, GCTs account for at least 2% of all primary intracranial neoplasms and as many as 15% of pediatric intracranial neoplasms. In Japan and Korea, GCTs represent 70–80% of pineal region tumors.[31] About 90% of these tumors occur in those 20 years of age and younger, with a peak incidence in the second decade of life. Less than 10% of these tumors occur in patients over age 20, and probably less than 2% in those over age 30. Overall, the tumors are 2–2.5 times more common in males than in females, with an even higher male-to-female ratio in the NGGCTs. There is also a sex predilection for location of GCTs: pineal tumors primarily occur in boys, and suprasellar tumors are more common in girls. In one series, 76/78 (97%) pineal region GCTs were found in males, whereas 25/46 (54%) suprasellar tumors were found in females.[29]

Etiology

Specific environmental risk factors have not been identified. There is an increased risk of intracranial GCTs in patients with Klinefelter's syndrome, a disorder characterized by 2 X chromosomes, i.e. a 47 XXY genotype. Such patients are also predisposed to mediastinal GCTs. Less well established are GCTs associated with Down's syndrome, neurofibromatosis type-1 (NF-1) and prior gonadal GCTs. Interestingly, 6/14 brain tumors reported in patients with Down's syndrome were GCTs. Chromosomal imbalances include losses of 13q, 18q, 9q, 11q and gains on 12p, 8q and 1q;[32] p53 mutations are absent,[33] but telomerase activity is present.[34]

Intracranial GCTs are believed by many to arise from embryonic cell rests that lie in the midline of the brain. However, unlike the epithelial cell rests of Rathke's pouch that are found in some normals and are believed to give rise to craniopharyngiomas (Chapter 10), no such embryonic germ cells have been found in the nervous system. Sano[35] has proposed that when the primitive streak begins to form, embryonic germ cells enter the primitive groove and migrate with the moving cells of the mesoderm to the neural plate. They may then be enfolded into the neuraxis.

The origin of the various kinds of intracranial GCTs is also in dispute. The germ cell theory of tumors posits that primordial germ cells give rise to either germinomas or totipotential cells, the latter giving rise to the NGGCTs. Sano has pointed out that such a scheme would make germinoma the most primitive, and therefore the most malignant, of GCTs, although its biological behavior is actually among the most benign. He has proposed the scheme outlined in Fig. 8.5, in which each of the various GCTs arises from a different stage of embryonic development.[35]

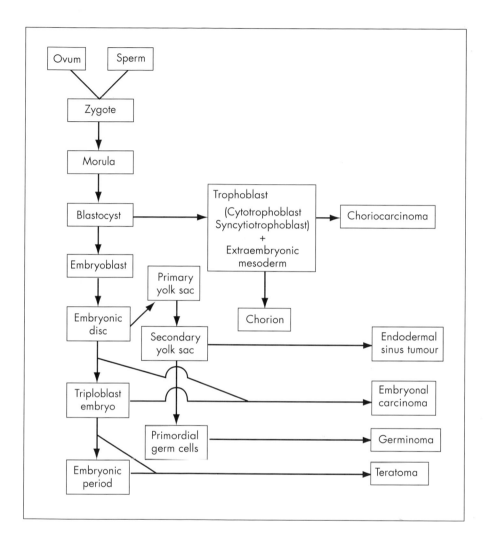

Figure 8.5
Hypothesis concerning the origin of germ cell tumors. Sano suggests that each of the individual tumors arises at a different site in the course of embryologic development; the most primitive arising from the blastocyst, forming choriocarcinoma; the most well-formed arising during the embryonic period, forming a teratoma. From Sano[35] with permission.

Pathology

GCTs are solid, although many, particularly the more malignant ones, show necrosis and hemorrhage. Microscopically, the germinoma is identical to the testicular seminoma and consists of large germ cells with a vesicular nucleus and prominent nucleoli. The cytoplasm is abundant and may appear pale or clear because of glycogen accumulation. The cells may appear as sheaths or lobules. Mitoses are frequent. Lymphocytes often infiltrate the tumor, giving it a granulomatous appearance. The inflammatory infiltrate may be so pronounced that it leads to a misdiagnosis of granuloma rather than neoplasm.[36] Most germinomas label with placental alkaline phosphatase but this may be hard to demonstrate in highly inflammatory tumors. Some germinomas contain syncytiotrophoblastic giant cells that produce human chorionic gonadotropin (HCG). The presence of these

257

cells and the concomitant elevation of CSF HCG is believed to diminish the usually excellent prognosis of germinoma,[37,38] although one study reports no difference in prognosis.[39]

Teratomas are composed of cells of different tissue types. Small uniform cells with inconspicuous nucleoli and moderate eosinophilic cytoplasm may differentiate along neuronal or, rarely, astrocytic lines, expressing appropriate immunohistochemical markers. Mitoses are rare or absent, but occasional multinucleated giant cells are identified. Mature teratomas contain fully differentiated tissue elements, and may contain cartilage, bone, hair or even teeth. Mitotic figures are sparse or absent. Immature teratomas show the same cell types but incompletely differentiated, resembling fetal tissues. Mitoses are common. Some teratomas undergo malignant degeneration, with evidence of a sarcoma or carcinoma within what would otherwise be a mature teratoma. Teratomas may be positive for α-fetoprotein or cytokeratins, the cytokeratin reactivity being a feature of the epithelial components and the α-fetoprotein of enteric-type glandular components.

The yolk sac or endodermal sinus tumor is composed of primitive epithelial-like cells, sometimes growing in a background of myxoid tissue. The tumor has eosinophilic inclusions within the cytoplasm that contain α-fetoprotein, a characteristic that distinguishes it from a germinoma or embryonal carcinoma. The tumors may also contain placental alkaline phosphatase and cytokeratins.

The embryonal carcinoma contains primitive epithelial cells, usually with a clear cytoplasm. Mitoses are frequent and necrosis is common. The cells stain for placental alkaline phosphatase but they also stain for cytokeratin, which distinguishes them from the sometimes similarly appearing germinomas. The choriocarcinomas consist of cells resembling embryonic trophoblast. The cells are positive for HCG, which distinguishes them from other GCTs; they may also be positive for placental alkaline phosphatase and cytokeratins.

Mixed tumors are relatively common and consist of cell types from any of the above-listed tumors. These tumors carry the prognosis of the most aggressive histology contained within the specimen. An accurate histopathologic diagnosis is essential to determine treatment. Only germinomas and teratomas usually occur as pure tumors, the others being mixed. The diagnosis is made both by routine histology and immunohistochemistry

Clinical findings

The symptoms and signs of GCTs depend on the location of the tumor (i.e. pineal or suprasellar).[40] Those tumors that arise in the pineal region present in a fashion similar to primary parenchymal pineal tumors (Table 8.5).

They usually present with a combination of the generalized symptoms of hydrocephalus and the focal symptoms of tectal compression, e.g. Parinaud's syndrome. Those tumors that arise in the suprasellar area have symptoms indistinguishable from those of pituitary region tumors (Chapter 10), e.g. bitemporal hemianopia, pituitary failure and often diabetes insipidus. Cognitive abnormalities (e.g. low IQ) are common in patients with suprasellar GCTs, but not in those with pineal region tumors.[41] Those tumors that arise within the parenchyma of the brain, particularly the basal ganglia, cause focal symptoms appropriate to their location (Fig. 8.5). One of our patients developed a spastic left hemiparesis associated with an enhancing lesion in the thalamus and internal capsule. The tumor was thought by clinical and MR criteria to be a glioma, but biopsy revealed a germinoma.

GCTs are occasionally associated with precocious puberty, in either girls or boys. This is

	Frequency (%)	
	Pineal	*Suprasellar*
Headache	47–78	21
Diplopia; visual deficits	33	33
Parinaud's syndrome	34–42	14
Papilledema; hydrocephalus	47–61	21
Lethargy; obtundation	22–26	15
Ataxia	20	9
Diabetes insipidus	10–18	41
Hypothalamic–pituitary dysfunction	19	33
Precocious puberty	6	3
Growth delay	4	9
Menstrual abnormalities	3–4	16

Table 8.5
Presenting symptoms and signs clustered by primary tumor location. From Kretschmar[27] with permission.

probably a result of tumor involvement of the hypothalamus, releasing the immature gonads from tonic inhibitory control. Alternatively, HCG, elaborated by the tumor, can act as a stimulant of testosterone production. This mechanism would explain precocious puberty in boys, but not girls, harboring HCG-producing intracranial germ cell neoplasms.

GCTs cannot be distinguished from other pineal region tumors on MR scan (Fig. 8.6).[42] They usually are iso- or hypointense on the T1-weighted image and isointense with brain

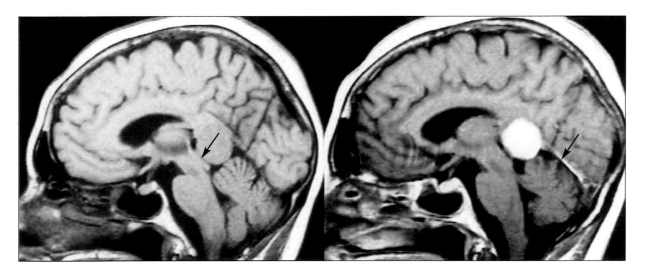

Figure 8.6
Meningioma of the pineal region. A large isointense mass on the T1-weighted image appears to be within the pineal region, compressing the tectum (left panel, arrow). The lesion contrast enhances and one sees a dural tail (right panel, arrow) which suggests a meningioma rather than a germ cell tumor.

259

Table 8.6
Biological tumor markers in germ cell tumors.

Tumor histology	α-Fetoprotein	β-Human chorionic gonadotropin	Human placental lactogen	Lactate dehydrogenase isoenzymes	Placental alkaline phosphatase	Cytokeratins
Teratoma	+/–	–	–	–	–	+
Germinoma	–	–	–	+	+	–
Embryonal carcinoma	+/–	+/–	–	–	+	+
Choriocarcinoma	–	++	+	–	+/–	+
Yolk sac tumor (endodermal sinus)	++	–	–	–	–	+

Modified from Kleihues et al.[45]

on the T2-weighted image with fairly intense homogeneous contrast enhancement. One radiographic feature that differentiates GCTs from primary pineal tumors is that the GCT appears to surround the pineal gland, compressing pineal calcifications, whereas parenchymal pineal tumors explode the pineal gland, dispersing pineal calcifications. Teratomas are often cystic and may have calcified regions as well as areas of lipid that are hyperintense on both T1- and T2-weighted images. When germinomas occur in the basal ganglia or thalamus, they are generally cystic and some are hemorrhagic. The signal intensity is heterogeneous on T1- and T2-weighted images and the tumor usually enhances.[43]

Examination of the CSF for biochemical markers often helps establish the diagnosis (Table 8.6). Cytologic examination demonstrates tumor cells in only 10–15% of patients.[44]

Important markers include α-fetoprotein, β-HCG and placental alkaline phosphatase. Lactate dehydrogenase isozymes are less important. As Table 8.6 indicates, germinomas normally do not excrete either α-fetoprotein or HCG. Low levels of HCG in the spinal fluid (< 2000 mIU/ml) may be seen in germinomas which contain syncytiotrophoblastic giant cells. However, the presence of detectable HCG in the CSF may predict a higher rate of recurrence than if no HCG is present.[37] Absence of all markers in the spinal fluid suggests that the lesion is a germinoma or a teratoma. A grossly elevated level of HCG establishes the diagnosis of choriocarcinoma; a grossly elevated α-fetoprotein suggests a yolk sac tumor, and an elevated placental alkaline phosphatase, a germinoma. These markers are quite reliable, but because of mixed tumors an accurate histopathologic diagnosis is essential to determine treatment.

Treatment

Treatment depends on the histologic type and stage of the disease (Fig. 8.7). Prior to therapy a spinal MR scan with contrast to search for subarachnoid metastases (mature teratomas do not require further imaging), lumbar and, if a shunt or ventriculostomy is present, ventricular CSF should be examined for malignant cells.

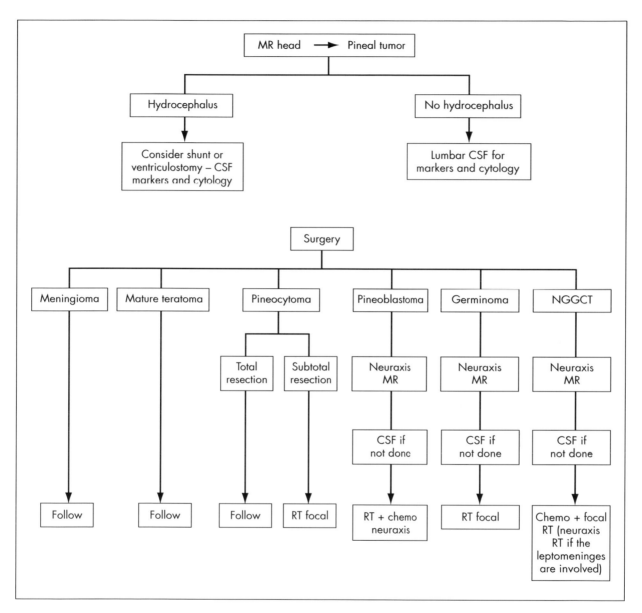

Figure 8.7
Approach to pineal region tumor. RT, radiation therapy.

Although some physicians will treat on the basis of imaging studies and spinal fluid examination, most require tumor histology to determine treatment. The larger the tissue sample the better, because mixed tumors are relatively common and a small sample may prevent accurate histologic identification of all components in a mixed tumor; the most aggressive histology identified in such a lesion determines the therapeutic approach.

We recommend a surgical approach to all pineal region tumors with the intent of achieving a maximally feasible resection, except for pure germinomas (see below). Pineal region tumors can be approached surgically in several ways.[20,22] They can be approached supratentorially via a parietal interhemispheric approach, or an occipital transtentorial approach. Tumors can also be approached via an infratentorial, supracerebellar approach; the technique is performed with the patient in the prone position, with the head lower than the heart. This avoids the complication of air embolism that can occur with patients in the sitting position. Some tumors can be approached endoscopically.[20] Most surgeons believe that radical debulking of the more malignant tumors leads to a better prognosis.[46] In one series of operations for pineal region tumors, gross total removal was possible in 90% of benign tumors and 25% of malignant tumors. Furthermore, for NGGCTs, survival depends on the extent of resection. In one series, the 3-year survival was 73% after complete resection, 32% after partial resection and 0% after biopsy.[46] Because germinomas are curable with radiation, radical resection is not required. If the diagnosis of germinoma is strongly suspected clinically and on the basis of pre-operative CSF data, and the diagnosis can be established by biopsy, many believe that no additional risks should be taken by continuing the resection.[47]

With modern techniques, operative mortality varies from 0%–8%, usually 1–2%, and permanent morbidity from 0%–12%, usually 5–6%. The common complications include ocular movement disorders, postoperative confusion that may precede permanent cognitive dysfunction, ataxia and aseptic meningitis (Chapter 7). Many of the neurologic deficits are transient. Hemorrhage into the tumor bed may occur up to several days postoperatively and is probably related to tumor vascularity and malignancy. Risk factors for neurologic deficit include highly malignant and vascular tumors, preoperative neurologic deficit and preoperative RT.

Diagnostic stereotactic needle biopsy is the preferred approach for some patients, such as those with basal ganglia or thalamic tumors, or with disseminated tumor, in whom CSF does not yield a definitive diagnosis. Stereotactic biopsies in the pineal region carry a greater risk of hemorrhage than in other areas of the brain, particularly when the tumor is highly vascular. However, both morbidity and mortality are low and there are times when stereotactic biopsy should be performed in preference to open surgery. Endoscopic biopsy via the 3rd ventricle may be safer in some tumors.

After the histologic diagnosis is established, patients can be divided into those with pure germinoma (Fig. 8.8), those with mature teratomas, and those with other NGGCTs. All patients, except those with pure mature teratomas, should have a complete staging evaluation if not performed preoperatively. This should include a complete spine MRI with gadolinium and a CSF examination. In those few patients with preoperative studies which show tumor dissemination, the diagnosis may be established by cytologic examination of ventricular or lumbar CSF. Furthermore, serum or CSF tumor markers may delineate the pathologic diagnosis, particularly when only a biopsy was obtained. For example, a biopsy demonstrating teratoma associated with a very high CSF α-fetoprotein level suggests that the tumor contains endodermal sinus components not sampled by biopsy, and the patient should be treated accordingly. Spinal MRI should be performed before CSF is obtained to avoid possible meningeal enhancement induced by the lumbar puncture, which can be confused with subarachnoid tumor dissemination. The

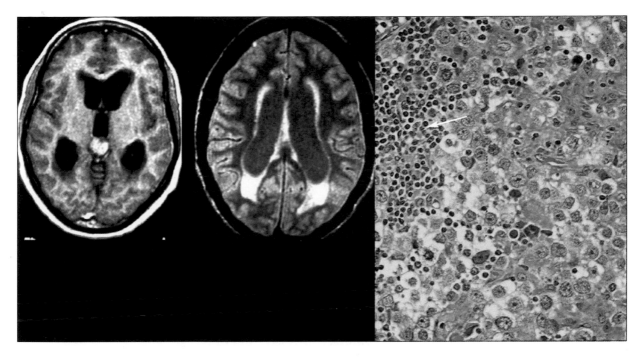

Figure 8.8
A pineal region germinoma. This 30-year-old man presented to medical attention with headache but no other symptoms. An MR scan revealed hydrocephalus with marked periventricular hyperintensity, indicating transependymal spinal fluid absorption (right panel). A uniformly contrast-enhancing tumor was found in the pineal region, obstructing the ventricular system (left panel). Biopsy revealed a pure germinoma. The tumor was treated with radiation therapy with complete resolution. This patient had an unusual but occasionally described symptom during radiation. Each time the beam was turned on, he was able to see blue light through his closed eyes in a darkened room. He was told by the technician and a junior radiation oncologist that it must be a psychological reaction, but the symptom is well-described in the literature.[65] Even rarer is the ability to smell the radiation beam, which this patient did not experience. The photomicrograph shows neoplastic germ cells with large vesicular nuclei and clear cytoplasm, interspersed with typical collections of mature T-cells (arrow).

CSF should be examined about 2 weeks postoperatively to allow time for biochemical markers and cells shed by the resected tumor but not representing dissemination to be cleared from CSF.

In patients with germinoma, surgery should be followed by RT to a portal that includes the site of the tumor, either pineal or suprasellar, and the lateral and 3rd ventricles. A total tumor dose of 50.4 Gy is usually sufficient. The usual dose of RT is 19.8 Gy delivered to the lateral 3rd and 4th ventricles, with an additional 30.6 Gy to the tumor bed in 1.8-Gy fractions (Fig. 8.9). Some advocate lower doses of radiation, either independently or combined with chemotherapy.[48,49] If either CSF cytology or a contrast-enhanced MRI of the spine suggests leptomeningeal dissemination, craniospinal irradiation is required.[50] Radiosurgery may have a role by providing a local boost to the pineal region tumor to reduce overall radiation exposure of the remainder of the brain. Rarely, transient spontaneous or steroid-induced regression of intracranial germinomas

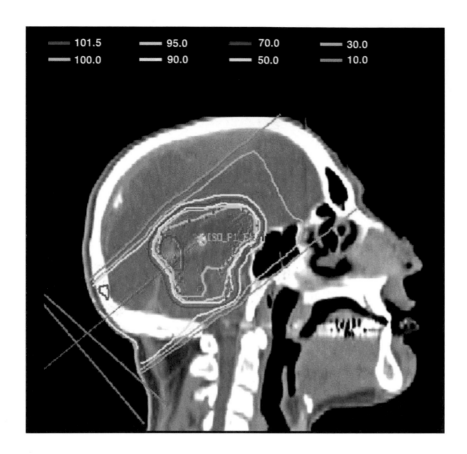

Figure 8.9
Radiation portal for treatment of a germinoma. Focal treatment to the pineal region alone is not sufficient to control tumor recurrence. A radiation portal that encompasses both the pineal and the supratentorial ventricular system, as seen in this illustration, cures more than 90% of patients. Whole-neuraxial radiation is unnecessary.

has been described;[51,52] steroid regression may be related to lymphocytic elements within the tumor[53] (Chapter 11).

Some investigators have recommended chemotherapy as the primary treatment for germinomas[54] in an effort to eliminate cranial RT and its potential for neurotoxicity. Most tumors respond, but the regimens are toxic and there is a 50% relapse rate within 2 years, requiring radiation.[55] RT is efficacious even after failed chemotherapy. Accordingly, in adolescents and adults, we recommend RT, which has a 10-year progression-free survival of about 90%. Furthermore, RT appears to be well tolerated in this population, with few significant long-term neurologic sequelae.[38] Chemotherapy may allow for a reduction in

radiation dosage, particularly in patients with leptomeningeal dissemination at diagnosis.[56]

NGGCTs require maximal surgical resection,[57] RT and chemotherapy in all cases.[57] RT is delivered to a total dose of 54 Gy to a focal field involving the 3rd and 4th ventricles. Any evidence of leptomeningeal dissemination mandates neuraxis RT. In these instances, pre-irradiation chemotherapy is probably indicated, using multiagent chemotherapy, usually cisplatin, etoposide, vincristine and cyclophosphamide.[46]

If there is a response after two cycles of chemotherapy, it should be continued for six cycles. Some suggest high-dose chemotherapy with stem cell or bone marrow rescue.[58] The efficacy of this approach is not known, because the number of patients so treated is

Table 8.7
Prognosis of intracranial germ cell tumors.

Histology	5-year survival (%)	10-year survival (%)
Good prognosis		
Pure germinoma	95	92
Mature teratoma	93	93
Intermediate prognosis		
Germinoma with STGC[a]	83	83
Immature teratoma	70	70
Mixed tumor[b]	53	35
Poor prognosis		
Choriocarcinoma		
Yolk sac tumor	9	–
Embryonal tumor		
Other mixed tumor		

Modified from Tagliabue et al,[3] with permission.
[a]STGC, syncytiotrophoblastic giant cell.
[b]Mainly germinoma or teratoma.

small but some reports are enthusiastic.[58] Whether or not successful, chemotherapy should be followed by RT. The dose of 54 Gy is the same as that for NGGCTs. Adjuvant chemotherapy is usually not well tolerated because of limited bone marrow reserve following neuraxis RT.

Mature teratomas require no treatment beyond surgery if they can be successfully resected. Some mature teratomas involve the hypothalamus or hypophyseal region, and only partial removal or biopsy is possible. In those cases, some have advocated adjuvant chemotherapy without radiation.[59] The recommended regimen is etoposide and cisplatin. Immature teratomas require postoperative RT combined with chemotherapy. One regimen includes ifosfamide, cisplatin, etoposide and local radiation to a dose of 50 Gy. The prognosis of immature teratomas is relatively good, with one series yielding 5- and 10-year survival rates of 70%.[60]

Prognosis

The major factor that determines prognosis is the tumor type (Table 8.7); a lesser factor is the extent of the surgical resection (Fig. 8.10).[38,46] For mixed tumors, the amount of malignant tissue is also prognostic. For example, a mature teratoma with a small amount of choriocarcinoma has a better prognosis than a mature teratoma containing a large amount of choriocarcinoma.[46]

Yolk sac tumors, embryonal carcinomas and choriocarcinomas have a poor prognosis; these tumors usually relapse within 2 years, and dissemination through the leptomeninges is common. Some children with pineal region tumors are at risk for cognitive deficits leading to school failure. The complications of irradiation are discussed in Chapter 4. However, recent evidence suggests that such children have an excellent quality of life as adults.[61] Because the cure rate for germinomas is also so

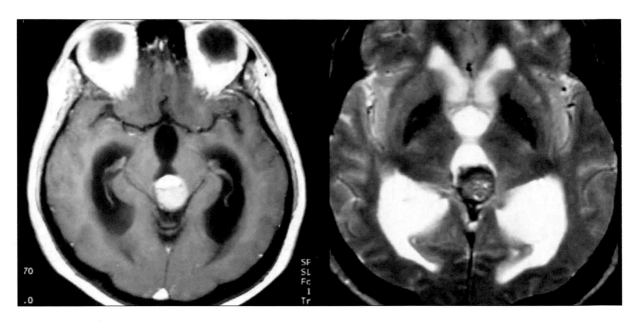

Figure 8.10
A pineal region primary central nervous system melanoma. This patient presented with headache and hydrocephalus. The tumor was a melanocytoma with elements of melanoma (Chapter 6). The CSF and spinal MRI were normal. Two years after focal radiation therapy, the patient is free of disease.

high, both these groups are at risk for very late complications (often greater than 20 years), including secondary tumors within the radiation portal. These include malignant meningiomas and malignant astrocytomas.

The prognosis for survival in patients with suprasellar germinomas is also excellent, but many suffer cognitive and endocrine dysfunction despite successful RT.[62] However, quality of life seems good; many patients go on to complete college and even graduate school.[63] The role that radiotherapy plays in causing cognitive dysfunction is unclear because many patients with suprasellar GCTs have cognitive abnormalities preceding treatment.[41] Other complications are seen rarely. One patient with a suprasellar germinoma developed a vascular malformation of the spinal cord 5 years after neuraxis RT.[64]

GCTs usually recur locally. Spinal dissemination may occur, but usually in the presence of local recurrence as well. Systemic metastases occur but are rare. Recurrent disease is treated with chemotherapy if the patient has not received chemotherapy before, or with different agents if the patient has received prior chemotherapy. Focal spinal RT may be an option for symptomatic spinal leptomeningeal metastases, depending upon prior neuraxis RT.

References

1. Mena H, Armonda RA, Ribas JL, Ondra SL, Rushing EJ. Nonneoplastic pineal cysts: a clinicopathologic study of twenty-one cases. Ann Diagn Pathol 1997; 1: 11–8.
2. Etzioni A, Luboshitzky R, Tiosano D et al. Melatonin replacement corrects sleep disturbances in a child with pineal tumor. Neurology 1996; 46: 261–3.

3. Tagliabue M, Lissoni P, Barni S et al. A radiologic study by CT scan of pineal size in cancer patients: correlation to melatonin blood levels. Tumori 1989; 75: 226–8.

4. Schild SE, Scheithauer BW, Haddock MG et al. Histologically confirmed pineal tumors and other germ cell tumors of the brain. Cancer 1996; 78: 2564–71.

5. Fauchon F, Jouvet A, Paquis P et al. Parenchymal pineal tumors: A clinicopathological study of 76 cases. Int J Radiat Oncol Biol Phys 2000; 46: 959–68.

6. Engel U, Gottschalk S, Niehaus L et al. Cystic lesions of the pineal region – MRI and pathology. Neuroradiology 2000; 42: 399–402.

7. Packer RJ, Cohen BH. Germ-cell tumors and pineal tumors. In: Vecht CJ, ed. Neuro-Oncology. Part II. Amsterdam: Elsevier 1997: 229–56.

8. Konovalov AN, Spallone A, Pitzkhelauri DI. Pineal epidermoid cysts: diagnosis and management. J Neurosurg 1999; 91: 370–4.

9. Kleihues P, Cavenee WK. World Health Organization Classification of Tumours: Tumours of the nervous system – pathology and genetics. Lyon: IRAC Press, 2000.

10. Kivela T. Trilateral retinoblastoma: a meta-analysis of hereditary retinoblastoma associated with primary ectopic intracranial retinoblastoma. J Clin Oncol 1999; 17: 1829–37.

11. Chang SM, Lillis-Hearne PK, Larson DA et al. Pineoblastoma in adults. Neurosurgery 1995; 37: 383–90.

12. Ito T, Takahashi H, Ikuta F, Sato H. Metastatic pineocytoma of the spinal cord after long-term dormancy. Pathol Int 1994; 44: 860–4.

13. Marcus DM, Brooks SE, Leff G et al. Trilateral retinoblastoma: insights into histogenesis and management. Surv Ophthalmol 1998; 43: 59–70.

14. Rickert CH, Simon R, Bergmann M, Dockhorn-Dworniczak B, Paulus W. Comparative genomic hybridization in pineal parenchymal tumors. Genes Chromosom Cancer 2001; 30: 99–104.

15. Fèvre-Montange M, Jouvet A, Privat K et al. Immunohistochemical, ultrastructural, biochemical and in vitro studies of a pineocytoma. Acta Neuropathol (Berl) 1998; 95: 532–9.

16. Schild SE, Scheithauer BW, Schomberg PJ et al. Pineal parenchymal tumors. Clinical, pathologic, and therapeutic aspects. Cancer 1993; 72: 870–80.

17. Jan JE, Tai J, Hahn G, Rothstein RR. Melatonin replacement therapy in a child with a pineal tumor. J Child Neurol 2001; 16: 139–40.

18. Kreth FW, Schatz CR, Pagenstecher A et al. Stereotactic management of lesions of the pineal region. Neurosurgery 1996; 39: 280–9.

19. Brandes AA, Pasetto LM, Monfardini S. The treatment of cranial germ cell tumours. Cancer Treat Rev 2000; 26: 233–42.

20. Oi S, Shibata M, Tominaga J et al. Efficacy of neuroendoscopic procedures in minimally invasive preferential management of pineal region tumors: a prospective study. J Neurosurg 2000; 93: 245–53.

21. Saenz A, Zamorano L, Matter A, Bucius R, Diaz F. Interactive image guided surgery of the pineal region. Minim Invasive Neurosurg 1998; 41: 27–30.

22. Fukui M, Natori Y, Matsushima T, Nishio S, Ikezaki K. Operative approaches to the pineal region tumors. Child Nerv Syst 1998; 14: 49–52.

23. Ziyal IM, Sekhar LN, Salas E, Olan WJ. Combined supra/infratentorial-transsinus approach to large pineal region tumors. J Neurosurg 1998; 88: 1050–7.

24. Kurisaka M, Arisawa M, Mori T et al. Combination chemotherapy (cisplatin, vinblastin) and low-dose irradiation in the treatment of pineal parenchymal cell tumors. Childs Nerv Syst 1998; 14: 564–9.

25. Sawamura Y, Ikeda J, Ozawa M et al. Magnetic resonance images reveal a high incidence of asymptomatic pineal cysts in young women. Neurosurgery 1995; 37: 11–5.

26. Kang HS, Kim DG, Han DH. Large glial cyst of the pineal gland: a possible growth mechanism. Case report. J Neurosurg 1998; 88: 138–40.

27. Kretschmar CS. Germ cell tumors of the brain in children: a review of current literature and new advances in therapy. Cancer Invest 1997; 15: 187–98.

28. Hooda BS, Finlay JL. Recent advances in the diagnosis and treatment of central nervous system germ-cell tumours. Curr Opin Neurol 1999; 12: 693–6.

29. Matsutani M, Sano K, Takakura K et al. Primary intracranial germ cell tumors: a clinical analysis of 153 histologically verified cases. J Neurosurg 1997; 86: 446–55.

30. Chandy MJ, Damaraju SC. Benign tumours of the pineal region: a prospective study from 1983 to 1997. Br J Neurosurg 1998; 12: 228–33.

31. Oi S, Matsuzawa K, Choi JU et al. Identical characteristics of the patient populations with pineal region tumors in Japan and in Korea and therapeutic modalities. Childs Nerv Syst 1998; 14: 36–40.

32. Rickert CH, Simon R, Bergmann M, Dockhorn-Dworniczak B, Paulus W. Comparative genomic hybridization in pineal germ cell tumors. J Neuropathol Exp Neurol 2000; 59: 815–21.

33. Nozaki M, Tada M, Matsumoto R et al. Rare occurrence of inactivating p53 gene mutations in primary nonastrocytic tumors of the central nervous system: reappraisal by yeast functional assay. Acta Neuropathol (Berl) 1998; 95: 291–6.

34. Hiraga S, Ohnishi T, Izumoto S et al. Telomerase activity and alterations in telomere length in human brain tumors. Cancer Res 1998; 58: 2117–25.

35. Sano K. Pathogenesis of intracranial germ cell tumors reconsidered. J Neurosurg 1999; 90: 258–64.

36. Kraichoke S, Cosgrove M, Chandrasoma PT. Granulomatous inflammation in pineal germinoma. A cause of diagnostic failure at stereotaxic brain biopsy. Am J Surg Pathol 1988; 12: 655–60.

37. Inamura T, Nishio S, Ikezaki K, Fukui M. Human chorionic gonadotrophin in CSF, not serum, predicts outcome in germinoma. J Neurol Neurosurg Psychiatry 1999; 66: 654–7.

38. Matsutani M, Sano K, Takakura K et al. Primary intracranial germ cell tumors: a clinical analysis of 153 histologically verified cases. J Neurosurg 1997; 86: 446–55.

39. Shin KH, Kim IH, Choe C. Impacts of elevated level of HCG in serum on clinical course and radiotherapy results in the histology-confirmed intracranial germinomas. Acta Oncol 2001; 40: 98–101.

40. Salzman KL, Rojiani AM, Buatti J et al. Primary intracranial germ cell tumors: clinicopathologic review of 32 cases. Pediatr Pathol Lab Med 1997; 17: 713–27.

41. Kitamura K, Shirato H, Sawamura Y et al. Preirradiation evaluation and technical assessment of involved-field radiotherapy using computed tomographic (CT) simulation and neoadjuvant chemotherapy for intracranial germinoma. Int J Radiat Oncol Biol Phys 1999; 43: 783–8.

42. Satoh H, Uozumi T, Kiya K et al. MRI of pineal region tumours: relationship between tumours and adjacent structures. Neuroradiology 1995; 37: 624–30.

43. Kim DI, Yoon PH, Ryu YH, Jeon P, Hwang GJ. MRI of germinomas arising from the basal ganglia and thalamus. Neuroradiology 1998; 40: 507–11.

44. Paulino AC, Wen B-C, Mohideen MN. Controversies in the management of intracranial germinomas. Oncology (Huntingt) 1999; 13: 513–30.

45. Kleihues P, Cavenee WK. Pathology and genetics of tumours of the nervous system. Lyons: International Agency for Research on Cancer, 1997.

46. Schild SE, Haddock MG, Scheithauer BW et al. Nongerminomatous germ cell tumors of the brain. Int J Radiat Oncol Biol Phys 1996; 36: 557–63.

47. Sawamura Y, de Tribolet N, Ishii N, Abe H. Management of primary intracranial germinomas: diagnostic surgery or radical resection? J Neurosurg 1997; 87: 262–6.

48. Shibamoto Y, Sasai K, Oya N, Hiraoka M. Intracranial germinoma: radiation therapy with tumor volume-based dose selection. Radiology 2001; 218: 452–6.

49. Brandes AA, Pasetto LM, Monfardini S. The treatment of cranial germ cell tumours. Cancer Treat Rev 2000; 26: 233–42.

50. Shibamoto Y, Oda Y, Yamashita J et al. The role of cerebrospinal fluid cytology in radiotherapy planning for intracranial germinoma. Int J Radiat Oncol Biol Phys 1994; 29: 1089–94.

51. Ide M, Jimbo M, Yamamoto M et al. Spontaneous regression of primary intracranial germinoma – a case report. Cancer 1997; 79: 558–63.

52. Fujimaki T, Mishima K, Asai A, Suzuki I, Kirino T. Spontaneous regression of a residual pineal tumor after resection of a cerebellar vermian germinoma. J Neurooncol 1999; 41: 65–70.

53. Mascalchi M, Roncaroli F, Salvi F, Frank G. Transient regression of an intracranial germ cell tumour after intravenous steroid administration: a case report. J Neurol Neurosurg Psychiatry 1998; 64: 670–2.

54. Balmaceda C, Heller G, Rosenblum M, et al. Chemotherapy without irradiation – a novel approach for newly diagnosed CNS germ cell tumors: results of an international cooperative trial. J Clin Oncol 1996; 14: 2908–15.

55. Merchant TE, Davis BJ, Sheldon JM, Leibel SA. Radiation therapy for relapsed CNS germinoma after primary chemotherapy. J Clin Oncol 1998; 16: 204–9.

56. Buckner JC, Peethambaram PP, Smithson WA et al. Phase II trial of primary chemotherapy followed by reduced-dose radiation for CNS germ cell tumors. J Clin Oncol 1999; 17: 933–40.

57. Robertson PL, DaRosso RC, Allen JC. Improved prognosis of intracranial non-germinoma germ cell tumors with multimodality therapy. J Neurooncol 1997; 32: 71–80.

58. Tada T, Takizawa T, Nakazato F et al. Treatment of intracranial nongerminomatous germ-cell tumor by high-dose chemotherapy and autologous stem-cell rescue. J Neurooncol 1999; 44: 71–6.

59. Sawamura Y, Kato T, Ikeda J et al. Teratomas of the central nervous system: treatment considerations based on 34 cases. J Neurosurg 1998; 89: 728–37.

60. Matsutani M, Sano K, Takakura K et al. Primary intracranial germ cell tumors: A clinical analysis of 153 histologically verified cases. J Neurosurg 1997; 86: 446–55.

61. Bamberg M, Kortmann R, Calaminus G et al. Radiation therapy for intracranial germinomas: results of the German Cooperative Prospective Trials MAKEI 83/86/89. J Clin Oncol 1999; 17: 2585–92.

62. Oka H, Kawano N, Tanaka T et al. Long term functional outcome of suprasellar germinomas: usefulness and limitations of radiotherapy. J Neurooncol 1998; 40: 185–90.

63. Sutton LN, Radcliffe L, Goldwein JW et al. Quality of life of adult survivors of germinomas treated with craniospinal irradiation. Neurosurgery 1999; 45: 1292–7.

64. Maraire JN, Abdulrauf SI, Berger S, Knisely J, Awad IA. De novo development of a cavernous malformation of the spinal cord following spinal axis radiation – case report. J Neurosurg 1999; 90: 234–8.

65. Steidley KD, Eastman RM, Stabile RJ. Observations of visual sensations produced by cerenkov radiation from high-energy electrons. Int J Radiat Oncol Biol Phys 1989; 17: 685–90.

9

Tumors of cranial nerves and skull base

Introduction

Several intracranial tumors cause their symptoms by invading or compressing cranial nerves (Fig. 9.1). These tumors fall into two large categories: tumors that arise from the nerve sheath and directly invade cranial nerves, and tumors that arise from bones or other structures at the skull base and compress cranial nerves either within the intracranial cavity or as they exit the skull to innervate the various cranial organs (Table 9.1).

Although the two groups of tumors differ with respect to histogenesis, biology, treatment and prognosis, they are both considered in this chapter because they often present to the physician with similar symptoms. Moreover, neither group is restricted to cranial nerves or the base of the skull. Nerve sheath tumors can arise anywhere in the body and are particularly common along spinal roots. Most of the tumors that affect the base of the skull can also

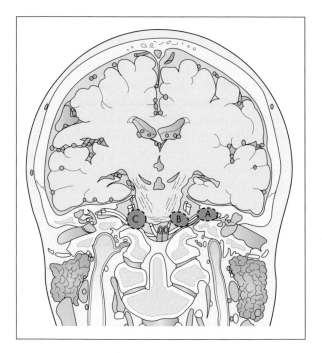

Figure 9.1
Location of cranial nerve tumors. Although any cranial nerve can be involved, the most common are the acoustic and trigeminal. (A) Vestibular schwannoma in internal auditory canal.
(B) Vestibular schwannoma in cerebellopontine angle.
(C) Trigeminal schwannoma.

Table 9.1
Tumors of cranial and spinal nerves and skull base.

> Nerve sheath tumors
>   Schwannoma (neurilemmoma, neurinoma)
>   Neurofibroma
>   Malignant schwannoma
> Skull base tumors
>   Paraganglioma (chemodectoma)
>   Chordoma
>   Chondroma or chondrosarcoma
>   Carcinoma/lymphoma of the paranasal sinuses
>   Esthesioneuroblastoma
>   Meningioma (see Chapter 6)
>   Sarcoma (Ewing's, rhabdomyosarcoma)

affect the calvarium or other bones. Nevertheless, cranial nerves are frequent targets, and this chapter is a convenient place to discuss the tumors as a group.

Nerve sheath tumors

Introduction

The WHO recognizes four groups of nerve sheath tumors: schwannomas, neurofibromas, malignant peripheral nerve sheath tumors, also called neurogenic sarcoma or malignant schwannoma, and the rare benign perineurinoma, not discussed here. Nerve sheath tumors can occur as sporadic tumors or as part of the familial tumor syndromes neurofibromatosis-1 (NF-1) and neurofibromatosis-2 (NF-2). When they occur sporadically, they are usually single and the vast majority are benign. When they occur as part of a familial syndrome, they are more likely to be multiple, and to undergo malignant degeneration (Chapter 12). Nerve sheath tumors can occur along any cranial or peripheral nerve root or nerve except the olfactory and optic nerves, which are not truly nerves but extensions of the brain, and thus not susceptible to the development of nerve sheath tumors. (Gliomas do arise in the optic nerve, particularly as part of the NF-1 syndrome.) Nerve sheath tumors are more common in the spinal canal and peripheral nerves than they are in the intracranial cavity. However, when they arise in the intracranial cavity, they are often responsible for significant symptoms. The major intracranial nerve sheath tumor is the vestibular schwannoma, also called acoustic neuroma or acoustic neurinoma (Fig. 9.2); it is a benign tumor that arises within the vestibular portion of the VIIIth cranial nerve. Pure schwannomas may also arise in other cranial nerves, particularly the trigeminal nerve. Schwannomas

account for 8% of intracranial tumors and represent about 30% of primary spinal tumors. Incidental acoustic neuromas found at autopsy from individuals dying of unrelated causes are even more common. One autopsy study suggests that acoustic neuromas may be present in over 2% of autopsies.[1] The incidence of vestibular schwannomas has increased from 7.8/10⁶ per year in 1976–83 to 12/10⁶ per year in 1990–95, probably a result of easier and better diagnosis with MRI. The peak age is between 40 and 60. Intracranial schwannomas are twice as common in women as in men.

Unilateral schwannomas are, for the most part, sporadic; bilateral vestibular schwannomas are pathognomonic of NF-2 (Chapter 12). All familial and 60% of sporadic schwannomas have a defect in the NF-2 tumor suppressor gene, but only patients with NF-2 have a germline mutation as well. The NF-2 gene is inactivated either by a point mutation leading to a truncated protein, or by loss of the short arm of chromosome 22 leading to complete loss of the protein. The NF-2 gene codes for a protein called 'merlin', a protein that regulates cell proliferation and motility.[2] Other common chromosomal abnormalities include a deletion at 1p.[3] No p53 mutations have been encountered.[4] Most acoustic neuromas express transforming growth factor beta-1 (TGF-β_1) in the cytoplasm of Schwann cells, tumor cells, blood vessel walls and the tumor capsule. This growth factor could promote tumor growth.[5] Other than NF-2, there are no established risk factors for vestibular schwannomas or other benign schwannomas of the peripheral or central nervous systems. In particular, head injury does not appear to be a risk factor.[6]

Vestibular schwannoma

Vestibular schwannomas are thought to arise near the zone of Obersteiner–Redlich. This is the area where oligodendroglial myelin gives way to Schwann cell myelin. The zone may occur near the exit of the vestibular nerve from the brain or further out laterally within the internal auditory canal. Current evidence suggests that about 50–60% of tumors arise from the superior vestibular nerve, 40–50% from the inferior vestibular nerve, and less than 10% from the cochlear nerve. Acoustic neuromas are classified by imaging into (1) small, less than 2-cm intracanalicular tumors, (2) medium-sized, extending beyond the internal auditory meatus but less than 3 cm, and (3) large, greater than 3 cm. Macroscopically, the tumors are typically firm, well-circumscribed and encapsulated. If they involve brain (i.e. cerebellum), they compress rather than invade it. They are relatively avascular, although on occasion they are hemorrhagic. The tumors are usually solid, although small cysts sometimes occur. Microscopically, the tumors are composed of what appear to be mature Schwann cells with relatively abundant, faintly eosinophilic cytoplasm. Nuclear pleomorphism and mitotic figures are sometimes seen but do not indicate malignancy. The tumors consist of so-called Antoni-A areas, represented by closely packed tumor cells, and Antoni-B areas, where cell density is much less. The Antoni-B areas dominate in vestibular schwannomas. Immunohistochemically, the tumors express S100 protein and sometimes glial fibrillary acidic protein (GFAP). MIB-1 labeling indices range from 0.3 to 6.6, with a mean of 1.7. In subtotally resected tumors there is a correlation between the labeling index and the rapidity of recurrence. Several variants have been described, including the cellular schwannoma, the plexiform schwannoma and the melanotic schwannoma. Although all three may occur in vestibular schwannoma, the cellular is the most common, and the histologic variant does not affect treatment or prognosis. However, these variants may occasionally be difficult to distinguish from other tumors, especially the melanotic schwannoma, and particularly when it occurs in the spinal canal.

The tumors are slow growing and, even if untreated, some may be stable or even regress over time.[7] On average, vestibular schwannomas are thought to increase at a rate of less than 2 mm per year, but growth can be slower or faster. Growth rate is usually slower in older than in younger patients. Serial imaging can sometimes predict growth rate. SPECT scanning using thallium chloride has been reported to be particularly useful in assessing tumor growth. It was found to be superior to MRI because it better quantifies tumor vascularity, essential for tumor growth.[8] Slow or absent growth over a period of 18 months to 3 years is said to make it unlikely that subsequent enlargement will be significant. Such patients can then be followed clinically and with scans at infrequent intervals, i.e. every 2 years.

Whether growth rate is controlled by hormones is unclear. Many of these tumors have estrogen and progesterone receptors and some are said to increase in size during pregnancy. Human vestibular schwannomas implanted into nude mice grew more rapidly when treated with estrogen, and this estrogen effect was blocked by tamoxifen.[9] Other growth factors may increase the tumor size by an autocrine mechanism.

Clinical findings

The symptoms and signs of a schwannoma depend on its location. The vestibular schwannoma (Fig. 9.2) usually presents with unilateral hearing loss, sometimes preceded or accompanied by tinnitus, and a vague feeling of 'dizziness' and unsteadiness when walking (Table 9.2).

In most patients, the symptoms of vestibular schwannoma begin with hearing loss without

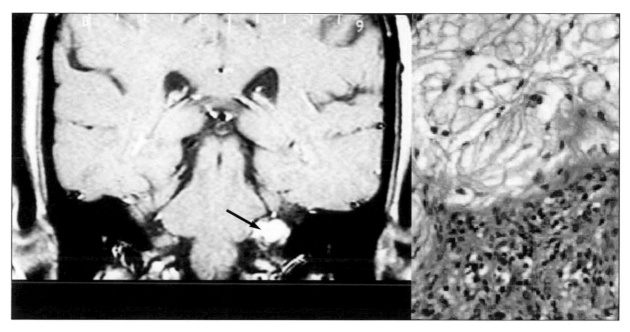

Figure 9.2
A vestibular schwannoma. This middle-aged woman presented with progressive hearing loss and mild tinnitus. She was an athlete and noticed that she was slightly more unsteady than she had been previously but not sufficient to interfere with function. Her neurologic examination was normal, save for hearing loss; at surgery, an acoustic neuroma was found (arrow). The photomicrograph shows the typical biphasic histological appearance with Antoni B-type loosely textured tissue (upper half) and Antoni A-type dense tissue (lower half).

Symptomatology	Percentage of patients	Average symptom duration (years)
Hearing loss		
Gradual	79	4.5
Sudden	10	2.0
Tinnitus	51	4.0
Dysequilibrium	41	3.6
Facial numbness	19	4.1
Headache	15	4.0
Facial weakness	9	6.0
Trigeminal neuralgia	5	8.8

From Janetta,[10] with permission.

Table 9.2
Presenting symptoms in 491 patients with vestibular schwannoma.[10]

other symptoms. The history is one of gradually declining hearing over many years. The patient may completely fail to notice the hearing loss until it is quite severe. If the schwannoma is on the left, the patient may recognize that he has unconsciously shifted the telephone from the accustomed left ear (to keep the dominant hand free for writing) to the right ear. Hearing loss usually begins in the high tones and often affects speech discrimination disproportionately. Accordingly, a few patients with even normal audiograms may complain of difficulty understanding what is said on the telephone. In about 10% of patients, the hearing loss begins suddenly and mimics the more common condition of idiopathic sudden hearing loss.[10] Accordingly, all patients with the sudden onset of unilateral hearing loss require evaluation for vestibular schwannoma.[11]

Because of the tumor's slow growth, the vestibular system is affected so slowly that central compensation for the peripheral vestibular loss often occurs without symptoms. In a minority of patients, the tumor may cause vertigo at onset or a feeling of dysequilibrium, as if being pushed to one side (away from the side of the lesion) when walking. Occasionally hyperventilation can induce nystagmus. Despite the lack of symptoms, by the time the patient presents for medical care, ipsilateral vestibular function, as tested by stimulating the semicircular canals, is usually absent. Other symptoms are extremely uncommon. About 1% of patients present with hemifacial spasm. About 10–20% complain of numbness in the face. Facial weakness, particularly a delayed blink response, may sometimes be apparent on examination but is rarely noticeable by the patient. Very large tumors have presented as contralateral facial numbness, facial pain, or facial spasm due to brainstem compression. Intratumoral hemorrhage or cyst formation may cause acute symptoms.

Table 9.3
Preoperative cranial nerve and other neurologic deficits in 190 patients with large vestibular schwannomas.

Cranial nerve abnormality	Percentage of patients
Vth nerve	
Corneal reflex	45.3
Facial numbness	31.6
VIIth nerve	4.7
IXth nerve	1.1
Xth nerve	1.6
Cerebellar ataxia	12.1
Nystagmus	20.0
Raised intracranial pressure	2.1
Neurofibromatosis type-2	14.2
Other diseases	8.4

From Lanman et al,[12] with permission.

Signs other than hearing loss and vestibular failure are associated with large tumors (> 3 cm) (Table 9.3). Ipsilateral decreased sensation in the face and particularly a decreased corneal reflex are common signs of a large tumor. Facial weakness, often subtle and manifested only by slowed or slightly decreased blinking on the involved side or failure of the ipsilateral platysma muscle to contract when the patient grimaces, occurs in some patients. Cerebellar ataxia, nystagmus and evidence of increased intracranial pressure occur as the tumors grow larger and compress the cerebellum and the IVth ventricle.

The diagnosis is established by MRI. The tumors are characteristically isointense with nerve on the T1-weighted image but they enlarge the involved nerve. They are isointense with cerebrospinal fluid (CSF) on the T2-weighted image and thus may not be visible. They contrast enhance intensely, making even small tumors clearly visible on most MR scans. **Magnetic resonance cisternography** using a heavily T2-weighted two-dimensional fast spin–echo technique allows one to see the internal auditory meatus and identify the spatial relationships between the facial nerve and the superior vestibular nerve as well as the relationship between blood vessels and cranial nerves in the internal auditory canal and in the cerebellopontine cistern. This technique should be of considerable benefit to the surgeon.[13,14] A recent report has suggested that screening by fast T2 magnetic resonance (MR) may be as efficacious and substantially cheaper than gadolinium-enhanced MR scan.[11] This is clinically relevant, because although about 10% of patients with vestibular schwannomas present with sudden deafness, far less than 1% of sudden deafness is caused by vestibular schwannomas. Thus, a large number of patients must be screened, to identify the rare patient with a tumor.

Several other laboratory tests are sometimes used in the diagnosis of vestibular schwannoma, including audiometry (which is usually abnormal but non-specific), caloric testing (also abnormal but non-specific), brainstem auditory evoked responses (which yield a pattern of retrocochlear loss with consistent abnormality of wave 5), stapedial reflex testing, electrocorticography and electroneuronography. Although all of these tests can be used to evaluate hearing function, none is as sensitive or specific for the diagnosis as the MR scan. Of patients with vestibular schwannomas, 4–5% have NF-2. About 10–20% of patients with NF-2 present with an apparently sporadic unilateral vestibular schwannoma. All patients with unilateral vestibular schwannomas require evaluation for other stigmata of NF-2 (Chapter 12)[15]

Differential diagnosis

The clinical differential diagnosis includes all causes of hearing loss, vestibular dysfunction or unilateral ataxia (Fig. 9.3). All of these are excluded by a high-resolution gadolinium-enhanced MR scan. Intracanalicular tumors are virtually always vestibular schwannomas. However, we recently encountered a patient with slowly progressive facial weakness and slight enhancement of the facial and acoustic nerve in the internal auditory canal. The tumor grew over 3 years and was believed to be an

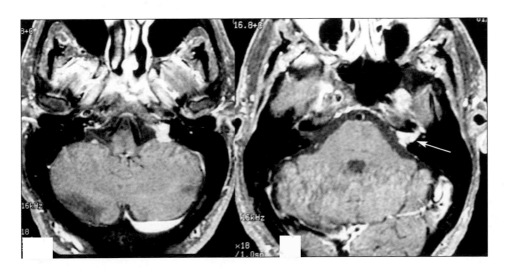

Figure 9.3
This patient presented with progressive facial weakness followed by hearing loss 2 years later (see text). Contrast enhancing tumor on the left involved the acoustic canal. A second tumor was found at the jugular foramen (arrow). Both turned out to be metastatic carcinomas.

unusual vestibular schwannoma (Fig. 9.3). At surgery, it turned out to be a carcinoma. The primary tumor was not identified but was believed by histologic characteristics to arise from an occult parotid or skin tumor that tracked back along the facial nerve into the internal auditory canal (neurotropic cancer).[16] Another patient with a similar clinical story had a lymphoma.

When the tumor is located more proximally near the cerebellum, the differential diagnosis includes other tumors that arise there, predominantly meningiomas and epidermoids (Chapter 12).[17] The distinction cannot always be made preoperatively between a cerebellopontine angle acoustic tumor or meningioma, but meningiomas are usually larger and do not track along the cranial nerve toward the internal auditory meatus. They do not enlarge the internal auditory meatus on CT scan, as do vestibular schwannomas. Symptoms of CPA meningiomas include ataxia and many present with hydrocephalus; only two-thirds have hearing loss.[17]

Treatment

The treatment of vestibular schwannomas has two goals. The first is to prevent the tumor from causing increased symptoms over time, i.e. cure the tumor. Unchecked, a tumor in the internal auditory canal that presents with hearing loss, with or without tinnitus, may later cause facial paralysis and eventually, as it grows more medially, dysfunction of other cranial nerves. A medially placed tumor will also compress the cerebellum, causing ataxia and eventually hydrocephalus. The larger the tumor, the more difficult the treatment.

The second goal is to preserve remaining intact neurologic function. Often, hearing loss is not complete and the goal is to maintain residual hearing function. In addition, preservation of facial nerve function is an important goal. These two goals are sometimes in conflict.

Although microsurgical techniques can frequently preserve hearing and facial nerve function, total extirpation of tumors, particularly large tumors, often requires sacrifice of the acoustic nerve and may damage the facial and trigeminal nerves. Total removal of a vestibular schwannoma cures the patient. A variety of surgical approaches have been recommended, including a translabyrinthine approach,[12] a middle cranial fossa approach,[18] and a suboccipital retrosigmoid approach for hearing preservation.[19,20] The approach depends largely on the location of the tumor and the presence or absence of preserved hearing. In expert hands, the size of the tumor is irrelevant and even large tumors can be resected in most instances. The operating microscope and more recently the endoscope[21] are useful tools. Sometimes the capsule is adherent to cranial nerves, making complete resection difficult. In those instances, a partial resection may preserve facial nerve function and the tumor may cease growing. Intraoperative monitoring of acoustic and facial nerves helps to preserve those functions.[22–25] Successful surgery does not improve hearing but, when hearing function is present, it can be preserved in approximately 50% of patients with small tumors. Facial nerve function can be preserved in up to 100% of patients with small tumors but in less than 50% of patients with tumors greater than 3 cm in size. Some patients develop severe facial paralysis despite anatomic preservation of the nerve. Most recover; if no recovery has occurred within a year, hypoglossal-facial anastomosis should be considered.[26]

Operative mortality is extremely low. Operative morbidity, however, is common. Headache, not present prior to surgery, occurs in about 50% of patients after vestibular schwannoma surgery and it can sometimes be quite severe and persistent.[27] Its cause is unknown.[28] The headache usually improves with time and responds to medical treatment that includes valproic acid and verapamil[29] but, if intractable, may be improved by a cranioplasty to repair the skull defect,[30] even in the absence of a CSF leak. Headache usually does not occur following a translabyrinthine approach. CSF leakage occurs in approximately 1–2% of patients, although figures vary from 1–20%.[31] Patients with CSF leakage, which is usually rhinorrhea, should be treated conservatively with a lumbar drain. If the leak is from the wound, additional sutures are placed. If the leakage does not repair itself by conservative treatment, re-exploration and occasionally CSF diversion may be necessary. Infectious meningitis is a very rare complication. It can occur either in the presence or absence of CSF leakage. Aseptic meningitis is more common; this complication is described in detail in Chapter 7. Decreased CSF pressure from the surgery or from lumbar drainage can cause transient low tone hearing loss, believed to be related to decreased perilymphatic pressure.[32] Patients generally recover spontaneously. Transverse sinus thrombosis leading to the syndrome of pseudotumor cerebri (increased venous and thus intracranial pressure resulting in headache, papilledema and visual obscuration) followed translabyrinthine or suboccipital craniectomy in 5% of 107 patients.[33] Two serious but rare complications of surgery are hematoma in the operative cavity and brainstem infarction. Infarction results from vasospasm of small vessels supplying the brainstem that are traumatized during the surgery. Less serious but common operative complications include tinnitus, not present preoperatively and rarely a significant problem,[34] taste dysfunction (reduced or distorted) and abnormal tearing (dry eye or tearing when eating – 'crocodile tears').[35]

In recent years, a number of physicians have recommended radiosurgery for acoustic neuromas smaller than 3 cm in diameter and some have suggested it is superior to surgery[36] as the preferred approach for most patients. A dose of 10–15 Gy is delivered to the tumor periphery and a maximum of 15–25 Gy to the center of the tumor. The entire dose can be delivered either as a single fraction or a few fractions. Radiosurgery has been delivered both by gamma knife and by linear accelerator,[37] the former giving a more restricted field. Local control, i.e. no growth of tumor, has been reported in over 90% of patients. Useful hearing has been preserved acutely in 75% of patients, a greater proportion than usual after surgery. Lower doses (14 Gy) improve hearing preservation.[36] Facial and trigeminal function are also reported to be better preserved after radiosurgery. However, acute hearing loss, delayed hearing loss, delayed facial paresis, either transient or permanent, and delayed trigeminal sensory loss occur in some patients within 2–3 years after the procedure, particularly with higher doses of radiation.[36] Fractionated stereotactic radiosurgery may be as effective as other treatments, with less cranial nerve dysfunction.[38] This approach may be most appropriate for patients with NF-2 and bilateral vestibular schwannomas, where even partial hearing preservation is a critical issue.

Undoubtedly, both surgery and radiosurgery will continue to play a role in the management of patients with vestibular schwannomas. Many tumors are too large to be treated by radiosurgery and demand a surgical approach. Sometimes surgery fails or the tumor regrows after surgery. Pathologic features including hyaline degeneration, cell density and the labeling index predict an increased likelihood of regrowth after surgery. In those instances, radiosurgery may be effective.[39] Conversely, radiosurgery sometimes fails, and those patients should be considered for surgery.[40] One note of caution is that tumors can temporarily expand after radiosurgery, and one must be certain that the tumor is increasing in size over time before approaching it surgically. Chemotherapy has no role to play in the treatment of these tumors.

Not all vestibular schwannomas grow. In one study, only half of the tumors grew over a 3-year period.[41] Thus, patients who refuse surgical or radiosurgical treatment, or who have a tumor in the sole hearing ear, or who are medically unable to undergo treatment, can be followed. No radiologic test, except perhaps SPECT scans,[8] predicts rate of growth.

Other schwannomas

Schwannomas can arise from other cranial nerves. Ocular nerve schwannomas are rare.[42,43] The most common involved nerve, other than the vestibular, is the trigeminal (Fig. 9.4), which represents only about 5% of all intracranial schwannomas and less than 1% of primary intracranial tumors (Fig. 9.4).[44] Like vestibular schwannomas, they occur during middle life and are slightly more common in

women than men. The schwannomas may arise from Schwann cells within the trigeminal (gasserian) ganglion, the nerve root, or one of the three divisions of the trigeminal nerve. About half are within the middle cranial fossa, 30% are within the posterior fossa, and 20% are dumbbell-shaped with extension into both cranial fossae.[45] Rarely, the tumor arises from extradural portions of the trigeminal nerve, presenting in the maxillary sinus, orbit or retropharyngeal space.[46]

Because the trigeminal nerve supplies somatic sensation, pain is much more common with schwannomas of the trigeminal than of the vestibular nerve. Most patients present with sensory loss or paresthesias in the face, usually involving all three divisions, although the sensory loss is not necessarily complete in the distribution of any of the divisions. In some patients, paroxysms of facial pain resembling trigeminal neuralgia are the presenting complaint.[47] Usually, such patients can be found to have sensory abnormalities on examination,

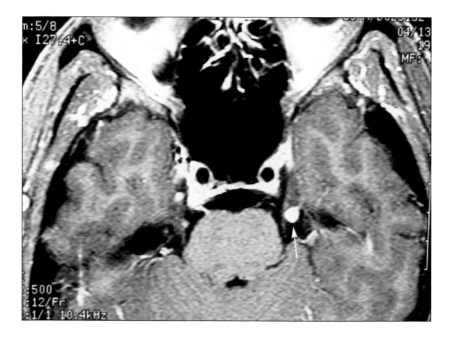

Figure 9.4
A trigeminal neurinoma (arrow). This 40-year-old man had an MRI after a mild concussion. He had no neurologic symptoms or signs. The tumor has not grown in 2 years.

Table 9.4
Symptoms and signs of trigeminal schwannomas.

Symptom	Percentage	Sign	Percentage
Trigeminal nerve dysfunction	55	Trigeminal nerve	
Numbness	27	Decreased sensation	74
Pain	23	Diminished or absent corneal reflex	68
Paresthesias	5	Pain	38
Headache	15	Motor weakness	39
Diplopia	10	Other cranial nerve deficits	
Hearing loss/tinnitus	8	II	10
Visual loss	5	III	14
Ear pain	3	IV	7
Other[a]	8	VI	35
		VII	23
		VIII	32
		IX, X	8
		XI	1

From Shrivastava et al,[49] with permission.
Only 27 patients (21%) had abnormal findings limited to the trigeminal nerve.
[a]Other symptoms, subarachnoid hemorrhage, vertigo, seizure, exophthalmus, gait difficulty, hemifacial spasm. Two patients had more than one initial symptom.

a finding not present with typical trigeminal neuralgia. Furthermore, the pain may persist between paroxysms and the pain usually lacks the trigger points characteristic of trigeminal neuralgia. Although sensory loss and pain limited to one division of the trigeminal nerve suggest that the lesion is within that division rather than the ganglion or the root, there is enough variability that the tumor cannot be localized by clinical examination alone.[48] As the tumor grows, it can compress other cranial nerves, causing diplopia, hearing loss, headache and ear pain (Table 9.4).

At the time of examination, most patients have sensory loss to a variable degree in all three sensory divisions of the trigeminal nerve, and about 40% of patients have some weakness of the muscles of mastication. As many as three-quarters of patients have findings referable to other cranial nerves (Table 9.4).

The diagnosis is made by MR scan.[48] The tumor is usually hyperintense on the T2-weighted image and hypo or isointense on the T1-weighted image with enhancement that is typically uniform but may show areas of necrosis, particularly in large tumors. The differential diagnosis includes other mass lesions that may arise along the distribution of the trigeminal nerve. In the posterior fossa and Meckel's cave, meningiomas, epidermoid tumors and aneurysms may mimic trigeminal schwannomas. In the cavernous sinus, meningiomas, lymphomas, metastases and aneurysms must be considered in the differential diagnosis. Neurotropic metastatic tumors (Chapter 13) may mimic peripheral trigeminal schwannomas, and other base of skull tumors may present with trigeminal symptoms (see below).[48]

Schwannomas of the trigeminal nerve do not differ in their pathologic findings from other schwannomas. The tumors are benign, but they may occasionally undergo malignant degeneration. Intratumoral hemorrhage can sometimes be found microscopically or grossly.

The treatment is surgical.[47] Total resection results in cure, whereas partial resection may be followed by tumor recurrence. The surgical mortality is low, less than 2%, but morbidity includes injury to other cranial nerves, CSF leak with meningitis, and sometimes, as in vestibular schwannomas, hydrocephalus, probably a consequence of blood spilled into the subarachnoid space. Most patients are left with permanent trigeminal dysfunction. Although experience is limited, radiosurgery has been reported to be safe and efficacious, and tumors may either cease growing or actually regress.[50,51]

Facial nerve schwannomas represent less than 2% of intracranial schwannomas. The patients present with facial weakness, tinnitus, hearing loss and, sometimes, vertigo (Table 9.5).

Because the facial nerve acquires its Schwann cell sheath closer to the brainstem than does the vestibular nerve, tumors can arise closer to the brainstem and cause brainstem compression as their initial symptom. The facial nerve also extends through the internal auditory canal along with the acoustic nerve, and these tumors can be mistaken for vestibular schwannomas when they arise intracanalicularly. The tumor can also present as a visible mass in the middle ear, causing conductive rather than sensorineural hearing loss. Otalgia and otorrhea may also be present.

The diagnosis is made by MR scan. The MR characteristics are the same as those of vestibular schwannomas. Because the facial nerve lies

Table 9.5

Signs and symptoms of facial nerve schwannomas.

Symptom	Percentage
Hearing loss	41–91
Tinnitus	60
Vertigo	34
Facial weakness	46–90
Sudden onset	20

From Shrivastava et al[49] with permission.

so close to the acoustic nerve through most of its course, it may be impossible to distinguish on scan whether the tumor has arisen in the facial or the vestibular nerve. However, clinical symptoms help the differentiation: vestibular schwannomas almost always begin with hearing loss, whereas facial schwannomas usually begin with facial weakness. The differential diagnosis includes meningiomas in the posterior fossa, vestibular schwannomas and other base of skull tumors.

Facial schwannomas, like vestibular schwannomas, may not enlarge over time and thus can be followed conservatively in some patients.[52] When appropriate, the treatment is surgical. Complete resection leads to cure. With modern microsurgical techniques, mortality is low. Facial paralysis is very common and hearing loss, either transient or permanent, occurs in about one-third of patients. The complications are similar to those of surgery for vestibular schwannomas. Because of the rarity of these tumors, the role of radiosurgery is not yet established. Some evidence suggests that radiosurgery is safe and efficacious.[50]

Schwannomas occasionally arise from the nerves exiting the **jugular foramen**.[53] This includes the glossopharyngeal, vagus and spinal accessory nerves. As with the facial nerve, these nerves acquire the Schwann cell sheath close to the brainstem (spinal cord in the case of the spinal accessory nerve), so the tumors may arise either within the posterior fossa or within the jugular foramen extracranially.[53] Posterior fossa tumors often present with hearing loss, facial numbness or occasionally hemifacial spasm resulting from compression of other cranial nerves. These tumors can grow to a large size and may cause brainstem or cerebellar dysfunction as their initial symptom. Cranial nerve dysfunction, including hoarseness, dysphagia, weakness or atrophy of the sternocleidomastoid and trapezius muscles, is more likely to occur from tumors within the jugular foramen than those nearer the brainstem. Unilateral tongue weakness and atrophy may occur from extracranial tumors compressing the hypoglossal nerve. Sometimes the jugular vein is compressed. Pressure on the vein can result in turbulent flow causing tinnitus,[54] or, if the compressed jugular vein is dominant, i.e. substantially larger than its partner, compression may sufficiently interfere with blood flow to cause increased intracranial pressure with papilledema.[55] The tumors are benign. Diagnosis by MR imaging and treatment are similar to those for vestibular schwannomas. The most serious postoperative complication is dysphagia, which may require a feeding tube, usually temporarily.[56] Dysphagia can follow either surgery or RT.[56]

Hypoglossal schwannomas are fairly rare (Table 9.6). Patients present with unilateral tongue dysfunction which may cause dysarthria but may also be asymptomatic. As the mass grows, it compresses brainstem, cerebellum or adjacent cranial nerves. Headache is common, along with dysfunction of adjacent vagus, glossopharyngeal and spinal accessory nerves. The diagnosis and treatment are similar to those of other schwannomas.

Table 9.6
Signs and symptoms of hypoglossal nerve schwannomas.

Major findings	Percentage	Less common findings
Headache	73	Tongue hemiatrophy
IX, X, XI nerve dysfunction	67	Vertigo
Limb weakness (spastic)	66	Nystagmus
Ataxia		Facial weakness
Dysarthria		Hearing loss

From Shrivastava et al[49] with permission.

Neurofibromas

Neurofibromas are not found in the intracranial cavity. They involve spinal or peripheral nerves but not cranial nerves. They are of interest when considering intracranial tumors because most are associated with NF-1 (Chapter 12). NF-1, in turn, is associated with a variety of intracranial tumors including schwannomas.

Malignant nerve sheath tumors

Malignant nerve sheath tumors, also called malignant schwannomas, are found primarily in peripheral nerves, including the brachial plexus and sciatic nerve. They may arise from a pre-existing neurofibroma or, much more rarely, a schwannoma, or they may arise de novo. Rarely, they are found in the intracranial cavity, involving cranial nerves.[57] The trigeminal nerve is most commonly affected, but the acoustic nerve, the facial nerve, including the nervus intermedius, and occasionally other cranial nerves can be involved. The tumors are often sporadic, but may be associated with NF-1, in which case they may be multiple. The tumors cannot be identified as malignant prior to surgery. They are treated with surgery followed by radiation but, unlike their more benign counterparts, they usually recur and may be responsible for the patient's death.

Skull base tumors

Introduction

Several tumors, both benign[58] and malignant, have a predilection to involve cranial nerves by affecting the base of the skull (Fig. 9.5). These include esthesioneuroblastomas (olfactory neuroblastoma), carcinomas or lymphomas of the paranasal sinuses, as well as paragangliomas that often arise from the glomus jugulare (glomus jugulare tumor) and rhabdomyosarcomas.[59] Chordomas characteristically arise either in the clivus, thus affecting cranial nerves, or in the sacrum, causing a cauda equina syndrome. They can, however, arise almost anywhere along the vertebral column, although less commonly than the two places cited above. Chondromas and chondrosarcomas, as well as tumors discussed elsewhere in this book, including meningiomas, schwannomas and pituitary adenomas, can also affect the skull base. Table 9.7 classifies these tumors by their relative incidence and common location.

Most skull base tumors are treated surgically if possible. All surgery of skull base tumors is difficult. The location of these tumors makes them hard to reach, and involvement of cranial

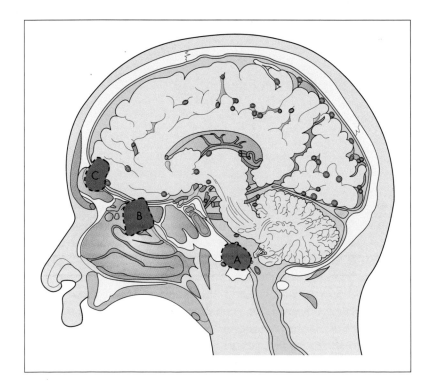

Figure 9.5
Some of the tumors that characteristically occur at the skull base. (A) Clivus chordoma. (B) Nasopharyngeal cancer. (C) Paranasal sinus (frontal) carcinoma.

Table 9.7
Cranial base tumors: type and relative occurrence.

Tumors	Percentage of intracranial tumors	Other data
Meningioma	20%	40–50% in cranial base
Vestibular schwannoma	6–8%	60–78% of cerebellopontine angle tumor
Trigeminal schwannoma	0.07–0.36%	0.8–8% of intracranial schwannomas
Jugular foramen schwannoma	< 1%	2.9% of intracranial schwannoma
Facial schwannoma	< 1%	0.8% of intrapetrous mass
		1.9% of all intracranial schwannomas
Other cranial nerve schwannoma	< 1%	Oculomotor, trochlear, abducens, hypoglossal: rare, case reports
Pituitary adenoma	7–15%	25% in autopsy of general population
Paraganglioma	0.01%	0.6% of all head–neck tumors
Chordoma	0.15–1%	3% of malignant bone tumors
Chondrosarcoma	< 1%	5% of cranial base tumors
Esthesioneuroblastoma		3% of all intranasal tumors
Nasopharyngeal carcinoma		3% of all head–neck cancers
Adenoid cystic carcinoma		1% of all head–neck cancers
		6% of salivary neoplasms
Primary sarcoma (rhabdomyosarcoma, Ewing's, fibrosarcoma, etc.)	4%	
Juvenile angiofibroma		< 0.5% of all head/neck neoplasms

From Morita and Piepgras with permission.

nerves makes increased dysfunction of those nerves a major operative risk. When the tumors are in the cavernous sinus, they can also involve the carotid artery, usually compressing rather than invading it. CSF leak after surgery represents another major risk because it is often hard to repair the bone and dura at the skull base. Nevertheless, there have been considerable advances in skull base surgery that have allowed neurosurgeons who specialize in that area to carry out substantial resection with reduced but still significant morbidity and mortality. In some instances of carotid artery involvement, a graft can be placed and the tumor better resected. Endoscopy of the posterior fossa sometimes allows tumor removal with minimal invasiveness, particularly for vestibular schwannomas.[61] The operating microscope has been a major advance in allowing neurosurgeons to separate tumor tissue from intertwined cranial nerves.

RT is also difficult for tumors at the skull base. Their intimate association with the cranial nerves and other intracranial structures sometimes prohibits the delivery of sterilizing doses to the tumor without side-effects. Often, these tumors appear to respond better and more safely to radiosurgery or heavy particle radiation. Chemotherapy plays an important role in some tumors, but most of the tumors that arise at the base of the skull are not sensitive to chemotherapy. However, the combination of surgery and RT has substantially improved survival in recent years.

Esthesioneuroblastoma (olfactory neuroblastoma)

Esthesioneuroblastoma is a rare malignant neuroectodermal tumor that is believed to originate from neurons of the olfactory epithelium high in the nasal cavity, usually involving the cribriform plate (Fig. 9.6). The tumor shows a slight male predominance and has a peak age at presentation in the second to fifth decades. However, small infants and elderly patients have occasionally been reported.

Little is known of the genetic alterations because of its rarity, but one study indicated multiple chromosomal changes with overrepresentation of chromosomes 4, 8, 11 and 14. Partial DNA gains on chromosomes 1 and 17, deletions of the entire chromosomes 16, 18, 19 and X, and partial losses of chromo-

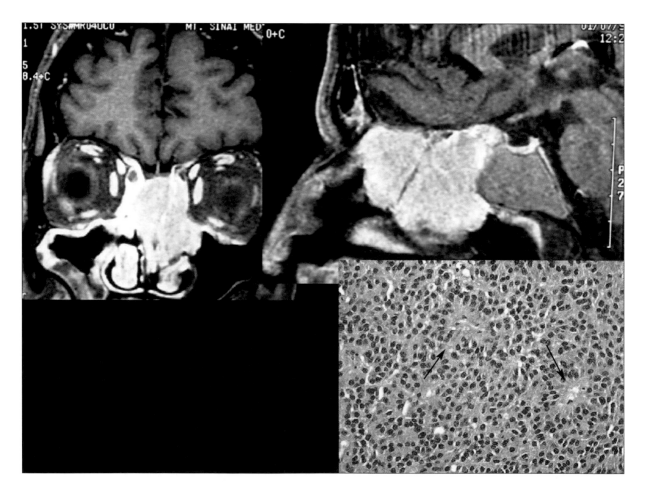

Figure 9.6
An esthesioneuroblastoma involving the cribriform plate. The patient did not have neurologic symptoms, only nasal obstruction and epistaxis. After surgery, he completely lost his sense of smell but was not particularly bothered by this. The photomicrograph shows monomorphic nests of round cells in a fibrillary background with occasional rosette formation (arrow).

somes 5q and 17p have been reported. These are unusual chromosomal aberrations.[62] Esthesioneuroblastomas do not have gene translocations similar to those that occur in Ewing's sarcoma, suggesting that the tumor is not a primitive neuroectodermal tumor.[63] Mutations in p53 have not been detected but there appears to be overexpression of wild-type p53 protein in subsets of the tumor that show aggressive behavior and a tendency for recurrence.[64]

Grossly, the tumor is highly vascular and may contain intratumoral hemorrhage. Microscopically, the tumor appears as a small round cell tumor, such as a poorly differentiated carcinoma, melanoma or other neuroectodermal tumor. Immunohistochemical stains are helpful because all of the neuroendocrine markers are positive. These include neuron-specific enolase, chromogranins, synaptophysin and the neuronal marker anti-Hu. Epithelial markers such as cytokeratin and epithelial membrane antigen (EMA) are absent. The MIB-1 index can be as high as 50%.

The tumor usually presents with nasal rather than neurologic symptoms. Patients complain of either nasal obstruction, epistaxis or both. Anosmia, either unilateral or bilateral, is present but the patient is often unaware of the symptom. As the tumor grows, it infiltrates adjacent structures, including the cribriform plate and base of the skull, sometimes compressing or invading the frontal lobes. It also invades paranasal sinuses and the oronasal pharynx. The tumor can metastasize to other organs and can seed the leptomeninges, in which case neurologic symptoms are inevitable.

CT, MR and radionuclide imaging are all helpful in the diagnosis. MRI gives the best estimate of tumor spread into the surrounding soft tissue areas and intracranial space. The tumor is hypo- or hyperintense on the T1-weighted image and usually hyperintense on the T2-weighted image. It uniformly contrast enhances. CT scan provides the best information concerning bone destruction, particularly of the cribriform plate and the orbit. Radionuclide scanning with octreotide, a somatostatin analog, shows uptake similar to that with other neural crest tumors, helping distinguish esthesioneuroblastoma from other neoplasms that may arise in the paranasal sinuses. The differential diagnosis includes all other tumors of the paranasal sinuses or nasal cavity, e.g. carcinomas and lymphomas.

Treatment includes radical surgical resection and postoperative RT.[65] Chemotherapy with cisplatin-based regimens improves survival, particularly in those with high-grade tumors.[66] Some investigators have advocated preoperative neoadjuvant therapy, including RT and chemotherapy prior to radical craniofacial resection. Such treatment has led to 5- and 10-year overall survival rates of 81% and 54.5% respectively.[67]

The prognosis is guarded. In most series, local recurrence appears in 30–70% of patients and regional lymph node or distant metastasis is as high as 40%. Recurrence may appear after many years in remission. Unfavorable prognostic factors include widespread or metastatic disease, a proliferative index greater than 10%, overexpression of wild-type p53, and aneuploid or polyploid chromosomes.

Paraganglioma

The paraganglioma is usually a benign tumor that originates in autonomic ganglia anywhere in the body. The cells are of neural crest origin and, pertinent to this book, can arise from paraganglionic tissues at the base of the skull.[68] The most common is the glomus jugulare tumor.[69] The tumors can arise from the glomus tympanicum and are found in the middle ear and mastoid; they can also arise from chemoreceptor cells in the adventitia of the jugular vein or the glomus intravagale, a collection of chemoreceptor cells on the auricular branch of the vagus nerve.

Paragangliomas are found largely in middle-aged women, with a peak incidence in the 5th decade. Bilateral glomus tumors occur in about 1–2% of patients. Familial occurrence is seen in about 10% of patients. In both familial and sporadic tumors, deletions occur on 11q.[70] In one study, mutations of p53 and p16 were noted at relapse but not in the initial tumor.[71]

Grossly, the tumors are red-brown, highly vascular and reasonably well-circumscribed. Histologically, they resemble a normal paraganglion and consist of pale 'chief' cells that are arranged in nests and lobules. Sustentacular (supporting cells – from Latin 'to hold upright') cells surround the lobules. Neuroendocrine markers, such as neuron-specific enolase and chromogranin, identify the chief cells. Sustentacular cells react with S-100 protein and sometimes show immunoreactivity with GFAP.

Tinnitus is the typical presenting complaint of the glomus jugulare tumor. The tinnitus is usually pulsatile and can often be heard by an observer who places a stethoscope over the mastoid or jugular vein. Other common findings include hearing loss and hoarseness due to involvement of the vagus nerve with vocal cord dysfunction. Ear pain occurs in a significant number of patients. In some individuals, a bluish tumor can be seen behind the eardrum on otoscopic inspection. The tumors are quite slow growing, and progression of symptoms is usually slow. About 1% of tumors may secrete catecholamines, causing palpitations, intermittent hypertension and anxiety. The tumor occasionally occludes the transverse sinus, but rarely presents as pseudotumor cerebri.

The diagnosis is suggested by MR scan. The lesions have variable intensity on the T1-weighted image but are hyperintense on the T2-weighted image; multiple flow voids and a heterogeneously contrast-enhancing mass are characteristic. An MR angiogram reveals the extreme vascularity of these tumors. Scintigraphy using either iodine-123-labeled metaiodobenzylguanidine or indium-111-labeled pentetreotide suggests a neuroendocrine tumor. In secreting tumors, the diagnosis can be suggested by a 24-h urinary assay for catechols. For such patients, catecholamine secretion must be blocked prior to surgery, usually by administration of α-adrenergic blocking agents before and during surgery. The differential diagnosis can include any tumor that involves the skull base, but the high vascularity and slow progression strongly suggest a glomus tumor.

Surgery and radiation are the modes of treatment. Total resection can sometimes be achieved and, if so, the patient is usually cured.[72] In lesions not amenable to surgery, local control can be achieved in over 90% of patients.[73] For subtotal resection, RT in the postoperative period delays recurrence. Embolization prior to surgery will decrease the vascularity and sometimes make total excision possible. Vocal cord paralysis, swallowing difficulty, facial paralysis, hearing loss and CSF leak are among the major complications of surgery.

The tumors are usually benign but recurrence is common after partial resection, even with postoperative RT. A few tumors become malignant and metastasize. Radiosurgery has been reported to decrease tumor volume and vascularity in some patients.

Chordoma

Chordomas are tumors of notochordal origin. They characteristically arise in the clivus (Fig. 9.7) or sacral spinal cord. Although benign and slow growing, they tend to recur and

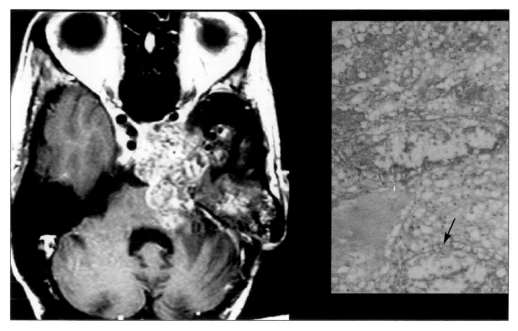

Figure 9.7
A clival chordoma. This young woman presented in 1979 with progressive quadriparesis. A clinical diagnosis of multiple sclerosis was made, but when CT scanning became available, a mass was revealed that was believed to be intrinsic to the brainstem. At exploration, nothing was found. Subsequently, as imaging improved, a mass was found to be compressing the brain from the clivus and was partially resected. It turned out to be a chordoma. She was treated with multiple operations, standard radiation therapy and finally proton beam radiation. She lived for over 20 years but suffered multiple recurrences. The photomicrograph shows nodules of vacuolated physaliphorous tumor cells (arrow).

sometimes late in their course may metastasize to bone or lungs. This tumor usually occurs in middle age without any specific sex preponderance.

Chordomas constitute less than 0.5% of intracranial tumors. They are believed to arise from vestigial remnants of the interosseous primitive notochord. Little is known about the genetics of chordomas. One study demonstrated loss of heterozygosity in intron 17 of the retinoblastoma (RB) gene in two of seven chordomas which may serve as a marker for aggressive behavior.[74] Another study of familial clivus chordomas (an exceedingly rare entity) demonstrated a rearrangement between chromosomes 1 and 9, with variable losses of chromosome 1p. Other cytogenetic abnormalities have been identified in sporadic chordomas; 1p appears to be involved frequently.

The tumor has a characteristic appearance consisting of lobules of pleomorphic, vacuolated, physaliphorous (from Greek for 'bubble' and 'bearing') cells scattered in a mucoid or myxoid matrix. Some workers have divided chordomas into typical chordomas and chondroid chordomas, the latter with some evidence of cartilage formation. Chondroid chordomas are believed to have a somewhat better prognosis. Histochemically, the tumors react with cytokeratin, S-100 protein and vimentin. The typical and chondroid tumors do not differ in labeling index. The MIB-1 index of recurrent tumors is considerably higher than that of primary tumors. p53 and cyclin D1 labeling, which indicate mutations in these genes, also correlate with recurrence and a high MIB-1 labeling index.[75]

The most common presenting symptoms of clival chordomas are diplopia, headache and, less commonly, visual disturbances and ataxia. Because the tumors often arise from the base of the clivus, bilateral VIth nerve palsies are a highly suggestive sign. Other lower cranial nerves can be affected, either singly or in combination. Symptoms are often subtle at onset and progress insidiously, so that tumors are usually large when the diagnosis is established.

Imaging usually establishes the diagnosis. The MR image varies on the T1-weighted scan but the tumor is hyperintense on the T2-weighted image and irregular enhancement is usually seen. Contrast material enhances chordomas more slowly than it does other tumors at the skull base, often taking several minutes to reach maximum enhancement.[76] Therefore, if the post-contrast images are obtained too quickly, the enhancement may be missed. On CT scan there is clear evidence of bone destruction and sometimes calcification in the lesion. Rarely, the bone is not involved. The location of the intracranial chordoma is characteristic. Other tumors of bone, however, can occur in a similar position (Table 9.8), and thus definitive diagnosis requires biopsy.

The primary treatment is surgical. Patients who undergo total or near-total resection survive substantially longer than patients with a partial resection. Whatever the degree of resection, RT is required in the postoperative period.

Table 9.8
Differential diagnosis of chordomas and chondrosarcomas.

- Pituitary adenoma
- Craniopharyngioma
- Meningioma
- Schwannoma
- Nasopharyngeal carcinoma
- Salivary gland tumors
- Metastasis

Women treated with radiation do less well than men. Radiosurgery has been suggested for small lesions.[77] Others have recommended charged particle radiation.[78] Ten-year control rates for skull base chordomas using mixed-beam proton–photon therapy are 65% for men and 42% for women.[79] Reoperation at recurrence sometimes helps but the tumors relentlessly recur, eventually causing death.

As indicated above, the prognosis is poor. Age is the most significant factor associated with longer overall and disease-free survival, with younger patients doing better than older patients. Diplopia is associated with longer survival, probably because it is a symptom which initiates early medical evaluation. The degree of resection and postoperative RT also predict longer survival.

Chondrosarcomas

Both the more benign chondroma and the more malignant chondrosarcoma can develop at the skull base. These are tumors of cartilage cells or their precursors. The chondrosarcomas are divided into two categories: myxoid and mesenchymal. The classic chondrosarcoma is composed of mature cartilage plus malignant chondrocytes that are frequently multinucleated. The de-differentiated chondrosarcoma is

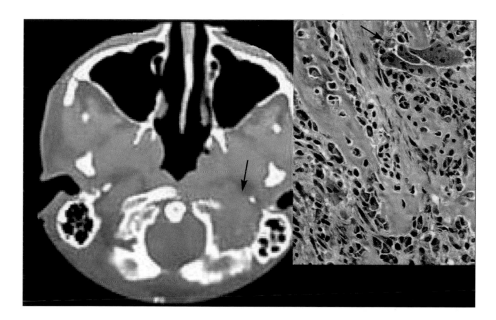

Figure 9.8
An osteoblastoma destroying the base of the skull and causing hearing loss. The tumor presented with tinnitus and hearing loss and progressed very slowly. The CT scan revealed bone destruction (arrow). Biopsy revealed an osteoblastoma, an unusual base of skull tumor. The photomicrograph shows an osteoid trabecula lined by uniform large osteoblasts, and stromal giant cells (arrow).

histologically indistinguishable from a malignant fibrohistiocytoma. The mesenchymal chondrosarcoma is composed of undifferentiated round or small cells which may be anti-Hu positive, suggesting neuronal differentiation; they tend to occur in younger people and often originate from the sphenoid or petrous bone. Chondrosarcomas may be subclassified histologically into grades I–III, with the higher grades behaving in a more aggressive fashion. Rarely, osteoblastomas also affect the skull base (Fig. 9.8).

Chondrosarcomas (and even osteogenic sarcomas) are occasionally found within the parenchyma of the brain or the dura.[80] They are usually a result of metastasis from a distant tumor but, rarely, they are primary brain tumors. Lower-grade chondrosarcomas are sometimes associated with Ollier's disease,[81] a rare syndrome characterized by multiple enchondromas; when Ollier's disease is associated with multiple hemangiomas, it is called Maffucci syndrome.[82] Both the enchondromas

and hemangiomas can become malignant, and Ollier and Maffucci syndromes have also been associated with gliomas.

The clinical picture depends on where the tumor arises. The middle and posterior fossae are common sites. MR images show high intensity on T2-weighted images, and enhancement is irregular. Chondrosarcomas differ from chordomas in that they tend to be more laterally placed. The lateral placement makes them more accessible to surgery and probably leads to a better prognosis than that of chordomas.

The treatment, whatever the grade, is surgery. The lowest-grade tumors are often cured by surgery alone. Partial resection or complete resection of a high-grade tumor requires postoperative RT. Charged particle radiation has been recommended, as it has for chordomas, because it can deliver highly focused radiation which will spare surrounding critical structures. Proton–photon therapy yields a 10-year control rate of 94%.[79] Because the tumor grows slowly, recurrences may be late. The 5-year recurrence-free survival rate may be as high as 90% following surgery and conventional RT. One study reports a 10-year local control rate of 98% after 64–80 Gy of conformal radiation therapy,[83] but not without hypothalamic/pituitary dysfunction.[84] There is no established chemotherapy for this tumor; one report describes a durable response to ifosfamide–doxorubicin chemotherapy.[85]

Tumors of nasopharynx and paranasal sinuses

A group of tumors arise in the nasopharynx or the paranasal sinuses and may involve the skull base, presenting with neurologic symptoms and signs (Fig. 9.9). The tumors vary in their histology and include squamous cell cancers, adenocarcinomas and nasopharyngeal cancers,

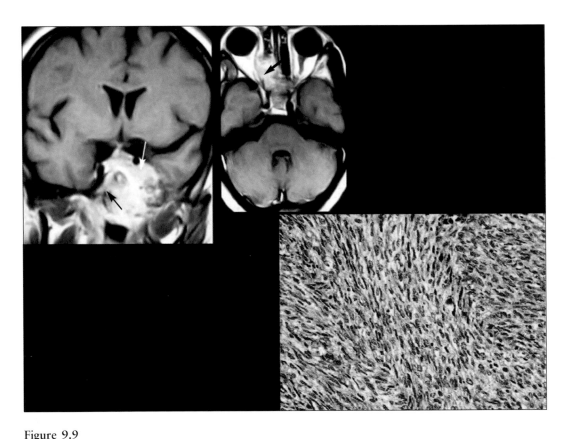

Figure 9.9
This 40-year-old woman developed left facial pain in 1993. She was treated for Lyme disease but the pain persisted and she developed left-sided headaches and eventually some hearing loss on the left, which was believed to be conductive. An MRI in 1995 (left) showed an enhancing tumor in the ethmoid sinus invading the base of the brain and surrounding the carotid arteries (arrows). The tumor was resected and she received postoperative radiation therapy. She was followed with serial scans and felt reasonably well until June 1998, when she began feeling face pain on the right side; again, diagnosis was delayed but, by December, she noticed that her right eye was bulging. There was no diplopia. A repeat scan at that time (right) showed recurrent tumor invading the orbit, causing proptosis and lateral deviation of the right eye (arrow). A reoperation was done. The tumor was a low-grade fibrosarcoma. It recurred several months later. The photomicrograph shows interlacing fascicles of spindle cells with atypical nuclei and low mitotic index.

including lymphoepithelial carcinoma and lymphoma. They also differ in their epidemiology. Tobacco plays a role in the pathogenesis of squamous cell cancers, as do some occupational hazards such as nickel refining. Asbestos inhalation and woodworking play a role in adenocarcinoma. Nasopharyngeal carcinoma is 20 times more common in Asians than in North Americans, and has a particular predilection in those of southern Chinese origin. Two major risk factors appear to be salted fish as a dietary staple and exposure to the Epstein–Barr virus (EBV). Interleukin-10, whose sequence is homologous to an open reading frame of EBV, is expressed in about one-half of nasopharyngeal carcinomas and is negatively associated with survival.[86] Genetic changes have been described and depend on the specific tumor.[87,88]

Most patients present with local symptoms, but involvement of cranial nerves can be the first symptom. Local symptoms depend on the tumor site. Paranasal sinus and nasal tumors cause nasal obstruction and epistaxis, as can nasopharyngeal carcinomas. If the tumor invades the orbit, proptosis can be an early symptom, usually associated with diplopia but not visual loss. These tumors affect the anterior base of the skull and, in addition to headache, can cause other neurologic symptoms such as anosmia, visual disturbances from compression of the optic nerves or diplopia from compression of ocular motor nerves in or near the cavernous sinus. Facial pain and sensory disturbance may also occur. Hearing loss with nasopharyngeal carcinoma is usually unilateral and can be conductive, due to occlusion of the eustachian tubes by the tumor.

The diagnosis is suggested by MR scanning. In those patients who present with cranial nerve palsies, a CT scan will often better identify bone destruction of the skull base. The diagnosis can only be established by biopsy.

Paranasal sinus carcinomas are best treated by surgery if possible.[89] In some individuals, preoperative radiation and/or chemotherapy may shrink the tumor sufficiently to make surgery feasible. If not administered prior to surgery, resection should be followed by RT and chemotherapy. Nasopharyngeal carcinomas are generally not surgically accessible. RT and chemotherapy are the treatment modalities of choice. Even when radiation is successful, several months may elapse before biopsies become negative.[90] Some have suggested that concurrent chemo-radiotherapy, followed by adjuvant chemotherapy, may be more effective.[91]

The prognosis depends upon the extent and degree of malignancy of the tumor. In nasopharyngeal carcinoma, disease-free survival can be as high as 65% with aggressive treatment.[92] It is substantially lower, about 35%, in paranasal sinus tumors. RT of nasal and paranasal tumors may lead to delayed retinopathy.[93] Conformal radiation therapy reduces the dose to optic nerves and chiasm, thus diminishing the risk of late complications.[94] Temporal lobe necrosis is a late complication of treatment of nasopharyngeal carcinoma. MRS may show temporal lobe abnormalities before the MRI does.[95]

References

1. Wiegand DA, Ojemann RG, Fickel V. Surgical treatment of acoustic neuroma (vestibular schwannoma) in the United States: report from the Acoustic Neuroma Registry. Laryngoscope 1996; 106: 58–66.
2. Reed N, Gutmann DH. Tumorigenesis in neurofibromatosis: new insights and potential therapies. Trends Mol Med 2001; 7: 157–62.
3. Leone PE, Bello MJ, Mendiola M et al. Allelic status of 1p, 14q, and 22q and NF2 gene mutations in sporadic schwannomas. Int J Mol Med 1998; 1: 889–92.

4. Monoh K, Ishikawa K, Yasui N et al. p53 tumor suppressor gene in acoustic neuromas. Acta Otolaryngol Suppl (Stockh) 1998; 537: 11–5.

5. Cardillo MR, Filipo R, Monini S et al. Transforming growth factor-beta1 expression in human acoustic neuroma. Am J Otol 1999; 20: 65–8.

6. Inskip PD, Mellemkjaer L, Gridley G, Olsen JH. Incidence of intracranial tumors following hospitalization for head injuries (Denmark). Cancer Causes Control 1998; 9: 109–16.

7. Charabi S, Tos M, Thomsen J, Charabi B, Mantoni M. Vestibular schwannoma growth: the continuing controversy. Laryngoscope 2000; 110: 1720–5.

8. Charabi S, Thomsen J, Tos M et al. Acoustic neuroma vestibular schwannoma growth: past, present and future. Acta Otolaryngol (Stockh) 1998; 118: 327–32.

9. Stidham KR, Roberson JBJ. Effects of estrogen and tamoxifen on growth of human vestibular schwannomas in the nude mouse. Otolaryngol Head Neck Surg 1999; 120: 262–4.

10. Jannetta PJ. Vestibular neurilemmomas. Clin Neurosurg 1997; 44: 529–48.

11. Daniels RL, Shelton C, Harnsberger HR. Ultra high resolution nonenhanced fast spin echo magnetic resonance imaging: cost-effective screening for acoustic neuroma in patients with sudden sensorineural hearing loss. Otolaryngol Head Neck Surg 1998; 119: 364–9.

12. Lanman TH, Brackmann DE, Hitselberger WE, Subin B. Report of 190 consecutive cases of large acoustic tumors (vestibular schwannoma) removed via the translabyrinthine approach. J Neurosurg 1999; 90: 617–23.

13. Kumon Y, Sakaki S, Ohue S et al. Usefulness of heavily T2-weighted magnetic resonance imaging in patients with cerebellopontine angle tumors. Neurosurgery 1998; 43: 1338–43.

14. Ryu H, Tanaka T, Yamamoto S et al. Magnetic resonance cisternography used to determine precise topography of the facial nerve and three components of the eighth cranial nerve in the internal auditory canal and cerebellopontine cistern. J Neurosurg 1999; 90: 624–34.

15. Evans DGR, Lye R, Neary W et al. Probability of bilateral disease in people presenting with a unilateral vestibular schwannoma. J Neurol Neurosurg Psychiatry 1999; 66: 764–7.

16. McCord MW, Mendenhall WM, Parsons JT, Flowers FP. Skin cancer of the head and neck with incidental microscopic perineural invasion. Int J Radiat Oncol Biol Phys 1999; 43: 591–5.

17. Mallucci CL, Ward V, Carney AS, O'Donoghue GM, Robertson I. Clinical features and outcomes in patients with non-acoustic cerebellopontine angle tumours. J Neurol Neurosurg Psychiatry 1999; 66: 768–71.

18. Gjuric M, Wigand ME, Wolf SR. Enlarged middle fossa vestibular schwannoma surgery: experience with 735 cases. Otol Neurotol 2001; 22: 223–30.

19. Magliulo G, Sepe C, Varacalli S, Fusconi M. Cerebrospinal fluid leak management following cerebellopontine angle surgery. J Otolaryngol 1998; 27: 258–62.

20. Irving RM, Jackler RK, Pitts LH. Hearing preservation in patients undergoing vestibular schwannoma surgery: comparison of middle fossa and retrosigmoid approaches. J Neurosurg 1998; 88: 840–5.

21. Göksu N, Bayazit Y, Kemaloglu Y. Endoscopy of the posterior fossa and dissection of acoustic neuroma. J Neurosurg 1999; 91: 776–80.

22. Mullatti N, Coakham HB, Maw AR, Butler SR, Morgan MH. Intraoperative monitoring during surgery for acoustic neuroma: benefits of an extratympanic intrameatal electrode. J Neurol Neurosurg Psychiatry 1999; 66: 591–9.

23. Roberson JB Jr, Jackson LE, McAuley JR. Acoustic neuroma surgery: absent auditory brainstem response does not contraindicate attempted hearing preservation. Laryngoscope 1999; 109: 904–10.

24. Axon PR, Ramsden RT. Intraoperative electromyography for predicting facial function in vestibular schwannoma surgery. Laryngoscope 1999; 109: 922–6.

25. Colletti V, Fiorino FG. Advances in monitoring of seventh and eighth cranial nerve function during posterior fossa surgery. Am J Otol 1998; 19: 503–12.

26. Kunihiro T, Kanzaki J, Shiobara R, Inoue Y, Kurashima K. Long-term prognosis of profound facial nerve paralysis secondary to acoustic

neuroma resection. ORL J Otorhinolaryngol Relat Spec 1999; 61: 98–102.

27. Levo H, Pyykkö I, Blomstedt G. Postoperative headache after surgery for vestibular schwannoma. Ann Otol Rhinol Laryngol 2000; 109: 853–8.

28. Levo H, Blomstedt G, Pyykkö I. Vestibular schwannoma surgery and headache. Acta Otolaryngol (Stockh) 2000; 23–5.

29. Hanson MB, Glasscock ME III, Brandes JL, Jackson G. Medical treatment of headache after suboccipital acoustic tumor removal. Laryngoscope 1998; 108: 1111–4.

30. Wazen JJ, Sisti M, Lam SM. Cranioplasty in acoustic neuroma surgery. Laryngoscope 2000; 110: 1294–7.

31. Brennan JW, Rowed DW, Nedzelski JM, Chen JM. Cerebrospinal fluid leak after acoustic neuroma surgery: influence of tumor size and surgical approach on incidence and response to treatment. J Neurosurg 2001; 94: 217–23.

32. Stoeckli SJ, Bohmer A. Persistent bilateral hearing loss after shunt placement for hydrocephalus. Case report. J Neurosurg 1999; 90: 773–5.

33. Keiper GL Jr, Sherman JD, Tomsick TA, Tew JM, Jr. Dural sinus thrombosis and pseudotumor cerebri: unexpected complications of suboccipital craniotomy and translabyrinthine craniectomy. J Neurosurg 1999; 91: 192–7.

34. Levo H, Blomstedt G, Pyykko I. Tinnitus and vestibular schwannoma surgery. Acta Otolaryngol Suppl 2000; 543: 28–9.

35. Irving RM, Viani L, Hardy DG, Baguley DM, Moffat DA. Nervus intermedius function after vestibular schwannoma removal: clinical features and pathophysiological mechanisms. Laryngoscope 1995; 105: 809–13.

36. Flickinger JC, Kondziolka D, Niranjan A, Lunsford LD. Results of acoustic neuroma radiosurgery: an analysis of 5 years' experience using current methods. J Neurosurg 2001; 94: 1–6.

37. Spiegelmann R, Lidar Z, Gofman J et al. Linear accelerator radiosurgery for vestibular schwannoma. J Neurosurg 2001; 94: 7–13.

38. Fuss M, Debus J, Lohr F et al. Conventionally fractionated stereotactic radiotherapy (FSRT) for acoustic neuromas. Int J Radiat Oncol Biol Phys 2000; 48: 1381–7.

39. Pollock BE, Lunsford LD, Flickinger JC, Clyde BL, Kondziolka D. Vestibular schwannoma management. Part I. Failed microsurgery and the role of delayed stereotactic radiosurgery. J Neurosurg 1998; 89: 944–8.

40. Pollock BE, Lunsford LD, Kondziolka D et al. Vestibular schwannoma management. Part II. Failed radiosurgery and the role of delayed microsurgery. J Neurosurg 1998; 89: 949–55.

41. Selesnick SH, Johnson G. Radiologic surveillance of acoustic neuromas. Am J Otol 1998; 19: 846–9.

42. Asaoka K, Sawamura Y, Murai H, Satoh M. Schwannoma of the oculomotor nerve: a case report with consideration of the surgical treatment. Neurosurgery 1999; 45: 630–3.

43. Kawasaki A. Oculomotor nerve schwannoma associated with ophthalmoplegic migraine. Am J Ophthalmol 1999; 128: 658–60.

44. Friedman RA, Pensak ML, Osterhaus D, Tew JMJ, van Loveren HR. Trigeminal schwannomas: the role of the neurotologist in multidisciplinary management. Otolaryngol Head Neck Surg 1999; 120: 355–60.

45. Yoshida K, Kawase T. Trigeminal neurinomas extending into multiple fossae: surgical methods and review of the literature. J Neurosurg 1999; 91: 202–11.

46. Krishnamurthy S, Holmes B, Powers SK. Schwannomas limited to the infratemporal fossa: report of two cases. J Neurooncol 1998; 36: 269–77.

47. Samii M, Migliori MM, Tatagiba M, Babu R. Surgical treatment of trigeminal schwannomas. J Neurosurg 1995; 82: 711–8.

48. Nemzek WR. The trigeminal nerve. Top Magn Reson Imaging 1996; 8: 132–54.

49. Shrivastava RK, Strauss R, Post KD. Other schwannomas of cranial nerves. In: Kaye AH, Laws Jr ER eds. Brain tumors: An encyclopedic approach. Edinburgh: Churchill Livingstone, 2001: 687–709.

50. Mabanta SR, Buatti JM, Friedman WA, Meeks SL, Mendenhall WM, Bova FJ. Linear accelerator radiosurgery for nonacoustic schwannomas. Int J Radiat Oncol Biol Phys 1999; 43: 545–8.

51. Huang CF, Kondziolka D, Flickinger JC, Lunsford LD. Stereotactic radiosurgery for trigeminal schwannomas. Neurosurgery 1999; 45: 11–16.

52. Van Den Abbeele T, Viala P, Francois M, Narcy P. Facial neuromas in children: delayed or immediate surgery? Am J Otol 1999; 20: 253–6.

53. Kanemoto Y, Ochiai C, Yoshimoto Y, Nagai M. Primary extracranial jugular foramen neurinoma manifesting with marked hemiatrophy of the tongue: case report. Surg Neurol 1998; 49: 534–7.

54. Meador KJ, Swift TR. Tinnitus from intracranial hypertension. Neurology 1984; 34: 1258–61.

55. Graus F, Slatkin NE. Papilledema in the metastatic jugular foramen syndrome. Arch Neurol 1983; 40: 816–18.

56. Périé S, Coiffier L, Laccourreye L et al. Swallowing disorders in paralysis of the lower cranial nerves: a functional analysis. Ann Otol Rhinol Laryngol 1999; 108: 606–11.

57. Akimoto J, Ito H, Kudo M. Primary intracranial malignant schwannoma of trigeminal nerve. A case report with review of the literature. Acta Neurochir (Wien) 2000; 142: 591–5.

58. Eisenberg MB, Al-Mefty O, DeMonte F, Burson GT. Benign nonmeningeal tumors of the cavernous sinus. Neurosurgery 1999; 44: 949–54.

59. Paulino AC. Role of radiation therapy in parameningeal rhabdomyosarcoma. Cancer Invest 1999; 17: 223–30.

60. Morita A, Piepgras DG. Tumors of the skull base. In: Vecht CJ, ed. Handbook of clinical neurology, Vol. 68: Neuro-oncology Part 2. Amsterdam: Elsevier Science, 1997: 465–96.

61. Jennings CR, O'Donoghue GM. Posterior fossa endoscopy. J Laryngol Otol 1998; 112: 227–9.

62. Szymas J, Wolf G, Kowalczyk D, Nowak S, Petersen I. Olfactory neuroblastoma: detection of genomic imbalances by comparative genomic hybridization. Acta Neurochir (Wien) 1997; 139: 839–44.

63. Mezzelani A, Tornielli S, Minoletti F et al. Esthesioneuroblastoma is not a member of the primitive peripheral neuroectodermal tumour Ewing's group. Br J Cancer 1999; 81: 586–91.

64. Papadaki H, Kounelis S, Kapadia SB et al. Relationship of p53 gene alterations with tumor progression and recurrence in olfactory neuroblastoma. Am J Surg Pathol 1996; 20: 715–21.

65. Eich HT, Staar S, Micke O et al. Radiotherapy of esthesioneuroblastoma. Int J Radiat Oncol Biol Phys 2001; 49: 155–60.

66. McElroy EA Jr, Buckner JC, Lewis JE. Chemotherapy for advanced esthesioneuroblastoma: The Mayo Clinic experience. Neurosurgery 1998; 42: 1023–7.

67. Polin RS, Sheehan JP, Chenelle AG et al. The role of preoperative adjuvant treatment in the management of esthesioneuroblastoma: The University of Virginia experience. Neurosurgery 1998; 42: 1029–37.

68. Reithmeier T, Gumprecht H, Stolzle A, Lumenta CB. Intracerebral paraganglioma. Acta Neurochir (Wien) 2000; 142: 1063–6.

69. Robertson JH, Gardner G, Cocke EWJ. Glomus jugulare tumors. Clin Neurosurg 1994; 41: 39–61.

70. Bikhazi PH, Messina L, Mhatre AN, Goldstein JA, Lalwani AK. Molecular pathogenesis in sporadic head and neck paraganglioma. Laryngoscope 2000; 110: 1346–8.

71. Gran S, Tali T. p53 and p16INK4A mutations during the progression of glomus tumor. Pathol Oncol Res 1999; 5: 41–5.

72. Sen C, Hague K, Kacchara R et al. Jugular foramen: Microscopic anatomic features and implications for neural preservation with reference to glomus tumors involving the temporal bone. Neurosurgery 2001; 48: 838–47.

73. Springate SC, Weichselbaum RR. Radiation or surgery for chemodectoma of the temporal bone: a review of local control and complications. Head Neck 1990; 12: 303–7.

74. Eisenberg MB, Woloschak M, Sen C, Wolfe D. Loss of heterozygosity in the retinoblastoma tumor suppressor gene in skull base chordomas and chondrosarcomas. Surg Neurol 1997; 47: 156–60.

75. Matsuno A, Sasaki T, Nagasima T et al. Immunohistochemical examination of proliferative potentials and the expression of cell cycle-related proteins of intracranial chordomas. Hum Pathol 1997; 28: 714–9.

76. Ikushima I, Korogi Y, Hirai T et al. Chordomas of the skull base: dynamic MRI. J Comput Assist Tomogr 1996; 20: 547–50.

77. Muthukumar H, Kondziolka D, Lunsford LD, Flickinger JC. Stereotactic radiosurgery for chordoma and chondrosarcoma: further

experiences. Int J Radiat Oncol Biol Phys 1998; 41: 387–92.

78. Hug EB, Loredo LN, Slater JD et al. Proton radiation therapy for chordomas and chondrosarcomas of the skull base. J Neurosurg 1999; 91: 432–9.

79. Munzenrider JE, Liebsch NJ. Proton therapy for tumors of the skull base. Strahlenther Onkol 1999; 175 Suppl 2: 57–63.

80. Oruckaptan HH, Berker M, Soylemezoglu F, Ozcan OE. Parafalcine chondrosarcoma: an unusual localization for a classical variant. Case report and review of the literature. Surg Neurol 2001; 55: 174–9.

81. Hofman S, Heeg M, Klein JP, Krikke AP. Simultaneous occurrence of a supra- and an infratentorial glioma in a patient with Ollier's disease: more evidence for non-mesodermal tumor predisposition in multiple enchondromatosis. Skeletal Radiol 1998; 27: 688–91.

82. Ramina R, Coelho NM, Meneses MS, Pedrozo AA. Maffucci's syndrome associated with a cranial base chondrosarcoma: case report and literature review. Neurosurgery 1997; 41: 269–72.

83. Rosenberg AE, Nielsen GP, Keel SB et al. Chondrosarcoma of the base of the skull: a clinicopathologic study of 200 cases with emphasis on its distinction from chrodoma. Am J Surg Pathol 1999; 23: 1370–8.

84. Pai HH, Thornton A, Katznelson L et al. Hypothalamic/pituitary function following high-dose conformal radiotherapy to the base of skull: demonstration of a dose-effect relationship using dose-volume histogram analysis. Int J Radiat Oncol Biol Phys 2001; 49: 1079–92.

85. La Rocca RV, Morgan KW, Paris K, Baeker TR. Recurrent chondrosarcoma of the cranial base: a durable response to ifosfamide-doxorubicin chemotherapy. J Neurooncol 1000; 41: 281–3.

86. Fijieda S, Lee K, Sunaga H et al. Staining of interleukin-10 predicts clinical outcome in patients with nasopharyngeal carcinoma. Cancer 1999; 85: 1439–45.

87. Hui AB, Lo KW, Leung SF et al. Detection of recurrent chromosomal gains and losses in primary nasopharyngeal carcinoma by comparative genomic hybridisation. Int J Cancer 1999; 82: 498–503.

88. Caruana SM, Zwiebel N, Cocker R et al. p53 alteration and human papilloma virus infection in paranasal sinus cancer. Cancer 1997; 79: 1320–8.

89. Le QT, Fu KK, Kaplan M et al. Treatment of maxillary sinus carcinoma – a comparison of the 1997 and 1977 American Joint Committee on Cancer staging systems. Cancer 1999; 86: 1700–11.

90. Kwong DLW, Nicholls J, Wei WI et al. The time course of histologic remission after treatment of patients with nasopharyngeal carcinoma. Cancer 1999; 85: 1446–53.

91. Tan EH, Chua ET, Wee J et al. Concurrent chemoradiotherapy followed by adjuvant chemotherapy in Asian patients with nasopharyngeal carcinoma: toxicities and preliminary results. Int J Radiat Oncol Biol Phys 1999; 45: 597–601.

92. Lin JC, Jan JS. Locally advanced nasopharyngeal cancer: long-term outcomes of radiation therapy. Radiology 1999; 211: 513–8.

93. Takeda A, Shigematsu N, Suzuki S et al. Late retinal complication of radiation therapy for nasal and paranasal malignancies: relationship between irradiated-dose area and severity. Int J Radiat Oncol Biol Phys 1999; 44: 599–605.

94. Brizel DM, Light K, Zhou SM, Marks LB. Conformal radiation therapy treatment planning reduces the dose to the optic structures for patients with tumors of the paranasal sinuses. Radiother Oncol 1999; 51: 215–8.

95. Chong VFH, Rumpel H, Aw YS et al. Temporal lobe necrosis following radiation therapy for nasopharyngeal carcinoma: ¹H MR spectroscopic findings. Int J Radiat Oncol Biol Phys 1999; 45: 699–705.

10

Pituitary and sellar region tumors

Introduction

The pituitary (Latin for 'phlegm') or hypophysis (Greek for 'undergrowth') sits in a bony indentation of the skull base called the sella turcica. Its superior surface is covered by dura called the diaphragma sella, through which passes the pituitary stalk connecting the pituitary gland with the hypothalamus (Fig. 10.1). The diaphragm sella is pain-sensitive; its nerve supply is from the ophthalmic division of the trigeminal nerve. In about 20% of individuals, the diaphragma sella is incompetent, potentially allowing cerebrospinal fluid (CSF) from the suprasellar cistern to enter the sella turcica. Lateral to the pituitary gland are the paired cavernous sinuses, which contain the carotid artery, the nerves to the extraocular muscles (oculomotor–cranial nerve III; trochlear–cranial nerve IV; and abducens–cranial nerve VI) and the first division of the trigeminal nerve–cranial nerve V. Below the floor of the sella is the

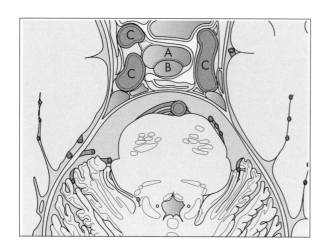

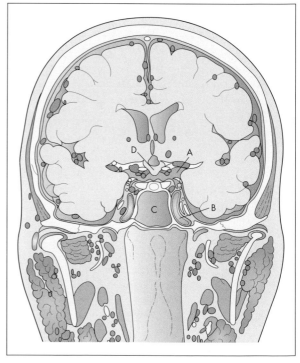

Figure 10.1
The pituitary gland and its relationships to surrounding structures. Left horizontal plane: (A) adenohypophysis, (B) neurohypophysis, (C) cavernous sinus with carotid artery. Right coronal plane: (A) optic chiasm, (B) cavernous sinus, (C) sphenoid sinus, (D) hypothalamus.

sphenoid sinus. Above the diaphragma sella and within the suprasellar cistern is the optic chiasm, which contains crossing fibers of the optic nerve from each of the retinas. Above the optic chiasm is the hypothalamus, that secretes the releasing factors that regulate pituitary function and are transmitted to the pituitary gland via the stalk.

The pituitary gland is actually two structures: an anterior portion (adenohypophysis), a true endocrine gland, and a posterior portion (neurohypophysis), an extension of the hypothalamus, i.e. neural tissue; both secrete hormones. The anterior pituitary secretes growth hormone (GH), prolactin (PRL), corticotropin (ACTH), thyroid-stimulating hormone (TSH) and the gonadotropins, luteinizing hormone (LH), and follicle-stimulating hormone (FSH). The posterior pituitary secretes arginine vasopressin, an antidiuretic hormone (ADH), and oxytocin, a regulator of smooth muscle contraction important for lactation and uterine contraction. Tumors of the anterior pituitary are common and almost uniformly benign.[1,2] Tumors of the posterior pituitary are rare[3] and, with few exceptions (e.g. granular cell tumors), do not differ from those that arise elsewhere in the brain. Tumors not of pituitary origin can affect either the gland itself (e.g. metastases) or areas in proximity to the sella (e.g. in the suprasellar cistern or the optic chiasm). These sellar region, but non-pituitary, tumors are also discussed in this chapter (Table 10.1).

Anterior pituitary tumors

Introduction

Pituitary tumors are the third most common primary intracranial neoplasms, exceeded only by gliomas and meningiomas; they account for 10–15% of all primary intracranial tumors encountered in clinical practice. Their incidence ranges from 1–14/100 000 annually in various clinical series, and their prevalence at autopsy varies from 5% to 25%. In one autopsy series, incidental pituitary adenomas larger than 2 mm, and thus identifiable on MR scan, were found in 1.7% of the population.[4] An additional 4.4% of pituitary glands had other lesions greater than 2 mm (i.e. focal hyperplasia, Rathke cysts). Another series reported a 9% incidence of lesions of unspecified size.[5] The most recent study reported adenomas in 24% of 100 glands, 10 of which were lactotrophs and 12 were nonfunctioning. Granular cell tumors were found in 9%.[6] Most of the tumors were < 3 mm. Thus, all pituitary lesions identifiable on MR scan are not necessarily symptomatic. Clinically, pituitary tumors are more common in women than in men, but in autopsy series they appear to be equally common in both sexes.

Pituitary tumors can be classified in several ways:

1. By size. Microadenomas are tumors less than 1 cm in diameter and macroadenomas are those larger than 1 cm. Microadenomas cause symptoms by excessive secretion of hormones not under normal feedback control from the hypothalamus. Macroadenomas cause their symptoms

Table 10.1
Classification of pituitary and sellar region tumors

I	Pituitary adenomas and carcinomas
II	Posterior pituitary tumors
III	Metastases to pituitary gland and stalk
IV	Germ cell tumors (Chapter 8)
V	Craniopharyngiomas
VI	Optic nerve and chiasm tumors (Chapter 5)
VII	Rathke cleft cysts

either by excessive hormone secretion or by compressing normal glandular or neural structures.

2. By endocrine function. Pituitary adenomas are divided into those that secrete hormones and those that are chemically inactive. Chemically inactive adenomas can cause symptoms only when they grow large enough to compress other structures, i.e. become macroadenomas.
3. By clinical findings.[1]
4. By histology.[7] Almost all pituitary adenomas are benign. They are identified microscopically by uniformity of cells with disruption of the normal acinar patterns. The tumors are usually well demarcated by a pseudocapsule consisting of reticulin and compressed normal gland. Mitoses and proliferative indices are usually low, but invasiveness is common. Dural invasion, cellular pleomorphism, increased cellularity, necrosis or aneuploidy do not necessarily imply aggressive biological activity.[9] Mitotic activity and p53 immunoreactivity may imply decreased likelihood of cure. Immunohistochemistry and electron

microscopy are very useful because they can define the hormones secreted by the tumor and thus allow for a functional classification.[7]

Pituitary tumors arise clonally from a single cell-type within the pituitary gland (Table 10.2). Some pituitary adenomas secrete the hormone(s) from their cell of origin, whereas others lose the capacity to secrete hormones. Virtually all pituitary adenomas escape feedback control and thus, if they secrete hormones, they do so excessively, leading to endocrine abnormalities.

Etiology

Pituitary adenomas are monoclonal tumors whose only established genetic defect occurs in patients with multiple endocrine neoplasia syndrome type I (MEN I).[2,10] This autosomal dominant condition is characterized by spontaneous development of tumors of the anterior pituitary, pancreatic islets and parathyroid glands. Pituitary adenomas,

Table 10.2
Classification of pituitary adenomas.

Cell type	Clinical prevalence[a] (%)	Hormone secreted	Endocrine syndrome
Lactotroph	27	Prolactin	Galactorrhea, amenorrhea (women) Impotence (men)
Somatotroph	21	Growth hormone ± prolactin	Acromegaly
Corticotroph	8	ACTH	Cushing's syndrome, ± Nelson's syndrome
Thyrotroph	1	Thyroid stimulating hormone	Hyperthyroidism
Gonadotroph	6	FSH, LH	None or hypogonadism
Null cell	35	None	Hypopituitarism

[a] Data from Thapar and Laws based on 3000 surgically treated pituitary adenomas.[9]

usually associated with GH, ACTH or PRL hypersecretion, occur in about 25% of such patients. MEN I is associated with both micro- and macroadenomas, mostly PRL secreting. The genetic abnormality is allelic loss of a tumor suppressor gene called menin at 11q13.[10] The function of the menin protein is unknown, but it reacts with the metastasis-suppressor nm23.[10] MEN I patients account for no more than a few percent of pituitary tumors, but deletions of the 11q13 locus, where menin resides, have been found in sporadic pituitary tumors.[9] The G-protein oncogene, GSPT1 is mutated in 30–40% of patients with acromegaly. This mutation in the α-chain of the G-protein results in constitutive activity of adenyl cyclase. Adenomas with G-protein mutations are significantly smaller than those without mutations and may be more sensitive to inhibitory factors such as somatostatin or dopamine. Amplification of C-fos and point mutations in H-ras oncogenes have been shown in isolated prolactinoma cases. A number of growth factors have been identified in the pituitary and it is believed that growth factor mediated autocrine and paracrine stimulation may be important in pituitary tumor development.

Clinical findings diagnosis

Pituitary adenomas cause their symptoms by abnormal hormone secretion (found in about 70% of pituitary adenomas) or by compression of normal glandular and neural structures.[11,12] As macroadenomas outgrow the sella turcica, they compress neural structures including ocular motor nerves laterally and the optic chiasm and hypothalamus superiorly. An occasional pituitary adenoma erodes the floor of the sella turcica and presents as a mass in the sphenoid sinus or nasopharynx.

Endocrine abnormalities

Table 10.2 lists the various syndromes caused by hypersecretion of particular hormones. The clinical symptoms are detailed in the paragraphs on specific tumor types (see below). Macroadenomas, by compressing surrounding normal glandular elements, can lead to hypo-secretion of one or more pituitary hormones (Table 10.3).

Gonadotrophs are most vulnerable to compression. Loss of libido, amenorrhea, and impotence are often the presenting symptoms in patients with large pituitary adenomas. TSH and GH are the next most vulnerable cell types.

Table 10.3
Some symptoms and signs of pituitary failure.

- Gonadotroph failure
  Loss of libido
  Impotence
  Osteoporosis
- Thyrotroph failure
  Fatigue, malaise
  Apathy, slow cognition
  Myalgias
  Carpal tunnel syndrome
  Constipation
  Delayed reflexes
  Weight gain
  Deep voice
- Somatotroph failure
  Reduced strength (muscle mass)
  Central obesity
  Premature atherosclerosis
  Depression, anxiety, emotional lability
- Corticotroph failure
  Fatigue
  Weight gain
  Hypoglycemia
- Vasopressin (posterior pituitary)
  Polydipsia
  Frequent urination (especially nocturia)
  Thirst

GH deficiency has subtle but important effects in adults,[13] and GH deficiency can mimic other diseases because of its psychiatric and cardiac manifestations. Hypothyroidism with its vague and protean symptoms of fatigue and malaise may be a confusing presenting complaint. Hypoadrenalism is rare. Prolactin levels may be elevated in patients with non-secreting pituitary adenomas, because the hypothalamus controls PRL by releasing inhibitors, of which dopamine is the most important. Thus, compression of the pituitary stalk by a macroadenoma decreases the output of most anterior pituitary hormones, but may increase output of PRL. PRL levels caused by stalk compression rarely rise above 200 ng/ml, which is easily distinguished from the usually high PRL levels (2500 ng/ml) seen with PRL-secreting adenomas. Diabetes insipidus, although a common finding in pituitary metastases and seen transiently after pituitary surgery, is almost never a presenting complaint of pituitary adenoma. Sudden pituitary failure may be caused by pituitary apoplexy (see below).

Non-endocrine findings (Table 10.4)

Headache is frequently an early symptom, probably due to stretching of the diaphragma sella. The headache is non-specific, usually felt as a dull bifrontal or vertex pain and, like headache from other brain tumors, is often more intense in the morning. In some patients, as the tumor grows and the diaphragma sella is ruptured, the headache disappears. As the tumor grows superiorly, above the diaphragma sella, it encounters the optic chiasm (Fig. 10.2). Compression of that structure may lead to bitemporal hemianopia of which the patient is often unaware. Thus, the first symptom of a pituitary tumor may be an automobile accident

Table 10.4
Non-endocrine signs and symptoms.

Symptoms	Signs
Headache	Extraocular muscle paresis
Peripheral visual loss	Bitemporal hemianopsia or unilateral optic neuropathy
Sudden blindness Loss of consciousness	Optic neuropathy

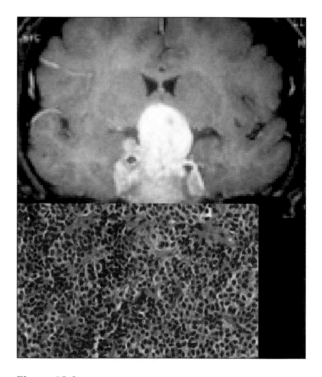

Figure 10.2
Large prolactin-secreting pituitary adenoma. The patient is a middle-aged physician who developed impotence but had no other symptoms. The tumor responded completely to bromocriptine. The photomicrograph shows loss of acinar architecture with sheets of neoplastic cells with round nuclei, basophilic cytoplasm and distinct cell borders.

because of the patient's lack of peripheral vision. Depending on the exact location of the optic structures and the site of suprasellar tumor growth, one optic nerve anterior to the chiasm may be compressed, causing unilateral visual loss with optic atrophy and rarely a temporal visual defect in the opposite eye, a junctional scotoma.[14] If the tumor grows laterally rather than anteriorly, it compresses the cavernous sinus, causing ptosis (oculomotor nerve), diplopia (oculomotor, trochlear or abducens nerve), or facial numbness (trigeminal nerve). Very large pituitary adenomas can compress the hypothalamus, causing dementia, drowsiness, hypo- or hyperphagia, emotional disturbances and obstructive hydrocephalus from compression of the 3rd ventricle.

For reasons not entirely understood, both large and small pituitary adenomas have a tendency to either bleed or infarct spontaneously, causing pituitary apoplexy.[15] The vascular insult usually occurs spontaneously but may result from cerebral angiography or during provocative endocrine testing; it also occurs with greater frequency during pregnancy. The result is sudden enlargement of the pituitary tumor and spillage of hemorrhagic or necrotic material into the suprasellar cistern and the subarachnoid space. The clinical symptoms include sudden onset of visual loss, ocular palsies, acute hypopituitarism, and alteration in consciousness varying from confusion to coma. Fever and nuchal rigidity may suggest the diagnosis of bacterial or viral meningitis. The CSF may contain blood or white cells, the latter in response to spilled necrotic material. Most patients respond to conservative treatment, replacing absent hormones and using corticosteroids to suppress inflammation. In some patients, emergency decompression of the enlarged pituitary is necessary to relieve symptoms. Untreated pituitary apoplexy can be fatal.

Laboratory evaluation

If a pituitary abnormality is suspected, high-resolution MRI with gadolinium enhancement and 1 mm sections through the pituitary fossa will establish the diagnosis in most instances, even when microadenomas are as small as 2–3 mm (Fig. 10.3). The physician who suspects a pituitary adenoma should tell the radiologist that he requires 'fine sections' and rapid imaging during bolus contrast administration, particularly for a suspected microadenoma. With macroadenomas, the MRI also establishes the spatial relationship between the tumor and important surrounding neural structures. Characteristically, the tumor is isointense on T1 and variably iso- to hypointense on T2. Immediately after injection of contrast, the tumor is hypointense on T1 compared to normal gland, which has no blood–brain barrier and therefore enhances diffusely. Later it becomes isointense with the contrast-enhanced normal gland. About 10% of prolactinomas calcify, which is best seen on CT scan. A CT scan of the pituitary fossa is particularly valuable in identifying acute hemorrhages in patients with pituitary apoplexy and may help with the differential diagnosis of pituitary tumor versus meningioma by identifying the hyperostosis of bone characteristic of a meningioma.

A second approach to diagnosis is measurement of hormones in the blood. Both hyper- and hyposecretion of pituitary hormones can be identified by blood measurement. Hormone levels not only help establish the diagnosis of the tumor cell type, but are also useful to follow tumor response to treatment and to identify post-treatment hypopituitarism. Careful neuro-ophthalmologic examination with special attention to visual fields and ocular movements will determine whether

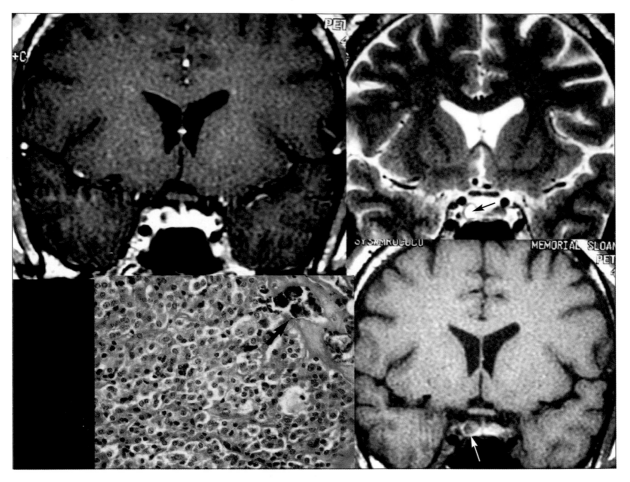

Figure 10.3
A prolactin-secreting microadenoma in an adult male with sexual difficulties. Microadenomas are generally found on MR scan by their failure to enhance as rapidly as normal pituitary during dynamic injection of contrast material. This particular prolactinoma, which responded to bromocriptine therapy with normalization of the prolactin level, was actually seen before contrast as a hypointense 5 mm lesion (arrow lower right). It was also hyperintense on the T2-weighted image (arrow upper right), possibly because of cystic degeneration. The photomicrograph shows a chromophobe adenoma. A psammomatous concretion is also present (arrow).

macroadenomas have substantially interfered with neurologic function. An occasional patient whose tumor has eroded the floor of the sella may develop a CSF leak. All patients with macroadenomas should be questioned concerning the presence of rhinorrhea. If rhinorrhea is present, measurement of the nasal fluid glucose is helpful and easily accomplished using urine dipsticks. If measurable glucose is present, the fluid is CSF; if absent, it may or may not be CSF. Transferrin, a protein present only in CSF, is more specific,[16] but requires collection of an adequate fluid specimen.

Differential diagnosis

In most instances, MR scans will distinguish pituitary neoplasms from other masses of the sella turcica (Table 10.5).

MRI cannot distinguish pituitary adenomas from the much rarer pituitary carcinomas;[9] that distinction requires biopsy. Tumors of neurohypophyseal origin, which are quite rare, may be hard to distinguish from those of adenohypophyseal origin. Tumors of non-pituitary origin, such as craniopharyngiomas, germ cell tumors, meningiomas and hypothalamic gliomas, are generally easily distinguishable because they either spare the pituitary fossa or invade it only after filling the suprasellar area. Dermoids and epidermoids, Rathke's cleft cysts and the empty sella syndrome (from CSF in the sella) have different signal intensity on MRI from pituitary tumors. Carotid aneurysms rarely mimic pituitary adenoma, and MR scan characteristics easily differentiate these.

One diagnostic problem involves metastasis to the pituitary gland (Fig. 10.4).[20] Carcinomas of the breast have a predilection to metastasize to the pituitary, but other cancers may also do this. Unlike pituitary adenomas, the first symptom is usually diabetes insipidus from

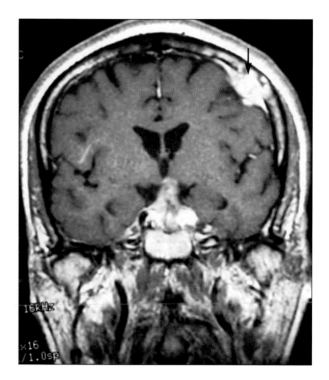

Figure 10.4
A pituitary metastasis in a man with advanced colon cancer. He presented with rapidly developing visual loss. A diagnosis of pituitary apoplexy was made. At surgery, both the pituitary tumor and the dural tumor (arrow) were metastases.

invasion of either the pituitary stalk or the neurohypophysis. Sometimes the tumor also invades the subarachnoid space, allowing one to make a diagnosis of metastatic tumor by examining the CSF. The clinical situation also helps establish the diagnosis of pituitary metastasis, which usually occurs in the setting of disseminated tumor. Occasionally a diagnosis is not possible on the basis of imaging or CSF examination, and biopsy is the only option.

The most difficult differential diagnosis is between certain inflammatory conditions and pituitary adenoma. Lymphocytic hypophysitis and giant cell granulomas of the pituitary often present with hypopituitarism, particularly

Table 10.5
Sellar and suprasellar masses: differential diagnosis.

- Pituitary adenoma
- Craniopharyngioma
- Meningioma
- Rathke cleft cyst
- Carotid aneurysm
- Langerhans' cell histiocytosis (see Chapter 11)
- Lymphocyte hypophysitis
- Pituitary granuloma
- Teratoma[17] (Chapter 9)
- Pituitary abscess[18]
- Pituitary lymphoma[19]

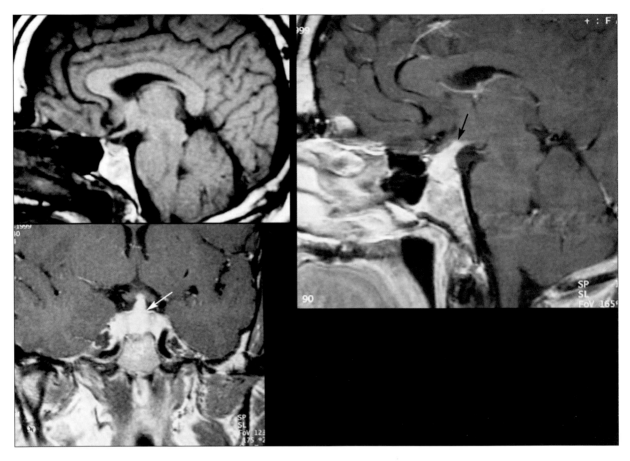

Figure 10.5
Lymphocytic hypophysitis mimicking a pituitary tumor. The intense enhancement of the infundibulum (arrows) was suggestive of inflammation rather than tumor, as was the fact that 2 months previously (upper left) the patient had a scan for non-specific headaches which was negative.

hypothyroidism; diabetes insipidus is common (Fig. 10.5).[21,22] A CSF pleocytosis may be present.[23] The inflammatory lesion enlarges the sella and mimics pituitary adenomas on MR scan; however, the frequent enhancement of the stalk and inferior hypothalamus is often a clue that the process is inflammatory and not an adenoma. Because their treatment is non-surgical, i.e. corticosteroid therapy,[24] the physician should consider all patients, particularly pregnant or postpartum young women, with rapidly developing hypothyroidism and an enlarging sella turcica to be suffering from a possible inflammatory condition and consider a trial of steroids.

Treatment

Surgery
For most pituitary adenomas, the treatment is surgical.[2,25] Microadenomas not causing symptomatic hormonal dysfunction may just be followed, and some prolactinomas[26] and GH secreting adenomas[27] may be successfully

treated with pharmacologic suppression of hormone hypersecretion (see below). For patients who require surgery, neurosurgeons with extensive experience in pituitary surgery have substantially better results than those who are less experienced. In most patients, the tumor can be reached from below through a transsphenoidal approach. Transsphenoidal surgery takes advantage of access to the skull base and sella turcica via the nose and air sinuses. The original early surgical approach to pituitary tumors via a frontal craniotomy was abandoned in the late 1950s because of its limited exposure and the inability of the surgeon to see the anatomy and pathology adequately. In the 1960s, the introduction of the operating microscope into neurosurgery, with its powerful illumination and magnification, made the transsphenoidal approach the procedure of choice for resection of pituitary tumors. A few very large tumors that do not enlarge the sella turcica to allow good surgical access, or that spill laterally and cannot be reached through the sella from below, may require a craniotomy and transfrontal approach. Surgery is both safe and efficacious. It has an additional advantage of establishing the correct diagnosis. In one study, a preoperative diagnosis of non-functioning pituitary adenoma was incorrect in 4 out of 22 patients.[28] Operative mortality and morbidity rates from several series are generally 0.5% and 2.2% respectively. The most common complication is CSF rhinorrhea predisposing to meningitis. Cognitive dysfunction has been reported to follow both transfrontal and transsphenoidal surgery, with the former associated with more severe impairment.[29] Rare complications include traumatic injury to the hypothalamus resulting in coma or death, laceration of the carotid artery and damage to the optic chiasm. These benign tumors may rarely seed the meninges after operation.[30]

Diabetes insipidus may also be a complication of surgery (usually transient) but is easily controlled by appropriate hormonal therapy. Postoperative hypopituitarism is uncommon and can also be controlled by hormonal therapy. About 50% of patients who have evidence of hypopituitarism preoperatively recover some endocrine function.[31] Persistent postoperative hormone hypersecretion, even if MRI demonstrates complete tumor removal, mandates additional pharmacologic therapy and/or radiotherapy.

Radiation therapy

Radiation therapy (RT) using doses of 45–50 Gy in 1.8-Gy fractions is also effective at reducing tumor growth.[32] Radiation is indicated for persistent or recurrent, medically refractory hypersecreting adenomas, or administered postoperatively to patients with invasive or large, incompletely removed tumors.[33] Late complications include hypopituitarism, and rarely with modern radiation techniques, optic nerve, hypothalamic or temporal lobe damage. These effects usually develop within a year or two. Years later, as a very late-delayed effect, secondary brain tumors may appear.[34] Excluding of the above complications, radiation therapy does not cause cognitive dysfunction.[29] Unlike surgery, radiation may take years to normalize elevated hormone levels. Radiosurgery may produce more rapid hormonal and clinical responses with similar or less toxicity than conventional RT,[35,36] but it cannot be used for large tumors or those < 3 mm from the optic nerve or chiasm. Charged particle beams have been advocated by some.[37]

Pharmacologic therapy

Some pituitary adenomas have proved sensitive to pharmacologic treatment.[38] PRL-secreting tumors that require therapy can be treated with dopamine agonists to inhibit the output of

PRL. These drugs substantially reduce the size of prolactinomas and control their growth. Bromocriptine and pergolide were the most frequently used agents, but cabergoline is more effective and better tolerated and is now the drug of choice.[26,39] The drug need be given only twice weekly. Somatostatin and its analogs, such as octreotide, have been used in the management of tumors associated with acromegaly.[27] However, the degree of tumor shrinkage is not as dramatic as with dopamine agonist therapy of prolactinomas. In selected patients, somatostatin analogs may be primary therapy, but they are usually reserved to control symptoms if surgery and radiotherapy fail. Gene therapy of pituitary tumors, still in its infancy, may hold hope for the future.[40]

Treatment complications

Aside from the usual complications of surgery and RT,[41] patients treated for pituitary adenomas are at increased risk of cerebral infarction, probably related to the combination of endocrine dysfunction and RT, both of which may accelerate atherosclerosis.[42]

Specific anterior pituitary tumors

Prolactinomas (Table 10.6)

PRL-secreting pituitary adenomas are the most common clinically recognized tumor of the pituitary gland, accounting for about one-third of symptomatic tumors. They occur in both sexes but are most common in young women and older men. Women usually present with amenorrhea and galactorrhea as a consequence of PRL excess; some present with infertility. Men present with headache and visual loss from the enlarging mass or sometimes with impotence or gynecomastia. The lack of early

Table 10.6
Signs and symptoms of prolactinomas.

Women	Men
Amenorrhea	Impotence
Galactorrhea	Decreased libido
Decreased libido	Gynecomastia
Infertility	

endocrine symptoms in men may explain why tumors in men are generally larger than those in women. Fewer than 10% of PRL-secreting microadenomas evolve into macroadenomas; the others seem not to grow after they are identified, or even regress spontaneously.[7] The diagnosis is made on the basis of MR imaging and PRL levels. A PRL level in excess of 200 ng/ml is, with rare exceptions,[43] diagnostic of a prolactinoma, while levels in excess of 1000 ng/ml suggest that the prolactinoma is invasive. The treatment of choice is pharmacologic.[26,39] PRL levels are controlled with dopamine agonists in almost all microadenomas;[44] about 60% of patients with macroadenomas respond with > 80% tumor shrinkage.[45] In women with the amenorrhea-galactorrhea syndrome, dopamine agonist therapy can restore appropriate hormonal levels and allow for pregnancy. PRL levels can be followed to determine the effectiveness of therapy. The drugs are discontinued during pregnancy and resumed after pregnancy. There is a risk, however, of accelerated tumor growth during pregnancy in patients with macroadenoma, so that one might consider surgery before pregnancy in such a patient.

In men with asymptomatic microadenomas, treatment is unnecessary. Macroadenomas can be treated successfully by dopamine agonist therapy. The treatment must be maintained for life and the lesion tends to scar. Some neuro-surgeons believe that the scarring makes subsequent surgery more difficult,[46] although the final results of surgery are usually the same whether treated with dopamine agonists or not. If drugs fail or cannot be tolerated by the patient, surgery is effective.[47] The surgical cure rate for microadenomas is as high as 75%, higher if PRL levels are < 100 ng/ml and lower if levels are > 200 ng/ml; it is about 30% for macroadenomas and even lower for invasive tumors. Patients whose prolactin levels fall 10% within 10 min after resection and reach < 20 ng/ml are probably cured.[48] Symptomatic recurrence is seen in about 25% of patients. Risk factors for recurrence include basal PRL levels > 400 ng/ml, macroadenoma, male sex, and prolonged preoperative dopamine agonist therapy.[49] RT or radiosurgery should be reserved for patients who fail both pharmacologic therapy and surgery.

Growth hormone-secreting adenomas (Table 10.7)

GH excess from pituitary adenomas results in pituitary gigantism in children[50] and acromegaly in adults. Coarsening of facial features, separation of teeth and enlargement of the hands and feet characterized by an increase in shoe and glove size are signs of acromegaly. Patients may develop diabetes mellitus. With further tumor growth, hypopituitarism and visual complaints develop. Headache, carpal tunnel syndrome and arthritic pain are common complications of acromegaly. The diagnosis can be made by inspection of the patient and is supported by elevation of GH following a glucose load, and by elevation of insulin-like growth factor-1 (IGF-1) in the serum when the pituitary tumor cannot be identified on MRI. The tumors are sometimes too small to be identified by MRI. If the pituitary MRI is

Table 10.7
Signs and symptoms of somatotroph adenomas.

Children	Adults
Tall	Hand, feet and jaw growth
Rapid growth	Deep voice
Joint pain	Joint pain
Increased sweating	Increased sweating
	Diabetes mellitus
	Renal stones
	Headache
	Cardiac disease

negative, ectopic acromegaly caused by carcinoids or small cell lung cancer must be considered in the differential diagnosis and a search for those lesions undertaken. The treatment of choice for most GH-secreting adenomas is surgery;[2] however, recent experience dictates that a trial of octreotide or slow release lanreotide[51] is warranted as primary therapy for some patients, giving response rates > 60%.[27] Dopamine agonists are effective in some patients, usually at high doses.[44] Biochemical cure, defined as normalization of IGF-1 levels or basal or glucose suppressed GH levels of 2 ng/ml or less, can be achieved in almost 90% of patients with microadenomas and 55% of patients with macroadenomas.[52] Tumor recurrence is uncommon in adults but more common in children.[50] Risk factors for recurrence include basal GH levels > 40 ng/ml, macroadenoma, invasive adenoma and an abnormal postoperative glucose tolerance test.[49] Radiation therapy can be delivered to invasive tumors or those that fail to achieve a biochemical cure. Within 10 years of RT, 80% of patients achieve GH levels below 5 ng/L, but IGF-1 levels remain elevated[53] and RT is rarely curative. Long-term treatment with a somatostatin analog is often required.

		Table 10.8
Weight gain	Diabetes mellitus	Signs and symptoms of
Abdominal striae (purple)	Hypertension	corticotrophic adenomas.
Increased hair growth (face, chest, abdomen)	Osteoporosis	
Depression	Proximal muscle weakness	
Easy bruising		

ACTH-secreting adenomas (Table 10.8)

About 15% of pituitary adenomas secrete ACTH. ACTH secretion leads to two distinct clinical syndromes: Cushing's disease and Nelson's syndrome. Seventy-five percent of patients with Cushing's disease are women, usually in the third and fourth decades. Patients characteristically develop deposition of fat in the face (moon facies), supraclavicular fossae, abdomen (central obesity) and back of the neck (buffalo hump). Muscle atrophy leads to thin extremities, accentuating the central obesity. Hirsutism, thinning and hyperpigmentation of the skin, and vascular fragility, lead to diffuse ecchymoses and purple abdominal striae. Proximal weakness is first characterized by difficulty in getting off the toilet seat and subsequently in climbing stairs. Patients may develop hypertension, glucose intolerance, and osteoporosis. The disorder, untreated, is life-threatening with a 5-year mortality of about 50%. The diagnosis is made by: (1) elevated levels of 24-hour urinary free cortisol, (2) loss of ACTH suppression by glucocorticoids and (3) elevated ACTH levels. Because some cancers (especially small cell lung cancer) secrete ACTH-like substances and cause Cushing's syndrome, and because ACTH-secreting pituitary adenomas are often too small to identify on MR scan, it is sometimes necessary to measure ACTH in each inferior petrosal sinus which drains the pituitary gland

to verify a pituitary origin of excessive ACTH secretion.[54] Rarely, the adenoma may be ectopic, e.g. in the cavernous sinus.[55] Transsphenoidal exploration of the pituitary gland can lead to curative resection of more than 70% of microadenomas and 30% of macroadenomas.[2] Most failures are a result of difficulty locating the tumor. Intraoperative ultrasound often helps.[56] However, transsphenoidal surgery for Cushing's disease has a higher complication rate than that for other pituitary adenomas, primarily related to more medical complications, especially deep vein thrombosis.[57] Prophylactic therapy for thrombosis in the postoperative period should be considered. Despite surgery, persistence or recurrence of tumor is common. Pharmacologic blocking agents such as mitotane, ketoconazole and metyrapone have some effect but probably should be used only after failure of surgical intervention. The same applies to RT, which controls more than 80% of patients who fail transsphenoidal surgery.[58] However, IGF-1, also elevated in patients with Cushing's disease as well as those with acromegaly, is not normalized by RT.[53] In some instances, bilateral adrenalectomy is necessary to ameliorate the potentially fatal hyperadrenocorticalism.

When patients with Cushing's disease are treated with bilateral adrenalectomy rather than hypophysectomy, Nelson's syndrome occurs in about 10–15% of these patients. The persistent high levels of ACTH stimulate melanocyte-stimulating hormone. The patients develop diffuse hyperpigmentation and expansion of the sella turcica, which can lead to compression of adjacent neural structures. Transsphenoidal surgery cures only 25%. RT may help control tumor growth, but some patients die of continued local growth and even metastases.[59]

Thyroid-stimulating adenomas (Table 10.9)

TSH-secreting adenomas account for about 1% of all pituitary tumors. Most patients who present with hyperthyroidism have TSH levels that are not repressed by the elevated thyroid hormone levels. TSH levels are normal or high and are accompanied by an increase in plasma alpha subunits,[60] indicating that the problem lies in the pituitary and not the thyroid. Except for TSH secretion, many tumors are silent so that by the time the diagnosis is recognized, often after thyroid ablation has been performed for presumed thyroiditis, the tumor is usually macroscopic in size. About 50% of large tumors demonstrate mitoses and nuclear atypia and have invaded parasellar structures. Most TSH-secreting tumors also secrete GH or PRL, also helping to establish the diagnosis of a pituitary rather than a thyroid lesion. The treatment is surgical, with adjunctive radiotherapy in cases of invasion. Surgery cures about 25% of tumors. In some instances, use

Table 10.9
Signs and symptoms of thyrotroph adenomas.

Tachycardia	Insomnia
Tremor	Anxiety
Weight loss	Diarrhea
Increased appetite	Enlarged thyroid
Heat intolerance	

of a somatostatin analog has reduced TSH levels,[61] but generally it does not reduce the tumor mass.

Gonadotropin-secreting pituitary adenomas

Gonadotropic adenomas secrete FSH and LH. They account for 5–15% of pituitary adenomas. They are usually macroadenomas[62] and present with visual loss and hypopituitarism. These hormones can cause hypogonadism with diminished libido in men and amenorrhea in premenopausal women, but are usually asymptomatic until they compress normal tissue. Microadenomas do not require treatment unless symptomatic, or if a woman wishes to become pregnant. Macroadenomas should be treated surgically. Persistence or recurrence of tumors occurs in about 40% of patients.[62] Residual tumor may respond to RT.

Non-secreting pituitary adenomas

Non-functioning pituitary adenomas account for about one-third of clinically recognized pituitary adenomas and most incidental tumors encountered at autopsy. The tumors present as macroadenomas with headache, visual disturbances and symptoms of pituitary failure. PRL may be elevated because of pituitary stalk compression. These tumors generally occur in the older age group, are diagnosed by MRI and are treated surgically. Visual abnormalities are reversed in most, and preserved if they are normal preoperatively; endocrine function is preserved. Symptomatic recurrence develops in fewer than 10% of patients after gross total resection.[33] Radiotherapy prevents tumor regrowth in about 90% of patients after subtotal resection.[63,64] Risk factors for recurrence include macroadenoma, invasive adenoma, plurihormonal adenoma, silent ACTH adenoma and oncocytoma.[49,65]

Pituitary carcinoma

Pituitary carcinoma is rare; fewer than 100 cases have been reported.[20] The diagnosis is made when tumors of anterior pituitary origin, believed to be adenomas, cause distant metastases or disseminate into the subarachnoid space. The tumors often declare themselves with clinical evidence of invasion of the intracranial or spinal leptomeninges. Extraneural metastases to the mediastinum and lymph nodes also occur. The tumors may be hormonally active or hormonally silent. Once distant metastases develop, standard anti-cancer chemotherapy may be tried but is usually ineffective. The metastatic disease is usually responsible for death.

Posterior pituitary tumors

Posterior pituitary tumors are rare. The most common primary posterior pituitary tumor is the granular cell tumor, usually an incidental finding at autopsy. If the tumor causes symptoms, diabetes insipidus is usually the first symptom, a rare finding with pituitary adenomas. Astrocytomas, usually low-grade, also occur in the posterior pituitary.

The most common tumor of the neurohypophysis is a metastasis, usually from breast cancer, with lung and prostate cancer being less common. In most, diabetes insipidus is the first symptom. About 20% of patients presenting to a general hospital with diabetes insipidus have metastatic breast cancer as the cause.

Craniopharyngiomas

Introduction

The craniopharyngioma is a low-grade suprasellar tumor believed to arise from remnants of Rathke's pouch, the embryologic precursor of the anterior pituitary gland, the oral mucosa and teeth (Fig. 10.6). The tumor has two histologic types. The adamantinomatous type, representing teeth primordia, is usually a calcified multicystic tumor of childhood with a peak age of onset of 5–9; it rarely occurs in adults. The squamous papillary type, representing oral mucosa primordia, is a tumor of adults and is rarely associated with macroscopic cysts, although microscopic cysts may sometimes be identified. Xanthogranulomatous change with cholesterol clefts, inflammatory infiltrates and necrosis is generally considered a variant of the adamantinomatous type, although some place it in a separate category.[66] The incidence of craniopharyngioma is 1.3 per million without gender or race specificity. Thus, approximately 338 cases occur annually in the USA.[67] Overall, about half of craniopharyngiomas occur in children or adolescents. No risk factors, either genetic or environmental, have been identified for this tumor. Abnormalities involving chromosomes 2 and 12 have been reported.

Pathology

The tumors are usually well-circumscribed, sometimes surrounded by a pseudocapsule. However, within this capsule there may be microscopic rests of tumor that can lead to recurrence after what is believed to be a gross total resection. Within the adamantinomatous tumors are so-called 'wet' or 'ghost cell' keratins. These consist of cells in which the nucleus is missing. The papillary type is associated with so-called dry keratin and is often located in the 3rd ventricle rather than the suprasellar cistern. It may be difficult to distinguish craniopharyngiomas from epidermoid cysts based on histology alone. Grossly, adamantinomatous craniopharyngiomas contain both solid and cystic components. Cystic tumors express vascular endothelial growth factor (VEGF); solid tumors do not.[68] The cysts,

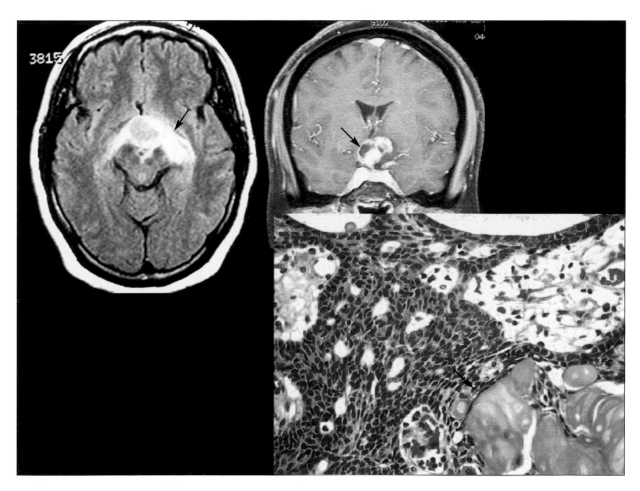

Figure 10.6
Craniopharyngioma. The MRI on the right is a contrast-enhanced scan showing a large suprasellar tumor with a cystic component (arrow). The lesion was originally misinterpreted as an optic glioma because of the apparent involvement of the optic tract on the T2-weighted image (left MRI). This is edema extending through the optic tracts, giving the 'mustache sign' characteristic of craniopharyngiomas. The photomicrograph shows epithelial sheets containing cysts with peripheral palisading and the typical 'wet keratin'.

which contain cholesterol, have a thick yellowish machine oil-like appearance and are filled with debris that may include keratin. Microscopically, the adamantinomatous type consists of stratified squamous epithelium, sometimes flattened when it lines the cyst. Compact wet keratin is more nodular and can calcify. Fibrosis and chronic inflammation are present in the cyst wall. The papillary craniopharyngioma lacks calcification but has cholesterol-filled cysts as well. The squamous cells are not columnar as they are in the adamantinomatous variety.

Keratins can be identified by immunohistochemistry (high molecular weight in adamantinomatous types and low molecular weight in papillary types). Intense gliosis and Rosenthal fibers are common; the MIB-1 index is usually less than 1%, but may be somewhat more active in recurrent tumors.

Clinical findings

Symptoms and signs

Craniopharyngiomas are located just above the sella (rare ectopic craniopharyngiomas have been reported in the optic nerve, sphenoid bone, pharynx and posterior fossa). Therefore, signs and symptoms are similar to those of pituitary tumors and include endocrine deficits and visual problems (Table 10.10).

In addition, because the tumors often compress the 3rd ventricle, increased intracranial pressure and hypothalamic dysfunction are also common. Endocrine dysfunction includes growth failure in children and impotence in adults. About 75% of patients have deficiencies of GH, 40% deficiencies of gonadotropins and about 25% deficiencies of ACTH or TSH.

Table 10.10
Craniopharyngioma: clinical findings.

I. Endocrine deficiency
Growth failure (children)
Impotence (adults)
Diabetes insipidus (20–30%)
II. Visual abnormalities
Bitemporal hemianopia
Blindness
III. Increased intracranial pressure (children)
Headache, vomiting
Papilledema (20%)
Cognitive dysfunction
Alterations of consciousness
IV. Hypothalamic dysfunction (23%)
Weight gain (or loss)
Behavioral problems
Memory loss

Unlike with pituitary tumors, diabetes insipidus is a common presenting complaint.

The tumor frequently compresses the optic chiasm, causing a bitemporal hemianopia, the characteristic visual abnormality. Neither adults nor children may be aware of the visual field defect. Adults may become aware of it when the failure of peripheral vision leads to automobile accidents. In one series of children, 5 of 75 children required emergency surgical decompression because they were virtually blind by the time of referral.[69] Other visual field abnormalities, including unilateral visual loss, are also occasional symptoms.

Increased intracranial pressure and hydrocephalus occur because the tumor often grows to a large size in both adults and children without earlier symptoms or signs having been recognized. Of 75 children, 25% required an emergency surgical procedure for relief of hydrocephalus, often presenting with acute alterations of consciousness.[69] About two-thirds of all children present with symptoms of increased intracranial pressure, including headache and vomiting. Papilledema occurs in 20% of children.

Hypothalamic dysfunction was reported in 23% of children and included weight gain resulting from hypothalamic hyperphagia or weight loss resulting from hypothalamic anorexia, in addition to behavioral, memory and cognitive changes. Deterioration in schoolwork may be an early symptom in children. Personality changes include psychomotor retardation, emotional immaturity, apathy and short-term memory losses.

In men, decreased libido or impotence occur in about 90% of patients. Premenopausal women often present with amenorrhea (80%). Pregnancy has been reported to exacerbate symptoms caused by a craniopharyngioma.[70] Signs of increased intracranial pressure are less common, although about half of adult patients have headaches. In rare instances, rupture of a craniopharyngioma may produce severe aseptic meningitis with severe headaches, stiff neck and alterations of consciousness.

Imaging

Craniopharyngioma is one tumor in which plain skull films may be useful. Suprasellar calcification is seen in over 75% of children and in somewhat less than half of adults. Enlargement of the sella with erosion of the anterior clinoids and dorsum sellae is also common. In the absence of calcification, plain skull films may show sellar enlargement, falsely suggesting a pituitary rather than a suprasellar tumor. CT scans are also sometimes useful, showing contrast enhancement of the solid portion of the tumor as well as identifying the typical calcifications, which are sometimes hard to see on MR scan. On MR, the cystic portion of the tumor may be either hyper- or hypointense on the T1-weighted image (cholesterol and keratin are hypointense on T1, whereas hemorrhage is hyperintense). On the T2-weighted image, cholesterol and hemorrhage are hyperintense and keratin hypointense. The solid portion of the tumor is usually hypointense on T1, hyperintense on T2, and contrast enhances. An MR angiogram may help the surgeon identify the relationship of the tumor to major vessels passing near the suprasellar cistern. An unusual sign of craniopharyngioma is the so-called 'mustache' sign.[71] This sign is related to vasogenic edema caused by increased permeability of the blood–brain barrier in the optic tracts and optic radiations (Fig. 10.6). Vasogenic edema is thought to result from leakage of the craniopharyngioma contents, causing swelling and blood–brain barrier breakdown in the optic pathways. It is usually asymptomatic but may be misinterpreted as representing an optic nerve tumor rather than a craniopharyngioma.

Treatment

The tumor is often adherent and difficult to separate from vascular structures, optic apparatus, and hypothalamus. When the tumor can be completely removed, surgery is often curative,[72] with a recurrence rate of 19% at 10 years. Rarely, the tumor will seed the leptomeninges postoperatively.[73] Unfortunately, the location of the tumor and its tenacious adherence to vital structures often makes complete removal either impossible or unacceptably dangerous. However, some reports suggest that as many as 90% of tumors can be totally removed using modern microsurgical techniques. In one series, 90% of the 144 patients who underwent microsurgical resection of craniopharyngioma were completely resected and only 7% had a recurrence.[74] Frontal or frontotemporal craniotomy is the most common exposure used to remove the tumor. Transnasal surgery for certain tumors that are infradiaphragmatic appears safe and effective.[75] Diabetes insipidus often follows surgery for craniopharyngioma, although anterior pituitary function may be retained.[76] If complete removal is not possible, postoperative radiotherapy appears to decrease considerably the incidence of recurrence.[72]

Radiosurgery is sometimes useful for the treatment of small solid craniopharyngiomas,[77] but most tumors are too large and their proximity to the optic tract (< 3 mm) prevents its use in most instances. Interstitial implantation of radionuclides, including phosphorus-32, yttrium-90, gold-198, and rhenium-186, all of which emit β-particles, has been recommended for some monocystic craniopharyngiomas; the target dose to the inner wall of the cyst is about 200–350 Gy. Only ^{32}P is available in the USA.[78]

Chemotherapy is not widely applied for craniopharyngiomas. Bleomycin has been directly injected into the tumor,[79] with encouraging results, but also sometimes with severe toxicity.[80] Despite multimodality treatment, about 25% of craniopharyngiomas recur, even some that have been 'totally' resected. At least one investigator reports the cumulative recurrence rate at 10 years as 33% and that after 15 years as 40%, not differing by age, radical surgery, or postoperative radiotherapy.[81] Repeat surgery should be the first consideration since total tumor resection can sometimes be accomplished even when the tumor has recurred. If radiation has not been used, it should be applied in the postoperative period. Other options as outlined above can also be considered.[82]

Prognosis

Total surgical removal results in about 80% cure.[72] About half of the patients with subtotal removal are also cured and many more can be salvaged after recurrence. However, a small but significant percentage of patients are damaged by treatment. Surgical mortality ranges from 0% to 15% in several surgical series, and surgical morbidity, including endocrine dysfunction, visual field abnormalities and chronic hypothalamic dysfunction, varies with preoperative status. The side effects can be obviated to a substantial degree by planned subtotal resection followed by RT. Risk factors for high morbidity include lethargy, visual deterioration, papilledema, hydrocephalus, tumor calcification or adhesiveness, adverse intraoperative events and age < 5 years at presentation.[72] Tumors impinging on the hypothalamus, patients with hypothalamic disturbance at diagnosis, and attempts to remove adherent tumors from the hypothalamus are likely to have a higher surgical morbidity.[69] Others believe that neuropsychological performance and quality of life are not impaired by radical

surgical removal.[83] Visual deterioration, hydrocephalus and cognitive dysfunction may develop during or within 2 months of postoperative RT due to cyst enlargement or hydrocephalus. Early detection and treatment of the enlarged cyst by drainage or placement of a ventriculoperitoneal (VP) shunt improves long-term outcome.[84] Late-delayed effects also develop as a consequence of RT, particularly memory dysfunction. Secondary glial tumors can also appear many years after successful RT for a craniopharyngioma.

Rathke cleft cyst

Arising from the epithelial remnants of Rathke's cleft, these cysts, which are found either in sellar or suprasellar areas, are usually small and asymptomatic. Symptomatic cysts are associated with symptoms similar to those of pituitary tumors, including pituitary dysfunction, visual disturbances and headache (Fig. 10.7). Sometimes they may grow large enough to cause symptoms comparable to those of a craniopharyngioma. The cyst has both an intrasellar and suprasellar location in at least 70% of patients, and symptoms are usually present for 3 years before the diagnosis is established. On MR scan, they may have either high or low intensity on both T1- and T2-weighted images, depending on cyst contents. Some cysts contain intracystic nodules, hyperintense on T1 and hypointense on T2.[85] Unlike craniopharyngiomas, the tumors are not calcified and when small and intrasellar may be confused with a microadenoma. They are best treated surgically, often by a transsphenoidal approach, which usually leads to both visual and hormonal recovery and appears to cure the tumor.[86] The recurrence rate is low.

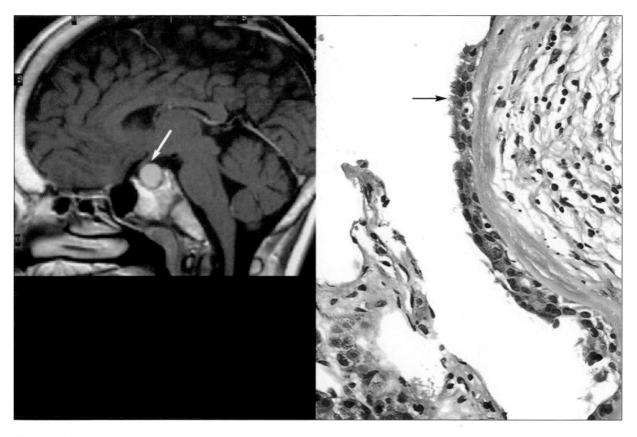

Figure 10.7
A Rathke pouch cyst (arrow). The symptoms in this 12-year-old boy were headache and visual loss. The photomicrograph shows a cyst lined by ciliated epithelium (arrow).

Germinomas

Germinomas usually occur in the pineal region in boys, in the suprasellar cistern in girls, and occasionally within the parenchyma of the brain, particularly in the thalamus, in either boys or girls (Chapter 8). When in the suprasellar area, they can produce hormonal or visual symptoms similar to those of a craniopharyngioma. However, germinomas have a different radiographic appearance with diffuse contrast enhancement and they do not calcify or have cysts.

References

1. Anderson JR, Antoun N, Burnet N et al. Neurology of the pituitary gland. J Neurol Neurosurg Psychiatry 1999; 66: 703–21.
2. Ciric I, Rosenblatt S, Kerr W, Jr et al. Perspective in pituitary adenomas: an end of the century review of tumorigenesis, diagnosis, and treatment. Clin Neurosurg 2000; 47: 99–111.
3. Brat DJ, Scheithauer BW, Staugaitis SM et al. Pituicytoma – a distinctive low-grade glioma of the neurohypophysis. Am J Surg Pathol 2000; 24: 362–8.
4. Teramoto A, Hirakawa K, Sanno N, Osamura Y. Incidental pituitary lesions in 1000

unselected autopsy specimens. Radiology 1994; 193: 161–4.

5. Sano T, Kovacs KT, Scheithauer BW, Young WF. Aging and the human pituitary gland. Mayo Clin Proc 1993; 68: 971–7.

6. Tomita T, Gates E. Pituitary adenomas and granular cell tumors – incidence, cell type, and location of tumor in 100 pituitary glands at autopsy. Am J Clin Pathol 1999; 111: 817–25.

7. Kovacs K, Scheithauer BW, Horvath E, Lloyd RV. The World Health Organization classification of adenohypophysial neoplasms. Cancer 1996; 78: 502–10.

8. Blevins LS. Aggressive pituitary tumors. Oncology 1998; 12: 1307–16.

9. Thapar K, Laws ER Jr. Pituitary tumors. In: Kaye AH, Laws ER Jr, eds. Brain tumors: an encyclopedic approach. New York: Churchill Livingstone, 2001: 803–56.

10. Ohkura N, Kishi M, Tsukada T, Yamaguchi K. Menin, a gene product responsible for multiple endocrine neoplasia type 1, interacts with the putative tumor metastasis suppressor nm23. Biochem Biophys Res Commun 2001; 282: 1206–10.

11. Lamberts SW, De Herder WW, Van der Lely AJ. Pituitary insufficiency. Lancet 1998; 352: 127–34.

12. Gsponer J, de Tribolet N, Déruaz JP et al. Diagnosis, treatment, and outcome of pituitary tumors and other abnormal intrasellar masses – retrospective analysis of 353 patients. Medicine 1999; 78: 236-69.

13. Wiren L, Bengtsson BA, Johannsson G. Beneficial effects of long-term GH replacement therapy on quality of life in adults with GH deficiency. Clin Endocrinol 1998; 48: 613–20.

14. Karanjia N, Jacobson DM. Compression of the prechiasmatic optic nerve produces a junctional scotoma. Am J Ophthalmol 1999; 128: 256–8.

15. Hanna FWF, Williams OM et al. Pituitary apoplexy following metastasis of bronchogenic adenocarcinoma to a prolactinoma. Clin Endocrinol 1999; 51: 377–81.

16. Roelandse FW, van der Zwart N, Didden JH, van Loon J, Souverijn JH. Detection of CSF leakage by isoelectric focusing on polyacrylamide gel, direct immunofixation of transferrins, and silver staining. Clin Chem 1998; 44: 351–3.

17. Nishioka H, Ito H, Haraoka J, Akada K. Immature teratoma originating from the pituitary gland: Case report. Neurosurgery 1999; 44: 644–7.

18. Somali MH, Anastasiou AL, Goulis DG, Polyzoides C, Avramides A. Pituitary abscess presenting with cranial nerve paresis. Case report and review of literature. J Endocrinol Invest 2001; 24: 45–50.

19. Landman RE, Wardlaw SL, McConnell RJ et al. Pituitary lymphoma presenting as fever of unknown origin. J Clin Endocrinol Metab 2001; 86: 1470–6.

20. Morita A, Meyer FB, Laws ER, Jr. Symptomatic pituitary metastases. J Neurosurg 1998; 89: 69–73.

21. Honegger J, Fahlbusch R, Bornemann A et al. Lymphocytic and granulomatous hypophysitis: Experience with nine cases. Neurosurgery 1997; 40: 713–22.

22. Thodou E, Asa SL, Kontogeorgos G et al. Clinical case seminar: lymphocytic hypophysitis: clinicopathological findings. J Clin Endocrinol Metab 1995; 80: 2302–11.

23. Cooper R, Belilos E, Drexler S et al. Idiopathic giant-cell granulomatous hypophysitis mimicking acute meningitis. Am J Med Sci 1999; 318: 339–42.

24. Kristof RA, Van Roost D, Klingmüller D, Springer W, Schramm J. Lymphocytic hypophysitis: non-invasive diagnosis and treatment by high dose methylprednisolone pulse therapy? J Neurol Neurosurg Psychiatry 1999; 67: 398–402.

25. Jho HD, Alfieri A. Endoscopic transsphenoidal pituitary surgery: various surgical techniques and recommended steps for procedural transition. Br J Neurosurg 2000; 14: 432–40.

26. Webster J, Piscitelli G, Polli A et al. A comparison of cabergoline and bromocriptine in the treatment of hyperprolactinemic amenorrhea. N Engl J Med 1994; 331: 904–9.

27. Newman CB, Melmed S, George A et al. Octreotide as primary therapy for acromegaly. J Clin Endocrinol Metab 1998; 83: 3034–40.

28. Mindermann T, Staub JJ, Probst A. High rate of unexpected histology in presumed pituitary adenomas. Lancet 1998; 352: 1445.

29. Peace KA, Orme SM, Padayatty SJ, Godfrey HP, Belchetz PE. Cognitive dysfunction in

patients with pituitary tumour who have been treated with transfrontal or transsphenoidal surgery or medication. Clin Endocrinol 1998; 49: 391–6.

30. Matsuki M, Kaji Y, Matsuo M, Kobashi Y. MR findings of subarachnoid dissemination of a pituitary adenoma. Br J Radiol 2000; 73: 783–5.

31. Webb SM, Rigla M, Wägner A, Oliver B, Bartumeus F. Recovery of hypopituitarism after neurosurgical treatment of pituitary adenomas. J Clin Endocrinol Metab 1999; 84: 3696–700.

32. Laws ER, Jr., Vance ML. Conventional radiotherapy for pituitary tumors. Neurosurg Clin N Am 2000; 11: 617–25.

33. Lillehei KO, Kirschman DL, Kleinschmidt-DeMasters BK, Ridgway EC. Reassessment of the role of radiation therapy in the treatment of endocrine-inactive pituitary macroadenomas. Neurosurgery 1998; 43: 432–8.

34. Simmons NE, Laws ER, Jr. Glioma occurrence after sellar irradiation: case report and review. Neurosurgery 1998; 42: 172–8.

35. Marcou Y, Plowman PN. Stereotactic radiosurgery for pituitary adenomas. Trends Endocrinol Metab 2000; 11: 132–7.

36. Izawa M, Hayashi M, Nakaya K et al. Gamma knife radiosurgery for pituitary adenomas. J Neurosurg 2000; 93: 19–22.

37. Levy RP, Schulte RWM, Slater JD, Miller DW, Stater JM. Stereotactic radiosurgery – the role of charged particles. Acta Oncol 1999; 38: 165–9.

38. Colao A, Di Sarno A, Marzullo P et al. New medical approaches in pituitary adenomas. Horm Res 2000; 53, S3: 76–87.

39. Cannavò S, Curtò L, Squadrito S et al. Cabergoline: a first-choice treatment in patients with previously untreated prolactin-secreting pituitary adenoma. J Endocrinol Invest 1999; 22: 354–9.

40. Castro MG, Southgate T, Lowenstein PR. Molecular therapy in a model neuroendocrine disease: developing clinical gene therapy for pituitary tumours. Trends Endocrinol Metab 2001; 12: 58–64.

41. Chong VFH, Rumpel H, Aw YS, Ho GL, Fan YF, Chua EJ. Temporal lobe necrosis following radiation therapy for nasopharyngeal carcinoma: ^{1}H MR spectroscopic findings. Int J Radiat Oncol Biol Phys 1999; 45: 699–705.

42. Brada M, Burchell L, Ashley S, Traish D. The incidence of cerebrovascular accidents in patients with pituitary adenoma. Int J Radiat Oncol Biol Phys 1999; 45: 693–8.

43. Albuquerque FC, Hinton DR, Weiss MH. Excessively high prolactin level in a patient with a nonprolactin-secreting adenoma – case report. J Neurosurg 1998; 89: 1043–6.

44. Muratori M, Arosio M, Gambino G et al. Use of cabergoline in the long-term treatment of hyperprolactinemic and acromegalic patients. J Endocrinol Invest 1997; 20: 537–46.

45. Colao A, Di Sarno A, Landi ML et al. Long-term and low-dose treatment with cabergoline induces macroprolactinoma shrinkage. J Clin Endocrinol Metab 1997; 82: 3574–9.

46. Bevan JS, Adams CBT, Burke CW et al. Factors in the outcome of transsphenoidal surgery for prolactinoma and non-functioning pituitary tumour, including pre-operative bromocriptine therapy. Clin Endocrinol 1997; 26: 541–56.

47. Tyrrell JB, Lamborn KR, Hannegan LT, Applebury CB, Wilson CB. Transsphenoidal microsurgical therapy of prolactinomas: Initial outcomes and long-term results. Neurosurgery 1999; 44: 254–61.

48. Guieu R, Dufour H, Grisoli F et al. An ultra-rapid prognostic index in microprolactinoma surgery. J Neurosurg 1999; 90: 1037–41.

49. Cheung AYC, Sligh T, Bauserman S, Schultz G. Evaluation of modern pathologic nomenclature, tumor imaging and treatment of pituitary adenomas in a recent surgical series. J Neurooncol 1998; 37: 145–53.

50. Abe T, Abou Tara L, Lüdecke DK. Growth hormone-secreting pituitary adenomas in childhood and adolescence: Features and results of transnasal surgery. Neurosurgery 1999; 45: 1–10.

51. Cannavò S, Squadrito S, Curtò L et al. Results of a two-year treatment with slow release lanreotide in acromegaly. Horm Metab Res 2000; 32: 224–9.

52. Kaltsas GA, Isidori AM, Florakis D et al. Predictors of the outcome of surgical treatment in acromegaly and the value of the mean growth hormone day curve in assessing post-operative disease activity. J Clin Endocrinol Metab 2001; 86: 1645–52.

53. Barkan AL, Halasz I, Dornfeld KJ et al. Pituitary irradiation is ineffective in normalizing plasma insulin-like growth factor I in patients with acromegaly. J Clin Endocrinol Metab 1997; 82: 3187–91.

54. Padayatty SJ, Orme SM, Nelson M, Lamb JT, Belchetz PE. Bilateral sequential inferior petrosal sinus sampling with corticotrophin-releasing hormone stimulation in the diagnosis of Cushing's disease. Eur J Endocrinol 1998; 139: 161–6.

55. Sanno N, Tahara S, Yoshida Y et al. Ectopic corticotroph adenoma in the cavernous sinus: Case report. Neurosurgery 1999; 45: 914–7.

56. Watson JC, Shawker TH, Nieman LK et al. Localization of pituitary adenomas by using intraoperative ultrasound in patients with Cushing's disease and no demonstrable pituitary tumor on magnetic resonance imaging. J Neurosurg 1998; 89: 927–32.

57. Semple PL, Laws ER, Jr. Complications in a contemporary series of patients who underwent transsphenoidal surgery for Cushing's disease. J Neurosurg 1999; 91: 175–9.

58. Estrada J, Boronat M, Mielgo M et al. The long-term outcome of pituitary irradiation after unsuccessful transsphenoidal surgery in Cushing's disease. N Engl J Med 1997; 336: 172–7.

59. Kemink SAG, Wesseling P, Pieters GFFM et al. Progression of a Nelson's adenoma to pituitary carcinoma; a case report and review of the literature. J Endocrinol Invest 1999; 22: 70–5.

60. Bertholon-Grégoire M, Trouillas J, Guigard MP, Loras B, Tourniaire J. Mono- and plurihormonal thyrotropic pituitary adenomas: pathological, hormonal and clinical studies in 12 patients. Eur J Endocrinol 1999; 140: 519–27.

61. Skoric T, Korsic M, Zarkovic K et al. Clinical and morphological features of undifferentiated monomorphous GH/TSH-secreting pituitary adenoma. Eur J Endocrinol 1999; 140: 528–37.

62. Young WF Jr, Scheithauer BW, Kovacs KT et al. Gonadotroph adenoma of the pituitary gland: a clinicopathologic analysis of 100 cases. Mayo Clin Proc 1996; 71: 649–56.

63. Gittoes NJ, Bates AS, Tse W et al. Radiotherapy for non-functional pituitary tumours. Clin Endocrinol 1998; 48: 331–7.

64. Tsang RW, Brierley JD, Panzarella T, Gospodarowicz MK, Sutcliffe SB, Simpson WJ. Radiation therapy for pituitary adenoma: treatment outcome and prognostic factors. Int J Radiat Oncol Biol Phys 1994; 30: 557–65.

65. Breen P, Flickinger JC, Kondziolka D, Martinez AJ. Radiotherapy for nonfunctional pituitary adenoma: analysis of long-term tumor control. J Neurosurg 1998; 89: 933–8.

66. Paulus W, Honegger J, Keyvani K, Fahlbusch R. Xanthogranuloma of the sellar region: a clinicopathological entity different from adamantinomatous craniopharyngioma. Acta Neuropathol (Berl) 1999; 97: 377–82.

67. Bunin GR, Surawicz TS, Witman PA et al. The descriptive epidemiology of craniopharyngioma. J Neurosurg 1998; 89: 547-51.

68. Vaquero J, Zurita M, De Oya S et al. Expression of vascular permeability factor in craniopharyngioma. J Neurosurg 1999; 91: 831–4.

69. De Vile CJ, Grant DB, Kendall BE et al. Management of childhood craniopharyngioma: can the morbidity of radical surgery be predicted? J Neurosurg 1996; 85: 73–81.

70. Aydin Y, Can SM, Gulkilik A et al. Rapid enlargement and recurrence of a preexisting intrasellar craniopharyngioma during the course of two pregnancies – Case report. J Neurosurg 1999; 91: 322–4.

71. Kearney D, Tay-Kearney ML, Khangure MS. Craniopharyngioma and the moustache sign. Australas Radiol 1993; 37: 370–1.

72. Duff JM, Meyer FB, Ilstrup DM et al. Long-term outcomes for surgically resected craniopharyngiomas. Neurosurgery 2000; 46: 291–302.

73. Ito M, Jamshidi J, Yamanaka K. Does craniopharyngioma metastasize? Case report and review of the literature. Neurosurgery 2001; 48: 933–5.

74. Yasargil MG, Curcic M, Kis M et al. Total removal of craniopharyngiomas. Approaches and long-term results in 144 patients. J Neurosurg 1990; 73: 3–11.

75. Abe T, Lüdecke DK. Transnasal surgery for infradiaphragmatic craniopharyngiomas in pediatric patients. Neurosurgery 1999; 44: 957–64.

76. Honegger J, Buchfelder M, Fahlbusch R. Surgical treatment of craniopharyngiomas: endocrinological results. J Neurosurg 1999; 90: 251–7.

77. Chung WY, Pan DH, Shiau CY, Guo WY, Wang LW. Gamma knife radiosurgery for craniopharyngiomas. J Neurosurg 2000; 93, S3: 47-56.

78. Pollock BE, Lunsford LD, Kondziolka D, Levine G, Flickinger JC. Phosphorus-32 intracavitary irradiation of cystic craniopharyngiomas: current technique and long-term results. Int J Radiat Oncol Biol Phys 1995; 33: 437–46.

79. Savas A, Arasil E, Batay F, Selcuki M, Kanpolat Y. Intracavitary chemotherapy of polycystic craniopharyngioma with bleomycin. Acta Neurochir (Wien) 1999; 141: 547–8.

80. Savas A, Erdem A, Tun K, Kanpolat Y. Fatal toxic effect of bleomycin on brain tissue after intracystic chemotherapy for a craniopharyngioma: case report. Neurosurgery 2000; 46: 213–6.

81. Bulow B, Attewell R, Hagmar L et al. Postoperative prognosis in craniopharyngioma with respect to cardiovascular mortality, survival, and tumor recurrence. J Clin Endocrinol Metab 1998; 83: 3897–904.

82. Caldarelli M, Di Rocco C, Papacci F, Colosimo CJ. Management of recurrent craniopharyngioma. Acta Neurochir (Wien) 1998; 140: 447–54.

83. Honegger J, Barocka A, Sadri B, Fahlbusch R. Neuropsychological results of craniopharyngioma surgery in adults: a prospective study. Surg Neurol 1998; 50: 19–28.

84. Rajan B, Ashley S, Thomas DG et al. Craniopharyngioma: improving outcome by early recognition and treatment of acute complications. Int J Radiat Oncol Biol Phys 1997; 37: 517–21.

85. Byun WM, Kim OL, Kim D. MR imaging findings of Rathke's cleft cysts: significance of intracystic nodules. Am J Neuroradiol 2000; 21: 485–8.

86. el-Mahdy W, Powell M. Transsphenoidal management of 28 symptomatic Rathke's cleft cysts, with special reference to visual and hormonal recovery. Neurosurgery 1998; 42: 7–16.

11

Primary central nervous system lymphoma and other hemopoietic tumors

Introduction

Leukemias, lymphomas, Hodgkin's disease and other tumors of hemopoietic origin, when found in the CNS, usually represent metastases of tumor that started systemically. The metastases mostly affect the meninges, causing either dural masses (e.g. plasmacytoma and Hodgkin's disease)[1] or diffusely seeding the leptomeninges (e.g. leukemia and lymphoma). Occasionally, hemopoietic tumors arise within the CNS (Fig. 11.1), with no systemic tumor being identified either at initial workup or, in most cases, even at autopsy.[2,3] The most

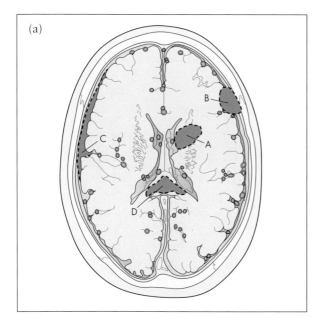
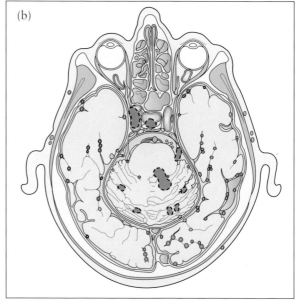

Figure 11.1
(a) The typical location of primary CNS lymphoma and of some other hemopoietic tumors. Primary CNS lymphomas tend to occur deep in the brain, usually near the ventricles (A,D). Plasmacytomas and other hemopoietic tumors are usually durally based (B). All of these lesions may involve the leptomeninges (C).
(b) Histiocytic lesions, especially Langerhans cell histiocytosis, may involve either the hypothalamic pituitary axis or brain parenchyma.

Table 11.1
Primary CNS lymphomas and hemopoietic neoplasms.

- Malignant lymphomas
    B-cell lymphomas
    T-cell lymphomas
    Intravascular lymphoma
- Plasmacytomas
- Granulocytic sarcomas
- Histiocytic tumors
    Langerhans cell histiocytosis
    Non-Langerhans cell histiocytosis
    Hemophagocytic lymphohistiocytosis

common hemopoietic tumor to arise within the CNS is the primary central nervous system lymphoma (PCNSL) (Table 11.1).

Primary CNS lymphoma
Introduction

Most textbooks indicate that PCNSLs represents 1–2% of primary brain tumors. Indeed, 20 years ago at MSKCC such tumors were encountered at the rate of approximately 1 every 2–4 years. Beginning in the mid-1980s, the incidence at MSKCC appeared to increase to the point where approximately 15% of the primary brain tumors encountered in immuno-competent hosts were PCNSL.[4] Although a few studies question whether an increase in PCNSLs is real,[5] most recognize a dramatic epidemiologic change over the past 20–30 years.[6,7] A substantial rise has also been noted in ocular lymphoma, a part of the spectrum of CNS lymphoma.

PCNSL occurs in two settings, the first in patients with known immune suppression and the second in immunocompetent patients.[8] The former are usually children or young adults, and the latter older adults and the elderly. Only PCNSL arising in the immunocompetent host is discussed in this chapter. Current estimates indicate that 6–7% of primary intracranial neoplasms are lymphomas, with an incidence of 0.3–0.4 per 100 000 in the immunocompetent population and 4.7 per 1000 person-years in the AIDS population – about 3600-fold higher than in the general population.[6,9] In the

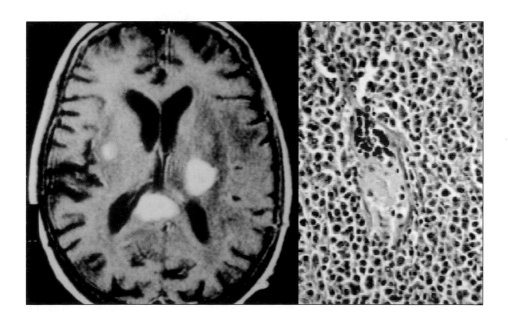

Figure 11.2
A patient with a typical primary CNS lymphoma. Note the uniform enhancement, the paucity of edema, the fuzzy tumor margins and the periventricular location of these multiple lesions. The photomicrograph shows infiltration of neoplastic large B-cells around a blood vessel.

immunocompetent population, the peak incidence is between 50 and 70 years,[10] with males slightly more likely to be involved than females.

PCNSL can arise anywhere in the nervous system, including the eyes, spinal cord and leptomeninges, but it primarily involves the periventricular areas of the brain and brainstem (Fig. 11.2). About 40% of PCNSLs are multiple in the immunocompetent population, whereas 50–70% of immunocompromised patients have multiple PCNSL lesions. Twenty percent of patients have ocular involvement at presentation and about 42% of patients have demonstrable leptomeningeal involvement at diagnosis.[11,12] At least an additional 40% of patients with PCNSL have an increased number of lymphocytes in the cerebrospinal fluid (CSF), which cannot be identified on cytologic examinations as malignant, but strongly suggest that leptomeningeal disease is present. In some patients, focal leptomeningeal infiltration is seen on a surgical specimen even with negative cytology on CSF examination, indicating that the incidence of subarachnoid involvement may be underestimated by CSF analysis alone.

Etiology

PCNSL is a typical non-Hodgkin's lymphoma. Non-Hodgkin's lymphoma has increased in incidence about 3–4% per year since the 1970s, with the greatest increase seen in extra-nodal lymphomas, particularly gastric and CNS. This increase cannot be accounted for by the number of AIDS patients who develop lymphoma, even though there is a marked overrepresentation of extranodal tumors in the AIDS population. Among the possible risk factors for the development of non-Hodgkin's lymphoma in general are immunosuppression including autoimmunity: the incidence of the

disorder is increased in patients with Sjogren's syndrome and rheumatoid arthritis, independent of therapy. Other established or putative risk factors include exposure to certain pesticides or hair dyes, infection with the HTLV-1 virus or Epstein–Barr virus (EBV) (see below) and old age, possibly a result of decreased immunity with aging. One kind of gastric lymphoma has been associated with chronic infection by *Helicobacter pylori*. An important risk factor is a history of a previous cancer. A previous or concomitant malignant neoplasm has been found in up to 15% of so-called immunocompetent patients with PCNSL.[3]

Because of the relatively small number of PCNSLs, the environmental factors that play a role in this disorder have not been established. A case–control study of PCNSL has suggested that lower education was associated with the disease and that PCNSL patients were less likely to have had tonsillectomy or use oral contraceptives.[13] However, these findings are preliminary and need to be confirmed.

The most important risk factor for PCNSL is immunosuppression. As many as 10–40% of patients infected with human immunodeficiency virus type 1 (HIV-1) have PCNSL at autopsy, although at least half are missed prior to death.[14,15] In the early days of transplantation, PCNSL was a common complication of renal and other organ transplants,[16] a result of the massive immunosuppression necessary to maintain the transplant. Fully half of the lymphomas arising in the post-transplantation period arose in the brain, an extraordinarily high proportion, given that < 1% of all lymphomas arise in brain in the immunocompetent population. PCNSL is also known to accompany congenital or other acquired immunodeficiency states, such as the Wiskott–Aldrich syndrome and collagen–vascular diseases. In most immunosuppressed states, PCNSL appears to be related to latent EBV infection.[16] After primary EBV infection, which usually occurs in youth, a small number of B-cells retain a latent infection, which immortalizes this tiny population of cells. Growth of these cells is kept under control by normal suppressor T-cells. Removal of T-cell control by immunosuppression allows these B-cells to grow, leading to lymphoma formation. Viral genome can be found within tumor tissue in 85–100% of patients with AIDS-related PCNSL.[17,18] On the contrary, in PCNSL arising in immunocompetent hosts, viral genome is rarely found within the tumor.

Approximately 15% of immunocompetent patients with PCNSL have had a prior malignancy.[3] Many of these cancers occurred decades previously and the patient is cured of their original primary. There is no specific tumor type which pre-dates the development of PCNSL; a variety of solid and hemopoietic tumors have been observed. Furthermore, treatment of the original tumor is not usually of the sort which predisposes to second malignancy formation; for example, abdominal resection of a colon cancer without alkylating agent chemotherapy would not be expected to lead to PCNSL years later. Whether the history of prior cancer reflects an underlying genetic abnormality is unknown.

Why hemopoietic tumors should arise within the nervous system is unknown, given the fact that the CNS is devoid of lymph nodes and deficient in lymphatics (see Chapter 2). Two hypotheses have been advanced. The first is that a hemopoietic tumor develops outside of the CNS. The tumor cells circulate in the blood and seed multiple organs, including the brain. The immune system has the capacity to find and eliminate tumor cells in most of the body, but the brain, being a relatively immunologically privileged site, gives sanctuary to lymphoma cells which grow and form a tumor in that organ. A second hypothesis suggests that lymphocytes traffic into the CNS as part of an inflammatory process and become transformed into malignant cells within the nervous system. Unfortunately, neither hypothesis is truly satisfying. Against the first is the failure to find deposits of lymphoma in other immunologically privileged sites, such as the testis, in patients with PCNSL. Against the second hypothesis is the fact that there appears to be no increased incidence of PCNSL in patients with inflammatory diseases of the nervous system that attract lymphocytes, such as multiple sclerosis or encephalitis. Furthermore, almost exclusively, T-cells are associated with inflammatory diseases, and PCNSL is usually a disease of B-lymphocytes.

Although only a few PCNSLs have been genetically analyzed, the genetics do not differ from the genetics of non-Hodgkin's lymphoma occurring elsewhere in the body.[19] Chromosomal abnormalities with gains of chromosomes 12q, 18q and 22q and loss of 6q have been described.[20,21] An analysis of cell surface markers, such as ICAM and integrins, fails to demonstrate any differences between systemic and cerebral lymphomas.[22] Telomerase activity and telomerase-related RNA are present in almost all PCNSLs.[23]

Pathology

Macroscopically, lymphomas tend to have a fleshy, granular appearance with ill-defined borders; hemorrhage and necrosis are rare except in AIDS patients, where they are seen commonly. Microscopically, the tumors generally exhibit an angiocentric growth pattern with multiple areas of perivascular lymphocytes, which eventually become confluent, producing a mass. The tumor may contain a prominent astrocytic and microglial response and a large number of reactive lymphocytes (T-cells) are common even in the B-cell lymphomas.[24] Microscopically, PCNSL is indistinguishable from high-grade non-Hodgkin's lymphomas occurring elsewhere in the body. They are identified both by their microscopic appearance and by their monoclonality, most frequently IgM kappa. PCNSLs are virtually all intermediate or high-grade subtypes, with approximately half of tumors having a diffuse large cell histology, with diffuse large cell immunoblastic subtype forming 20%, diffuse small cleaved cell 10%, and others in lesser quantities. In AIDS patients, there is a much higher incidence of the diffuse large cell immunoblastic subtype. It is unknown whether the subtypes carry different prognoses, because there have been too few patients in most categories to analyze. T-cell lymphomas represent about 2% of all PCNSLs;[25] one Japanese series reports that 8.5% of 466 patients with PCNSL had T-cell lymphoma.[2]

The vasculature of PCNSL differs from that of gliomas. Like gliomas, the tumors are highly vascular, but endothelial proliferation is absent. Electron microscopy reveals two distinct populations of cells: electron-dense endothelial cells that give evidence of apoptosis, and electron-lucent cells that give evidence of cellular regeneration. These findings are not present in the endothelial cells of gliomas. Investigators interpret these changes to represent apoptosis induced by cytokines released from necrotic or apoptotic tumor lymphocytes. If so, the findings may partially explain so-called 'ghost tumors', PCNSLs that regress in response to corticosteroids (see below).[26]

Clinical findings

Symptoms and signs
As indicated in Chapter 3, the signs and symptoms depend on the tumor site. Because the tumors are often deep, seizures are less common than in other primary brain tumors but behavioral changes and focal signs are more common than in gliomas.[27] Common

findings include headache, personality and cognitive changes, and progressive hemiparesis. The symptoms usually progress over weeks or months, more like glioblastoma multiforme than lower-grade gliomas. The median time from symptom onset to diagnosis is 3–5 months in immunocompetent patients, and longer when personality change is the only symptom.[27] Leptomeningeal involvement is usually asymptomatic until late in the course of the disease.

Because ocular involvement is common,[28] patients may present with visual symptoms. Usually the patient complains of floaters or visual blurring. A misdiagnosis of uveitis is common, particularly in those patients who have isolated ocular disease as the first manifestation of PCNSL. The ocular findings on slit-lamp exam resemble vitreitis or uveitis and the patient may be so treated, often initially successfully because of the response of lymphoma to corticosteroids. However, such patients ultimately become refractory to corticosteroid therapy, often precipitating consideration of lymphoma as the diagnosis. The diagnosis may then be difficult to establish because of the chronic steroid treatment (see below). In about half of the patients, ocular involvement is asymptomatic and detectable only on slit-lamp examination.

Imaging
MR is far superior to CT scan for delineating the extent of PCNSL involvement; however, the contrast-enhanced images of either modality reveal similar characteristic findings. The tumors are usually supratentorial and periventricular (Fig. 11.2). They are hypointense on the MR T1-weighted image and hypo- to isointense relative to gray matter on T2-weighted images with variable surrounding edema.[29] The T2 signal reflecting dense cellularity helps to differentiate

lymphomas from gliomas that are hyper-intense on T2. Lymphomas enhance homogeneously after contrast administration and have rather indistinct borders. Ring enhancement is uncommon. Even more than gliomas, lymphomas may widely infiltrate the nervous system without causing a change in signal on MR scan. When patients are treated with corticosteroids, PCNSL will sometimes show a rapid complete disappearance of contrast enhancement. This response has been called a 'ghost tumor' and may result from cytokine-induced apoptosis as seen in PCNSL endothelial cells, and a direct response of lymphoma cells that contain corticosteroid receptors.[26]

Hypointense lesions, or T2 hyperintense lesions that do not contrast enhance on MR scan, are occasionally found in both immuno-competent and immunosuppressed patients, but they are more common among the immunosuppressed population.[16,30] Ring-enhancing lesions similar to those of toxoplasmosis are characteristic of PCNSL in the AIDS patient, making the differential diagnosis difficult, whereas ring enhancement is uncommon in the immunocompetent population. In addition, the lesions are more frequently located in the subcortical white matter in AIDS patients. Perfusion MRI suggests that most PCNSLs have a low cerebral blood volume, similar to lower-grade gliomas and in contrast to high-grade gliomas.[29] PET scanning reveals a hypermetabolic lesion but this is non-specific and not helpful in the immuno-competent population; however it may help distinguish tumor from toxoplasmosis (hypometabolic) in AIDS patients.[31] Single-photon emission tomography may help distinguish PCNSL from other lesions.[32] In PCNSL uptake of [123]IMP is delayed, whereas it occurs early in other brain tumors. MRS may also help.[33]

Other diagnostic tests

Unlike most intracranial tumors, where cranial imaging will suffice to reveal the full extent of disease, patients with PCNSL should undergo a neurologic staging evaluation including an ocular examination and slit-lamp, and a lumbar puncture for CSF analysis (Table 11.2).

If a lumbar puncture is performed before biopsy in a patient suspected of having a PCNSL, a diagnosis of lymphoma can be made in up to 15% of patients (see below). In patients whose cranial MRI suggests PCNSL, if the ocular examination shows inflammatory infiltrates in the vitreous, a vitrectomy may be performed and the material examined for malignant lymphocytes. If lymphoma is identified, a brain biopsy can be avoided. However, if a patient has biopsy-proven PCNSL and cells are identified on slit-lamp examination in the vitreous, this is presumptive evidence of lymphoma involving the eye, and a vitrectomy is not essential for pathologic confirmation.

When trying to establish the diagnosis of PCNSL, the presence of lymphocytes in a CSF or vitreous sample is not always sufficient to distinguish inflammatory infiltrates from lymphoma. In both CSF and vitreous specimens, immunohistochemical staining may establish the diagnosis; if a substantial percentage of the cells

Table 11.2
Diagnostic evaluation of PCNSL patients.

1. Cranial MRI
2. Spinal MRI (enhanced) if spinal symptoms are present
3. Lumbar puncture
4. Ophthalmologic examination including slit lamp
5. Bone marrow
6. Abdominal-pelvic CT scan

are B-cells, lymphoma is strongly suggested. If the cells demonstrate a monoclonal population, this confirms the malignant nature of the lymphocytes even when they appear histologically benign. Like many systemic non-Hodgkin's lymphomas, PCNSL may be accompanied by an inflammatory infiltrate composed of T-cells. These reactive cells can infiltrate tumor tissue in the brain and can also accompany malignant lymphocytes in CSF or the vitreous complicating the cytologic diagnosis.

A strong clinical suspicion of PCNSL on imaging, or by examination of the vitreous, or spinal fluid, should lead one to consider a stereotactic needle biopsy rather than an open craniotomy with attempt at surgical removal. As indicated below, corticosteroids should be withheld until just before or immediately after the needle biopsy is performed. Optimally CSF, and, if appropriate, a vitreous specimen should be obtained prior to the start of corticosteroids as well.

PCNSL rarely metastasizes outside the nervous system, although, as indicated above, it may spread widely within the nervous system, including the eyes, leptomeninges and rarely spinal cord. Metastasis of systemic lymphoma to the CNS usually occurs late in the course of the disease, after the diagnosis of systemic lymphoma is evident and treatment is

underway. When CNS metastases are present at initial diagnosis of systemic lymphoma, the systemic manifestations are usually obvious clinically. It is extremely rare to have systemic non-Hodgkin's lymphoma present as an intracranial mass. Thus, an extensive systemic work-up in a patient believed to have PCNSL is usually unrewarding. However, an occasional patient presents with what appears to be PCNSL and is discovered subsequently to have systemic lymphoma.[34] Because the yield is so low, not all investigators believe a systemic workup is necessary in patients with presumed PCNSL. However, we suggest a limited workup to include CT of abdomen and pelvis and bone marrow examination for all patients with PCNSL.

Differential diagnosis

Table 11.3 lists the differential diagnosis of PCNSL in immunocompetent and immunosuppressed patients. In immunocompetent patients, lymphoma must be distinguished from other CNS tumors, particularly gliomas and metastases. As indicated above, clinical findings and imaging usually suggest the diagnosis, but only biopsy will unequivocally establish the diagnosis and dictate treatment. Rarely, lymphoma may either mimic a benign

Immunocompetent patients	Immunosuppressed patients
Glioma	Toxoplasmosis
Metastases	Fungal infection
Other hemopoietic tumors	Brain abscess(es)
Schwannoma[35]	Pituitary adenoma[36]
Multiple sclerosis	Progressive multifocal leukoencephalopathy
Sarcoid	Glioma
Inflammatory pseudotumor[37,38]	Metastases

Table 11.3
Differential diagnosis of PCNSL.

brain tumor[35] or even develop within a benign intracranial tumor.[36] Other hemopoietic tumors, as indicated later in this chapter, may mimic non-Hodgkin's lymphoma, and discriminating between these entities may be difficult even with biopsy. Especially important is distinguishing non-neoplastic lesions from PCNSL. Such lesions include multiple sclerosis, sarcoid and inflammatory pseudotumors. Inflammatory pseudotumor or plasma cell granuloma may be difficult to distinguish from lymphoma histologically; genetic studies may be required to demonstrate a clonal origin of the plasma or B-cells or identify gene rearrangements, indicating that the lesion is neoplastic rather than inflammatory.

In immunosuppressed patients, opportunistic infections such as toxoplasmosis, aspergillosis, progressive multifocal leukoencephalopathy and bacterial brain abscesses may mimic lymphoma. Gliomas, metastases and other lesions that also occur in immunocompetent patients may occasionally mimic lymphoma.

Treatment

Corticosteroids

Unlike their use in other brain tumors, where they control edema, corticosteroids also function as oncolytic agents for PCNSL. Steroid-induced apoptosis of lymphoma cells does not require wild-type p53 activity or caspase activation, but the apoptosis is inhibited by the bcl-2 oncogene.[39] In about 60% of patients treated with corticosteroids alone, there is substantial regression of the tumor within days to the point where the tumor may completely disappear. A needle biopsy performed after several days of corticosteroid treatment may reveal either normal brain tissue or evidence of necrosis without lymphocytes being present. In patients who have a prominent reactive lymphocytosis

accompanying their PCNSL, the tumor cells may be gone and the reactive T-lymphocytes persist, giving the false impression that this was an inflammatory process and not a neoplasm. Because the differential diagnosis includes a variety of inflammatory disorders of the nervous system that can also be suppressed by corticosteroids (e.g. multiple sclerosis), the clinician cannot tell whether the original lesion was tumor or inflammation. However, corticosteroids are not curative and the patient usually relapses within a matter of months, often with more aggressive disease, although we have seen occasional long-term remissions. One of our patients went 7 years while being treated with two courses of corticosteroids alone before developing a recurrence, which proved to be PCNSL on biopsy. Spontaneous remissions lasting as long as 4 years have also been reported,[40] perhaps representing the ability of the patient's immune system to partially control the tumor.

Surgery

The correct surgical approach to PCNSL is a stereotactic needle biopsy. Because PCNSL infiltrates so widely and is usually in a deep location, surgery does not increase survival and often results in worse neurologic deficits. If PCNSL was not suspected prior to craniotomy and a diagnosis is made on frozen section, further resection should be abandoned and the patient treated as indicated below. Surgical resection should be reserved for only those patients whose tumor mass is producing herniation leading to imminent death. Unlike most other primary brain tumors, extirpation is an unfavorable prognostic factor, perhaps because these patients are in poor neurologic condition preoperatively.[10] Hemorrhage, sometimes fatal, may complicate biopsy in more than 10% of immunosuppressed patients.[16]

Radiation therapy

For reasons that are unclear, radiation therapy (RT) that usually provides excellent local control in systemic non-Hodgkin's lymphoma, does not in PCNSL. Whereas non-CNS diffuse large cell lymphoma has a 75–90% local control rate in Stage I, the local control rate is only 39% in the brain, and most recurrences appear in regions of the brain that have received 60 Gy of irradiation.[41] A complete response to RT has been reported in most patients with PCNSL, over 80% in one series.[42] However, relapse is generally early and the median survival is only 12–18 months, with fewer than 5% of patients surviving 5 years after RT. Whole-brain RT is the treatment of choice, because of the widespread nature of PCNSL, even in those patients who have a single lesion on MRI. A number of RT protocols have been proposed. The Radiation Therapy Oncology Group (RTOG) conducted a prospective study using 40-Gy whole-brain RT plus a 20-Gy boost to the tumor site. Median survival was only 12.2 months.[43] Age and Karnofsky performance status (KPS) were important prognostic factors. Patients over 60 had a median survival of 7.6 months, compared to 23.1 months for those younger than 60. Those with a KPS ≥ 70 had a median survival of 21.1 months versus 5.6 months for those with a KPS of 40–60. Increasing the dose to 60 Gy in the boosted field did not improve survival or local control. We have also found that, despite a whole-brain dose of 40 Gy and a 14.40-Gy boost, recurrences developed with equal frequency both within and outside the boosted area.[44] Therefore, there was no added benefit with dose escalation beyond 40–50 Gy. Our approach now is to use 45-Gy whole-brain RT without a boost, recognizing that cerebral, leptomeningeal or even spinal recurrences are possible.

The eyes are not included in the radiation portal unless ocular lymphoma is present, in which case both eyes are radiated to a total of 36–40 Gy. RT is effective in controlling ocular lymphoma, although ocular relapse can occur after RT. In addition, up to 80% of patients who present with isolated ocular lymphoma eventually develop cerebral involvement if followed for up to 10 years, and most develop CNS disease within 3 years of their ocular diagnosis. Because there is occult involvement of the leptomeninges in virtually all PCNSL patients, craniospinal RT has been used in a small number of patients.[45] However, neuraxis RT did not improve survival over whole-brain RT alone and it is associated with significant morbidity, particularly myelosuppression, which can compromise the subsequent administration of chemotherapy. Radiation toxicity, especially dementia, is common in those who are over 60 (Fig. 11.3).[46] Leukoencephalopathy on MRI without evident dementia is frequent in younger patients (Fig. 11.4).

Chemotherapy

The initial treatment of choice for PCNSL is chemotherapy.[47,48] Whether RT is required after successful chemotherapy is not established. The standard chemotherapeutic approach to the treatment of systemic non-Hodgkin's lymphoma, cyclophosphamide, doxorubicin, vincristine and prednisone (CHOP), is not successful in treating PCNSL.[49–51] Complete remissions are achieved in only a few patients, and early relapse is common. The reported median survival is only 9.5–16 months when CHOP is combined with whole-brain RT, no improvement over that seen with RT alone. These agents, which effectively treat systemic lymphoma, prednisone excepted, cross the blood–brain barrier poorly. Because PCNSL widely and microscopically infiltrates the brain, infiltrative disease in every patient is protected by the blood–brain barrier. Although

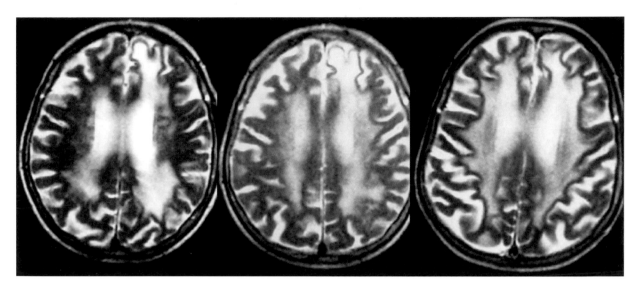

Figure 11.3
Complications of radiation therapy for the treatment of primary CNS lymphoma. This 84-year-old woman developed a lesion deep in the left parietal lobe in December 1996. The lesion responded completely to 50-Gy whole-brain radiation and did not recur. However, as scans in December 1996 (left), April 1997 (middle), and September 1998 (right) show, there is progressive hyperintensity in the white matter associated with loss of normal cognitive function.

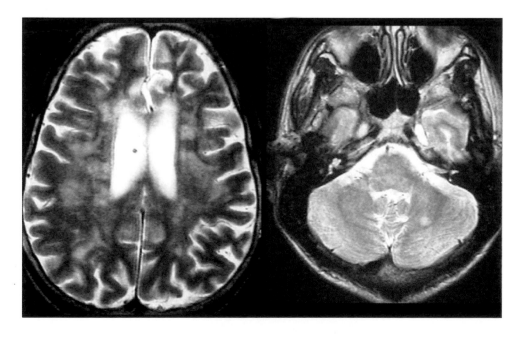

Figure 11.4
Younger people tolerate radiation better than older people. This scan is of a 35-year-old man 8 years post-radiation and chemotherapy for primary CNS lymphoma. The tumor has not recurred. There is a great deal of white matter hyperintensity but he functions at a very high level without evident cognitive difficulty.

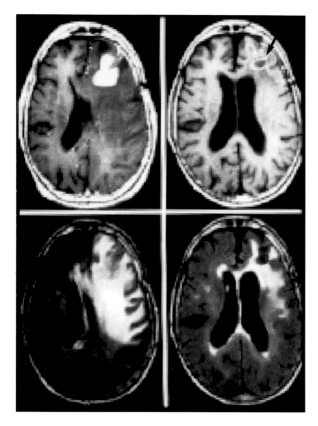

Figure 11.5
Response of primary CNS lymphoma to
methotrexate. The left scan show the typical lesion
prior to treatment. The right scans are after two
courses of high-dose methotrexate. The mass has
reduced (arrow), and ventricular compression and
shift has returned to normal.

enhancing lesions may respond to CHOP
because of focal disruption of the barrier, microscopic tumor, which is protected by an intact
blood–brain barrier, continues to grow. When
drugs which cross the blood–brain barrier and
are effective against lymphoma are used the
outcome is much better.

High-dose methotrexate is recognized as the
single most active agent against PCNSL (Fig.
11.5).[52,53] Methotrexate in standard doses does
not cross the blood–brain barrier in sufficient

quantity to treat the tumor. However, if high
doses (> 1 g/m²) are used, adequate concentration of drug reach and kill tumor cells protected
by the blood–brain barrier. The rest of the body
is protected by leucovorin, a folate analog that
reverses the effect of methotrexate but does not
reach the CNS. Accordingly, most protocols
now call for high-dose methotrexate with
leucovorin rescue, sometimes in association
with other drugs given in high enough doses to
cross the blood–brain barrier, e.g. cytarabine, or
lipid-soluble agents such as procarbazine. Rapid
infusion of methotrexate over 3 h, rather than
the conventional 6–24 h, significantly increases
levels of the drug in CSF and presumably
brain.[54] Some investigators have used intra-
arterial hyperosmolar agents to open the
blood–brain barrier, followed by intra-arterial
methotrexate,[55] but there is no evidence that
this technique is better than forcing water-
soluble agents across the blood–brain barrier by
using high intravenous doses. Moreover, the
intra-arterial method is associated with unique
acute toxicities including seizures, strokes,
arterial dissections and cerebral swelling.[56]
Several protocols based on high-dose methotrexate have reported complete remission rates
of 80–90% and event-free survival rates of
greater than 5 years. Our long-term follow-up
reveals a 22% 5-year survival rate with some
patients 12 years from diagnosis; these patients
are probably cured of their PCNSL.[57]

Age and performance status are important
prognostic factors.[58] Not only do patients over
60 years old have a poor prognosis, regardless
of treatment, but they are also more likely to
suffer neurotoxicity, usually dementia, from
combined modality therapy if they survive more
than a year.[57] Accordingly, several protocols
call for treatment with chemotherapy alone in
patients over 60, reserving RT for relapse.
Although overall survival for patients treated in
this fashion is comparable to those treated with

up-front chemotherapy and RT, CNS relapse occurs earlier after chemotherapy alone.[47,59]

Several other chemotherapy regimens, some of which incorporate high-dose methotrexate, have been tried but none has been shown to be superior.[60,61] In some relapsed patients who achieve a complete remission from induction chemotherapy, high-dose chemotherapy with bone marrow or stem cell rescue without cranial RT is being tried as experimental treatment.[62] A major effort in the design of new regimens is not only to improve efficacy but also to reduce the risk of delayed cognitive impairment.

'Salvage' therapy, given when patients fail first-line treatment, significantly improves survival and probably improves quality of life. Injection of methotrexate and thiotepa directly into the vitreous can successfully treat recurrent ocular lymphoma.[63] Biological treatment of non-CNS lymphomas is becoming increasingly successful.[64] Such approaches include the anti-CD-20 monoclonal antibody (Rutuximab), radioimmune conjugates and patient-specific vaccination. Preliminary evidence with Rutuximab suggests that it may have activity against PCNSL.[65] Whether these techniques will prove useful in PCNSL is unknown.

Prognosis

Regardless of treatment, the prognosis is worse in patients over 60 than in those who are younger, and is much poorer in patients who are immunocompromised than in those who are immunocompetent. Patients in poor condition at diagnosis also fare worse than those in good condition. Telomerase activity predicts a shorter interval to relapse and shorter survival.[23]

Median survival is only 1–2 months with supportive care alone. With surgery alone, the median survival is about 3 months, little longer than with no treatment at all (Table 11.4).

Patients treated with RT alone have a median survival of about 12–18 months with relapse usually occurring 12–14 months after treatment. The high-dose methotrexate-based chemotherapeutic regimens yield an overall survival of about 40–60 months. Some patients may be secondarily salvaged by additional chemotherapy or, if they have not received it, RT. Approximately 50% of patients can achieve a second remission with salvage treatment and 25% have prolonged survival for many years after reinduction.

Late neurotoxicity can limit survival and quality of life for some patients after successful treatment of their PCNSL. Progressive memory impairment, ataxia and eventually urinary incontinence are the major clinical manifestations of leukoencephalopathy. While elderly patients are particularly vulnerable, even young patients can occasionally develop this irreversible complication. The symptoms

Treatment	Median survival (months)
Surgery alone	3–4
Whole-brain RT	12–18
CHOP + Whole-brain RT	9.5–16
HD-MTX[a] + Whole-brain RT	40–60

aHD-MTX = high-dose methotrexate

Table 11.4
Treatment and median survival rates.

often appear months after completion of treatment. There is no good treatment for delayed neurotoxicity although ventriculoperitoneal shunt can sometimes ameliorate symptoms, especially ataxia and urinary incontinence.[66] The main objective is to prevent the sequelae of therapy by designing effective but less toxic regimens.

Other hemopoietic tumors

Plasmacytomas[67,68] (Fig. 11.6), Hodgkin's disease[69,70] and granulocytic sarcomas[71] (myelogenous leukemia chloroma) occasionally arise in the CNS. Most are dural-based, although a few are parenchymal.[72,73] When these tumors develop in the absence of systemic disease, they are difficult to distinguish from non-hemopoietic tumors. Their diagnosis depends on biopsy, and treatment is similar to that of their systemic counterparts.

Intracranial disease may be a manifestation of widespread metastases, or can occur as an isolated site of disease, particularly with plasmacytomas or granulocytic sarcomas. Neurologic symptoms and signs are related to tumor location. These tumors often invade or compress cerebral cortex. Therefore, seizures and lateralizing signs, such as hemiparesis and confusion, are common at presentation. Neuroimaging, either CT or MRI, typically reveals a dural-based, prominently enhancing mass. It may be difficult to distinguish such lesions from a meningioma except that significant edema of the underlying brain is more common with hemopoietic tumors. A dural tail may also be evident with these lymphoid tumors. CT usually reveals any accompanying underlying bone destruction better than MRI. Magnetic resonance venography (MRV) should be performed for any lesion located close to the superior sagittal sinus to assess its patency.

Surgical resection is often the principal treatment, and also enables accurate histologic diagnosis. Unless a patient has known active systemic disease, the identification of one of these intracranial lesions should prompt a

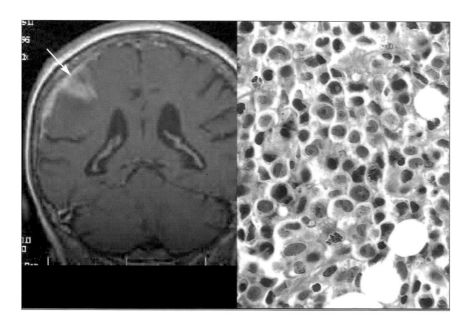

Figure 11.6
Plasmacytoma involving the dura. This 65-year-old woman presented with headache and some changes in behavior. A scan revealed an enhancing dural-based mass (arrow) that on biopsy was a plasmacytoma. Local radiation therapy was delivered. The mass disappeared and she has been well in the ensuing 5 years. The photomicrograph shows dense sheets of abnormal plasma cells, some with intranuclear inclusion bodies.

comprehensive evaluation to determine whether there is evidence of a systemic malignancy. Post-surgical therapy is often determined by the need for generalized systemic treatment, but focal RT may be used to control CNS disease. If such a lesion is identified radiographically in a patient with known or active systemic tumor, such as a dural granulocytic sarcoma in a patient with documented acute myelogenous leukemia, then focal RT alone may be used since surgery is not essential for diagnosis and these lesions are usually radiosensitive. In addition, patients with these lesions should have a lumbar puncture to assess whether there is also involvement of the subarachnoid space. In operated patients, the lumbar puncture should be done a few weeks post-operatively unless done prior to surgery to avoid confusion with surgically-related shedding of tumor cells in the CSF. Demonstration of leptomeningeal metastases is rare but would necessitate intrathecal chemotherapy as well as cranial RT.

Histiocytic disorders

A heterogeneous group of tumor and tumor-like masses composed of histiocytes, including Langerhans cell histiocytosis and non-Langerhans cell histiocytosis, sometimes occur in isolation within the nervous system (Fig. 11.7). These lesions are usually not malignant and all are very rare (Table 11.5).

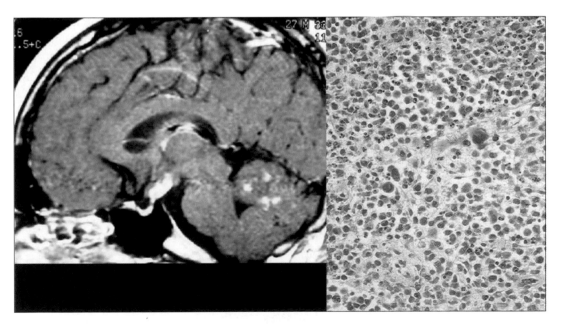

Figure 11.7
Langerhans cell histiocytosis. This 25-year-old man developed diabetes insipidus followed by pituitary failure. He had no neurologic complaints but an MR scan of the head revealed multiple contrast enhancing masses in the cerebellum. Cerebellar biopsy was consistent with Langerhans cell histiocytosis. After endocrine replacement, he had no neurologic complaints nor has he developed any in the past 7 years. The photomicrograph shows a mixed cellular infiltrate composed of eosinophils, plasma cells, and the characteristic Langerhans cells.

Table 11.5
Histiocytic disorders affecting the CNS.

- Dendritic cell-related disorders
  Langerhans cell histiocytosis
  Solitary histiocytomas of various dendritic
    cell phenotypes
- Macrophage-related disorders
  Hemophagocytic lymphohistiocytosis[74]
- Rosai–Dorfman disease (sinus histiocytosis
  with massive lymphadenopathy)[75]
- Erdheim–Chester syndrome[76]
- Malignant histiocytosis[77]

Langerhans cell histiocytosis (from Greek histio meaning 'web' or 'tissue' and kytos meaning 'cell') is a rare disorder characterized by proliferation of cells similar to the Langerhans cell, a dendritic cell of the epidermis.[78] Langerhans cell histiocytosis is the accurate classification for disorders previously called histiocytosis X, eosinophilic granuloma, Hand–Schuller–Christian disease and Abt–Letterer–Siwe disease. Neurologic dysfunction occurs in about 1–6% of patients with Langerhans cell histiocytosis. The hypothalamic–pituitary axis, the hypothalamus and the cerebellum are the sites most commonly involved. Occasionally, mass lesions are found elsewhere in the brain. CNS lesions may occur either in the presence or the absence of the characteristic bony lesions in the skull. Because of its predilection for the hypothalamic–pituitary axis, diabetes insipidus is the most common neurologic manifestation. Diabetes insipidus may precede other neurologic or systemic symptoms by months or years (Table 11.6).

MR images generally reveal infundibular thickening or an enhancing suprasellar or hypothalamic mass lesion. Occasionally, space

Table 11.6
Langerhans cell histiocytosis: 38 patients at diagnosis.

Systemic involvement	Per cent	CNS involvement/MRI	Per cent
Multisystem disease	72	White matter lesions, no enhancement	55
Single-system bone disease	18	White matter lesions with enhancement	24
Single-system skin, lymph node	0	Gray matter lesions, no enhancement	50
Primary CNS disease	10	Gray matter lesions with enhancement	8
Bone	84	Extraparenchymal, dural based	32
Skull	74	Extraparenchymal, arachnoidal based	5
Temporal bone	34	Extraparenchymal, choroid plexus based	8
Skin	58	Infundibular thickening	21
Diabetes insipidus	31	(Partial) empty sella	37
Orbits	24	Hypothalamic mass lesions	10
Endocrinopathies	18	Atrophy, diffuse	26
Lungs	16	Atrophy, localized	16
Gastrointestinal tract	10	Therapy-related enhancement and localized atrophy	15
Liver	10		
Spleen	10		

Modified from Grois et al,[79] with permission.

occupying lesions are found elsewhere in the brain. The symptoms are location specific. MRI usually reveals a contrast enhancing mass that can be in the parenchyma of the brain or can involve the meninges or choroid plexus. In the absence of other systemic lesions the diagnosis can be made only by biopsy.

The cerebellum and brainstem can be involved in one of two ways. The patient may present with a contrast-enhancing mass in the posterior fossa similar to those seen in the suprasellar or hypothalamic regions. Other patients present with progressive cerebellar signs associated with a normal MR scan or with non-enhancing white matter hyperintensity on the T2-weighted image. This phenomenon appears to be a reaction to systemic Langerhans cell histiocytosis and has been described in several patients as a paraneoplastic syndrome.[80]

The pathology of Langerhans cell histiocytosis in the brain differs from that elsewhere in the body and often lacks features that are specifically diagnostic of the disease, making isolated CNS disease difficult to diagnose. The paraneoplastic cerebellar and brainstem syndrome may show only destruction of Purkinje cells and demyelination with an absence of histiocytes.

Single-mass lesions respond to surgery.[81] RT is useful in some instances, although it does not appear to reverse diabetes insipidus. Some patients have responded to systemic chemotherapy.[81]

Several non-Langerhans cell histiocytic lesions can also involve the nervous system (Table 11.5). Hematophagocytic lymphohistiocytosis is generally a lethal disease characterized by a hemophagocytic syndrome including high fever, hemophagocytic cells, pancytopenia, low fibrinogen level, hemodilution, elevation of liver enzymes and hypertriglyceridemia. The cause of the disorder is unknown, but the CNS is affected in about 75% of patients. The disorder can appear either as an isolated lymphocytic meningitis or with parenchymal symptoms including seizures, ataxia[74] and brainstem abnormalities. When the brain itself is involved, CT scan may show calcifications. On MR scan, white matter hyperintensity is evident on T2-weighted images; lesions occasionally contrast enhance. Although CNS signs may appear early, most patients have evidence of systemic disease. The diagnosis is suggested by the presence of hemophagocytic cells within the spinal fluid. Although the disease is usually lethal, some patients respond to bone marrow transplantation.[74]

Other non Langerhans cell histiocytoses that may present with CNS involvement include the Rosai–Dorfman syndrome[75] and the Erdheim–Chester syndrome.[76] The diagnosis of these disorders can be made only by biopsy. These syndromes may present with dural or brain masses. Diagnosis is established radiographically if systemic disease is known; however, in those instances where no systemic disease is present, CNS biopsy may be required. The Erdheim–Chester disease, like Langerhans cell histiocytosis, may present with cerebellar signs, apparently as a paraneoplastic effect of the disorder on the nervous system.

References

1. Recht L, Straus DJ, Cirrincione C et al. Central nervous system metastases from non-Hodgkin's lymphoma: treatment and prophylaxis. Am J Med 1988; 84: 425–35.
2. Hayabuchi N, Shibamoto Y, Onizuka Y et al. Primary central nervous system lymphoma in Japan: a nationwide survey. Int J Radiat Oncol Biol Phys 1999; 44: 265–72.
3. DeAngelis LM. Primary central nervous system lymphoma. J Neurol Neurosurg Psychiatry 1999; 66: 699–701.

4. DeAngelis LM. Primary central nervous system lymphoma: a new clinical challenge. Neurology 1991; 411: 619–21.

5. Hao D, DiFrancesco LM, Brasher PM et al. Is primary CNS lymphoma really becoming more common? A population-based study of incidence, clinicopathological features and outcomes in Alberta from 1975 to 1996. Ann Oncol 1999; 10: 65–70.

6. Corn BW, Marcus SM, Topham A, Hauck W, Curran WJ Jr. Will primary central nervous system lymphoma be the most frequent brain tumor diagnosed in the year 2000? Cancer 1997; 79: 2409–13.

7. O'Neill BP, Janney CA, Olson J et al. The continuing increase in primary central nervous system non-Hodgkin's lymphoma (PCNSL): a surveillance epidemiology, and end results (SEER) analysis. Proc Am Soc Clin Oncol 2001; 2: 53.

8. Schabet M. Epidemiology of primary CNS lymphoma. J Neurooncol 1999; 43: 199–201.

9. CBTRUS (2000). Statistical report: primary brain tumors in the United States, 1992–1997. Central Brain Tumor Registry of the United States, 2000.

10. Bataille B, Delwail V, Menet E et al. Primary intracerebral malignant lymphoma: report of 248 cases. J Neurosurg 2000; 92: 261–6.

11. Peterson K, Gordon KB, Heinemann M-H, DeAngelis LM. The clinical spectrum of ocular lymphoma. Cancer 1993; 72: 843–9.

12. Balmaceda C, Gaynor JJ, Sun M, Gluck JT, DeAngelis LM. Leptomeningeal tumor in primary central nervous system lymphoma: recognition, significance, and implications. Ann Neurol 1995; 38: 202–9.

13. Schiff D, Suman VJ, Yang P, Rocca WA, O'Neill BP. Risk factor for primary central nervous system lymphoma. Cancer 1998; 82: 975–82.

14. Loureiro C, Gill PS, Meyer PR et al. Autopsy findings in AIDS-related lymphoma. Cancer 1988; 62: 735–9.

15. Cornford ME, Holden JK, Boyd MC, Berry K, Vinters HV. Neuropathology of the acquired immune deficiency syndrome (AIDS): report of 39 autopsies from Vancouver, British Columbia. Can J Neurol Sci 1992; 19: 442–52.

16. Phan TG, O'Neill BP, Kurtin PJ. Posttransplant primary CNS lymphoma. Neuro-Oncol 2000; 2: 229–38.

17. MacMahon EME, Glass JD, Hayward SD et al. Epstein–Barr virus in AIDS-related primary central nervous system lymphoma. Lancet 1991; 338: 969–73.

18. Rouach E, Rogers BB, Wilson DR, Kirkpatrick JB, Byffone GJ. Demonstration of Epstein–Barr virus in primary central nervous system lymphomas by the polymerase chain reaction and in situ hybridization. Hum Pathol 1990; 21: 545–50.

19. Paulus W. Classification, pathogenesis and molecular pathology of primary CNS lymphomas. J Neurooncol 1999; 43: 203–8.

20. Weber T, Weber RG, Kaulich K et al. Characteristic chromosomal imbalances in primary central nervous system lymphomas of the diffuse large B-cell type. Brain Pathol 2000; 10: 73–84.

21. Harada K, Nishizaki T, Kubota H et al. Distinct primary central nervous system lymphoma defined by comparative genomic hybridization and laser scanning cytometry. Cancer Genet Cytogenet 2001; 125: 147–50.

22. Bashir R, Coakham H, Hochberg F. Expression of LFA-1/ICAM-1 in CNS lymphomas: possible mechanism for lymphoma homing into the brain. J Neurooncol 1992; 12: 103–10.

23. Harada K, Kurisu K, Arita K et al. Telomerase activity in central nervous system malignant lymphoma. Cancer 1999; 86: 1050–5.

24. Bashir R, Chamberlain M, Ruby E, Hochberg FH. T-cell infiltration of primary CNS lymphoma. Neurology 1996; 46: 440–4.

25. Gijtenbeek JM, Rosenblum MK, DeAngelis LM. Primary central nervous system lymphoma. Neurology 2001; 57(4): 716–8.

26. Molnar PP, O'Neill BP, Scheithauer BW, Groothuis DR. The blood–brain barrier in primary CNS lymphomas: ultrastructural evidence of endothelial cell death. Neuro-Oncol 1999; 1: 89–100.

27. Herrlinger U, Schabet M, Bitzer M, Petersen D, Krauseneck P. Primary central nervous system lymphoma: From clinical presentation to diagnosis. J Neurooncol 1999; 43: 219–26.

28. Herrlinger U. Primary CNS lymphoma: Findings outside the brain. J Neurooncol 1999; 43: 227–30.

29. Sugahara T, Korogi Y, Shigematsu Y et al. Perfusion-sensitive MRI of cerebral lymphomas: a preliminary report. J Comput Assist Tomogr 1999; 23: 232–7.

30. DeAngelis LM. Cerebral lymphoma presenting as a nonenhancing lesion on computed tomographic/magnetic resonance scan. Ann Neurol 1993; 33: 308–11.

31. Roelcke U, Leenders KL. Positron emission tomography in patients with primary CNS lymphomas. J Neurooncol 1999; 43: 231–6.

32. Yoshikai T, Fukahori T, Ishimaru J et al. ^{123}I-IMP SPET in the diagnosis of primary central nervous system lymphoma. Eur J Nucl Med 2001; 28: 25–32.

33. Kuhlmann T, Schröter A, Dechent P et al. Diagnosis of a multifocal B cell lymphoma with preceding demyelinating central nervous system lesions by single voxel proton MR spectroscopy. J Neurol Neurosurg Psychiatry 2001; 70: 259–62.

34. Schwarz S, Schwab S, Harms W, Hacke W. Systemic lymphoma in patients with the initial diagnosis of primary central nervous system lymphoma: a report of two cases. J Neurol 1999; 246: 855–7.

35. Aziz KMA, van Loveren HR. Primary lymphoma of Meckel's cave mimicking trigeminal schwannoma: case report. Neurosurgery 1999; 44: 859–62.

36. Kuhn D, Buchfelder M, Brabletz T, Paulus W. Intrasellar malignant lymphoma developing within pituitary adenoma. Acta Neuropathol (Berl) 1999; 97: 311–6.

37. Postler E, Bornemann A, Skalej M et al. Intracranial inflammatory tumors: A survey of their various etiologies by presentation of 5 cases. J Neurooncol 1999; 43: 209–17.

38. Makino K, Murakami M, Kitano I, Ushio Y. Primary intracranial plasma-cell granuloma: a case report and review of the literature. Surg Neurol 1995; 43: 374–8.

39. Weller M. Glucocorticoid treatment of primary CNS lymphoma. J Neurooncol 1999; 43: 237–9.

40. Al-Yamany M, Lozano A, Nag S, Laperriere N, Bernstein M. Spontaneous remission of primary central nervous system lymphoma: report of 3 cases and discussion of pathophysiology. J Neurooncol 1999; 42: 151–9.

41. Nelson DF. Radiotherapy in the treatment of primary central nervous system lymphoma (PCNSL). J Neurooncol 1999; 43: 241–7.

42. Corn BW, Dolinskas C, Scott C et al. Strong correlation between imaging response and survival among patients with primary central nervous system lymphoma: A secondary analysis of RTOG studies 83-15 and 88-06. Int J Radiat Oncol Biol Phys 2000; 47: 299–303.

43. Nelson DF, Martz KL, Bonner H et al. Non-Hodgkin's lymphoma of the brain: can high dose, large volume radiation therapy improve survival? Report on a prospective trial by the Radiation Therapy Oncology Group (RTOG): RTOG 8315 Int J Radiat Oncol Biol Phys 1992; 23: 9–17.

44. DeAngelis LM, Yahalom J, Thaler HT, Kher U. Combined modality therapy for primary CNS lymphoma. J Clin Oncol 1992; 10: 635–43.

45. Brada M, Dearnaley D, Horwich A, Bloom HJG. Management of primary cerebral lymphoma with initial chemotherapy: preliminary results and comparison with patients treated with radiotherapy alone. Int J Radiat Oncol Biol Phys 1990; 18: 787–92.

46. Schlegel U, Pels H, Oehring R, Blümcke I. Neurologic sequelae of treatment of primary CNS lymphomas. J Neurooncol 1999; 43: 277–86.

47. Abrey LE, Yahalom J, DeAngelis LM. Treatment for primary CNS lymphoma: the next step. J Clin Oncol 2000; 18: 3144–50.

48. Schlegel U, Schmidt-Wolf IGH, Deckert M. Primary CNS lymphoma: clinical presentation, pathological classification, molecular pathogenesis and treatment. J Neurol Sci 2000; 181: 1–12.

49. O'Neill BP, Wang CH, O'Fallon JR et al. Primary central nervous system non-Hodgkin's lymphoma (PCNSL): Survival advantages with combined initial therapy? A final report of the North Central Cancer Treatment Group (NCCTG) study 86-72-52. Int J Radiat Oncol Biol Phys 1999; 43: 559–63.

50. Schultz C, Scott C, Sherman W et al. Preirradiation chemotherapy with cyclophosphamide, doxorubicin, vincristine and dexamethasone for primary CNS lymphomas: initial report of Radiation Therapy Oncology Group protocol 88-06. J Clin Oncol 1996; 14: 556–64.

51. Mead GM, Bleehen NM, Gregor A et al. A medical research council randomized trial in patients with primary cerebral non-Hodgkin lymphoma – cerebral radiotherapy with and without cyclophosphamide, doxorubicin, vincristine, and prednisone chemotherapy. Cancer 2000; 89: 1359–70.

52. Reni M, Ferreri AJM, Garancini MP, Villa E. Therapeutic management of primary central nervous system lymphoma in immunocompetent patients: results of a critical review of the literature. Ann Oncol 1997; 8: 227–34.

53. Blay JY, Conroy T, Chevreau C et al. High-dose methotrexate for the treatment of primary cerebral lymphomas: analysis of survival and late neurologic toxicity in a retrospective series. J Clin Oncol 1998; 16: 864–71.

54. Hiraga S, Arita N, Ohnishi T et al. Rapid infusion of high-dose methotrexate resulting in enhanced penetration into cerebrospinal fluid and intensified tumor response in primary central nervous system lymphomas. J Neurosurg 1999; 91: 221–30.

55. Kraemer DF, Fortin D, Doolittle ND, Neuwelt EA. Association of total dose intensity of chemotherapy in primary central nervous system lymphoma (Human non-acquired immunodeficiency syndrome) and survival. Neurosurgery 2001; 48: 1033–40.

56. Doolittle ND, Miner ME, Hall WA et al. Safety and efficacy of a multicenter study using intraarterial chemotherapy in conjunction with osmotic opening of the blood–brain barrier for the treatment of patients with malignant brain tumors. Cancer 2000; 88: 637–47.

57. Abrey LE, DeAngelis LM, Yahalom J. Long-term survival in primary CNS lymphoma. J Clin Oncol 1998; 16: 859–63.

58. Corry J, Smith JG, Wirth A, Quong G, Liew KH. Primary central nervous system lymphoma: Age and performance status are more important than treatment modality. Int J Radiat Oncol Biol Phys 1998; 41: 615–20.

59. Sandor V, Stark-Vancs V, Pearson D et al. Phase II trial of chemotherapy alone for primary CNS and intraocular lymphoma. J Clin Oncol 1998; 16: 3000–6.

60. Shibamoto Y, Sasai K, Oya N, Hiraoka M. Systemic chemotherapy with vincristine, cyclophosphamide, doxorubicin and pred-nisolone following radiotherapy for primary central nervous system lymphoma: a phase II study. J Neurooncol 1999; 42: 161–7.

61. Cheng AL, Yeh KH, Uen WC, Hung RL, Liu MY, Wang CH. Systemic chemotherapy alone for patients with non-acquired immunodeficiency syndrome-related central nervous system lymphoma – a pilot study of the BOMES protocol. Cancer 1998; 82: 1946–51.

62. Soussain C, Suzan F, Hoang-Xuan K et al. Results of intensive chemotherapy followed by hematopoietic stem-cell rescue in 22 patients with refractory or recurrent primary CNS lymphoma or intraocular lymphoma. J Clin Oncol 2001; 19: 742–9.

63. De Smet MD, Vancs VS, Kohler D, Solomon D, Chan CC. Intravitreal chemotherapy for the treatment of recurrent intraocular lymphoma. Br J Ophthalmol 1999; 83: 448–51.

64. Bendandi M, Longo DL. Biologic therapy for lymphoma. Curr Opin Oncol 1999; 11: 343–50.

65. Raizer JJ, DeAngelis LM, Zelenetz AD, Abrey LE. Activity of Rituximab in primary central nervous system lymphoma (PCNSL). Proc Am Soc Clin Oncol 2000;19: 166a.

66. Thiessen B, DeAngelis LM. Hydrocephalus in radiation leukoencephalopathy – results of ventriculoperitoneal shunting. Arch Neurol 1998; 55: 705–10.

67. Vaicys C, Schulder M, Wolansky LJ, Fromowitz FB. Falcotentorial plasmacytoma – case report. J Neurosurg 1999; 91: 132–5.

68. Vujovic O, Fisher BJ, Munoz DG. Solitary intracranial plasmacytoma: case report and review of management. J Neurooncol 1998; 39: 47–50.

69. Herrlinger U, Klingel K, Meyermann R et al. Central nervous system Hodgkin's lymphoma without systemic manifestation: case report and review of the literature. Acta Neuropathol (Berl) 2000; 99: 709–14.

70. Biagi J, MacKenzie RG, Lim MS, Sapp M, Berinstein N. Primary Hodgkin's disease of the CNS in an immunocompetent patient: a case study and review of the literature. Neuro-oncol 2000; 2: 239–43.

71. Byrd C, Edenfield JW, Shields DJ, et al. Extramedullary myeloid tumours in acute nonlymphocytic leukaemia: a clinical review. J Clin Oncol 1995; 13: 1800–16.

72. Klein R, Mullges W, Bendszus M et al. Primary intracerebral Hodgkin's disease: report of a case with Epstein–Barr virus association and review of the literature. Am J Surg Pathol 1999; 23: 477–81.

73. Clark WC, Callihan T, Schwartzberg L, Fontanesi J. Primary intracranial Hodgkin's lymphoma without dural attachment. Case report. J Neurosurg 1992; 76: 692–5.

74. Haddad E, Sulis ML, Jabado N et al. Frequency and severity of central nervous system lesions in hemophagocytic lymphohistiocytosis. Blood 1997; 89: 794–800.

75. Andriko JA, Morrison A, Colegial CH, Davis BJ, Jones RV. Rosai-Dorfman disease isolated to the central nervous system: a report of 11 cases. Mod Pathol 2001; 14: 172–8.

76. Wright RA, Hermann RC, Parisi JE. Neurological manifestations of Erdheim-Chester disease. J Neurol Neurosurg Psychiatry 1999; 66: 72–5.

77. Gogusev J, Nezelof C. Malignant histiocytosis. Histologic, cytochemical, chromosomal, and molecular data with a nosologic discussion. Hematol Oncol Clin N Am 1998; 12: 445–63.

78. Howarth DM, Gilchrist GS, Mullan BP et al. Langerhans cell histiocytosis – Diagnosis, natural history, management, and outcome. Cancer 1999; 85: 2278–90.

79. Grois NG, Favara BE, Mostbeck GH, Prayer D. Central nervous system disease in Langerhans cell histiocytosis. Hematol Oncol Clin N Am 1998; 12: 287–305.

80. Goldberg-Stern H, Weitz R, Zaizov R, Gornish M, Gadoth N. Progressive spinocerebellar degeneration 'plus' associated with Langerhans cell histiocytosis: a new paraneoplastic syndrome? J Neurol Neurosurg Psychiatry 1995; 58: 180–3.

81. Hund E, Steiner HH, Jansen O, Sieverts H, Sohl G, Essig M. Treatment of cerebral Langerhans cell histiocytosis. J Neurol Sci 1999; 171: 145–52.

12

Miscellaneous central nervous system neoplasms and 'tumors'

Introduction

In this chapter, we discuss a number of intracranial mass lesions not considered elsewhere in this book (Table 12.1). Included are familial intracranial tumors, cystic tumors and some other rare tumors.

Familial central nervous system tumors

Introduction

Table 1.7 lists some of the hereditary syndromes associated with brain tumors and the genetic defects that underlie each syndrome. In this chapter, we will emphasize the associated non-central nervous system (CNS) findings that should lead one to suspect the possibility of a hereditary brain tumor syndrome. Most of these syndromes are autosomal dominant, indicating that a careful family history will often identify the patient at risk. However, in many the penetrance is incomplete, and family members affected with the gene may not show clinical stigmata. In some, such as neurofibromatosis-1 (NF-1), tuberous sclerosis and retinoblastoma, the mutation rate is so high that the disorder often occurs in the absence of family history as a sporadic new mutation.

Table 12.1
Miscellaneous CNS neoplasms and 'tumors'

* Hereditary syndromes
  Neurofibromatosis-1 (NF-1)
  Neurofibromatosis-2 (NF-2)
  von Hippel–Lindau
  Tuberous sclerosis
  Li–Fraumeni
  Cowden
  Turcot
  Nevoid basal cell carcinoma syndrome (Gorlin)
  Retinoblastoma
  Bloom syndrome
  Fanconi anemia
  Familial melanoma
  Rhabdoid predisposition syndrome
* Cysts and tumor-like lesions
  Rathke cleft cyst (Chapter 10)
  Epidermoid cyst
  Dermoid cyst
  Colloid cyst of the 3rd ventricle
  Enterogenous cyst
  Neuroglial cyst
  Arachnoid cyst
  Granular cell tumor (Chapter 10) (choristoma, pituicytoma)
  Hypothalamic neuronal hamartoma
  Nasal glial heterotopia
  Plasma cell granuloma (Chapter 11)

A careful search for associated non-CNS findings may assist in making the diagnosis, and also identify lesions outside the nervous system

Table 12.2
Skin and other organ involvement in familial brain tumor syndromes.

Syndrome	Skin	Other tissues
Neurofibromatosis-1	Café-au-lait spots, axillary freckling, (cutaneous) neurofibromas	Iris hamartomas, osseous lesions, pheochromocytoma, leukemia
Neurofibromatosis-2	None	Posterior lens opacities, retinal hamartoma
von Hippel–Lindau	None	Retinal hemangioblastomas, renal cell carcinoma, pheochromocytoma, visceral cysts, endolymphatic sac tumor
Tuberous sclerosis	Cutaneous angiofibroma ('adenoma sebaceum'), peau chagrin, subungual fibromas	Cardiac rhabdomyomas, adenomatous polyps of the duodenum and small intestine, cysts of the lung and kidney, lymphangioleiomyomatosis, renal angiomyolipoma
Li–Fraumeni	None	Breast carcinoma, bone and soft tissue sarcomas, adrenocortical, lung and GI carcinomas, leukemia
Cowden	Multiple trichilemmomas, fibromas	Hamartomatous polyps of the eye, colon, and thyroid; breast carcinoma and thyroid cancer
Turcot syndrome	Café-au-lait spots	Colorectal polyps, colon carcinoma
Nevoid basal cell carcinoma syndrome (Gorlin)	Multiple basal cell carcinomas, palmar and plantar pits	Jaw cysts, ovarian fibromas, skeletal abnormalities
Bloom	Sun sensitivity, patches of hyper- and hypopigmentation	Characteristic face and voice, gonadal failure, diabetes, immunodeficiency
Fanconi anemia	Café' au-lait spots, hyper- and hypopigmentation	Anemia, skeletal malformations, enlarged cerebral ventricles, gastrointestinal malformations
Multiple endocrine neoplasia (MEN-1)	Facial angiofibroma, lipomas, collagenomas	Hyperparathyroidism, gastrinoma, insulinoma, thyroid/bronchial carcinoid
Retinoblastoma	None	Retinal tumors, osteosarcomas and other tumors
Familial melanoma	Patches of hyperpigmentation	None
Rhabdoid predisposition syndrome	None	Renal tumors, extrarenal malignant rhabdoid tumors

that can be treated before they become symptomatic. These findings are outlined in Table 12.2 and detailed in the paragraphs below.

Most hereditary neoplasms arise from abnormalities of tumor suppressor genes. The 'two-hit' theory proposed by Knudson to explain the different clinical patterns of hereditary and sporadic retinoblastomas can be applied to a number of other hereditary syndromes. That theory posits that the patient is born with a germline mutation deleting one allele of a tumor suppressor gene. When an environmental event deletes the second allele in a single cell, both tumor suppressor genes are then non-functional, the cell is released from normal growth controls, and a tumor develops. In hereditary retinoblastoma, there is a much higher likelihood that an environmental event will delete the remaining normal allele in each eye, explaining why most hereditary retinoblastomas appear bilaterally. Conversely, the low likelihood that an environmental event will delete both alleles in multiple retinal cells explains why most sporadic retinoblastomas are unilateral.

Tumor suppressor gene abnormalities can cause tumors even in the absence of deletion of both alleles. Mutations in tumor suppressor genes may lead the mutated gene to have a dominant negative effect; that is, the protein product of the mutated gene preferentially binds its receptor but does not function normally, thus leading to unrestrained growth. Some p53 mutations in brain tumors function in this way.

Most familial or hereditary syndromes associated with brain tumors result from loss of tumor suppressor genes along the lines of Knudson's two-hit hypothesis (Chapter 1). There are two different kinds of tumor suppressor genes that can be implicated in familial cancers.[1] These have been termed 'gatekeepers' and 'caretakers'. Gatekeepers are genes that directly inhibit tumor growth, i.e. tumor suppressor genes. In most instances, these genes are rate-limiting for cell growth and both copies must be inactivated for a tumor to develop. In familial cancers, one gene is inactivated in the germ line and environmental factors inactivate the second allele leading to tumor development. In sporadic cancers, both alleles must be inactivated by environmental factors for a tumor to develop. Examples of gatekeeper genes causing familial brain tumors are NF-1 and NF-2.

Caretaker gene inactivation does not directly promote tumor growth; instead, it leads to genetic instability that promotes other somatic gene mutations that in turn lead to cancer growth. In familial cancers, caretaker mutations in the germ line occur in two different forms. In the autosomal dominant syndromes, one mutant allele of the caretaker is inherited and the remaining allele is mutated by environmental factors. In other cases, both alleles of the gene must be inherited in mutant form to cause susceptibility. An example of a caretaker gene is the gene causing Fanconi anemia, associated with medulloblastomas and astrocytomas. The genetic defect results in hypersensitivity to DNA cross-linking agents and defects in the repair of the cross-linked DNA. A second abnormality is that associated with hereditary non-polyposis colorectal cancer. The gene hMSH2 is involved in repair of DNA mismatches. Loss of both alleles of the gene results in complete loss of DNA mismatch repair activity and in subsequent hypermutability of the cell.

Genetic testing is available for all the familial syndromes associated with brain tumors. This provides specific information for each family and allows for the identification of new mutations in a family. Genetic counseling is essential for all patients with familial germline syndromes, to enable them to understand the complexities of these inherited conditions.[2]

Neurofibromatosis-1

NF-1 (Fig. 12.1)[3–5] is an autosomal dominant disorder[4] caused by an abnormality of the NF-1 gene at chromosome 17q 11.2. The disorder

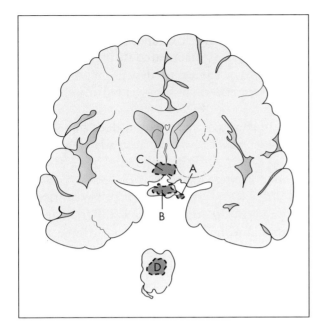

Figure 12.1
The common sites of intracranial lesions in patients with NF-1. (A) Optic nerve. (B) Optic chiasm. (C) Hypothalamus. Brainstem gliomas (D) are more common in patients with NF-1 and have a more benign prognosis.

is also called von Recklinghausen's disease. The disorder is frequent, with an incidence of about 1 in 3000 people, 30–50% of whom represent new mutations, predominantly in the paternal germ line. Genomic imprinting may also play a role in this disease. Genomic imprinting is a phenomenon where only one of the two alleles, either the maternal or paternal allele, is expressed in the cells of the offspring; the other allele is suppressed. If the expressed allele is mutated, the heterozygotic cell will behave like it has a homozygous mutation because of suppression of the normal non-mutated allele.

Imprinting may play an important role in other familial cancer syndromes as well.

The NF-1 gene is large, spanning at least 350 kilobases. The gene for oligodendrocyte myelin glycoprotein is embedded within intron 27b of the NF-1 gene, perhaps explaining the occasional occurrence of multiple sclerosis in NF-1 patients.[6] Genetic inactivation of the NF-1 gene can be accomplished by single base pair mutations, deletions of the entire gene, single or multiple exon deletions, insertions or chromosome rearrangement. The protein product of the gene, neurofibromin, is a 220-kDa protein consisting of 2818 amino acids. Neurofibromin is found in high levels in neurons, non-myelinated Schwann cells and testis, and at low levels in adult astrocytes and myelinated Schwann cells. A developmentally regulated isoform found in forebrain neurons may be relevant to learning disabilities found in some NF-1 children.[7] Neurofibromin is a Ras guanidine triphosphate-activating protein (GTPase) that promotes the conversion of the Ras oncoprotein from the active to the inactive form. Inactivation of neurofibromin may lead to stimulation of the Ras signal transduction pathway which controls cell division, resulting in unrestrained cell proliferation. Hyperactivity of the Ras pathway is characteristic of, and possibly necessary for, glioma formation. It is observed in all sporadic malignant gliomas as well as those found in patients with NF-1. The mutation rate of the gene may be 100 times higher than the usual mutation rate for a single locus. The reason for the high mutation rate is not clear. Other genes may also play a modifying role in NF-1, explaining why the phenotype is so variable from patient to patient even in the same family. Mutations of hMLH DNA mismatch repair genes, the genetic defect in one form of Turcot's syndrome (see below), predispose patients to hematologic malignancies, i.e. leukemia or lymphoma, and to NF-1. These

Table 12.3
Clinical diagnostic criteria for NF-1.

The presence of two or more of the following is diagnostic:

1. Six or more café-au-lait spots, greater than 5 mm in diameter in prepubertal and over 15 mm in postpubertal individuals
2. Two or more neurofibromas of any type, or one plexiform neurofibroma
3. Axillary and/or inguinal freckling
4. Optic nerve glioma
5. Two or more small elevated hamartomas of the iris (Lisch nodules)
6. A distinctive osseous lesion, such as sphenoid wing dysplasia or thinning of long bone cortex, with or without pseudoarthrosis
7. A first-degree relative (parent, sibling, or offspring) with NF-1 according to the above criteria

abnormalities of DNA mismatch repair apparently leave uncorrected mutations in neurofibromin, leading to an NF-1 gene phenotype.[8]

Table 12.3 outlines the diagnostic criteria for NF-1 as delineated by the NIH Consensus Conference on Neurofibromatosis in 1987. Minor disease features, including macrocephaly ($\geq$ 97th percentile), short stature ($\leq$ 3rd percentile), hypertelorism (clinical impression) and thoracic abnormalities such as pectus excavatum, assist in the diagnosis in young children.[9] A wide variety of tumors and other lesions occur in NF-1. Furthermore, the phenotype of the disease can vary widely; some patients are asymptomatic throughout life and others die from malignant neural tumors. Café-au-lait spots are generally the earliest manifestation and are present in almost all adults with the disease. However, many normal individuals have two or three café-au-lait spots and even

the presence of six is only suggestive of the disorder. Axillary freckling and small raised pigmented hamartomas of the iris, Lisch nodules, which originate from melanocytes, are a more specific sign. They generally appear late in childhood or in adulthood, and, by age 60, all patients have these nodules. Axillary and inguinal freckling usually develop during late childhood or puberty.

The common tumors of NF-1 are circumscribed and plexiform neurofibromas arising from Schwann cells of the peripheral nervous system (Fig. 12.2). The circumscribed neurofibromas can present either cutaneously (Fig. 12.3) or subcutaneously and are not a specific sign of NF-1. They are, as their name indicates, well circumscribed and, if symptomatic, can be resected. Plexiform neurofibromas are irregular, thickened and non-circumscribed, often extending long distances along the nerve. NF-1 expression is reduced or absent[10] in these tumors. These can involve the orbit and extend from the orbit into the brain or into the spinal cord from a paraspinal lesion, but otherwise do not affect the CNS. More commonly, they can involve the brachial or lumbosacral plexuses or viscera. In a small percentage of patients (less than 15%), the tumors may undergo malignant degeneration and become neurofibrosarcomas. Patients may also have neuroendocrine tumors, including pheochromocytomas and carcinoids, and they are at increased risk for leukemia. A number of osseous, vascular and nervous system lesions, as indicated in Table 12.4, can also be found.

Most CNS tumors associated with NF-1 are pilocytic astrocytomas (Chapter 5). They are located in the optic nerve,[11] hypothalamus or brainstem of children. There is also an increased frequency of diffuse astrocytomas and glioblastomas but these are much rarer.

Brainstem gliomas are associated with neurofibromatosis. These tumors generally run

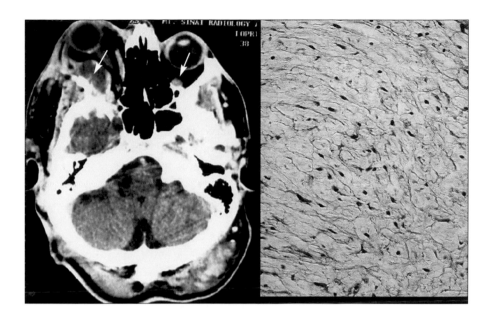

Figure 12.2
Multiple neurofibromas in a patient with NF-1. This CT scan shows bilateral orbital lesions (arrows). The lesion on the right is causing proptosis and deviation of the eye. The patient's complaint was diplopia. The photomicrograph shows bland spindle-shaped cells in a loose mucoid interstitial matrix.

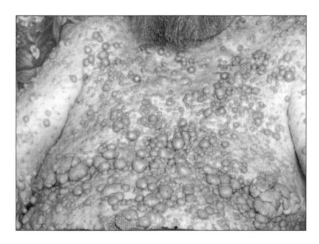

Figure 12.3
Multiple neurofibromas in a 55-year-old man with NF-1. The lesions began appearing at age 14. There was no family history of NF-1.

lesions are rarely biopsied, those associated with NF-1 could be hamartomas, which do not require treatment, rather than neoplasms. Furthermore, patients with NF-1 are at increased risk for leukemia,[14] making chemotherapy with potentially leukemogenic agents, such as alkylating agents, risky. MRS can help distinguish benign pontine lesions associated with NF-1 from brainstem gliomas.[15] However, asymptomatic brainstem gliomas should be followed and do not require immediate treatment. The lesions most likely to progress are those that are focal rather than diffuse and non-enhancing. If treatment is required, one might consider chemotherapy, particularly in young children;[16] focal radiation therapy (RT) is also useful, particularly for older children or adults.

Optic gliomas are also associated with NF-1 and most but not all reports suggest that the prognosis is better in NF-1 patients.[17,18] However, once optic gliomas progress, survival rates of NF-1 patients do not differ from those of others. Almost all symptomatic optic

a more benign course than in patients without NF-1 and have even been known to regress spontaneously.[13] Neuroimaging cannot definitively distinguish malignant from benign lesions in the brainstem and because brainstem

Table 12.4
Major manifestations of NF-1.

Tumors	
Neurofibromas	Dermal
	Nodular/circumscribed
	Plexiform
Gliomas	Optic nerve glioma
	Pilocytic astrocytoma
	Astrocytoma
	Glioblastoma multiforme
Sarcomas	Malignant peripheral nerve sheath tumor
	Triton tumor
	Rhabdomyosarcoma
Neuroendocrine tumors	Pheochromocytoma
	Carcinoid tumor
Hemopoietic tumors	Juvenile chronic myeloid leukemia
Other features	
Osseous lesions	Scoliosis
	Height reduction
	Macrocephaly
	Pseudoarthrosis
	Sphenoid wing dysplasia
	Limb hypertrophy
Nervous system	Intellectual handicap
	Epilepsy
	Neuropathy
	Hydrocephalus (aqueductal stenosis)
	Choroidal abnormalities[12]
Vascular lesions	Fibromuscular hyperplasia

gliomas develop before age 6. Optic nerve gliomas are found in about 15% of patients with NF-1, but at least one-half are asymptomatic. Similarly, about 15% of optic gliomas in most series occur in patients with NF-1. However, a recent series of 21 children with visual pathway gliomas found NF-1 in 62%. The tumor usually develops by the time the child is 10, but it may be asymptomatic for a long period. When symptoms develop, they include decreased visual acuity in one eye if the tumor is in the optic nerve or in both eyes if the lesion is chiasmal. The tumor may produce proptosis and, if it involves the hypothalamus, precocious puberty as well as other endocrine abnormalities. Since many optic gliomas involve the optic chiasm and hypothalamus, making surgery difficult, it is often wise to follow without therapy if the patient is not showing progressive symptoms.[19] If symptoms develop and the tumor is surgically inaccessible, RT and/or chemotherapy are useful.[16,19] Radiotherapy is effective but the response may take several years.[20] RT complications are more common and more severe in patients with NF-1,[21] including radiation-induced vascular disorders and cognitive dysfunction.[22]

If the patient is known to have neurofibromatosis and develops CNS symptoms, MR scan generally establishes the diagnosis. When the patient is not known to have neurofibromatosis and the MR scan reveals an optic glioma, a careful search for the stigmata of NF-1 in both the patient and first degree relatives is warranted. Brainstem gliomas are less likely to be caused by NF-1, but because of the hereditary and prognostic implications, a search is warranted under these conditions as well. NF-1 should be identified early in life and the patient followed lifelong in order to detect and treat complications in their early stages. Guidelines for surveillance at various ages have been published.[23,24] One caution: headache, particularly tension-type headache in children under age 10, is more common in patients with NF-1 than in the general population.[25] Headache alone is not an indication for MRI. Malignant neoplasms and hypertension are the major causes of the decreased life expectancy of NF-1 patients.[26]

Neurofibromatosis-2

NF-2 is an autosomal dominant disorder characterized by bilateral vestibular schwannomas, meningiomas and gliomas.[5,27] The disorder is also called central neurofibromatosis and is entirely different from NF-1, von Recklinghausen's disease. The incidence is much lower than that of NF-1, about 1 per 40 000, but new mutations are so frequent that about half of the patients have no family history.

The NF-2 gene has been mapped to chromosome 22q11. The gene product, called merlin, binds to components of the cytoskeleton and is believed to help organize membrane proteins. The protein is involved in cell proliferation and motility,[28] perhaps by interacting with CD44.[29] The most frequent germline mutations are point mutations that can be found in many parts of the gene and probably result in a truncated protein. A mutation at intron 15 splice donor site results in a mutation that causes a mild

Table 12.5
Diagnostic criteria for NF-2.

The following are diagnostic:

1. Bilateral vestibular schwannomas; or
2. A first-degree relative with NF-2, and either
   (a) a unilateral vestibular schwannoma, or
   (b) two of the following: meningioma, schwannoma, glioma, neurofibroma, posterior subcapsular lens opacity, or cerebral calcification; or
3. Two of the following
   (a) Unilateral vestibular schwannoma
   (b) Multiple meningiomas
   (c) Either schwannoma, glioma, neurofibroma, posterior subcapsular lens opacity, or cerebral calcification

form of the disease with very slow growing vestibular schwannomas with a late onset.[30]

Table 12.5 outlines the diagnostic criteria from the 1987 NIH Consensus Conference on Neurofibromatosis. About 95% of NF-2 patients have bilateral vestibular schwannomas (Chapter 9). Other tumors involving the CNS include meningiomas, gliomas, schwannomas other than on the vestibular nerve, and glial microhamartomas. Glial microhamartomas, also called 'hamartias', are circumscribed clusters of cells with large atypical nuclei that react strongly for S-100 protein. These lesions found within the cortex by microscopic examination are asymptomatic, but are pathognomonic of NF-2.

Approximately 5% of patients with unilateral vestibular schwannomas have NF-2. Multiple meningiomas are also common in NF-2 (Fig. 12.4). Meningioangiomatosis, a proliferation of meningothelial cells surrounding small vessels, occurs as a single intracortical lesion in some patients with NF-2 and may

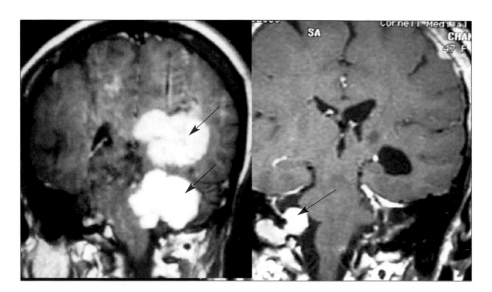

Figure 12.4
A patient with NF-2. This 45-year-old woman with known hearing loss in the left ear developed headache. A scan revealed bilateral acoustic schwannomas as well as a large meningioma both above and below the tentorium (arrows left). The meningioma was successfully removed (right). She continues to have bilateral hearing loss although non-progressive.

occur independently of a meningioma;[31] the disorder is usually asymptomatic. Intracerebral calcifications are also relatively frequent. They occur in the cerebral and cerebellar cortices, in paraventricular areas and in the choroid plexus. They are usually asymptomatic. Peripheral neuropathy, not due to detectable tumor, may be a rare manifestation of NF-2.[32]

Patients with NF-2 can present either with unilateral or bilateral hearing impairment or other symptoms anywhere along the neuraxis related to meningiomas or schwannomas (Chapters 6 and 9). The diagnosis should be suspected in any patient with bilateral vestibular schwannomas or with multiple meningiomas. Patients at risk for NF-2 should have audiologic or MR evaluation every year or two during late adolescence and early adulthood. Early detection of vestibular schwannomas is important, because treatment of small lesions may preserve hearing.[33] The treatment of vestibular schwannomas is outlined in Chapter 9. Criteria for long-term surveillance and management of NF-2 patients have been published.[23]

von Hippel–Lindau disease

von Hippel–Lindau (VHL) disease is an autosomal dominant illness characterized by hemangioblastomas of the brain and spinal cord, retinal angiomas, renal cell carcinomas, pheochromocytoma, and cysts and tumors of other viscera, including the endolymphatic sac.[34] Only about 25% of cerebellar hemangioblastomas occur in VHL patients, the others being sporadic (Fig. 6.10). The incidence of VHL is about 1 in 36 000, similar to NF-2 and much less common than NF-1. Unlike NF-1 and NF-2, new VHL mutations are rare, as is incomplete penetrance. Thus, in most patients a family history or examination of the parents establishes the familial nature of the illness. While penetrance is complete, expression is highly variable, ranging from a mild symptom (e.g. retinal angioma) to a lethal illness (renal cancer).

The mean age of VHL patients with cerebellar hemangioblastomas is significantly lower than that of sporadic patients. This finding, along with the functional loss of both alleles at the VHL locus, is consistent with the two-hit hypothesis. The locus for the VHL gene is on chromosome 3p25–26. The protein encoded by the gene is a 213 amino acid protein that binds to the protein elongen, which regulates elongation of an mRNA transcript. The protein is a component of a ubiquitin ligase, necessary for the oxygen-dependent degradation of hypoxia inducible factor (HIF); thus, when the VHL protein is absent, vascular endothelial growth factor (VEGF) is unregulated.[35] Germline mutations include large deletions, or frame shifts, as well as a variety of missense mutations and other small intragenic mutations. Most families with pheochromocytomas have missense mutations whereas those without pheochromocytomas have deletions or premature termination mutations.[34]

The disorder is usually recognized when a patient develops cerebellar signs and a typical hemangioblastoma is identified on MR scan. When a hemangioblastoma is identified, one should look for other CNS and extracranial manifestations of VHL disease[36] (Table 12.6). Early identification of spinal hemangioblastomas, renal cell carcinomas or pheochromocytomas may allow one to cure a disease which could become lethal if untreated. Retinal angiomas will be found in about 60% of VHL patients. Although they occur throughout life, they are typically the earliest finding of VHL disease, and are sometimes present in infancy. The angiomas are bilateral in about 50% of patients and may cause profound visual loss due to hemorrhage, retinal detachment, glaucoma and cataract. Cerebellar hemangioblastomas occur in 50–70% of patients but may be symptomatic in only half. Although they can occur in childhood, they usually occur in early middle age, between 30 and 40 years. The diagnosis and treatment of cerebellar hemangioblastomas are described in Chapter 6, and are no different in VHL patients.

Table 12.6
Manifestations of VHL disease.

Organ	Lesion
Retina	Angioma
Kidney	Cysts
	Renal cell carcinoma
Pancreas	Cysts
	Adenomas
	Islet cell tumors
Adrenal gland	Pheochromocytomas
Epididymis	Cysts
	Cystadenomas
Inner ear	Endolymphatic sac tumor
Other organs	Visceral cysts
	Adenomas
CNS	Hemangioblastoma of spinal cord, cerebellum

Tuberous sclerosis

The tuberous sclerosis complex (TSC) is an autosomal dominant disorder characterized by benign tumors of the nervous system, including hamartomas and subependymal giant cell astrocytomas.[37] Although usually an inherited disease, in many patients the disorder arises from a spontaneous mutation. The disorder is relatively common with an incidence between 1 in 5000 and 1 in 10 000. There are two distinct tuberous sclerosis genes, both of which function as tumor suppressor genes; tuberous sclerosis complex 1 (TSC1) on chromosome 9q34 and tuberous sclerosis complex 2 (TSC2) on chromosome 16p13.[38] The protein product of the TSC1 gene is called hamartin. Its function is not known; it has been localized to cytoplasmic vesicles and it interacts with tubulin, the protein product of the TSC2 gene. Germ line mutations of either gene are inactivating, and loss of heterozygosity at either region occurs in tuberous sclerosis tumors, indicating that both genes are tumor suppressor genes. NF-1 and TSC, although distinctive phenotypically, have molecular similarities. The genes of both syndromes are hypothesized to function as growth regulators by modulating the activity of small GTPase molecules.[39] Tuberin, which has a GTPase activating domain is localized to the Golgi apparatus and may be involved in vesicular transport. Mosaicism, a phenomenon in which a fraction of germline and somatic cells contain a mutation or chromosomal abnormality, occurs in a number of genetic disorders, including TSC. Somatic mosaicism, in which only some somatic cells are affected, may lead to a milder phenotype. Germ cell mosaicism may cause the disease in children of apparently unaffected parents.[37] Mosaicism is usually associated with a less severe form of the dis-

order, but it may be a potential cause of failure of molecular diagnosis.[40] The clinical syndrome of the TSC is identical regardless of which gene is dysfunctional. Most patients with TSC are mentally retarded. Those with TSC1 mutations are less likely to be retarded than those with TSC2 mutations. Cortical tubers can be identified on MR scan and are thought to be the cause of epilepsy, including infantile spasm (Fig. 12.5).[41] Hamartin and tuberin are coexpressed in the tubers.[42] Most patients develop facial angiofibromas, so-called adenoma sebaceum. These characteristic lesions, along with others outlined in Table 12.7, allow one to identify the syndrome. Imaging generally reveals subependymal nodules in the walls of the lateral ventricle. In neonates the lesions are hyperintense on T1 and hypointense on T2; the opposite findings occur in older children and adults. The hamartomas often calcify and rarely may hemorrhage. The tumors may grow large enough to obstruct the ventricular system,

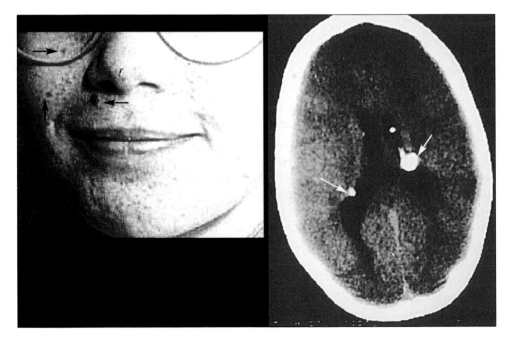

Figure 12.5
Tubers in a patient with tuberous sclerosis. The face was marked with typical 'adenoma sebaceum' (arrows). Note the 'candle-guttering' of the ventricular system (left arrow). This patient was asymptomatic with respect to the tubers.

Table 12.7
Major manifestations of the tuberous sclerosis complex (TSC).

Manifestation	Frequency (%)
CNS	
Cortical tuber	90–100
Subependymal nodule	90–100
White matter hamartoma	90–100
Subependymal giant cell astrocytoma	6–16
Skin	
Facial angiofibroma (adenoma sebaceum)	80–90
Hypomelanotic macule	80–90
Shagreen patch	20–40
Forehead plaque	20–30
Peri- and subungual fibroma	20–30
Eyes	
Retinal hamartoma	50
Retinal giant cell astrocytoma	20–30
Hypopigmented iris spot	10–20
Kidney	
Angiomyolipoma	50
Heart	
Cardiac rhabdomyoma	50
Digestive system	
Microhamartomatous rectal polyp	70–80
Liver hamartoma	40–50

leading to hydrocephalus. Tumors over 5 mm in diameter that are incompletely calcified and enhance on MRI are at higher risk of continued growth.[43] If they cause symptoms, the tumors can be resected, and total resection usually cures. Rare tumors undergo malignant degeneration and may recur. In addition to benign tumors of the brain, children and adults with TSC are at risk for developing a number of malignant tumors including renal cell carcinomas, malignant angiomyolipomas and glioblastoma multiforme.[44] Recent consensus conferences have outlined recommendations for diagnostic criteria and evaluation.[37] These include cranial MR scans every 1–3 years during childhood.

Other hereditary syndromes

The Li–Fraumeni syndrome is a rare autosomal dominant disorder leading to multiple different tumors in affected patients, often children and young adults.[2] The common tumors are breast cancer, osteosarcoma and brain tumors. Other tumors include soft tissue sarcomas, leukemia and lung, adrenal, gastric and colon cancers. Approximately 10% of patients suffer gliomas, most of which occur in young adulthood, usually before age 45. Some develop medulloblastomas and supratentorial PNETs.[45] Overall, penetrance of the gene is about 50% by age 30 and 90% by age 60. The disorder is usually caused by germline mutations in the p53 gene,[46] most of which are base–pair substitutions that result in missense mutations in the conserved domain and are similar to p53 mutations occurring in sporadic tumors. Some families with the clinical syndrome do not have p53 germline mutations and their genetic defect is unknown (see below, 'rhabdoid predisposition syndrome'). Brain tumors cluster in individual families, suggesting that some specific p53 mutations may be relatively organ specific. In addition to gliomas, medulloblastomas and PNETs, choroid plexus tumors, ependymomas and schwannomas have been reported. Except for the generally younger age of patients with brain tumors and the slightly higher male/female ratio compared to sporadic tumors, the brain tumors in these patients do not differ clinically from their sporadic counterparts.

The diagnosis is suspected in a patient with a brain tumor who either has a previous history of extraneural tumors, especially an osteosarcoma, or has a strong family history of brain or extraneural tumors. The treatment is the same as that for sporadic brain tumors but patients with Li–Fraumeni syndrome success-fully treated for a brain tumor should be carefully followed for the development of other cancers.

Lhermitte–Duclos disease is a rare autosomal dominant disorder usually presenting in early adulthood as a cerebellar hemispheric mass.[47] The estimated gene frequency is about 1 per million, although others believe it is under-recognized and thus substantially more frequent. Lhermitte–Duclos disease was thought to be a sporadic, isolated condition, but recently many cases have been reported in association with *Cowden's disease*,[48] an autosomal dominant disorder also called the multiple hamartoma syndrome which includes multiple facial trichilemmomas (a benign tumor of the outer root sheath of hair follicles), oral mucosal papillomas, palmoplantar kerato-sis, dysmorphic anomalies and hamartomas of the thyroid, breast, gastrointestinal tract, and eye. The hamartomas may become malignant, leading to fibroadenomatous or fibrocystic disease in 75% of patients, and breast cancer in 25–50% of patients. Thyroid abnormalities occur in more than half of patients, but thyroid cancer in less than 10%. The diagnosis is made by pathognomonic mucocutaneous lesions, trichilemmomas and papillomatous papules, which are present in all individuals by age 30.[49] Other neurologic disorders in addition to the Lhermitte–Duclos lesion include megencephaly, a bridged sella turcica, mental retardation, gliomas, meningiomas and neuromas.

Cowden's disease has been mapped to chromosome 10q23. The gene involved is the PTEN gene[50] which has a tyrosine phosphatase domain as well as a tensin-homology domain; it is involved in regulation of cell growth and differentiation. PTEN mutations have also been reported in sporadic glioblastomas (Chapter 5). In Cowden's disease men and women are affected equally. The Lhermitte–Duclos lesion is characterized by diffuse enlargement of cerebellar folia containing large ganglion cells that are probably Purkinje cells which expand and replace the granular and molecular layers. The lesion develops slowly, producing ataxia and symptoms of increased intracranial pressure. On MR scan, a characteristic sign is the presence of 'tiger stripes' or parallel linear striations on the T2-weighted image. The tumors do not enhance.

Turcot's syndrome refers to several different disorders which have in common multiple colorectal neoplasms, either polyps or carcino-mas, and neuroepithelial tumors including glioblastomas, medulloblastomas, astrocy-tomas and ependymomas.[45,51] Some cases are variants of the familial adenomatous polyposis syndrome or hereditary non-polyposis colorec-tal carcinoma syndrome.[52] The brain tumors do not differ from the sporadic variety, except that the gliomas generally occur before age 30 and the medulloblastomas often occur after age 10. The diagnosis and treatment are the same as for sporadic brain tumors, except that younger patients with a strong family history of colon polyps or carcinoma should undergo examina-tion of the colon.

Several genetic abnormalities have been identified. In those patients with the familial adenomatosis polyposis syndrome, germline mutations in the APC gene located on chromo-some 5q21 lead to failure of function of the APC gene product. This protein interacts with β-catenin and appears to modify its association with the E-cadherin cell adhesion molecule. Its exact role in the production of either colon cancers or brain tumors is not clear. Other families do not have germline mutations of the

APC gene but appear to have DNA replication errors in their tumors similar to those found in patients with hereditary non-polyposis colorectal cancer. These patients carry mutations of hMLH-1 or hPMS-2[53] genes. The hMLH-1 gene on chromosome 3p21 encodes a protein responsible for strand-specific DNA mismatch repair. The hPMS-2 gene at chromosome 7p22 interacts with the hMLH-1 protein in forming a mismatch protein complex. These gene mutations are associated with microsatellite instability in tumors. This abnormality is rare in brain tumors in the absence of Turcot's syndrome.

Gorlin syndrome, also called the nevoid basal cell carcinoma syndrome, is a rare autosomal dominant disorder in which patients develop multiple basal cell carcinomas at an early age. The incidence is about 1 in 50 000. Additional extraneural lesions include jaw keratocysts, pitting of the palms and soles, and skeletal deformities. Intracranial lesions include falx calcifications, hydrocephalus, dysgenesis of the corpus callosum and medulloblastomas.[45] Medulloblastoma occurs in 5–10% of patients with the syndrome. Conversely, among patients with medulloblastoma, only 1–2% have Gorlin syndrome.

The medulloblastoma develops around 2 years of age, younger than for sporadic medulloblastomas, and frequently has a desmoplastic phenotype. Treatment may lead to a more favorable outcome in these patients than in patients with sporadic medulloblastomas. However, basal cell carcinomas are likely to develop in the irradiated skin, and patients should be followed carefully for the late development of these skin cancers. The genetic abnormality is in the PTCH gene on chromosome 9q31.[54] The gene encodes a protein necessary for the intracellular signaling pathway of the Sonic hedgehog gene, necessary for normal development of several organs including the brain.[55] The protein is probably a transcriptional repressor which, when absent, leads to uncontrolled transcription. Similar mutations are infrequently found in sporadic medulloblastomas.[54]

Fanconi anemia (FA) is an autosomal recessive disorder that confers a predisposition to bone marrow failure and leukemia. Several other congenital abnormalities are present as well, as indicated in Table 12.2. The disorder is found in all races and ethnic groups and has a carrier frequency of about 1 in 300. This may be a low estimate because of poor ascertainment of cases. As many as 0.5% of all people may be heterozygous for an FA gene.[56] There are at least 7 distinct FA genes. They are believed to be 'caretaker' genes but their exact function is unknown.[57]. The basic defect in FA is believed to result in abnormalities in DNA repair, growth factor homeostasis and cell cycle regulation. It is probably the abnormality of DNA repair that leads to malignancy. The most common malignancy is leukemia, particularly acute myelogenous leukemia, but other cancers including medulloblastomas and astrocytomas have been reported.[58]

Bloom syndrome is an autosomal recessive disorder characterized by dwarfism, sun sensitivity and a characteristic facial appearance.[59] A variety of tumors have been recorded in patients with Bloom syndrome, including medulloblastoma, meningioma and retinoblastoma. The disorder is common in Ashkenazi Jews and is a result of mutation in a single locus, BLM, which maps to chromosome 15q26. The gene product is homologous to other proteins that function as DNA helicases.[60] A DNA helicase (helix is from the Greek for coil) is a repair enzyme which uncoils DNA. The disorder leads to unstable DNA in the somatic cells of those who inherit the disease, leading in turn to spontaneous hypermutability which is probably responsible for the development of neoplasms. The disease is rare and only a few patients with brain tumors have been reported.

Familial melanoma. About 51 000 people developed melanoma in 2001[61] in the USA, an impressive increase in frequency in melanoma in recent decades, probably related to sun exposure. Perhaps as many as 10% of all cases of melanoma are familial. Individuals who have a first-degree relative who has developed melanoma under the age of 50 have a relative risk of 6.5 fold of developing melanoma compared to the general population. Germ line mutations in the locus that encodes p16 (INK4A) and p14 ARF are associated with melanoma susceptibility in familial melanoma.[62] Other genetic abnormalities may exist as well.

Multiple endocrine neoplasia type I (MEN-1) is an autosomal dominant disorder that leads to a variety of endocrine tumors, including pituitary adenomas. About 15% of patients have prolactinomas, 5% other hormone-producing pituitary adenomas, and 2% non-secreting tumors. The tumors are benign. Associated endocrine disorders include primary hyperparathyroidism, gastrinoma and insulinoma. The MEN-1 gene maps to chromosome 11q13; its protein product is called menin.

Retinoblastoma is the prototypic example of a familial cancer. It is the most common intra-ocular malignancy in children, with a worldwide incidence of about 1 in 20 000 live births. Sixty percent of the tumors are non-hereditary and unilateral, and 40% are hereditary, most of which are bilateral. The gene maps to chromosome 13q14 and is called RB-1. Its protein product is 110 kDa in size and is a classic tumor suppressor. The tumors rarely involve the CNS but occasionally are associ-ated with pineal region or suprasellar tumors, so-called trilateral retinoblastoma.[45,63]

Rhabdoid predisposition syndrome is a recently described autosomal dominant disease characterized by malignant rhabdoid tumors involving the kidney and other organs including the brain. In addition, a number of patients have choroid plexus carcinomas, medulloblastomas and central PNETs. The disorder is associated with a germline mutation of the hSNF5/INI1 gene localized on chromosome 22. The penetrance of the syndrome is high and most tumors occur in children below the age of 3. The gene encodes a member of the SW1/SNF ATP-dependent chromatin-remodeling complex. Its exact role in the causation of the renal and extrarenal tumors is unknown. Because some of the multiple tumors are similar to those of the Li–Fraumeni syndrome, it is possible that some cases of apparent Li–Fraumeni syndrome without p53 germline mutations belong to this syndrome.[64]

Other familial brain tumors are undoubtedly more common than can be encompassed by the known genetic syndromes. A population-based study indicates that about 5% of gliomas are familial.[65] Further investigation of the genetics of brain tumors may lead to the identification of more familial syndromes.[66] Some clearly represent failure to diagnose the syndromes described above, making each of them more common than currently recognized. Others are a result of hereditary gene defects not yet identified. Careful attention to the possible familial occurrence of such tumors will not only allow for appropriate genetic counseling but may identify new genetic defects that may be a site for therapeutic intervention. Figure 12.6 shows an algorithm for patients with CNS tumors that might be potentially familial in origin.

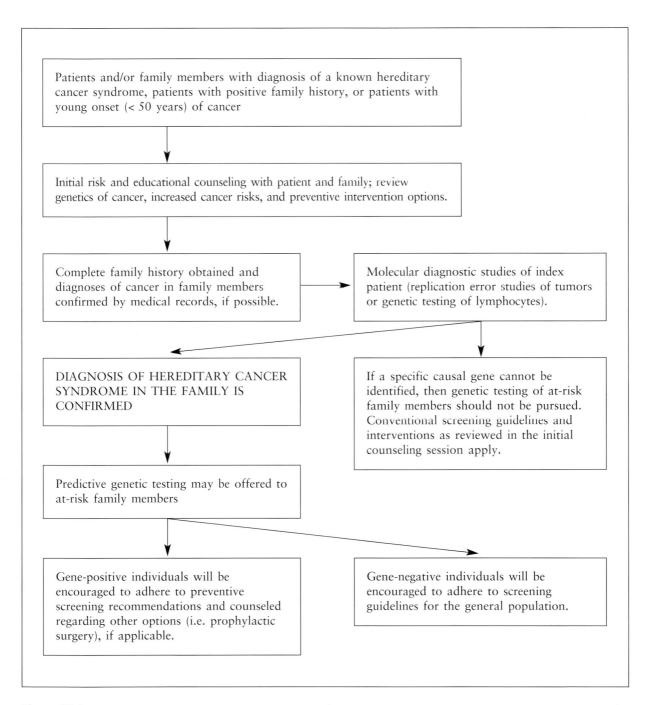

Figure 12.6
Cancer risk assessment and gene testing algorithm from Peterson and Cordori[94] with permission.

Neoplastic cysts and cyst-like tumors

In some patients, mass lesions of the brain cause their symptoms not by growth of tumor cells but by enlargement of a fluid-filled cyst. Some of these cysts are associated with neoplasms; others are not but must be considered in the differential diagnosis of neoplasm. Table 12.8 classifies these cysts. Many such cysts that accompany brain tumors, such as pilocytic astrocytomas and hemangioblastomas, are discussed in the chapters on those primary neoplasms. Cysts of infectious origin, such as cysticercosis and ex-vacuo cysts, i.e. those that result from loss of brain substance, are not discussed in this book except in the context of differential diagnosis. The cysts discussed here fall into two large categories, those lined by neuroepithelium which secretes CSF and those that have a non-neuroepithelial lining secreting a fluid different from CSF; some of these latter lesions occasionally become true neoplasms. Lesions in these two categories can often be distinguished by MR scan (see below).

Dermoids and epidermoids

These tumors account for only about 1% of all intracranial neoplasms, the epidermoid being three or four times more frequent than the dermoid.[68,69] Both tumors are probably malformations originating from incomplete cleavage of neural from fetal cutaneous ectoderm during the fourth week of gestation. Thus, fetal epiblasts are not excluded from the nervous system during development when the neural tube closes. The tumors usually occur in the midline along the base of the brain and the spinal canal, including fourth ventricle, suprasellar and parasellar cisterns. They may or may not communicate with the skin surface through a midline dermal tract. The epidermoid cyst is lined by keratin-producing squamous epithelial cells and may occur laterally in the skull or cerebellopontine angle. When these tumors are found in the middle ear, they are called cholesteatomas. Although congenital, epidermoids generally make their appearance in adulthood. Spinal epidermoids are sometimes associated with lumbar puncture, particularly those done early in life.[70]

The dermoid cyst is lined by squamous epithelium and underlying dermal appendages including hair follicles and adnexa. The cystic contents may include hair or primordial teeth. Dermoid cysts are commonly found within the midline of the cerebellum, usually in association with a dermal sinus, and usually present

Table 12.8
Intracranial cysts.

Cysts with CSF-like fluid
  (a) Ex vacuo
      Leptomeningeal cysts
      Cysts after surgical resection
      Cysts after cerebral infarction or trauma
      Porencephalic cysts
      Virchow–Robin spaces
  (b) Cysts with fluid-secreting walls
      Arachnoid cysts
      Neuroepithelial cysts
      Choroid plexus cyst
  (c) Midline cysts of dysgenetic origin
      Cysts arising from cavum septi pellucidi, cavum vergae and cavum veli interpositi
      Dandy–Walker cysts
Cysts with non-neuroepithelial lining
  Pineal cysts
  Rathke's cleft cysts (Chapter 10)
  Colloid cysts
  Epidermoid cysts
  Dermoid cysts
Cysts associated with brain neoplasms
Cysts associated with infections

Modified from Mooij and Go[63] with permission.

in childhood. Suprasellar dermoids in connection with dermal sinuses can also occur. Dermoids are common in the spinal canal where they may be associated with a sinus tract and a bony malformation.

The clinical presentation depends on the location of the tumor. They expand slowly, usually through desquamation of epithelial cells, and may become quite large before signs and symptoms develop (Fig. 12.7). The

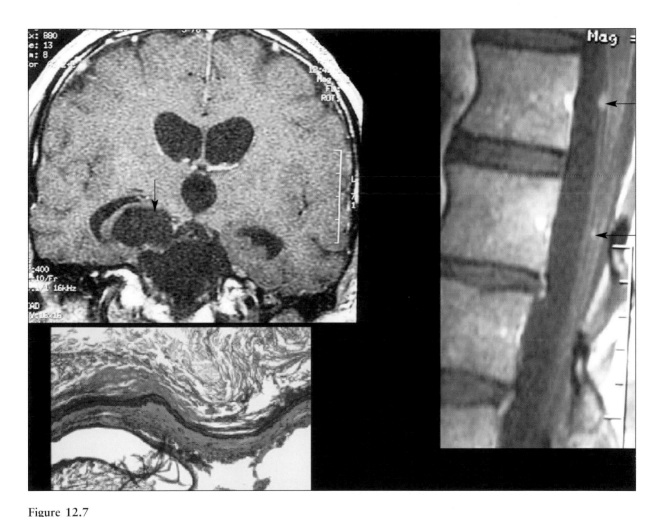

Figure 12.7
An epidermoid cyst of the posterior fossa. This 50-year-old man presented with mild headache. A scan revealed a large epidermoid cyst in the posterior fossa (arrow left upper). The cyst was believed to be asymptomatic. A year elapsed without any significant change in his symptoms, when he developed severe headache, diplopia, difficulty swallowing and some weakness in one lower extremity. A scan of the head revealed hydrocephalus but no change in the size of the epidermoid cyst. A scan of the spine revealed contrast enhancing nodules on lumbar roots (arrows, right). Although the CSF did not show abnormal cells, biopsy of the lumbar meninges revealed squamous cell carcinoma. The patient died and an autopsy revealed that the epidermoid contained squamous cell carcinoma both within it and involving the meninges. The photomicrograph shows the benign keratin-filled cyst lined by well-differentiated squamous epithelium.

supratentorial lesions may present with headaches, seizures or visual field defects. Tumors in the cerebellopontine angle present with hearing loss. Other posterior fossa symptoms include trigeminal neuralgia and hemifacial spasm. Pineal region epidermoids present with a headache, diplopia and vertigo.[71] Occasionally, rupture of the cyst structure may spill irritating contents into the subarachnoid space, causing an aseptic meningitis. Repetitive episodes of aseptic meningitis, sometimes associated with focal neurologic signs, have been reported as the presenting manifestation of these lesions.[72] At least one of our patients carried a diagnosis of multiple sclerosis for many years before the cyst was found. Recurrent infectious meningitis may be a presenting symptom if the dermoid communicates with the surface.

The diagnosis is made radiographically.[73] Epidermoids are hypointense on T1-weighted images but more intense than CSF, and iso- to hyperintense on T2-weighted images but isointense relative to CSF. There may be rim enhancement. Dermoids are often hyperintense on T1-weighted images and relatively hypointense on T2-weighted images (Fig. 12.8). Signal void may represent some calcification and hyperintensity may represent fat deposition. The difference between signal intensity in dermoids and that in epidermoids is probably explained by cholesterol, which, in its solid, crystalline state, is hypointense on T1, but in the liquid state appears hyperintense. CT scans of either epidermoids or dermoids show a lesion without enhancement. In some patients with recurrent aseptic meningitis, the ruptured cyst may not be seen on scan during an acute

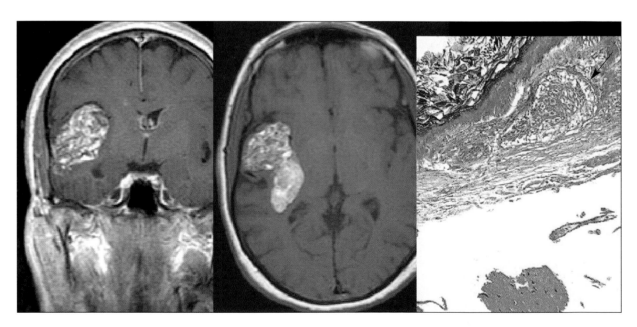

Figure 12.8
A dermoid cyst. This 56-year-old woman presented with partial complex seizures and was found to have this intracranial lesion that was hyperintense before contrast and did not enhance. Note the absence of edema around this large extraaxial mass. The photomicrograph shows the cyst wall is lined by squamous epithelium with an underlying stroma containing a sebaceous gland (arrow).

episode; subsequent imaging may be required to establish the diagnosis. Rupture may lead to subarachnoid seeding of the cyst contents and cells.[74] Rarely, the cysts may undergo malignant degeneration to squamous cell carcinoma; in one of our patients carcinoma seeded the leptomeninges and was the presenting manifestation of the epidermoid.[75]

Both dermoids and epidermoids are grossly well-defined masses with smooth, lobulated, somewhat irregular surfaces and a pearly appearance. Dermoids are filled with hair and keratinized debris. Microscopically, the tumors are lined by simple stratified squamous epithelium with a variable degree of keratinization. The presence of dermal appendages in the cyst wall, such as sebaceous glands, sweat glands and hair follicles or fatty tissue, defines the tissue as a dermoid (Fig. 12.8).

When the tumors are found incidentally, they may be followed without specific therapy unless they become symptomatic. In symptomatic patients, surgical removal is the treatment of choice. Using microsurgical techniques, total resection and cure is possible in some instances, but total resection is often difficult because the tumor capsule adheres to cranial nerves, blood vessels and other vital structures. However, even subtotal resection may yield a prolonged remission of symptoms. Mortality is quite low, but morbidity, including aseptic meningitis and transient cranial nerve palsies as well as hydrocephalus, may occur, particularly in surgery of posterior fossa masses. Sometimes the cyst wall cannot be totally eradicated. Such patients should be followed by serial MR scans. Radiotherapy and chemotherapy are not useful.

Colloid cysts

These non-neoplastic lesions located in the 3rd ventricle and attached to the choroid plexus produce their symptoms by obstructing the foramen of Monro and causing hydrocephalus (Fig. 12.9).[76] Colloid cysts are so named

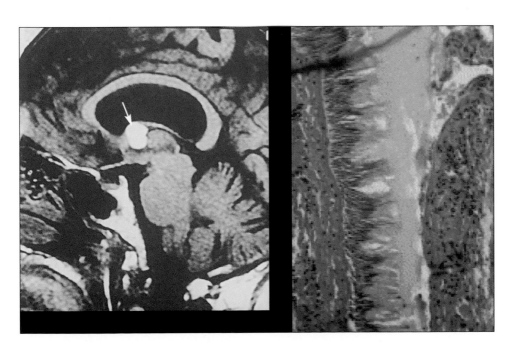

Figure 12.9
A colloid cyst of the 3rd ventricle (arrow). Note the hydrocephalus. The photomicrograph shows amorphous cyst contents with a lining of columnar ciliated epithelium.

because of the glue-like nature of the cyst contents (colloid from the Greek for 'glue' and 'appearance'). The cyst is lined by cuboidal to columnar ciliated epithelial and/or goblet cells, thought to be endodermal in origin. Characteristically, the patient suffers from headaches due to the hydrocephalus. At one time it was believed that colloid cysts would intermittently obstruct the ventricular system by a ball valve mechanism, producing sudden increased intracranial pressure (ICP), occasionally leading to herniation and death.[76] The choroidal attachment of the colloid cyst renders the mass sessile and makes a ball valve mechanism impossible. Sudden symptoms in patients with colloid cysts are caused by pressure waves (Chapter 3) developing in a setting of chronically elevated ICP.

The diagnosis is made by MR scan, showing a cyst within the 3rd ventricle at the level of the foramen of Monro. The cyst is iso- to hyperintense on the T1-weighted image and hypo- to isointense on T2.[77] Colloid cysts can range from a few millimeters to several centimeters in diameter. They are spherical or ovoid and have a smooth, semi-translucent wall. The viscosity of the cyst content varies from fluid to solid. The mucin-like cyst contents contain sulfonated carbohydrate epitopes. The carbohydrate epitopes are similar to those reported for mucins of the salivary gland and other peripheral cysts believed to be of endodermal origin.[78]

In some asymptomatic patients, particularly older patients without hydrocephalus, the cysts do not grow and need no treatment.[79] Two types of treatment have been recommended for symptomatic patients. One is drainage of the cyst via stereotactic needle placement. Although this relieves symptoms temporarily, the cyst usually reaccumulates. The best approach is surgical removal. Some surgeons have recommended shunting both ventricles and not

attacking the tumor, but shunt malfunction, leading to sudden recurrence of hydrocephalus, and the slit ventricle syndrome causing severe headache[80] make this a problematic treatment. Surgery through either a transcallosal or transcortical approach is the treatment of choice, but it may be associated with morbidity. Many neurosurgeons accomplish this by endoscopy.[81] Transient memory deficits from traction on the fornix have been noted in 26% of patients after a transcallosal approach. In a few, there was permanent memory difficulty.[82] Patients fare better when the operation is done by a surgeon experienced in approaching third ventricular tumors.[76] Removal of the cyst cures the patient, but asymptomatic patients can safely be followed without surgery.[83] RT and chemotherapy have no role to play.

Intracranial arachnoid cysts

These are CSF-filled cystic structures lined with a transparent membrane resembling the arachnoid. They are a congenital malformation and not a response to cerebral atrophy. They are often found in the middle cranial fossa[84] (Fig. 12.10) compressing the temporal lobe, at the cerebral convexity, the suprasellar area, the quadrigeminal area and the posterior fossa, particularly the cerebellopontine angle. They are occasionally intraventricular, arising from the arachnoid in the choroidal fissure.[85] Most are asymptomatic but some may cause headache, dizziness or seizures; some may grow large enough to produce substantial compression of the brain and elevate intracranial pressure. The cyst may bleed into itself or rupture into the subdural space, causing an effusion that is symptomatic and requires drainage.[86,87]

The diagnosis is made on MR scan. The lesion has signal characteristics similar to those of CSF, sometimes deeply indenting but not

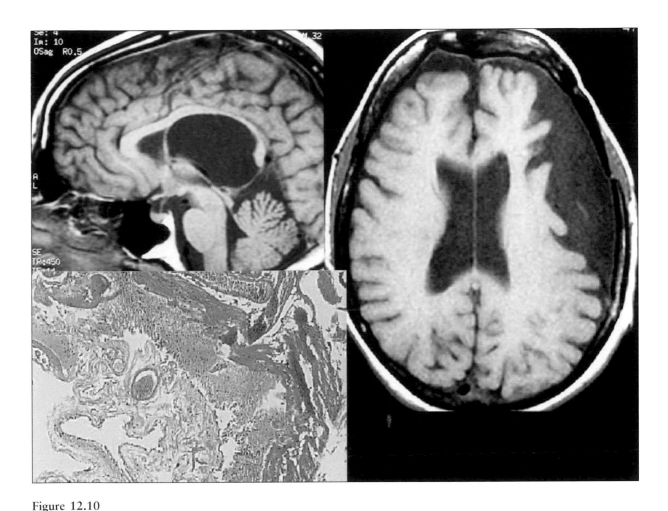

Figure 12.10
Two symptomatic arachnoid cysts. Left MRI: a 25-year-old university teacher complained of new-onset headache and difficulty in concentrating. Several physicians believed that the cyst of the cavum velum interpositum was coincidental and not responsible for the symptoms. However, after a year of symptoms, endoscopic evacuation of the cyst abolished all symptoms. Right MRI: a 30-year-old woman presented with headache. A scan revealed a large arachnoid cyst. Note that the cyst and the spinal fluid have the same signal intensity and that the gyri and sulci of the brain have a normal configuration, indicating that they are not compressed. The headache was relieved by analgesics and eventually disappeared. The photomicrograph shows an arachnoid cyst with a delicate fibrous connective tissue membrane lined by meningothelial cells.

invading brain parenchyma. Intrathecal injection of contrast material usually demonstrates slow if any communication between the cyst and the subarachnoid space. However, the fact that the membrane secretes fluid but the cyst does not grow suggests that there is enough loss of fluid from the cyst into the subarachnoid space to balance fluid production within the cyst.

The problem in diagnosis is to determine which cysts are symptomatic and which are discovered incidentally in the workup of a patient for headache or seizures. Most patients with seizure disorders do improve after treatment of an arachnoid cyst, suggesting that the cortical gliosis caused by the cyst may be a source of seizures and may improve after the cyst is treated. Many headaches improve as well. Nonetheless, in some instances, the headache is due to another cause and treatment of the cyst will not help. As with brain tumors, new onset headaches, change in headache frequency or intensity and focal headache at the site of the cyst suggest that the cyst is symptomatic. Arachnoid cysts that are asymptomatic should just be followed. Symptomatic arachnoid cysts should be drained by creating a communication between the cyst and the ventricular system or subarachnoid space, depending on the location of the cyst. In some instances, communication can be established by puncturing the wall of the cyst directly or endoscopically. In some instances, communication requires a cyst–peritoneal shunt. Stereotactic intracavitary irradiation by injection of ^{32}P has proved safe and effective.[88]

Hypothalamic neuronal hamartomas

These neuroepithelial masses are composed of mature and often clustered neurons and glial stroma. Most occur at the base of the brain, attached to the floor of the fourth ventricle, or within the hypothalamus (Fig. 12.11). The tumors are hamartomas but sometimes they expand. They are usually asymptomatic but may cause endocrine disorders or seizures, particularly gelastic seizures[89,90] (inappropriate sudden laughter, from Greek 'to laugh') or ictal autonomic dysfunction e.g. hypertension, tachycardia, bradycardia.[91] They can cause precocious puberty in both sexes. Children may be larger than normal with advanced bone age; hormonal dysfunction on laboratory tests is

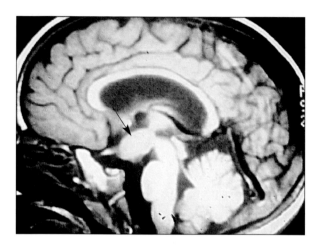

Figure 12.11
A hypothalamic hamartoma in a young boy with gelastic seizures (arrow) (see text).

also common. Mental retardation is common. MR scan reveals a non-enhancing mass lesion involving the hypothalamus, isointense with brain. On the T2-weighted images, the tumors are isointense or slightly hyperintense.

Differential diagnosis includes hypothalamic astrocytoma, optic glioma and germinoma. In the asymptomatic patient, no treatment is necessary. Hormonal abnormalities can often be corrected with appropriate agents. Surgery[92] and RT[93] have been reported to control seizures in some patients; radiofrequency ablation helped one patient.[94]

References

1. Vogelstein B, Kinzler KW. The genetic basis of human cancer. New York: McGraw–Hill, 1998.
2. Tomlinson GE. Familial cancer syndromes and genetic counseling. Cancer Treat Res 1997; 92: 63-97.
3. Pollack IF, Mulvihill JJ. Neurofibromatosis 1 and 2. Brain Pathol 1997; 7: 823–36.
4. Feldkamp MM, Gutmann DH, Guha A. Neurofibromatosis type 1: piecing the puzzle together. Can J Neurol Sci 1998; 25: 181–91.

5. Karnes PS. Neurofibromatosis: a common neurocutaneous disorder. Mayo Clin Proc 1998; 73: 1071–6.

6. Johnson MR, Ferner RE, Bobrow M, Hughes RA. Detailed analysis of the oligodendrocyte myelin glycoprotein gene in four patients with neurofibromatosis 1 and primary progressive multiple sclerosis. J Neurol Neurosurg Psychiatry 2000; 68: 643–6.

7. Gutmann DH, Zhang YJ, Hirbe A. Developmental regulation of a neuron-specific neurofibromatosis-1 isoform. Ann Neurol 1999; 46: 777–82.

8. Wang Q, Lasset C, Desseigne F et al. Neurofibromatosis and early onset of cancers in hMLH1-deficient children. Cancer Res 1999; 59: 294–7.

9. Cnossen MH, Moons KG, Garssen MP et al. Minor disease features in neurofibromatosis type 1 (NF1) and their possible value in diagnosis of NF1 in children < or = 6 years and clinically suspected of having NF1. Neurofibromatosis team of Sophia Children's Hospital. J Med Genet 1998; 35: 624–7.

10. Peters N, Waha A, Wellenreuther R et al. Quantitative analysis of *NF1* and *OMGP* gene transcripts in sporadic gliomas, sporadic meningiomas and neurofibromatosis type 1-associated plexiform neurofibromas. Acta Neuropathol (Berl) 1999; 97: 547–51.

11. Listernick R, Louis DN, Packer RJ, Gutmann DH. Optic pathway gliomas in children with neurofibromatosis 1. Consensus statement from the NF1 optic pathway glioma task force. Ann Neurol 1997; 41: 143–9.

12. Yasunari T, Shiraki K, Hattori H, Miki T. Frequency of choroidal abnormalities in neurofibromatosis type 1. Lancet 2000; 356: 988–92.

13. Perilongo G, Moras P, Carollo C et al. Spontaneous partial regression of low-grade glioma in children with neurofibromatosis-1: a real possibility. J Child Neurol 1999; 14: 352–6.

14. Stiller CA, Chessells JM, Fitchett M. Neurofibromatosis and childhood leukaemia/lymphoma: a population-based UKCCSG study. Br J Cancer 1994; 70: 969–72.

15. Broniscer A, Gajjar A, Bhargava R et al. Brain stem involvement in children with neurofibromatosis type 1: role of magnetic resonance imaging and spectroscopy in the distinction from diffuse pontine glioma. Neurosurgery 1997; 40: 331–7.

16. Packer RJ, Ater J, Allen J et al. Carboplatin and vincristine chemotherapy for children with newly diagnosed progressive low-grade gliomas. J Neurosurg 1997; 86: 747–54.

17. Deliganis AV, Geyer JR, Berger MS. Prognostic significance of type 1 neurofibromatosis (von Recklinghausen disease) in childhood optic glioma. Neurosurgery 1996; 38: 1114–8.

18. Chan MY, Foong AP, Heisey DM et al. Potential prognostic factors of relapse-free survival in childhood optic pathway glioma: a multivariate analysis. Pediatr Neurosurg 1998; 29: 23–8.

19. Shuper A, Horev G, Kornreich L et al. Visual pathway glioma: an erratic tumour with therapeutic dilemmas. Arch Dis Child 1997; 76: 259–63.

20. Tao ML, Barnes PD, Billett AL et al. Childhood optic chiasm gliomas: Radiographic response following radiotherapy and long-term clinical outcome. Int J Radiat Oncol Biol Phys 1997; 39: 579–87.

21. Grill J, Couanet D, Cappelli C et al. Radiation-induced cerebral vasculopathy in children with neurofibromatosis and optic pathway glioma. Ann Neurol 1999; 45: 393–6.

22. Cappelli C, Grill J, Raquin M et al. Long term follow up of 69 patients treated for optic pathway tumours before the chemotherapy era. Arch Dis Child 1998; 79: 334–8.

23. Gutmann DH, Aylsworth A, Carey JC et al. The diagnostic evaluation and multidisciplinary management of neurofibromatosis 1 and neurofibromatosis 2. JAMA 1997; 278: 51–7.

24. Huson SM. What level of care for the neurofibromatoses? Lancet 1999; 353: 1114–6.

25. DiMario FJ Jr, Langshur S. Headaches in patients with neurofibromatosis-1. J Child Neurol 2000; 15: 235–8.

26. Zoller ME, Rembeck B, Oden A, Samuelsson M, Angervall L. Malignant and benign tumors in patients with neurofibromatosis type 1 in a defined Swedish population. Cancer 1997; 79: 2125–31.

27. Bondy M, Ligon BL. Epidemiology and etiology of intracranial meningiomas: a review. J Neurooncology 1996; 29: 197–205.

28. Reed N, Gutmann DH. Tumorigenesis in neurofibromatosis: new insights and potential therapies. Trends Mol Med 2001; 7: 157–62.

29. Morrison H, Sherman LS, Legg J et al. The NF2 tumor suppressor gene product, merlin, mediates contact inhibition of growth through interactions with CD44. Genes Dev 2001; 15: 968–80.

30. Sainio M, Jaaskelainen J, Pihlaja H, Carpen O. Mild familial neurofibromatosis 2 associates with expression of merlin with altered COOH-terminus. Neurology 2000; 54: 1132–8.

31. Wiebe S, Munoz DG, Smith S, Lee DH. Meningioangiomatosis – A comprehensive analysis of clinical and laboratory features. Brain 1999; 122: 709–26.

32. Trivedi R, Byrne J, Huson SM, Donaghy M. Focal amyotrophy in neurofibromatosis 2. J Neurol Neurosurg Psychiatry 2000; 69: 257–61.

33. Subach BR, Kondziolka D, Lunsford LD et al. Stereotactic radiosurgery in the management of acoustic neuromas associated with neurofibromatosis Type 2. J Neurosurg 1999; 90: 815–22.

34. Friedrich CA. Von Hippel–Lindau syndrome – a pleomorphic condition. Cancer 1999; 86: 1658-62.

35. Kondo K, Kaelin WG, Jr. The von Hippel–Lindau tumor suppressor gene. Exp Cell Res 2001; 264: 117–25.

36. Richard S, Campello C, Taillandier L, Parker F, Resche F. Haemangioblastoma of the central nervous system in von Hippel–Lindau disease. French VHL Study Group. J Intern Med 1998; 243: 547–53.

37. Sparagana SP, Roach ES. Tuberous sclerosis complex. Curr Opin Neurol 2000; 13: 115–9.

38. Cheadle JP, Reeve MP, Sampson JR, Kwiatkowski DJ. Molecular genetic advances in tuberous sclerosis. Hum Genet 2000; 107: 97–114.

39. Gutmann DH. Parallels between tuberous sclerosis complex and neurofibromatosis 1: common threads in the same tapestry. Semin Pediatr Neurol 1998; 5: 276–86.

40. Kwiatkowska J, Wigowska-Sowinska J, Napierala D, Slomski R, Kwiatkowski DJ. Mosaicism in tuberous sclerosis as a potential cause of the failure of molecular diagnosis. N Engl J Med 1999; 340: 703–7.

41. Hancock E, Osborne JP. Vigabatrin in the treatment of infantile spasms in tuberous sclerosis: literature review. J Child Neurol 1999; 14: 71–4.

42. Johnson MW, Emelin JK, Park SH, Vinters HV. Co-localization of TSC1 and TSG2 gene products in tubers of patients with tuberous sclerosis. Brain Pathol 1999; 9: 45–54.

43. Nabbout R, Santos M, Rolland Y et al. Early diagnosis of subependymal giant cell astrocytoma in children with tuberous sclerosis. J Neurol Neurosurg Psychiatry 1999; 66: 370–5.

44. Al-Saleem T, Wessner LL, Scheithauer BW et al. Malignant tumors of the kidney, brain, and soft tissues in children and young adults with the tuberous sclerosis complex. Cancer 1998; 83: 2208–16.

45. Taylor MD, Mainprize TG, Rutka JT. Molecular insight into medulloblastoma and central nervous system primitive neuroectodermal tumor biology from hereditary syndromes: a review. Neurosurgery 2000; 47: 888–901.

46. Akashi M, Koeffler HP. Li–Fraumeni syndrome and the role of the p53 tumor suppressor gene in cancer susceptibility. Clin Obstet Gynecol 1998; 41: 172–99.

47. Tuli S, Provias JP, Bernstein M. Lhermitte–Duclos disease: literature review and novel treatment strategy. Can J Neurol Sci 1997; 24: 155–60.

48. Robinson S, Cohen AR. Cowden disease and Lhermitte–Duclos disease: Characterization of a new phakomatosis. Neurosurgery 2000; 46: 371–83.

49. Chapman MS, Perry AE, Baughman RD. Cowden's syndrome, Lhermitte–Duclos disease, and sclerotic fibroma. Am J Dermatopathol 1998; 20: 413–6.

50. Eng C. Genetics of Cowden syndrome: through the looking glass of oncology. Int J Oncol 1998; 12: 701–10.

51. McLaughlin MR, Gollin SM, Lese CM, Albright AL. Medulloblastoma and glioblastoma multiforme in a patient with Turcot syndrome: a case report. Surg Neurol 1998; 49: 295–301.

52. Foulkes WD. A tale of four syndromes: familial adenomatous polyposis, Gardner syndrome, attenuated APC and Turcot syndrome. QJM 1995; 88: 853–63.

53. Taylor MD, Perry J, Zlatescu MC et al. The *hPMS2* exon 5 mutation and malignant glioma. J Neurosurg 1999; 90: 946–50.

54. Vortmeyer AO, Stavrou T, Selby D et al. Deletion analysis of the adenomatous polyposis coli and *PTCH* gene loci in patients with sporadic and nevoid basal cell carcinoma syndrome-associated medulloblastoma. Cancer 1999; 85: 2662–7.

55. Ming JE, Roessler E, Muenke M. Human developmental disorders and the Sonic hedgehog pathway. Mol Med Today 1998; 4: 343–9.

56. Garcia-Higuera I, Kuang Y, D'Andrea AD. The molecular and cellular biology of Fanconi anemia. Curr Opin Hematol 1999; 6: 83–8.

57. Joenje H, Patel KJ. The emerging genetic and molecular basis of Fanconi anaemia. Nat Rev Genet 2001; 2: 446–57.

58. Alter BP, Tenner MS. Brain tumors in patients with Fanconi's anemia. Arch Pediatr Adolesc Med 1994; 148: 661–3.

59. German J. Bloom syndrome: a mendelian prototype of somatic mutational disease. Medicine (Baltimore) 1993; 72: 393–406.

60. Neff NF, Ellis NA, Ye TZ et al. The DNA helicase activity of BLM is necessary for the correction of the genomic instability of bloom syndrome cells. Mol Biol Cell 1999; 10: 665–76.

61. Greenlee RT, Hill-Harmon MB, Taylor M, Thum M. Cancer Statistics, 2001. Ca Cancer J Clin 2001; 51: 15–36.

62. Kaufman DK, Kimmel DW, Parisi JE, Michels VV. A familial syndrome with cutaneous malignant melanoma and cerebral astrocytoma. Neurology 1993; 43: 1728–31.

63. Paulino AC. Trilateral retinoblastoma – is the location of the intracranial tumor important? Cancer 1999; 86: 135–41.

64. Sévenet N, Sheridan E, Amram D et al. Constitutional mutations of the *hSNF5/INI1* gene predispose to a variety of cancers. Am J Hum Genet 1999; 65: 1342–8.

65. Malmer B, Iselius L, Holmberg E et al. Genetic epidemiology of glioma. Br J Cancer 2001; 84: 429–34.

66. Chène P, Ory K, Rüedi D, Soussi T, Hegi ME. Functional analyses of a unique *p53* germline mutant (Y236Delta) associated with a familial brain tumor syndrome. Int J Cancer 1999; 82: 17–22.

67. Mooij JJ, Go KG. Cysts, cyst-like tumors and other maldevelopmental tumors. In: Vecht C, ed. Handbook of clinical neurology vol 68 Neuro-oncology part 2. Amsterdam: Elsevier, 1997: 309–42.

68. Gormley WB, Tomecek FJ, Qureshi N, Malik GM. Craniocerebral epidermoid and dermoid tumours: a review of 32 cases. Acta Neurochir (Wien) 1994; 128: 115–21.

69. Iaconetta G, Carvalho GA, Vorkapic P, Samii M. Intracerebral epidermoid tumor: a case report and review of the literature. Surg Neurol 2001; 55: 218–22.

70. Potgieter S, Dimin S, Lagae L et al. Epidermoid tumours associated with lumbar punctures performed in early neonatal life. Dev Med Child Neurol 1998; 40: 266–9.

71. Konovalov AN, Spallone A, Pitzkhelauri DI. Pineal epidermoid cysts: diagnosis and management. J Neurosurg 1999; 91: 370–4.

72. Aristegui FJ, Delgado RA, Oleaga ZL, Hermosa CC. Mollaret's recurrent aseptic meningitis and cerebral epidermoid cyst. Pediatr Neurol 1998; 18: 156–9.

73. Kallmes DF, Provenzale JM, Cloft HJ, McClendon RE. Typical and atypical MR imaging features of intracranial epidermoid tumors. Am J Roentgenol 1997; 169: 883–7.

74. Miyagi Y, Suzuki SO, Iwaki T et al. Magnetic resonance appearance of multiple intracranial epidermoid cysts: intrathecal seeding of the cysts? Case report. J Neurosurg 2000; 92: 711–4.

75. Khan RB, Giri DD, Rosenblum MK, Petito FA, DeAngelis LM. Leptomeningeal metastasis from an intracranial epidermoid cyst. Neurology 2001; 56: 1419–20.

76. Mathiesen T, Grane P, Lindgren L, Lindquist C. Third ventricle colloid cysts: a consecutive 12-year series. J Neurosurg 1997; 86: 5–12.

77. Urso JA, Ross GJ, Parker RK, Patrizi JD, Stewart B. Colloid cyst of the third ventricle: radiologic–pathologic correlation. J Comput Assist Tomogr 1998; 22: 524–7.

78. Veerman EC, Go KG, Molenaar WM, Amerongen AV, Vissink A. On the chemical characterization of colloid cyst contents. Acta Neurochir (Wien) 1998; 140: 303–6.

79. Pollock BE, Schreiner SA, Huston J III. A theory on the natural history of colloid cysts

of the third ventricle. Neurosurgery 2000; 46: 1077–81.

80. Stoeckli SJ, Bohmer A. Persistent bilateral hearing loss after shunt placement for hydrocephalus. Case report. J Neurosurg 1999; 90: 773–5.

81. Rodziewicz GS, Smith MV, Hodge CJ, Jr. Endoscopic colloid cyst surgery. Neurosurgery 2000; 46: 655–60.

82. Aggleton JP, McMackin D, Carpenter K et al. Differential cognitive effects of colloid cysts in the third ventricle that spare or compromise the fornix. Brain 2000; 123: 800–15.

83. Pollock BE, Houston J, III. Natural history of asymptomatic colloid cysts of the third ventricle. J Neurosurg 1999; 91: 364–9.

84. Wester K. Peculiarities of intracranial arachnoid cysts: Location, sidedness, and sex distribution in 126 consecutive patients. Neurosurgery 1999; 45: 775–9.

85. Maiuri F, Iaconetta G, Gangemi M. Arachnoid cyst of the lateral ventricle. Surg Neurol 1997; 48: 401–4.

86. Albuquerque FC, Giannotta SL. Arachnoid cyst rupture producing subdural hygroma and intracranial hypertension: case reports. Neurosurgery 1997; 41: 951–5.

87. Parsch CS, Krauss J, Hofmann E, Meixensberger J, Roosen K. Arachnoid cysts associated with subdural hematomas and hygromas: analysis of 16 cases, long-term follow-up, and review of the literature. Neurosurgery 1997; 40: 483–90.

88. Thompson TP, Lunsford LD, Kondziolka D. Successful management of sellar and suprasellar arachnoid cysts with stereotactic intracavitary irradiation: An expanded report of four cases. Neurosurgery 2000; 46: 1518–22.

89. Striano S, Meo R, Bilo L et al. Gelastic epilepsy: Symptomatic and cryptogenic cases. Epilepsia 1999; 40: 294 302.

90. Sturm JW, Andermann F, Berkovic SF. 'Pressure to laugh': an unusual epileptic symptom associated with small hypothalamic hamartomas. Neurology 2000; 54: 971–3.

91. Kahane P, Di Leo M, Hoffmann D, Munari C. Ictal bradycardia in a patient with a hypothalamic hamartoma: a stereo-EEG study. Epilepsia 1999; 40: 522–7.

92. Rosenfeld JV, Harvey AS, Wrennall J, Zacharin M, Berkovic SF. Transcallosal resection of hypothalamic hamartomas, with control of seizures, in children with gelastic epilepsy. Neurosurgery 2001; 48: 108–18.

93. Régis J, Bartolomei F, de Toffol B et al. Gamma knife surgery for epilepsy related to hypothalamic hamartomas. Neurosurgery 2000; 47: 1343–51.

94. Parrent AG. Stereotactic radiofrequency ablation for the treatment of gelastic seizures associated with hypothalamic hamartoma – case report. J Neurosurg 1999; 91: 881–4.

95. Petersen GM, Codori A-M. Genetic testing for familial cancer. In: Vogelstein B, Kinzler KW, eds. The genetic basis of human cancer. New York: McGraw-Hill, 1998: 591-9.

13

Intracranial metastases

Introduction

Patients with intracranial metastases far outnumber those who suffer from primary intracranial tumors. In the USA new symptomatic primary intracranial tumors do not exceed 30 000 per year, whereas symptomatic intracranial metastases number greater than 100 000 per year. The diagnosis of a brain metastasis may be difficult for several reasons. (1) Metastases can affect any central nervous system (CNS) location, mimicking both the clinical and imaging findings of primary intracranial tumors (Fig. 13.1). (2) Metastases are increasing in frequency as the first site of relapse in patients whose cancers have apparently been 'cured'[1] or are under good systemic control.[2] (3) Symptoms and signs of brain metastases may appear before the primary tumor has been discovered.[3] In some instances, a patient may suffer multiple symptomatic intracranial metastases but the primary cancer is never found even after an extensive search.[3] (4) Primary brain tumors are more common in patients who have suffered other cancers than they are in the general population. Examples include meningiomas in patients with breast cancer (Chapter 6) and gliomas in patients with Li–Fraumeni syndrome (Chapter 12). (5) Other CNS processes, such as brain abscesses, can mimic brain metastases and occur with increased frequency in patients with cancer. Radiographic

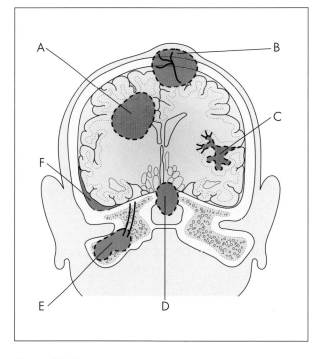

Figure 13.1
Cranial metastases. Most metastases affect the brain directly by hematogenous spread to the white matter of the cerebral hemispheres (A) (see also Fig. 1.2). The brain may be affected secondarily by a skull metastasis that invades the epidural space and compresses the brain. The skull metastasis may also compress the sagittal sinus (B). The tumor may involve the cranial leptomeninges and invade the brain by growing down the Virchow–Robin spaces (C). A metastasis to the base of the skull may affect the pituitary gland (D) or cranial nerves (E) as they exit from the skull. Subdural metastasis may cause effusions (F) that compress the brain. (Redrawn from Posner[4] with permission).

Table 13.1
Frequency of symptomatic intracranial metastases from systemic cancers.

Primary tumors	New cases USA 2001	No. of deaths USA 2001	Percentage with estimated intracranial tumor at autopsy, MSKCC	Total no. of deaths with symptomatic intracranial metastases
Lung	169 500	157 400	34	37 461
Breast	193 700	40 600	30	8 526
Colon and rectum	135 400	56 700	7	2 778
Urinary organs	87 500	25 000	23	4 025
Melanoma	51 400	7 800	72	3 931
Prostate	198 100	31 500	31[a]	6 835
Pancreas	29 200	28 900	7	1 416
Leukemia	31 500	21 500	23[b]	3 461
Lymphoma (non-Hodgkin's)	63 600	26 300	16[b]	2 945
Female genital tract	80 300	26 300	7	1 288
Brain and CNS	17 200	13 100	100	13 100
All sites	**1 268 800**	**553 400**	**24**	**92 971**

[a]Largely skull and dura.
[b]Largely leptomeningeal.
CNS, central nervous system; MSKCC, Memorial Sloan-Kettering Cancer Center.

images often do not differentiate metastases from infection and diagnosis must be based upon the clinical situation and occasionally requires biopsy. For all these reasons, diagnoses other than metastases must be considered in cancer patients who develop intracranial mass lesions and, conversely, metastases must be considered in patients without known cancer who develop intracranial mass lesions. A comprehensive review of neurologic complications of cancer is available.[4]

Table 13.1 uses extant data to estimate the frequency of symptomatic intracranial metastases in the USA. The first two columns of figures are taken from American Cancer Society 2001 data, indicating the number of new patients with specific cancers and the number of deaths expected.[5] The third column estimates the percentage of patients in whom

intracranial metastases, excluding calvarial tumors that do not invade or compress underlying brain, are found at autopsy.[6] Clinical data from Memorial Sloan-Kettering Cancer Center (MSKCC) indicate that patients with an intracranial metastasis identified at autopsy had an approximately 70% chance of having suffered neurologic symptoms during life.[7] Using the 70% factor, the final column indicates the number of patients with each primary tumor likely to suffer neurologic symptoms from an intracranial metastasis during their lifetime. Overall, we estimate that over 70 000 of the patients who die of cancer in 2001 will have had neurologic symptoms from intracranial metastases during life.

No epidemiologic studies describe the lifetime risk of either symptomatic or asymptomatic intracranial metastases in patients with

Table 13.2
Site of primary tumors in patients with CNS metastases.

Primary tumor	Percentage of brain metastases	
Lung	38	
Non-small cell		34
Small cell		4
Breast	19	
Melanoma	13	
Renal	4	
Unknown primary	1	
Other	25	
Total	100	

cancer. Furthermore, the incidence varies with the location and histology of the primary neoplasm, for example CNS metastases from lung cancer are common; while those from ovarian cancer are rare. The most common source of a brain metastasis is lung cancer, particularly from non-small cell lung cancer. However, small cell lung cancer, a less common tumor, is more likely to metastasize to the CNS than non-small cell lung cancer (Table 13.2). The second most common source of CNS metastasis is breast cancer,[8] both because it is a common tumor and it often metastasizes to the brain. Melanoma is an **uncommon** cancer that very often metastasizes to the brain.

Intracranial metastases differ by sex. Lung cancer is now the most common primary tumor in both men and women. Only about 1% of breast cancers occur in men. Thus, intracranial metastases from breast cancer in men are rare. Melanoma is more likely to metastasize to the brain in men than women, probably due to the greater incidence of truncal melanomas in men and appendicular melanomas in women. The risk of melanoma

spreading to the CNS increases with closer proximity of the primary to the cranium.

The age at which patients develop brain metastases is similar to the average age of the primary cancer with the exception that for a given cancer, young people are more likely to develop intracranial metastases than the elderly. Whether this is due to ascertainment or is a real finding is uncertain.

The numbers from Tables 13.1 and 13.2 are clinically important for several reasons:

(1) When one encounters a patient with an intracranial mass, it is statistically more likely to be metastatic than primary. The exact likelihood is difficult to calculate. Because 50% of metastatic lesions are multiple (the figures vary depending on the primary tumor), and 5% of gliomas are multiple, the presence of more than one lesion suggests but does not prove metastases. An exception is lymphoma, where about 40% of lesions are multiple (Chapter 11). When one encounters one or more brain lesions in a patient with no history of cancer, the likelihood of metastasis is still relatively high. For example, as many as 10% of patients with lung cancer come to initial medical attention with neurologic symptoms from a brain metastasis; this phenomenon occurs less frequently with other primary cancers. In one series, a single supratentorial brain lesion in a patient not known to have cancer was metastatic in 15% of patients.[9] Conversely, 5% of patients with a single supratentorial brain tumor and a history of cancer had a new primary brain tumor. Accordingly, even in the absence of a history of cancer, if the clinical evaluation suggests the possibility of metastasis, e.g. either multiple lesions or a single spherical lesion with a regular rim of contrast

enhancement, a focused search for a primary tumor with body CT scan is warranted before directly attacking the brain lesion.

(2) Intracranial metastases often cause devastating symptoms even when the patient's systemic cancer is asymptomatic. Thus, the development of a symptomatic intracranial metastasis substantially diminishes the patient's quality of life, regardless of its effect on the duration of life.

(3) Brain metastases are treatable. Even in patients with far advanced cancer, early detection and effective treatment of intracranial metastases may restore quality of life even if survival is not increased.

(4) The biology of metastases differs from that of primary brain tumors: most primary brain tumors are diffusely infiltrating, whereas metastases are usually well-circumscribed. Consequently, metastases are more likely to respond to focal therapy than are primary brain tumors. In addition, brain tumors rarely metastasize so that organ transplantation from a donor with a primary brain tumor, benign or malignant, has an extremely low risk of that tumor developing in the immunosuppressed recipient. However, glioblastoma has rarely been transmitted from a liver graft.[10] Thus, some investigators believe that patients with primary brain tumors can serve as organ donors, unlike patients with other systemic cancers.[11]

(5) The figures in Table 13.1 come from autopsy data at a cancer hospital where the ascertainment of both symptomatic and asymptomatic brain metastases is complete. In epidemiologic studies reported in the literature, primary CNS tumors equal or exceed intracranial metastases.[12] However, these studies grossly underestimate the incidence of

symptomatic metastatic brain tumors because in patients with extensive systemic cancer, neurologic symptoms are often ignored and not evaluated. The incidence of brain metastasis at autopsy is also often underestimated because careful neuropathologic studies were not carried out in many series. Although the data from Table 13.1 were published in 1978, they are not likely to be replicated because of the current low autopsy rate.

(6) Brain metastases can appear at any time in the course of a systemic cancer. In some patients, the brain metastasis is the presenting symptom and may even be responsible for death before the primary tumor can be identified. In others, an isolated metastasis may appear in the brain 20 or more years after treatment and apparent cure of the primary tumor. The first situation is particularly characteristic of lung cancer, and the second of melanoma and occasionally breast cancer. Routine brain scans of newly diagnosed patients with lung cancer demonstrate an asymptomatic brain metastasis in 3–5% of patients.[13] One series reports a figure of 22% occult brain metastases at initial evaluation for lung cancer.[14] Usually, brain metastases in the setting of known cancer typically occur 6 months to 2 years after diagnosis and are usually associated with systemic tumor progression.

Pathophysiology of the metastatic process

To reach the brain, a tumor that arises elsewhere in the body must undergo a complicated and arduous series of steps.[15,16] This is so difficult that only a small number of tumor cells ever complete the process illustrated in

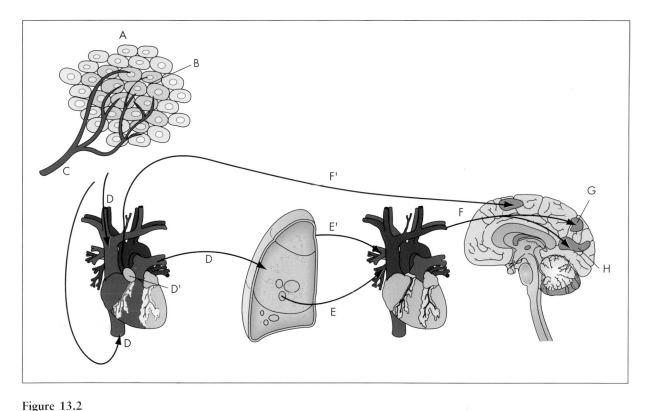

Figure 13.2

Pathophysiology of the metastatic process. Metastasis is a multistep process. In this schematic illustration: (A) a malignant neoplasm arises in an organ distant from the CNS and as it grows, it develops its own vascular supply. (B) Clones of malignant cells with metastatic potential enter blood or lymph channels and eventually reach the venous circulation. (C) The malignant cells enter the right heart with the venous circulation and either exit through the pulmonary artery to the lung (D) or cross a patent foramen ovale (D') to enter the systemic circulation. Most tumors that enter the lung either arrest in the pulmonary capillary bed, grow as pulmonary metastases and subsequently seed the pulmonary venous circulation, or (E) alternatively transverse the pulmonary vascular bed without arresting (E') to enter the pulmonary venous circulation. Malignant clones in the pulmonary venous circulation then enter the left heart and exit into the systemic circulation (F), along with those cells that may have crossed a patent foramen ovale (F'). Once in the systemic circulation, the likelihood of entering the cerebral circulation is high because, in the resting state, 15–20% of cardiac output supplies the CNS. (G, H) Tumor cells entering the cerebral circulation must then arrest in brain capillaries or venules, cross the vessel wall, and grow within the brain. (Redrawn from Posner[4] with permission.)

Fig. 13.2. A systemic cancer begins in the body by a series of genetic steps not dissimilar from those that occur in primary brain tumors (Chapter 1). Once established, the tumor grows, develops its own blood supply (angiogenesis – Chapter 2), invades local tissues and enters the circulation by invading venules or lymph channels that eventually reach the venous circulation. Because systemic tumors enter the venous circulation and ultimately the right side of the heart, the first capillary bed they encounter is in the lung. Accordingly, many patients with brain metastases either have primary lung tumors or lung metastases at the time the brain lesions become symptomatic. To reach the arterial circulation, the tumor must either: (1) grow in the lung and seed the pulmonary venous circulation, (2) traverse the lung capillary bed to enter the left side of the heart, or (3) cross a patent foramen ovale to enter the left heart directly where tumor cells can then enter the arterial circulation (an extraordinary case report illustrates a tumor embolus that occluded the middle cerebral artery and a second embolus within an open foramen ovale).[17]

Two factors promote intracranial metastases: (1) In the resting state, the brain receives 15–20% of the body's blood flow, thus making it likely that circulating tumor cells will reach the brain. (2) Certain tumor cells find the brain a propitious place for arrest and growth: the seed and soil hypothesis posits that tumor cells (the seed) must find an organ (the soil) that supports their growth in order to become a metastasis. This is one of the reasons that the probability of brain metastasis varies among tumor types and that the site of a brain metastasis may vary depending on the histology of the primary tumor. For example, certain primary tumors such as those from the kidney and colon are more likely to metastasize to the cerebellum than are lung cancers or those arising elsewhere in the body[18] (Fig. 13.3), although other reports disagree with this reported preferential distribution.[19] Once in the intracranial cavity, the tumor must arrest within the capillary bed, cross the capillary bed, grow within the organ, vascularize itself through the process of angiogenesis, and then grow large enough to cause symptoms. At each step in the metastatic process, the tumor cells may fail, so that only 0.01% of cells that reach the circulation ever become metastases.[16]

Tumors may metastasize to virtually any portion of the intracranial cavity (Fig. 13.1). The most common site is the brain parenchyma

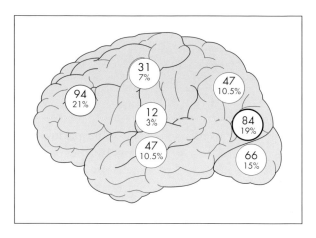

Figure 13.3
Schematic drawing showing the distribution of single metastases to the brain. The posterior fossa is significantly overrepresented in patients with pelvic (prostate or uterus) tumors and gastrointestinal primary tumors (left), compared with patients with other primary tumors (right) ($p < 0.001$). (Redrawn from Delattre et al[18] with permission.)

itself but dura, leptomeninges, pituitary and pineal glands can also develop metastases. Although, as indicated above, certain primary tumors have a predilection to metastasize to certain portions of the nervous system, the overall distribution of brain metastasis is also determined by the size of the region and its vasculature. Thus, about 85% of brain metastases are found in the cerebral hemispheres, usually in the posterior portion of the hemispheres at the watershed between the middle and posterior cerebral arteries. There is also an overrepresentation in the anterior border zone between the anterior and middle cerebral arteries. About 10–15% of metastases are found in the cerebellum, a number somewhat larger than might be expected on the basis of blood supply and probably representing the predilection for some pelvic tumors to metastasize to the cerebellum. Only about 3% of metastases are found in the brainstem.

Several unusual properties of the metastatic process can confuse and confound the physician. For example: (1) The intracranial tumor may be large but the primary tumor small or undetectable. Several reports describe metastatic brain tumors whose primary was undetectable even at autopsy.[3] The pathogenesis is believed to be secretion by the primary tumor of both angiogenic and anti-angiogenic factors (Chapter 2). Antiangiogenic factors in the primary tumor may control its growth whereas angiogenic factors secreted by the tumor may accelerate the growth of metastases. (2) Metastases may be biologically different from the primary tumor. Although metastatic tumors are usually histologically and biologically similar to the primary, this is not always true. Even two metastases to the same organ may differ somewhat in their biologic properties. For example, markers such as estrogen receptors may be present in the primary tumor but not the metastasis. Genetic differences between a primary tumor and its metastasis often exist.[20–22] For example, transforming growth factor (TGF) inhibits metastatic ovarian cancer more than it does the primary tumor.[23] The explanation is that metastases represent clones of the primary tumor that may differ from the bulk of the primary. Telomerase, an enzyme present in most primary cancers, is also expressed in most brain metastases, but the concentration varies markedly. No correlation exists between telomerase concentration and survival.[24] (3) In patients whose systemic tumor is otherwise controlled, the brain seems to be a more common site for isolated metastatic disease. This cannot be explained by either blood flow or the nature of the CNS microenvironment. The blood–brain barrier probably explains this phenomenon: in the first half of the 20th century, when no treatment was available for acute leukemia, CNS involvement was rare as patients died from uncontrolled systemic leukemia. As chemotherapeutic agents became effective in controlling systemic disease, the incidence of CNS involvement began to rise to the point where it reached almost 50% in patients with acute lymphoblastic leukemia. The chemotherapeutic agents used to treat leukemia were largely water-soluble and did not cross the blood–brain barrier; the few leukemic cells that reached the CNS were protected behind the blood–brain barrier where they could proliferate until they produced neurologic symptoms. 'Prophylactic' treatment of the CNS by radiation therapy and/or intrathecal drugs has again decreased the incidence of CNS metastases from leukemia to under 10%. This does not mean that leptomeningeal tumor, once established, cannot be treated by systemic water-soluble agents. Once tumor is established, the blood–CSF barrier is disrupted (Chapter 2) and the CNS becomes accessible to treatment with agents that do not normally cross the blood–brain barrier. Furthermore, some systemic agents can penetrate an intact blood–brain barrier when given in high doses. Accordingly, high-dose methotrexate delivered systemically for prophylaxis can, in patients with acute leukemia, prevent the development of CNS metastatic disease.

The CNS as a sanctuary site for microscopic disease now appears to apply to breast cancer, small cell lung and perhaps other cancers.[25–27] The CNS is becoming an important site of isolated relapse in patients with these tumors.[2] When a chemosensitive tumor has relapsed in the CNS, it does not necessarily mean that the CNS disease is resistant to the chemotherapeutic agents that controlled the systemic tumor. The blood–brain barrier may have prevented those tumor cells from ever seeing a significant concentration of the drug, thus preserving the tumor cells' intrinsic chemosensitivity to that agent.[28]

Pathology

Most metastases differ from diffuse gliomas in that they form discrete, well-circumscribed spherical masses. The center of large metastases is often necrotic. The tumors may be cystic or hemorrhagic and occasionally even calcify. Intraparenchymal brain metastases usually arise just below the cortex at the gray matter–white matter junction and expand by pushing normal brain aside rather than invading it. A pseudo-capsule can be identified in some tumors. Leptomeningeal tumors may appear only as thickening or as a decrease in translucency of the arachnoid membrane. Dural tumors may form dural plaques or nodules.

Histopathologically, metastatic intracranial tumors recapitulate the phenotype of the primary from which they arose. Mitoses are usually present and may be more striking in the metastasis than in the primary tumor. In a few instances, immunohistochemistry and genetic changes in the metastasis may differ somewhat from the primary. The capillaries of brain metastases resemble those of the primary tumor rather than those of the brain. They have gap rather than tight junctions and fenestrated rather than continuous endothelial cell membranes. These vessels form in tumors only a few millimeters in diameter, disrupting the blood–brain barrier and making even small lesions visible on contrast MR scans.

Clinical findings

Signs and symptoms

The symptoms and signs of brain metastasis do not differ significantly from those of most primary brain tumors (Chapter 3). There is a proportionately greater amount of edema surrounding brain metastases, which often causes increased intracranial pressure despite

Table 13.3
Signs and symptoms of brain metastases at presentation.

	Percentage of patients
Headache	24
Hemiparesis	20
Cognitive and behavioral disturbances	14
Seizures (focal or generalized)	12
Ataxia	7
Other	16
No symptoms	7

Data from Posner[29] with permission.

relatively small metastatic lesions. Table 13.3 lists the major symptoms of brain metastases at presentation.[29]

The major difference between the clinical signs of primary and metastatic brain tumors is that metastases usually grow more rapidly than even malignant primary brain tumors, causing subacute symptoms that evolve over a few weeks rather than months. Sometimes, as in primary brain tumors, the symptoms are acute in onset and then either improve or grow progressively worse. Acute symptoms may be caused by hemorrhage into the metastasis or by a seizure with a prolonged postictal state. Any intracranial metastatic tumor can bleed, but certain primary tumors, such as melanoma, thyroid, renal and choriocarcinoma, have a propensity to bleed. Because the most common source of brain metastasis is lung cancer, the most common hemorrhagic metastases are from lung primaries. When multiple metastases are present, it is common to see simultaneous hemorrhage into many of the lesions; the mechanism for this is unclear. When a patient presents with what appears to be a simple cerebral hemorrhage, one can suspect an underlying tumor when prominent edema surrounds the hemorrhagic mass early in its course, an unusual finding in primary hemorrhages. Likewise, prominent contrast enhancement immediately after the onset of hemorrhage strongly indicates an underlying metastasis. However, in some instances, even at surgery, the hemorrhage has destroyed the tumor so that one cannot identify the original hemorrhagic nidus.

On occasion, focal seizures can cause neurologic signs that do not resolve. The seizure probably causes ischemia in the brain immediately surrounding the tumor by stealing its blood supply. Metastatic tumors, primarily cause their symptoms by compressing surrounding brain. Consequently, symptoms caused by metastasis usually respond better to corticosteroids than those caused by primary brain tumors.

One rare but unique presentation of a brain metastasis is a three-phase presentation: a patient has sudden neurologic symptoms that quickly resolve, as in a transient ischemic attack. The MR scan is usually normal. Several months elapse without symptoms, then the patient, in a subacute or gradual fashion, develops symptoms recapitulating the so-called transient ischemic attack. A scan now reveals a metastasis in the area. The pathophysiology is believed to be a tumor embolus transiently occluding a brain vessel, causing reversible ischemia. The embolus breaks up and enters the capillary bed, where some tumor cells are able to extravasate into the brain and grow as a metastasis. The phenomenon is common in cardiac myxoma.[30]

Multiple bilateral brain metastases can have a unique presentation. These patients can develop a subacute confusional state without any evidence of lateralizing signs. Clinically, these patients are identical to those with a toxic/metabolic encephalopathy and can only be distinguished by neuroimaging. Conversely, some patients with brain metastases are completely asymptomatic. Because of the propensity for asymptomatic metastases, patients with lung cancer or melanoma should be evaluated with a brain MRI prior to definitive surgery of the primary tumor.[13,14] When tumor is found only in the brain and one suspects that it is a metastasis, whole-body FDG PET scans may aid in locating a small primary.[31]

Imaging

The most important and usually the only necessary diagnostic test is an MRI (Fig. 13.4). Although the scan cannot unequivocally differentiate metastases from other lesions, certain abnormalities suggest metastases. Metastases are usually spherical and have more regular margins than primary tumors. They are usually found at gray–white matter junctions in watershed areas of brain.[18] When small, they uniformly contrast enhance, and when larger, they may ring enhance. The ring is usually more regular than in a primary tumor but thicker than in an abscess. The tumor is usually surrounded by a substantial amount of edema, frequently more than one sees with comparably sized primary brain tumors. Very small metastases may appear as small dots of contrast enhancement with or without hyperintensity on the T2-weighted image; they usually lack surrounding edema.

One-half of patients have a single identifiable brain metastasis, 20% two metastases and 13% three metastases.[18] Thus, approximately 80% of patients are potential candidates for focal therapy. There is some variation in the number of intracranial metastases by primary tumor type. For example, melanomas are more likely to cause multiple

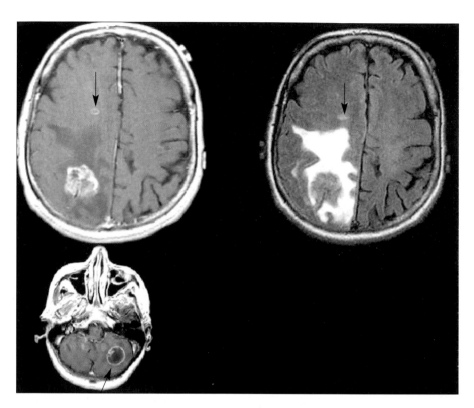

Figure 13.4
Multiple metastases from lung adenocarcinoma. Notice the ring-like enhancement of the metastasis in the cerebellum (lower right, arrow). A massive amount of edema appears as hypointensity on T1 (upper left) and hyperintensity on FLAIR (upper right) surrounding the contrast-enhancing lesion in the right frontal lobe. A small, contrast-enhancing lesion more anteriorly in the right frontal lobe is not surrounded by edema (arrow).

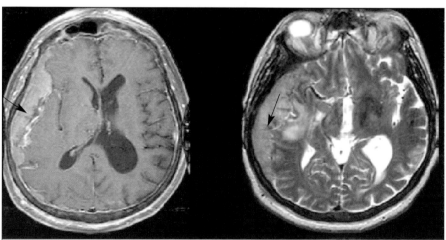

Figure 13.5
A dural metastasis (arrow) compressing the brain in a patient with prostate cancer.

brain metastases than are renal cancers. However, these data are not consistent enough to allow reliable predictions.

Skull and dural metastases are particularly common in breast and prostate cancers (Fig. 13.5). Most are asymptomatic but some may cause symptoms from sagittal sinus compression or subdural effusion. Dural metastasis may be difficult to distinguish from a meningioma (Chapter 6), particularly in women with breast cancer who have an increased incidence of meningiomas.[32] Other tumors, particularly subtypes of breast cancer and acute leukemia, have a predilection to seed the leptomeninges. Leptomeningeal (LM) tumor is identified by leptomeningeal enhancement of the cerebral and spinal meninges.[33] Sometimes LM metastases are suggested on MRI in patients whose brain metastases are multiple, small and located immediately adjacent to CSF, such as at the base of sulci or in a subependymal location. However, even in patients with predominantly cerebral symptoms from leptomeningeal metastases, enhancement of the cerebral leptomeninges may be sparse. It is often useful in such patients to scan the spine looking for nodules within the spinal subarachnoid space, particularly on the cauda equina. In addition, many such patients suffer hydrocephalus from obstruction of CSF pathways by tumor within the subarachnoid space and this is also visualized on cranial MRI.

Differential diagnosis

Table 13.4 lists some considerations in the differential diagnosis of a metastatic intracranial tumor.

In the appropriate setting, i.e. a patient with a cancer known to metastasize to the brain and one or more spherically shaped contrast-enhancing lesions surrounded by edema, the diagnosis is virtually certain and requires little further workup. In a patient without known cancer, but the typical appearance of a metastasis on MR of the brain, a CT of the chest, abdomen and pelvis or a PET scan may reveal a primary lesion. If this test, along with biochemical markers of systemic cancer, e.g. CEA, PSA and CA-125,[3] fail to suggest a primary tumor, further search is likely to be fruitless and the brain lesion should be

Table 13.4
Differential diagnosis of brain metastases.

Primary intracranial tumor
Glioma
Meningioma
Lymphoma
Infection
Brain abscess
Bacterial
Fungal
Parasitic (e.g. toxoplasmosis)
Viral encephalitis (e.g. progressive multifocal leukoencephalopathy, herpes zoster)
Demyelinating disease
Multiple sclerosis
Chemotherapy-induced
Cerebral infarction
Cerebral hemorrhage

attacked directly. A note of caution: secretory meningiomas can synthesize CEA and raise serum levels.[34]

In patients with a cancer that is known to cause immunosuppression but rarely metastasizes to the nervous system, e.g. Hodgkin's disease, one should suspect infection with an opportunistic organism such as Nocardia or Toxoplasma rather than cancer metastasis (Fig. 13.6). Lymphoreticular neoplasms, including Hodgkin's disease, some leukemias and lymphomas, characteristically cause immune suppression, particularly depression of cell-mediated immunity, leading to CNS infection. Patients with solid tumors do not become immunosuppressed until after treatment with either corticosteroids or immunosuppressing chemotherapeutic agents. In patients with solid tumors being treated with chemotherapy, brain infections with fungi, Gram-negative bacteria and viruses must be considered. Viral infections, particularly herpes simplex encephalitis, appear to be more common in patients with

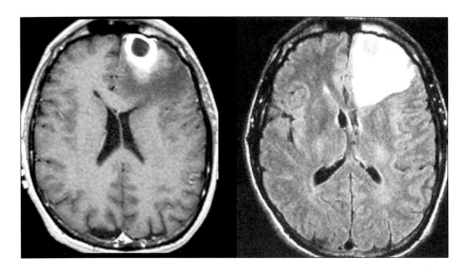

Figure 13.6
A brain abscess mistaken for a metastasis. This man with esophageal cancer had received immunosuppressive chemotherapy. He developed a headache and was found to have a contrast-enhancing mass in the frontal lobe. The lesion was believed to be a metastasis. Craniotomy revealed a bacterial abscess. No source was found.

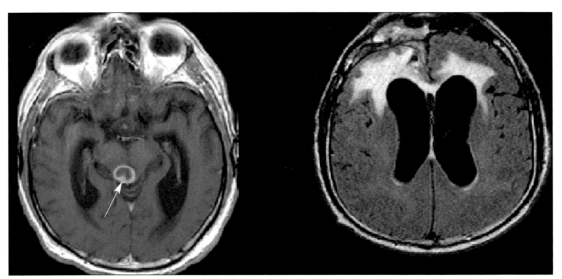

Figure 13.7
A primary tumor mistaken for a metastases. A 60-year-old man with a known history of renal cell carcinoma but without prior evidence of metastatic disease presented with headache and was found to have a ring-enhancing lesion in the tectum of the midbrain compressing the aqueduct (arrow). The hyperintensity surrounding the anterior horns of the ventricles (right MRI) is believed to represent transependymal absorption of spinal fluid resulting from the hydrocephalus. A needle biopsy of the tumor revealed not a metastatic renal cancer but a glioblastoma multiforme.

brain tumors and systemic cancer than in the general population and must always be considered in the differential diagnosis of an acute neurologic disorder in a cancer patient.[35]

Herpes zoster may cause an encephalitic disorder associated with immunosuppressing cancers and characterized by multiple areas of contrast-enhancing leukoencephalopathy. The disorder may follow herpetic skin infection by months or years and may even occur in patients who did not have prior skin lesions or in whom skin lesions were unrecognized.[36]

Demyelinating disease may occasionally mimic cerebral metastases. Although there are isolated reports of multiple sclerosis and primary brain tumor coexisting,[37] there is no evidence of an increased incidence of multiple sclerosis in patients with systemic cancer. However, because acute demyelinating lesions may contrast enhance, a patient who has multiple sclerosis and a coincidental cancer may occasionally present with neurologic signs and an enhancing lesion(s) in the brain. If the radiographic diagnosis is unclear, the diagnosis can usually be established by following the MR scan. A metastatic tumor will grow, whereas a multiple sclerosis lesion will disappear in several weeks. Figure 13.8 illustrates the problem. This patient with known breast cancer treated previously with chemotherapy presented with neurologic symptoms and a contrast-enhancing lesion in the brainstem. The lesion could not be distinguished from a breast metastasis. However, the patient had a past history of neurologic episodes, and a number of non-enhancing lesions were found in the brain consistent with demyelinating disease but not with metastases. The question then was whether she had two diseases, multiple sclerosis and metastatic cancer. Her symptoms did

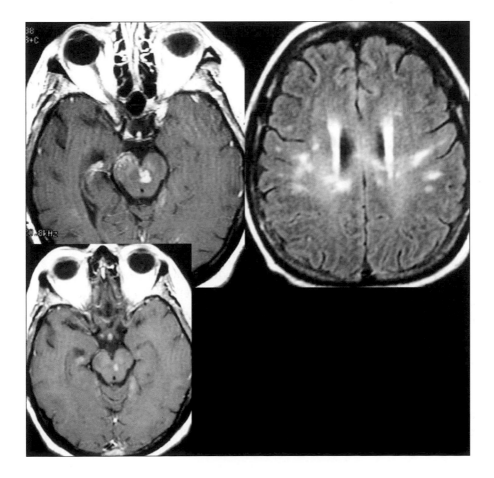

Figure 13.8
Multiple sclerosis mistaken for a metastasis. A patient with known breast cancer developed brainstem signs. An MR showed an enhancing lesion in the brainstem (top left) but there were multiple non-enhancing lesions in the cerebral hemispheres. Because of the possibility that the brainstem lesion was due to multiple sclerosis rather than metastatic tumor, the patient was followed. Two months later, the enhancement had largely disappeared (bottom left).

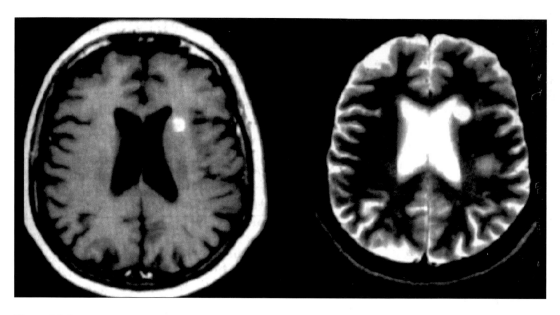

Figure 13.9
Encephalopathy caused by 5-FU–levamisole. This patient with Duke's B colon cancer developed a mild hemiparesis and underwent an MR scan (left) that showed a contrast enhancing lesion in the left hemisphere. Several other lesions did not contrast-enhance but were apparent as hyperintensity on the T2-weighted image (right). After a diagnosis of metastatic tumor, the patient received 3000 cGy to the whole brain. She became demented and bedridden. The needle biopsy specimen of the lesion following the radiation therapy revealed the typical demyelination reported as a side-effect of 5-FU-levamisole therapy. Metastatic disease was not present.

not progress and a repeat scan showed disappearance of the enhancement, indicating that the entire process was related to demyelination.

Another problem occurs in patients receiving chemotherapy with 5-FU and levamisole, or sometimes with levamisole alone.[38] This regimen, once commonly used for colon cancer, can cause multiple contrast enhancing demyelinating lesions in the brain which resolve with discontinuation of the drugs (Fig. 13.9). Patients with demyelinating disease, from either multiple sclerosis or chemotherapy, appear to be more susceptible to radiation neurotoxicity.[39] One of our patients with chemotherapy-induced demyelination received standard whole-brain RT for presumed metastases. She rapidly became severely demented,

despite the fact that the lesions themselves disappeared when the chemotherapy was discontinued. A stereotactic needle biopsy done after the fact revealed demyelination and no metastatic tumor. Therefore, this distinction is critical since premature diagnosis and treatment of brain metastasis can result in severe neurologic damage.[39]

Overall, cerebrovascular disease is much more common than brain tumors, either primary or metastatic. Accordingly, patients who present with acute lesions are often thought to have cerebral infarcts or hemorrhages. These disorders are more likely to occur in patients with cancer, for several reasons. Patients with cancer usually suffer from a hypercoagulable state. Deep vein thromboses, extremely common in patients with systemic cancer, can cause brain infarction by paradoxical embolization.[40] The most common symptomatic complication of cancer-induced nonbacterial thrombotic endocarditis is brain infarction.[41] Lung cancer itself or pulmonary metastases can embolize to brain, producing infarction and later brain metastases.[42] RT for head and neck tumors may accelerate arteriosclerosis and can lead to carotid occlusion and stroke.

The diagnosis of infarction is generally not difficult. A scan during the acute episode of cerebral infarction does not contrast enhance and the lesion may be visible only on diffusion-weighted MR images, a pattern very sensitive for the diagnosis of stroke. The lesion itself is far more diffuse than one sees with well-circumscribed brain metastases. Cerebral hemorrhage may be more difficult. Patients receiving chemotherapy for cancer are often thrombocytopenic and susceptible to brain hemorrhage. Others may be hypercoagulable and suffer venous sinus occlusion, leading to hemorrhagic infarction.

If there is any question about the diagnosis, a biopsy is essential. The most telling finding comes from the controlled trial of brain metastases conducted by Patchell et al.[43] A series of patients with known cancer and a single contrast-enhancing lesion of the brain were randomized to receive either surgical resection or stereotactic biopsy followed by RT. Despite the presence of cancer (usually lung cancer) and careful examination by experienced neuro-oncologists, 11% of the patients were discovered not to have metastatic lesions on pathologic examination. These lesions included high-grade and low-grade primary brain tumors and inflammatory or immune-mediated lesions. Accordingly, when there is any question about the diagnosis, a biopsy is essential.

Treatment

General considerations

The diagnostic and therapeutic approach to patients with brain metastases depends on the number and location of metastases, on the biology of the primary tumor, and on the extent of systemic disease.[19,44] Obviously, different approaches are required in patients known to have cancer from those not known to have cancer. Algorithms outlining the diagnostic and therapeutic approaches in some of these situations are presented in Figs 13.10 and 13.11. The therapeutic approach to patients with brain metastases is similar to that of primary brain tumors, and is divided into supportive and definitive treatments (Table 13.5) (Chapter 4).

Supportive therapy

As indicated in Chapter 4, supportive therapy may include corticosteroids, anticonvulsants, psychotropic drugs and anticoagulants. Corticosteroids are necessary only for symptomatic metastases, where they usually produce a dramatic response, and are also

Table 13.5
Treatment of brain metastases.

Supportive	Definitive
Corticosteroids	Surgery
Antibiotics	Radiation
Anticonvulsants	Whole-brain RT (WBRT)
Anticoagulants	Radiosurgery
Antidepressants	Whole-brain
	RT + radiosurgery
	Chemotherapy
	Systemic
	Local

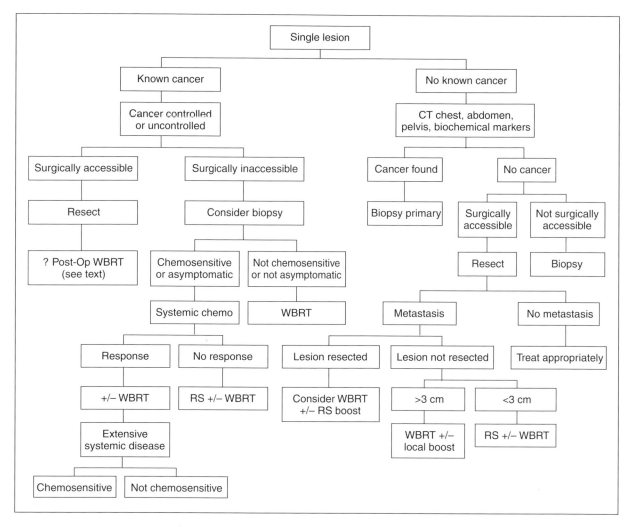

Figure 13.10
Approach to the patient with a single lesion. RS, Radiosurgery; WBRT, whole-brain radiation therapy.

indicated during the course of definitive treatment with surgery or radiation. Corticosteroids are not required for asymptomatic patients with small metastases unless RT or surgery is imminent. We do not routinely use gastric protection for patients receiving corticosteroids. In patients expected to be on corticosteroids for a prolonged period, e.g. more than 6 weeks, prophylactic antibiotics to prevent *Pneumocystis carinii* infection are indicated. However, these drugs often cause side-effects, particularly platelet suppression. Also, as indicated in Chapter 4, anticonvulsants are not used prophylactically. We recommend them only if the patient has had a seizure. Deep vein thrombosis is a common complication of patients with cancer, particularly those with brain metastases. Prophylactic treatment is

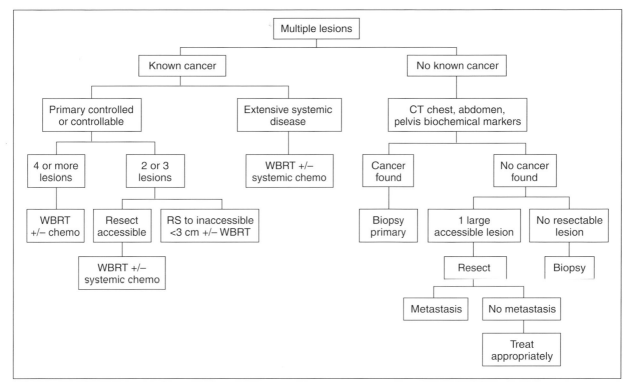

Figure 13.11
Approach to the patient with multiple lesions. RS, Radiosurgery; WBRT, whole-brain radiation therapy; chemo, chemotherapy.

probably not indicated, but patients must be followed carefully for symptoms and treated promptly. Psychologic complications of metastatic cancer are common; antidepressants are effective in relieving depression. Even when the physician believes that the depression is 'rational and justified', these drugs should be utilized as they effectively ameliorate 'reactive' depression.

Definitive treatment

Surgery
Two controlled trials clearly indicate that for patients with single brain metastases, surgical removal followed by whole-brain radiotherapy is superior to whole-brain RT alone, both in preventing brain relapse and in improving quality of life[43,45] (Fig. 13.12). A third trial[46] found no benefit. In our opinion, in patients whose systemic disease is quiescent or controllable, surgical removal of a single brain metastasis substantially improves survival. Two-year survivals are 15–20%, depending on the primary tumor; 5-year survivals are about 10%, and occasional 'cures' are reported.[47] There are now retrospective data to support the resection of two or even three metastases, with the outcome comparable to a surgically treated single brain metastasis. The operative mortality is 1–3%; neurologic worsening, often transient, occurs in 5–10%. Patients with

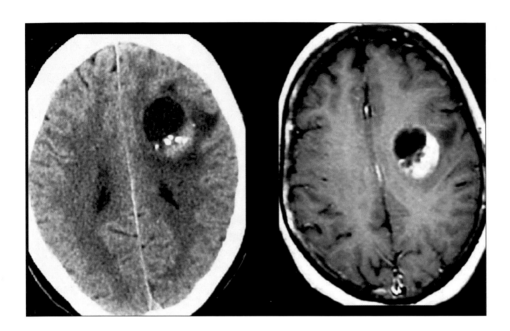

Figure 13.12
A single brain metastasis with both cyst and calcification in a patient with ovarian cancer. The tumor responded to surgical resection. Note that the calcium is hyperdense on CT and hypointense on MRI.

cerebellar lesions have a worse prognosis than those with hemispheral lesions,[48] and are at increased risk for subsequent leptomeningeal metastases.

A recent controlled trial indicates that patients with a single metastasis who receive postoperative radiotherapy have fewer recurrences of cancer in the brain and are less likely to die of neurologic causes than similar patients treated with surgical resection alone.[49] However, overall survival was comparable between the groups because patients with controlled cerebral disease died of progressive systemic tumor. Accordingly, the best extant data suggest that a patient with a single, surgically accessible brain metastasis, whose systemic disease is not imminently terminal, should have that metastasis removed and receive postoperative whole-brain RT. However, because of the toxicity of whole-brain RT, particularly in the older age group, many physicians do not use it in the immediate postoperative period, but reserve radiation until relapse.

Radiation therapy

The time-honored treatment of brain metastases has been whole-brain radiation, delivering 30 Gy in 10 fractions. For patients with extensive systemic disease or multiple brain metastases, this still remains the best option. Most patients have at least a transient response to radiation; they symptomatically improve with steroids and radiotherapy, and are less likely to die of their neurologic disease than are patients who do not receive this treatment (Fig. 13.13). Survival remains short, with a median of 4–6 months, because most patients die of uncontrolled systemic tumor. Even those patients who respond to RT and whose tumors are controlled, however, are at risk for reseeding of the brain from the systemic cancer. In occasional patients, RT actually sterilizes the brain metastases and they do not recur. Because of late-delayed radiation toxicity in those patients whose systemic prognosis is more than a year, particularly after resection of a single brain metastasis, we recommend a dose of 40–50 Gy given in 1.8–2.0-Gy fractions.[50] The lower dose per fraction diminishes radiation toxicity. Cognitive deficits from RT are more severe in the very young, the elderly and those who receive extensive chemotherapy. Nevertheless, even young adults often complain of memory loss after whole-brain RT.

The reason for using whole-brain RT in brain metastases as opposed to focal RT is because micrometastases may be present elsewhere in the brain, even when one can visualize only one or two metastatic tumors. Whole-brain radiation will prevent the growth of these microscopic as well as macroscopic tumors. Evidence for this

comes from two sources. First, prophylactic irradiation of the brain in patients with small cell lung cancer substantially decreases the subsequent development of CNS metastases. This is because micrometastases were present at the time of radiation and were eliminated by it. Second, a controlled trial demonstrated that postoperative whole-brain RT decreases relapse in the brain not only at the surgical site but throughout the brain, indicating that small metastatic deposits were eliminated by the radiation.[49]

Radiosurgery
Radiosurgery is increasingly being used instead of surgery for the treatment of single or even multiple brain metastases.[51–53] The treatment

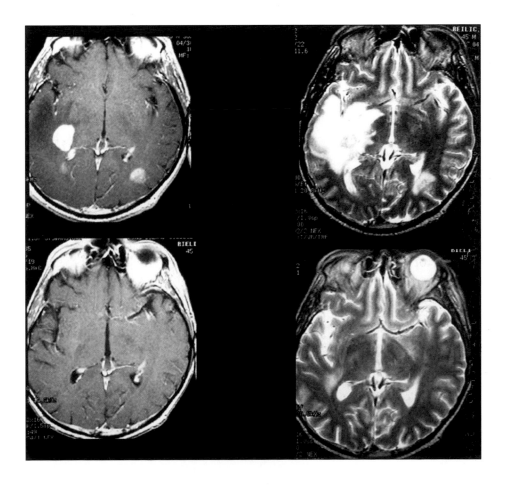

Figure 13.13 Response of a small cell lung cancer to whole-brain radiation therapy. The patient had multiple metastases, one of which was surrounded by a massive amount of edema (top panels). Two months after radiation therapy, the tumors had disappeared and the edema had largely cleared (bottom panels).

appears to be most effective against those tumors that are relatively resistant to conventional external beam radiation therapy, such as melanoma[54] and renal cell carcinoma.[55,56] The reason is unclear, but the higher dose per fraction may eliminate otherwise resistant tumor cells. Some report 78% tumor control with < 10% complications.[52] Tumor control is defined as disappearance, decrease in size or stability of the lesion. Other reports indicate that local control is maintained over 2 years in 61% of patients.[57] MRI may show a transient increase in tumor enhancement which does not necessarily indicate tumor growth.[57] Radiosurgery has advantages over surgery in that it is relatively non-invasive, not even requiring hospitalization in most instances, and can often reach areas that are surgically inaccessible. Radiosurgery has the disadvantage that it is not useful for tumors larger than 3–4 cm. Theoretically, radiosurgery should be a much better technique for brain metastases than gliomas, because metastases are well circumscribed and do not infiltrate widely into normal brain. At least one non-randomized comparative study of surgery versus radiosurgery suggests that survival is equal.[58] However, a case-control retrospective trial of the two modalities found that patients lived longer and did better with surgical resection. This was partially attributed to the propensity for radiosurgery to cause brain necrosis that in itself is symptomatic and may require surgery as treatment. A recent retrospective study comparing radiosurgery with surgery plus whole-brain RT yielded similar periprocedure morbidity (7.7% versus 8.9%), mortality (1.6% versus 1.2%) and 1-year survival (53% versus 43% not statistically significant) rates. Local control rates were also similar at 1 year (75% versus 83%).[58] The report suggests that whole-brain RT may not be necessary after radiosurgery. Others agree,[58,59] although this contradicts the controlled trial of RT after surgery.[49] A randomized trial is necessary to resolve this question. Until randomized trials prove the superiority of one treatment over the other, we believe that surgery is the preferred treatment for accessible lesions in good-prognosis patients. Surgery not only treats the lesion, but it also establishes the diagnosis, which has a 10% error rate[43] based on neuroimaging alone. However, there are situations in which radiosurgery is the therapy of first choice, e.g. elderly patients with multiple lesions which cannot all be resected (e.g. three or four), or patients with brainstem metastases.[60]

Chemotherapy

Chemotherapy is increasingly being recognized as efficacious for brain metastases from chemosensitive systemic cancers (Fig. 13.14). These include germ cell tumors, breast cancer, small cell lung cancer and some others.[61,62] Chemotherapy can be applied either systemically or locally into the brain tumor bed.[63] The latter approach is still highly experimental and its efficacy is unclear. In appropriate patients, one should probably use chemotherapy to treat brain metastases that have disrupted the blood–brain barrier, i.e. contrast enhance, before RT is applied. In addition, systemic chemotherapy is probably best used in patients who do not require corticosteroids, since those drugs restore blood–brain barrier function and decrease the amount of water-soluble drug that can reach the tumor. There are several reasons for administering chemotherapy before radiation: (1) it is useful to be able to judge tumor response to chemotherapy before initiating RT – if the tumor is responsive, the chemotherapy can be continued even after radiation is given. (2) After RT the blood supply to the tumor is disrupted and may decrease the access of

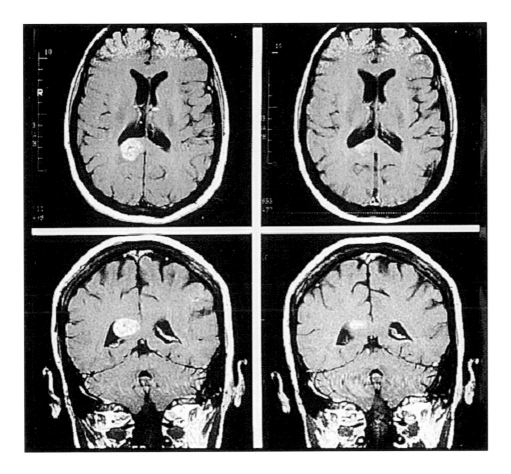

Figure 13.14
Response to chemotherapy. A patient with known ovarian cancer developed a brain metastasis with only mild headache as the symptom, but because she was about to undergo systemic chemotherapy, it was elected to follow her on treatment. The pre-chemotherapy (left panels) and post-chemotherapy images show a clear response of the tumor. The tumor was well controlled for about 2 years before her systemic disease and brain metastasis escaped treatment.

chemotherapy to the metastases. (3) Some evidence suggests that chemotherapy delivered before radiation is less neurotoxic than the converse. The evidence is best for methotrexate but may apply to other drugs as well.

Usually, the chemotherapeutic agent is chosen based on the underlying primary. However, there are circumstances in which there appears to be a good response of a variety of metastatic tumor types to a single protocol. Among 56 patients with brain metastases from breast cancer, cisplatin and etoposide gave a complete response in 7 (13%) and a partial response in 14 (21%). Among 43 patients with measurable non-small cell lung cancer, 3 (7%) had a complete response and 10 (25%) a partial response. None of 8 melanomas responded.[64]

Chemotherapy is not without its neurologic complications. A recent study of women receiving adjuvant chemotherapy for breast cancer indicated that there was a risk of late cognitive impairment when compared with patients not receiving such chemotherapy. The cognitive impairment was not caused by anxiety, depression or fatigue or related to time since treatment; only some patients were aware of their neuropsychological disorder.[65]

Specific treatment situations

The number of variables both within the CNS and outside the CNS is so great that each patient is unique. Nevertheless, a number of common scenarios are outlined and guidelines suggested for each. What follows are tentative recommendations based on the current state of knowledge.

(1) The patient's systemic tumor has been successfully treated or has a relatively good prognosis (more than 1 year). The patient has either a single, surgically accessible brain metastasis or, in especially good-risk patients, two or rarely three accessible metastatic lesions. Such patients have the best prognosis for preserved nervous system function and survival if focal therapy is delivered to the brain metastases. No controlled trials have yet addressed whether surgical removal of the tumor or radiosurgery is the superior modality. Surgery is more costly and the morbidity is similar; however, most complications occur early after surgery and later after radiosurgery.[66] If the lesion is greater than 3–4 cm in diameter, it should probably be removed. One report indicates that in patients with one large metastasis and one or more small lesions (< 2 cm), surgery of the large lesion followed by whole-brain RT yields results equal to surgery of a single metastasis followed by RT.[67] In one randomized trial, postoperative whole-brain RT improved control of the CNS disease, but did not improve overall survival.[49] However, not all patients relapse after surgery and the cognitive side-effects of whole-brain RT require one to give each patient individual consideration.

(2) A good-risk systemic patient with 1–3 small but surgically inaccessible (i.e. basal ganglia) lesions. Such patients are reported to have excellent local control of tumor with radiosurgery. Current data would suggest that if local control is achieved with radiosurgery, patients should also receive whole-brain RT to help prevent the appearance of tumors in other areas of the brain. However, whole-brain RT is often withheld in older patients because of the high incidence of cognitive impairment. For asymptomatic patients, particularly those with evidence of disease elsewhere in the body, and with relatively chemosensitive tumors (e.g. breast cancer, small cell lung cancer), systemic chemotherapy may be useful as initial treatment. Systemic chemotherapy may achieve control of the brain and systemic tumors without resorting to radiation. If chemotherapy succeeds, it can be continued. If it fails, radiosurgery can be substituted. We do not use chemotherapy as the first treatment in symptomatic brain metastases, because surgery and radiotherapy control symptoms much faster than chemotherapy and with greater reliability.

(3) The patient has poor-prognosis systemic disease and multiple brain metastases. In this situation, whole-brain RT, 30 Gy in 10 fractions, along with corticosteroids, will usually control brain symptoms for the duration of the patient's life. If one of the multiple brain lesions is large and symptomatic, removal of the mass may improve the patient's quality of life even though it may not extend the duration of survival.

(4) A patient previously treated for a brain metastasis improves and then relapses after several months to a year. All of the treatment modalities and considerations that apply to the initial treatment of a CNS metastasis also apply to recurrence.

In general, treatment after recurrence is less effective than initial treatment, but nonetheless may improve both quality and length of life. A patient in good systemic condition with a single surgically accessible brain metastasis that recurs either at the site of initial craniotomy or at a distance should be considered for a second craniotomy. In rare instances, even a third operation for a locally recurrent tumor may help the patient. However, long-term survival after a second resection is rare. In patients with surgically inaccessible lesions who are poor candidates for surgery, radiosurgery can be used for lesions not previously treated with radiosurgery. Prior whole-brain RT does not preclude the use of radiosurgery in selected instances. A second course of whole-brain RT, if brain metastases have been stable for 6 months or longer and then recur, may also be beneficial and usually can be administered safely. In some patients who fail chemotherapy, retreatment with different chemotherapeutic agents may give a response. With a repeat course of whole-brain RT, 20–25 Gy in 1.8–2.0-Gy fractions, most patients improve at least transiently, and occasional patients survive 6 months to a year. The likelihood of patients developing cognitive dysfunction or other signs of radiation toxicity are increased by the second course of radiation, but most patients do not live long enough to suffer this side effect.

(5) The patient has small cell lung cancer or another cancer with a high propensity for brain metastases. A staging cranial MR scan is negative. A number of studies have addressed the question of prophylactic brain RT in this situation. Strong evidence suggests that prophylactic radiation of the brain of patients with small cell lung cancer substantially diminishes the likelihood of subsequent brain metastases. Some studies suggest that, despite this, there is no increase in overall survival; other studies demonstrate that survival is prolonged.[68] Unfortunately, prophylactic brain irradiation comes at a cost, particularly in patients who have received or will receive systemic chemotherapy, which includes all patients with small cell lung cancer. Many patients suffer significant cognitive dysfunction, although not always to a disabling degree. The longer the patient survives, the more likely it is that cognitive dysfunction will become manifest since this is often a delayed complication of treatment.[69]

(6) Malignant germ cell tumors may present with brain metastases, although other disease, especially bulky thoracic disease, is always present.[70] Chemotherapy may be effective and sufficient treatment for the brain metastasis.

Complications of treatment

The neurologic complications that result from treatment of intracranial metastases are in general the same as those resulting from treatment of primary intracranial tumors (Chapter 4). Operative mortality from craniotomy for treatment of brain metastases is under 3%, usually occurring only in patients debilitated from their primary cancer. Many patients with CNS metastases have advanced systemic disease, are immunosuppressed from prior chemotherapy and may be poorly nourished. Thus, wound healing and postoperative infections are somewhat more common following surgery for CNS metastases than for primary tumors. Furthermore, hypercoagulability caused by the underlying cancer or hypocoagulability caused by prior treatment predisposes such patients to clotting disorders, e.g. venous thrombosis, and bleeding from thrombocytopenia. The operative morbidity, including worsening of neurologic symptoms (mostly transient) is about 5–10%. Because the majority of tumors are well demarcated from surrounding normal brain, neurologic worsening is less commonly encountered after surgery for metastasis than for glioma. Thus, most patients tolerate craniotomy well and leave the hospital within 4 or 5 days. Even patients debilitated with widespread systemic disease often respond well to craniotomy. However, the local recurrence rate of 30% without postoperative whole-brain RT suggests that, despite gross total resection, microscopic tumor often remains after surgery.[49]

Radiosurgery also has its complications. Headache, nausea, vomiting, seizures and even transient worsening of neurologic symptoms may follow within hours of radiosurgery. The symptoms are usually easily controlled with steroids. Local tumor control is defined by radiation oncologists as cessation of tumor growth; tumor shrinkage is not required. Accordingly, the residual tumor, or the necrosis produced by radiosurgery, may lead to edema with symptoms that are not easily controlled. Radionecrosis typically becomes symptomatic several weeks to months following radiosurgery. This may require further surgery to alleviate symptoms or chronic corticosteroid use with its own attendant complications. This is one of the disadvantages of radiosurgery when compared with surgical removal, where there is no gross tumor tissue left behind.

Whole-brain RT has few immediate side-effects, but in patients who survive more than a year or in those who have been heavily pretreated with chemotherapy, dementia is a common delayed side-effect. In addition, older patients are at greater risk than younger

patients for cognitive impairment. Accordingly, we divide patients who are to receive whole-brain RT into prognostic groups: those with a good systemic prognosis, i.e. likely to live more than 1 year, are treated in 1.8–2.0-Gy fractions to a total dose of 40–50 Gy; those who have a poor prognosis (less than 6 months) are treated in 3-Gy fractions to a total of 30 Gy. However, even the smaller dose fractions may cause cognitive dysfunction in some patients.

Prognosis

Untreated symptomatic brain metastases usually cause death within 1 or 2 months. Corticosteroids can control symptoms for several weeks to a few months. Whole-brain RT yields a median survival of 4–6 months with 80% or more having neurologic improvement. Patients with a single brain metastasis treated with surgery and whole-brain RT have a median survival of 40 weeks and some live longer than a year. Prolonged survival can also be seen after radiosurgery. Rarely, patients have long survivals and appear to be cured.

The prognosis depends in part on the histology of the primary tumor, on the stage of systemic disease, and on the number and location of CNS metastases. Chemo- and radiosensitive tumors have a better prognosis than chemo- and radioresistant tumors. Patients with single brain metastases that are surgically removed and whose systemic disease is well controlled have a 10–15% 5-year survival and an occasional apparent cure. Whether radiosurgery can also give such long survival is unclear. Accordingly, good-risk patients should be approached aggressively in an attempt to eliminate the focal disease and prevent recurrence elsewhere in the brain.

In a recent study of over 1000 patients with brain metastases,[71] the overall median survival was 3.4 months, with a 1-year survival of 12% and a 2-year survival of 4%. Steroids only yielded a median survival of 1.3 months, which increased to 3.6 months in patients treated with RT and to 8.9 months in patients treated with surgery followed by radiotherapy. In addition to treatment, performance status, response to steroids and systemic tumor activity were important prognostic factors. Somewhat less important were the site of the primary tumor, the age of the patient and the number of brain metastases. Treatment data must be interpreted carefully, particularly with respect to the poor-prognosis patients who receive less aggressive treatment. Many patients receive less aggressive treatment because they are substantially less well than those patients who are treated vigorously. Sometimes, statistical analysis does not fully account for these differences.

References

1. Boogerd W, Hart AAM, Tjahja IS. Treatment and outcome of brain metastasis as first site of distant metastasis from breast cancer. J Neurooncol 1997; 35: 161–7.
2. Robnett TJ, Machtay M, Stevenson JP, Algazy KM, Hahn SM. Factors affecting the risk of brain metastases after definitive chemoradiation for locally advanced non-small-cell lung carcinoma. J Clin Oncol 2001; 19: 1344–9.
3. Giordana MT, Cordera S, Boghi A. Cerebral metastases as first symptom of cancer: a clinico-pathologic study. J Neurooncol 2000; 50: 265–73.
4. Posner JB. Neurologic Complications of Cancer. Philadelphia: FA Davis, 1995.
5. Greenlee RT, Hill-Harmon MB, Taylor M, Thum M. Cancer Statistics, 2001. Ca Cancer J Clin 2001; 51: 15–36.
6. Posner JB, Chernik NL. Intracranial metastases from systemic cancer. Adv Neurol 1978; 19: 575–87.
7. Cairncross JG, Kim J-H, Posner JB. Radiation therapy of brain metastases. Ann Neurol 1980; 7: 529–41.
8. Lentzsch S, Reichardt P, Weber F, Budach V, Dörken B. Brain metastases in breast cancer: Prognostic factors and management. Eur J Cancer [A] 1999; 35: 580–5.
9. Voorhies RM, Sundaresan N, Thaler HT. The single supratentorial lesion. An evaluation of preoperative diagnostic tests. J Neurosurg 1980; 53: 364–8.
10. Jonas S, Bechstein WO, Lemmens HP et al. Liver graft-transmitted glioblastoma multiforme. A case report and experience with 13 multiorgan donors suffering from primary cerebral neoplasia. Transpl Int 1996; 9: 426–9.
11. Chui AK, Herbertt K, Wang LS et al. Risk of tumor transmission in transplantation from donors with primary brain tumors: an Australian and New Zealand registry report. Transplant Proc 1999; 31: 1266–7.
12. Counsell CE, Grant R. Incidence studies of primary and secondary intracranial tumors: a systematic review of their methodology and results. J Neurooncol 1998; 37: 241–50.
13. Yokoi K, Kamiya N, Matsuguma H et al. Detection of brain metastasis in potentially operable non-small-cell lung cancer – a comparison of CT and MRI. Chest 1999; 115: 714–9.
14. Earnest F, Ryu JH, Miller GM et al. Suspected non-small cell lung cancer: Incidence of occult brain and skeletal metastases and effectiveness of imaging for detection – pilot study. Radiology 1999; 211: 137–45.
15. Fidler IJ. The Paget–Ewing Award Lecture – The seed and soil hypothesis at the millennium: Recent advances in the pathogenesis of cancer metastasis. Clin Exp Metastasis 1999; 17: 731.
16. Liotta LA, Kohn EC. Invasion and Metastases. In: Bast RC, Kufe DW, Pollock RE et al, eds. Cancer Medicine. Hamilton: BC Decker, 2000: 121–31.
17. Kearsley JH, Tattersall MH. Cerebral embolism in cancer patients. Q J Med 1982; 51: 279–91.
18. Delattre J-Y, Krol G, Thaler HT, Posner JB. Distribution of brain metastases. Arch Neurol 1988; 45: 741–4.

19. Graf AH, Buchberger W, Langmayr H, Schmid KW. Site preference of metastatic tumours of the brain. Virchows Arch A Pathol Anat Histopathol 1988; 412: 493–8.

20. Morita R, Fujimoto A, Hatta N, Takehara K, Takata M. Comparison of genetic profiles between primary melanomas and their metastases reveals genetic alterations and clonal evolution during progression. J Invest Dermatol 1998; 111: 919–24.

21. Ruan S, Fuller G, Levin V, Bruner JM, Zhang W. Detection of p21[WAF1/Cip1] in brain metastases. J Neurooncol 1998; 37: 223–8.

22. Hampl M, Hampl JA, Schwarz P et al. Accumulation of genetic alterations in brain metastases of sporadic breast carcinomas is associated with reduced survival after metastasis. Invasion Metastasis 1999; 18: 81–95.

23. Hurteau JA, Allison B, Sutton GP et al. Transforming growth factor-β differentially inhibits epithelial ovarian carcinoma cells from primary and metastatic isolates without up-regulation of p21[WAF1]. Cancer 1999; 85: 1810–5.

24. Kleinschmidt-DeMasters BK, Shroyer AL, Hashizumi TL et al. Part I. Telomerase levels in human metastatic brain tumors show four-fold logarithmic variability but no correlation with tumor type or interval to patient demise. J Neurol Sci 1998; 161: 116–23.

25. Freilich RJ, Seidman AD, DeAngelis LM. Central nervous system progression of metastatic breast cancer in patients treated with paclitaxel. Cancer 1995; 76: 232–6.

26. Dhote R, Beuzeboc P, Thiounn N et al. High incidence of brain metastases in patients treated with an M–VAC regimen for advanced bladder cancer. Eur Urol 1998; 33: 392–5.

27. Kramer K, Kushner B, Heller G, Cheung NKV. Neuroblastoma metastatic to the central nervous system – The Memorial Sloan-Kettering Cancer Center experience and a literature review. Cancer 2001; 91: 1510–9.

28. Castiglione-Gertsch M, Tattersall M, Hacking A et al and the International Breast Cancer Study Group. Retreating recurrent breast cancer with the same CMF-containing regimen used as adjuvant therapy. Eur J Cancer [A] 1997; 33A: 2321–5.

29. Posner JB. Brain metastases: 1995. A brief review. J Neurooncol 1996; 27: 287–93.

30. Alvarez-Sabín J, Lozano M, Sastre-Garriga J et al. Transient ischaemic attack: A common initial manifestation of cardiac myxomas. Eur Neurol 2001; 45: 165–70.

31. Lassen U, Daugaard G, Eigtved A, Damgaard K, Friberg L. 18F-FDG whole body positron emission tomography (PET) in patients with unknown primary tumours (UPT). Eur J Cancer [A] 1999; 35: 1076–82.

32. Markopoulos C, Sampalis F, Givalos N, Gogas H. Association of breast cancer with meningioma. Eur J Surg Oncol 1998; 24: 332–4.

33. Freilich RJ, Krol G, DeAngelis LM. Neuroimaging and cerebrospinal fluid cytology in the diagnosis of leptomeningeal metastasis. Ann Neurol 1995; 38: 51–7.

34. Buhl R, Hugo HH, Mihajlovic Z, Mehdorn HM. Secretory meningiomas: clinical and immunohistochemical observations. Neurosurgery 2001; 48: 297–301.

35. Schiff D, Rosenblum MK. Herpes simplex encephalitis (HSE) and the immunocompromised: a clinical and autopsy study of HSE in the settings of cancer and human immunodeficiency virus-type 1 infection. Hum Pathol 1998; 29: 215–22.

36. Weaver S, Rosenblum MK, DeAngelis LM. Herpes varicella-zoster encephalitis in immunocompromised patients. Neurology 1999; 52: 193–5.

37. Khan OA, Bauserman SC, Rothman MI, Aldrich EF, Panitch HS. Concurrence of multiple sclerosis and brain tumor: clinical considerations. Neurology 1997; 48: 1330–3.

38. Figueredo AT, Fawcet SE, Molloy DW, Dobranowski J, Paulseth JE. Disabling encephalopathy during 5-fluorouracil and levamisole adjuvant therapy for resected colorectal cancer: A report of two cases. Cancer Invest 1995; 13: 608–11.

39. Peterson K, Rosenblum MK, Powers JM, Alvord EC, Walker RW, Posner JB. Effect of brain irradiation on demyelinating lesions. Neurology 1993; 43: 2105–12.

40. Yeung M, Khan KA, Shuaib A. Transcranial Doppler ultrasonography in the detection of venous to arterial shunting in acute stroke and transient ischaemic attacks. J Neurol Neurosurg Psychiatry 1996; 61: 445–9.

41. Rogers LR, Cho E-S, Kempin S, Posner JB. Cerebral infarction from non-bacterial thrombotic endocarditis. Clinical and pathological study including the effects of anticoagulation. Am J Med 1987; 83: 746–56.

42. Graus F, Rogers LR, Posner JB. Cerebrovascular complications in patients with cancer. Medicine 1985; 64: 16–35.

43. Patchell RA, Tibbs PA, Walsh JW. A randomized trial of surgery in the treatment of single metastases to the brain. N Engl J Med 1990; 322: 494–500.

44. Nieder C, Nestle U, Motaref B et al. Prognostic factors in brain metastases: Should patients be selected for aggressive treatment according to recursive partitioning analysis (RPA) classes? Int J Radiat Oncol Biol Phys 2000; 46: 297–302.

45. Vecht CJ, Haaxma-Reiche H, Noordijk EM, et al. Treatment of single brain metastasis: Radiotherapy alone or combined with neurosurgery? Ann Neurol 1993; 33: 583–90.

46. Mintz AH, Kestle J, Rathbone MP et al. A randomized trial to assess the efficacy of surgery in addition to radiotherapy in patients with a single cerebral metastasis. Cancer 1996; 78: 1470–6.

47. Arbit E, Wronski M. The treatment of brain metastases. Neurosurgery Quarterly 1995; 5: 1–17.

48. Wronski M, Arbit E. Resection of brain metastases from colorectal carcinoma in 73 patients. Cancer 1999; 85: 1677–85.

49. Patchell RA, Tibbs PA, Regine WF et al. Postoperative radiotherapy in the treatment of single metastases to the brain: a randomized trial. JAMA 1998; 280: 1485–9.

50. DeAngelis LM. Management of brain metastases. Cancer Invest 1994; 12: 156–65.

51. Seung SK, Sneed PK, McDermott MW et al. Gamma knife radiosurgery for malignant melanoma brain metastases. Cancer J Sci AM 1998; 4: 103–9.

52. Loeffler JS, Barker FG, Chapman PH. Role of radiosurgery in the management of central nervous system metastases. Cancer Chemother Pharmacol 1999; 43: S11–14.

53. Kondziolka D, Patel A, Lunsford LD, Kassam A, Flickinger JC. Stereotactic radiosurgery plus whole brain radiotherapy versus radiotherapy alone for patients with multiple brain metastases. Int J Radiat Oncol Biol Phys 1999; 45: 427–34.

54. Lavine SD, Petrovich Z, Cohen-Gadol AA et al. Gamma knife radiosurgery for metastatic melanoma: An analysis of survival, outcome, and complications. Neurosurgery 1999; 44: 59–64.

55. Mori Y, Kondziolka D, Flickinger JC, Logan T, Lunsford LD. Stereotactic radiosurgery for brain metastasis from renal cell carcinoma. Cancer 1998; 83: 344–53.

56. Becker G, Duffner F, Kortmann R et al. Radiosurgery for the treatment of brain metastases in renal cell carcinoma. Anticancer Res 1999; 19: 1611–7.

57. Peterson AM, Meltzer CC, Evanson EJ, Flickinger JC, Kondziolka D. MR imaging response of brain metastases after gamma knife stereotactic radiosurgery. Radiology 1999; 211: 807–14.

58. Muacevic A, Kreth FW, Horstmann GA et al. Surgery and radiotherapy compared with gamma knife radiosurgery in the treatment of solitary cerebral metastases of small diameter. J Neurosurg 1999; 91: 35–43.

59. Sneed PK, Lamborn KR, Forstner JM et al. Radiosurgery for brain metastases: Is whole brain radiotherapy necessary? In: J Radiat Oncol Biol Phys 1999; 43(3): 549–58.

60. Huang CF, Kondziolka D, Flickinger JC, Lunsford LD. Stereotactic radiosurgery for brainstem metastases. J Neurosurg 1999; 91: 563–8.

61. Cormio G, Gabriele A, Maneo A et al. Complete remission of brain metastases from ovarian carcinoma with carboplatin. Eur J Obstet Gynecol Reprod Biol 1998; 78: 91–3.

62. Franciosi V, Cocconi G, Michiara M et al. Frontline chemotherapy with cisplatin and etoposide for patients with brain metastases from breast carcinoma, non small cell lung carcinoma, or malignant melanoma. A prospective study. Cancer 1999; 85(7): 1599–605.

63. Ewend MG, Sampath P, Williams JA, Tyler BM, Brem H. Local delivery of chemotherapy prolongs survival in experimental brain metastases from breast carcinoma. Neurosurgery 1998; 43: 1185–93.

64. Franciosi V, Cocconi G, Michiara M et al. Front-line chemotherapy with cisplatin and etoposide for patients with brain metastases from breast carcinoma, non-small cell lung carcinoma, or malignant melanoma: a prospective study. Cancer 1999; 85: 1599–605.

65. Schagen SB, Van Dam FSAM, Muller MJ et al. Cognitive deficits after postoperative adjuvant chemotherapy for breast carcinoma. Cancer 1999; 85: 640–50.

66. Mehta M, Noyes W, Craig B et al. A cost-effectiveness and cost-utility analysis of radiosurgery vs. resection for single-brain metastases. Int J Radiat Oncol Biol Phys 1997; 39: 445–54.

67. Iwadate Y, Namba H, Yamaura A. Significance of surgical resection for the treatment of multiple brain metastases. Anticancer Res 2000; 20: 573–7.

68. Auperin A, Arriagada R, Pignon JP et al. Prophylactic cranial irradiation for patients with small-cell lung cancer in complete remission. Prophylactic Cranial Irradiation Overview Collaborative Group. N Engl J Med 1999; 341: 476–84.

69. Fonseca R, O'Neill BP, Foote RL et al. Cerebral toxicity in patients treated for small cell carcinoma of the lung. Mayo Clin Proc 1999; 74: 461–5.

70. Mahalati K, Bilen CY, Özen H, Aki FT, Kendi S. The management of brain metastasis in nonseminomatous germ cell tumours. Br J Urol 1999; 83: 457–61.

71. Lagerwaard FJ, Levendag PC, Nowak PJ et al. Identification of prognostic factors in patients with brain metastases: a review of 1292 patients. Int J Radiat Oncol Biol Phys 1999; 43: 795–803.

Index